Review in
PEDIATRICS

for all POSTGRADUATE ENTRANCE EXAMINATIONS

All references based on the latest editions of International Textbooks as well as Ghai's Essential Pediatrics, and standard pediatric journals

OTHER CBS BOOKS FOR PG ENTRANCE EXAMINATION PREPARATION

Review in PEDIATRICS

for all POSTGRADUATE ENTRANCE EXAMINATIONS

Ranjan Kumar Patel MBBS MD

UCMS and GTB Hospital
Delhi

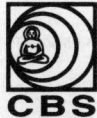

CBS

CBS Publishers & Distributors Pvt Ltd

New Delhi • Bengaluru • Chennai • Kochi • Mumbai • Pune
Hyderabad • Kolkata • Nagpur • Patna • Vijayawada

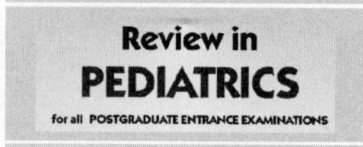

Review in PEDIATRICS
for all POSTGRADUATE ENTRANCE EXAMINATIONS

ISBN: 978-81-239-2396-3

Copyright © Author and Publishers

First Edition: **2014**

Published by Satish Kumar Jain for
CBS Publishers & Distributors Pvt Ltd
4819/XI Prahlad Street, 24 Ansari Road, Daryaganj, New Delhi 110 002, India.
Ph: 23289259, 23266861, 23266867   Fax: 011-23243014   Website: www.cbspd.com
                                                                                                    e-mail: delhi@cbspd.com; cbspubs@airtelmail.in.
Corporate Office: 204 FIE, Industrial Area, Patparganj, Delhi 110 092
Ph: 4934 4934   Fax: 4934 4935   e-mail: publishing@cbspd.com; publicity@cbspd.com

Branches

- **Bengaluru:** Seema House 2975, 17th Cross, K.R. Road,
  Banasankari 2nd Stage, Bengaluru 560 070, Karnataka
  Ph: +91-80-26771678/79   Fax: +91-80-26771680   e-mail: bangalore@cbspd.com
- **Chennai:** 20, West Park Road, Shenoy Nagar, Chennai 600 030, Tamil Nadu
  Ph: +91-44-26260666, 26208620   Fax: +91-44-42032115   e-mail: chennai@cbspd.com
- **Kochi:** 36/14 Kalluvilakam, Lissie Hospital Road, Kochi 682 018, Kerala
  Ph: +91-484-4059061-65   Fax: +91-484-4059065   e-mail: kochi@cbspd.com
- **Mumbai:** 83-C, Dr E Moses Road, Worli, Mumbai-400018, Maharashtra
  Ph: +91-22-24902340/2341   Fax: +91-22-24902342   e-mail: mumbai@cbspd.com
- **Pune:** Bhuruk Prestige, Sr. No. 52/12/2+1+3/2 Narhe, Haveli
  (Near Katraj-Dehu Road Bypass), Pune 411 041, Maharashtra
  Ph: +91-20-64704058, 64704059, 32392277 Fax: +91-20-24300160   e-mail: pune@cbspd.com

Representatives

- **Hyderabad**   0-9885175004   • **Kolkata**   0-9831437309, 0-9051152362
- **Nagpur**   0-9021734563   • **Patna**   0-9334159340   • **Vijayawada**   0-9000660880

Printed at : India Binding House, Noida

to

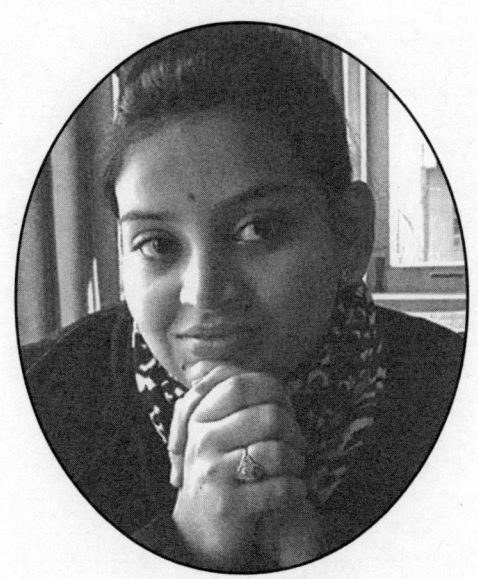

my late wife

Ranjeeta Nayak Patel

Without her I would not have been doing anything, that I am capable of today.

*Her love and inspiration always enlightened my darker days of life, even when I was away from her.
I just wish her peace, wherever she is and will always seek her love. She is related to each and
every line of this book. From the second of conception of this book's idea, till the completion of
pen ultimate chapter, she was always with me and this book. I had to write the last chapter alone and
honestly it was the longest chapter for me.*

She helped me not only to edit, but also gifted me her hours to write.

*Now that she has gone to a different world, this is the most precious memory that
I am sharing with this world. I hope she is watching from up and smiling at the release of her book.*

Preface

When we start talking about the PG examination preparation, one point is invariably said by all that the standard textbooks should be referred. Well when I say standard textbooks, I mean either Nelson or Rudolph for this particular subject, Pediatrics. But how many of us have studied these books in our UG days? All of you know the answer. Now if I tell you to open Nelson and prepare pediatrics in the very limited time that you have for PG exam, then it will not be practical.

This book has been written after critical analysis of the topics from various standard textbooks like Nelson, Rudolph, CPDT, Ghai and IAP Textbook of Pediatrics, and standard journals of pediatrics have been referred, if required. From the student's point of view, the most important aspect is not only good concept and understanding of topic but also tools to recall the same in the examination hall. For the first part, detailed care has been taken to give you the best possible explanation of various pathophysiological processes and disorders by flowcharts, diagrams and tables to help you build up on your concept. At the same time mnemonics have been supplemented to each topic, wherever possible to make your life easy in remembering and recalling the facts in these disorders.

After every chapter all the multiple choice questions that have been asked in various PG examinations like AIIMS, PGI, AIPG, DNB and State PG examinations from their day of conception till date have been included. They are not arranged topic-wise, rather chapter-wise, so that you can cruise through them after completing the theory of each chapter. When MCQs are solved in a random fashion for a given chapter, it challenges our memory and understanding to the deepest level. This is beneficial for the end result, i.e. in our desired PG examination. Explanations to the MCQs have been included as well, so that you do not have to turn back pages, in case of difficulty in understanding particular question.

As all of you are aware of the recent changes in the examination pattern, some changes in approach to the preparation is also required. No matter, who conducts the exam or whatever is the pattern, the best preparation is to build your concepts and understanding of the subject. Solve MCQs to consolidate the theory and have a feel of the ways MCQs can be asked from a particular topic. If you follow this path, no one in this world can deny you a branch and place of choice. My best wishes to all the PG aspirants.

Whenever a book is written, every possible effort is done to make it error free. However, wherever human work lies, errors are bound to be there. I would request you to point out if any present and not only me, but also your juniors will be grateful to you for this. You can contact me in case of any error found or doubt in the email given below.

Ranjan Kumar Patel
ranjankumarpatel@yahoo.com

Acknowledgements

Respect is something that cannot be described in words, as it is a feeling. Still I would like to reconstruct my respect in this form of acknowledgement to all the important figures who have influenced my life in some form or the other.

First of all I would like to thank Dr SK Bhattacharya, Prof and Head, Department of Pharmacology, UCMS and GTB Hospital, Delhi. He is like a father-figure to me and his guidance and kindness have helped me not only to evolve as a specialist but also as a human being.

I would also like to thank all Asst Professors, SRs and PGs in the Department of Pharmacology, UCMS and GTB Hospital, for their unconditional support and presence at every step of my life.

I would like to pay my respect to Dr KS Anand, Prof and Head, Department of Neurology, Dr RML Hospital. He holds an important position in my life and without his suggestions I would not have been anywhere nearby, where I am today.

I would like to thank Dr GR Garg, Asst Prof of Pharmacology, for his guidance. Forget about completion of this book, it would have never started without him. He knows what I am talking about.

School days lay down our foundation. I would never forget to thank Shri BK Singh, chemistry teacher, DAV Public School, Bandhabahal. He is the only person I would like to thank and appreciate his job as a teacher for guiding thousands of students through the right path in life.

I do believe in God and those are my parents, Shri Ashok Kumar Patel and Smt Tapaswini Patel. I would never be able to thank them enough for their love and sacrifices; I would always seek their blessing and love. I would like to thank my sister Ranjeeta Nayak, brother-in-law Shusil Nayak and nieces Sneha and Snitee for blessing my life with their presence.

I would like to mention all the people who had any role, at any moment in my life.

Prashanta Kumar Nayak, Prof History at Jamenkira; Late Mrs Nina Nayak; Manjeeta Nayak, BTech; Narendra Patel, MVI; Pushpanjali Patel; Anil Patel; Subrata Patel; Deepak Jaiswal, MBA; Sunil Rai, IMS, BHU, Varanasi; Devendra Dubey; Miss Tatyana Kuznetcova; Uden Dukpa; Dr BK Bajaj, Asst Prof Neurology, Dr RML Hospital; Dr Samir Kumar Patel, MS Surgery, Maysore; Dr Anamika Patel, MD Anaesthesia, Ahmedabad; Dr Dilip Kumar Nayak, MD Medicine, Bhubaneswar; Dr Raghvendra Singh, MD Medicine, Baradwar; Dr Updesh Singh Hora, MD Radiodiagnosis, Tashkent; Dr Kamaljeetsingh Hora, MD Pediatrics, Raipur; Dr Zulfiqar Ahmed Khan, MD Medicine, Moradabad; Dr AnjanaToley, DGO, Vardha; Dr Amit Jain, MS Surgery, Delhi; Dr Namita Kaul, DNB Neurology, INMAS; Dr Rietesh Aggarwal, MD Medicine, RML; Dr Jyoti Garg, Asst Prof Neurolgy, Dr RML Hospital; Dr Mahinda Chalwadi, MD Pharmacology; Dr Umesh Suranagi, MD Pharmacology, LHMC; Dr Vijay Chamle, MD Pharmacology; Dr Proteesh Rana, MD Pharmacology, MAMC; Dr Abhisek Kumar, MD Pharmacolgy, IHBAS; Dr Naveen Rathore, MD Pharmacology; Dr Amit Sharma, Asst Prof Pharmacology, Hindu Rao; Dr Tultul, MD Pharmacology; Dr Satbir Singh Madad, MD Medicine, Ismailabad; Dr Deepak Puri, MD Medicine, Gurgaon; Dr Deepak Sharma, DNB Surgery, Dr Ambedkar Hospital, Delhi; Dr Pulin Gupta, Asst Prof Medicine, Dr RML Hospital; Dr Prateek Upadhyay, MD, PSM, VMMC and Safdurjang Hospital; Dr Shivan Duggal Bharadwaj, MD Medicine, Delhi, Dr Toffique Ahmed, MD Medicine, Delhi; Dr Chandan Vishen, MD Medicine, Mau; Dr Faisal Khan, MD Medicine, Mau; Dr Sheetal Subba, MD Medicine.

Ranjan Kumar Patel
ranjankumarpatel@yahoo.com

Contents

Contents

Growth and Development

- The beginning of a new life takes place, when a sperm penetrates an ovum and thereby starting **fertilization**, a process by which male and female gametes fuse in the **ampullary region of uterine tube.** This follows a continuous process of cell division and growth passing through various stages of development.
- **Various stages of growth and development:**

Prenatal period	
Embryo	**From day of fertilization(generally 14th day post ovulation) to 9 weeks**
Fetus	9 weeks to birth
Perinatal period	**22 weeks of gestation to 7 days after birth**
Postnatal period	
Neonatal	**First 4 weeks or 28 days after birth**
Infancy	**First year**
Toddler	1–3 years
Preschool child	3–6 years
School age child	6–12 years
Adolescence	
Early	10–13 years
Middle	14–16 years
Late	17–19 years

EMBRYOGENESIS

Oogenesis and Spermatogenesis

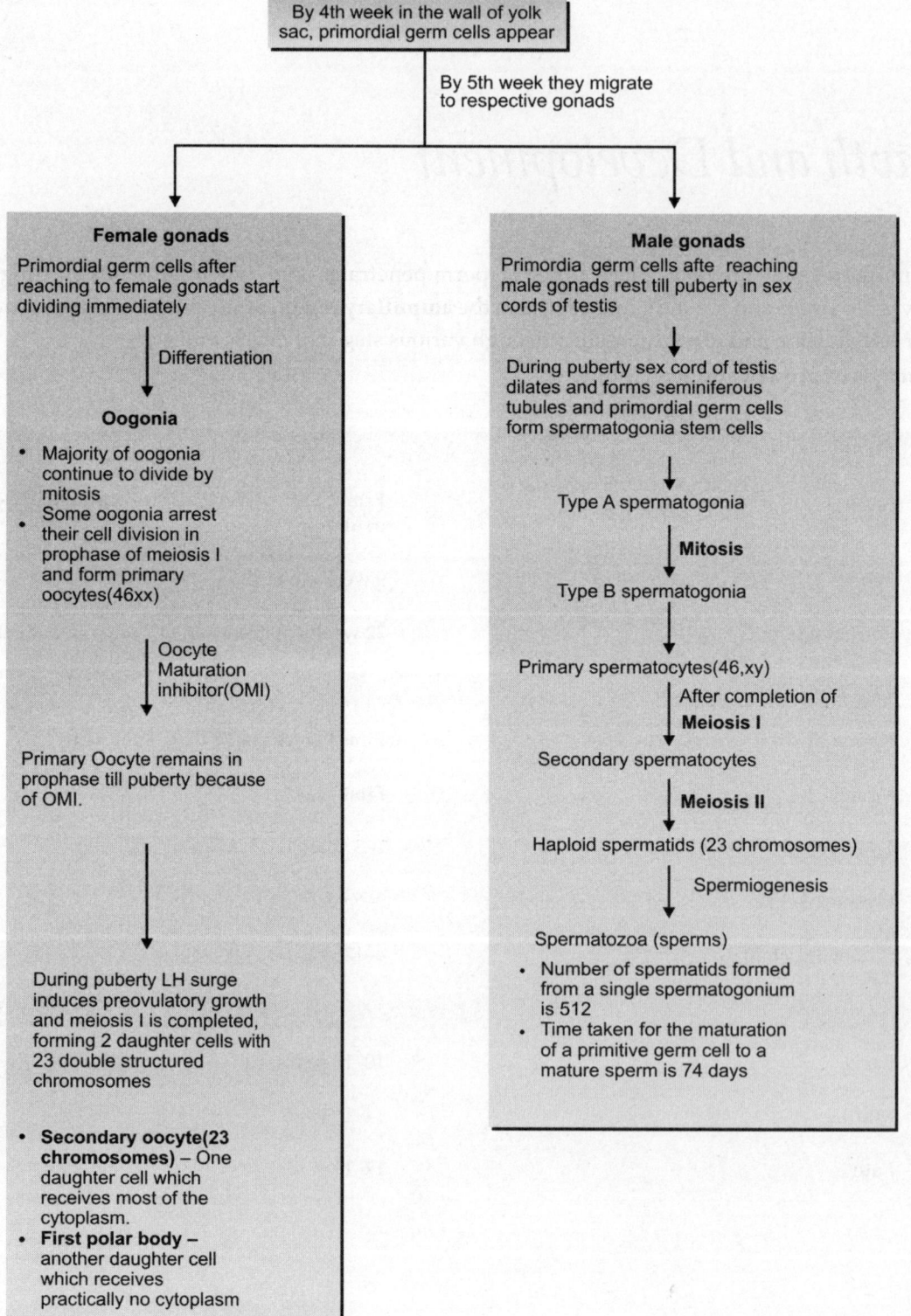

Fig. 1

Fertilization and Development of Embryo

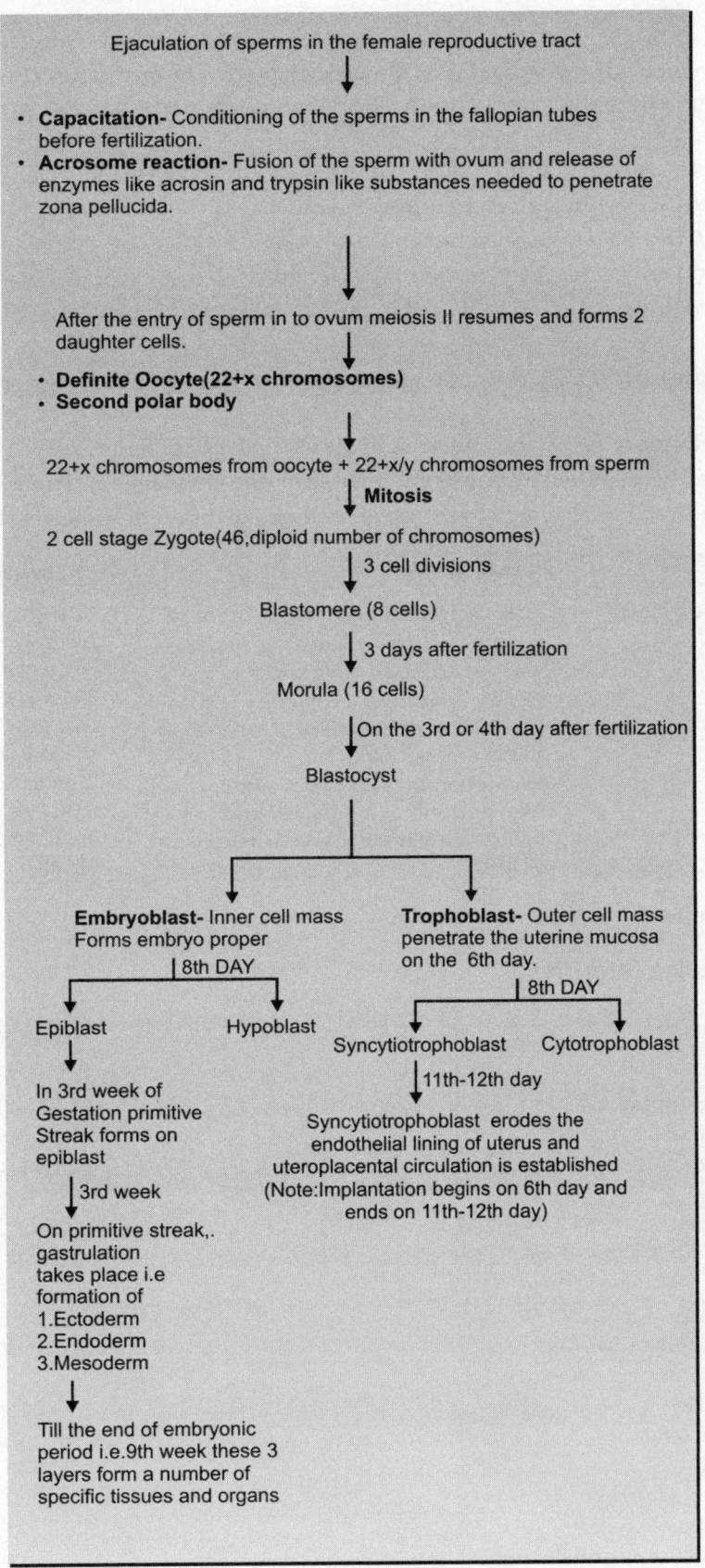

Ejaculation of sperms in the female reproductive tract

- **Capacitation-** Conditioning of the sperms in the fallopian tubes before fertilization.
- **Acrosome reaction-** Fusion of the sperm with ovum and release of enzymes like acrosin and trypsin like substances needed to penetrate zona pellucida.

After the entry of sperm in to ovum meiosis II resumes and forms 2 daughter cells.

- **Definite Oocyte(22+x chromosomes)**
- **Second polar body**

22+x chromosomes from oocyte + 22+x/y chromosomes from sperm

Mitosis

2 cell stage Zygote(46,diploid number of chromosomes)

3 cell divisions

Blastomere (8 cells)

3 days after fertilization

Morula (16 cells)

On the 3rd or 4th day after fertilization

Blastocyst

Embryoblast- Inner cell mass Forms embryo proper

8th DAY

Epiblast   Hypoblast

Trophoblast- Outer cell mass penetrate the uterine mucosa on the 6th day.

8th DAY

Syncytiotrophoblast   Cytotrophoblast

11th-12th day

Syncytiotrophoblast erodes the endothelial lining of uterus and uteroplacental circulation is established (Note:Implantation begins on 6th day and ends on 11th-12th day)

In 3rd week of Gestation primitive Streak forms on epiblast

3rd week

On primitive streak,. gastrulation takes place i.e formation of
1.Ectoderm
2.Endoderm
3.Mesoderm

Till the end of embryonic period i.e.9th week these 3 layers form a number of specific tissues and organs

Fig. 2

FETAL PERIOD

Gestational Age of Fetus

- The duration of fetal period is from beginning of **9th week till birth**. The growth of fetus is maximum in the first half of gestation; however maternal undernutrition before and during **any stage of pregnancy** can affect the fetal growth.
- The length of the fetus is usually indicated as crown rump length and crown heel length.
- **Crown - rump length (CRL)= Sitting height (upper segment).**
- **Crown -heel length (CHL)** = Standing height.
  - **Hasse's rule** is used to calculate age of fetus from its length:
  - **In first 5 months** of pregnancy CHL = (No of lunar months of pregnancy / Age of fetus in month)^2, so **Age in months** = $\sqrt{CHL}$.
  - **In second half of pregnancy** CHL = 5× (No of lunar months in pregnancy / Age of fetus in months), so **Age in months = CHL/5.**
- The **length is more reliable** criterion than the weight to calculate age of fetus.
- The gestational sac may be identified by transabdominal scanning at **5 weeks** and transvaginal scanning at **4 weeks**.
- Gestational age of fetus can be calculated by different methods in different trimesters by USG.

First trimester	Second trimester	Third trimester
• CRL is the most accurate method of pregnancy dating.	• BPD (Biparietal diameter) is the most accurate method of pregnancy dating, when **skull shape is normal**. • Head circumference is more accurate predictor of gestational age, **when skull shape is abnormal**. • **Femur length** is used for assessment of fetal age only when **fetal head is in a position unsuitable for measurement of BPD.**	• BPD (Biparietal diameter) is the most accurate method of pregnancy dating, when **skull shape is normal**. • Head circumference is more accurate predictor of gestational age, **when skull shape is abnormal**. • *Femur length** is used for assessment of fetal age only when **fetal head is in a position unsuitable for measurement of BPD.**

*David Sutton's Radiology, page no 1042, Volume 2, 7th edition.

Developmental Events During Fetal Life

Events	Age in weeks
Taste bud appears	7
First centers of ossification appear	8
Muscle contraction first appear	8
Breathing and swallowing	13–14
Grasp reflex appears	17
Grasp reflex is well developed	27
Suckling movements	24
Eye opening	26
Appearance of lanugo hair	20
Testes descend in to internal inguinal ring	28
One testicle descends to scrotum	36
Disappearance of lanugo hair	36
Both testicles descend in to scrotum	40
Posterior fontanel is closed	40
Fetal movement felt	20
Primary ossification centers are present	12
***Gender of external genitals are clearly distinguishable**	12

*Nelson 19th Ed / P27

Growth in Length and Weight during Fetal Period

Age(in weeks)	CRL(cm)	Weight(g)
9 12	5 8	10 45
21 24	20 23	500 820
37 38	**35 36 (CHL = 50)**	3250 ≅ **3 Kg**

DEVELOPMENT OF INFANTS AND CHILDREN

Weight

Weight of children is an important criterion of development and hence should be measured in every visit. The newborn may lose 10% of weight in the first week of life; however it is regained in following weeks.

Formulas for approximate average weight of normal infants and children:

Weight	Kilograms
At birth	3
3 12 months	$\dfrac{\text{Age (months)} + 9}{2}$
1 6 years	Age (years) $\times$ 2 + 8
7 12 years	$\dfrac{\text{Age (months)} \times 7 - 5}{2}$

Approximate weight in different ages calculated by above formulas:

Age	Weight (Kg)
Birth	3
6 months	**6**
1 year	**9**
2 years	**12**
3 years	14
4 years	16
12 years	39

Birth weight approximately
- **Doubles by 6 months**
- **Triples by 1 year**
- **Quadruples by 2 years**

Height

Height is also an important criterion of child growth and hence **serial measurement is required** in each visit. Usually Herpendens stadiometer is used for measurement of height.

After birth the baby grows faster in the **first year of life**; however another phase of accelerated growth is seen during puberty. From 4-12 years child grows at the rate of **6 cm/year**. The normal range of variation in the height and weight lies in between **3rd and 97th percentile**. The normal range of target height for a male is ± 8.5 cm and for female is ± 7 cm form the normal value.

The upper segment and lower segment should be separately measured for its clinical significance. The upper segment is measured from vertex to pubic symphysis and lower segment is measured from pubic symphysis to sole of foot.

Normal upper segment to lower segment ratio in children:

Age	Upper segment to lower segment ratio
Birth	3
Newborn	1.8
3 4 years	**1.3**
9 years	1

- Formulas for approximate average height of normal infants and children:

Height	Centimeters
At birth	50
At 1 year	75
2–12 years	Age (years) × 6 + 77

- Approximate height in different ages calculated by above formulas:

Age	Height(cm)
Birth	50
1 year	75
2 years	89
3 years	95
4 years	**101**
12 years	**149**

- Height approximately
  - **Doubles by 4 years**
  - **Triples by 12 years**

Head Circumference

- Head circumference measurement is an important part of neurological examination in the infants. It is important to add to the diagnosis of **neurological dysfunction** and **microcephaly**. A head circumference of **2 SD** below the mean or less than 5th percentile for age and sex is diagnostic of microcephaly. A rapid increase in head circumference suggests a tumor or **hydrocephalus**. A head circumference of more than 95th percentile for age and sex is diagnostic of macrocephaly.
- It is measured in every visit and a growth chart of head is prepared. A plastic tape is used to measure the greatest circumference through the **occipital protuberance** and **supraorbital ridge**.
- The head circumference grows by 0.5 cm in first 2 weeks, 0.75 cm in 3rd week and thereafter 1 cm/week till birth.

Age	Head circumference in cm
Newborn	35
3 months	40
6 months	**43**
1 year	46-47
2 years	48
12	52

Chest Circumference

- The chest circumference is usually measured at the level of nipples.
- **Chest circumference at birth is usually 3 cm less than head circumference.**
- Both are equal by the age of 9 months to 1 year. If chest circumference persists to be lower than head circumference after 1 year it indicates malnutrition.

Mid Arm Circumference

- Mid arm circumference (MAC) is measured in the middle of upper hand i.e. between the acromion and olecranon with the arm hanging by side.
- MAC is measured by **Shakir's tape** which can be even used by illiterate people. The tape is divided in to 3 coloured zones, the green zone located above 13.5 cm is normal MAC, yellow-orange zone from 12.5–13.5 cm represents borderline malnutrition and red zone i.e. below 12.5 cm represents severe malnutrition.
- The **MAC is usually constant in the age group of 2–5 years** and lies in between 16–17 cm, i.e. in the green zone.
- **Kanawati index** is calculated by multiplying MAC and head circumference. It is used for diagnosis of malnutrition. A value of >0.32 is normal and any lesser value indicates malnutrition.

Developmental Events of Children

Events	Age
Maximum growth	1st year of life
Head is 90% of adult brain	2nd year of life
Maximum lymphoid tissue growth	4–8 years of life
Gonadal growth	During puberty

Selected Primitive and Postural Reflexes

Reflex	Emerges	Disappears
Crossed extensor	28 weeks of gestation	1–2 months
Grasp	28 weeks of gestation	2–3 month
Rooting	32 weeks of gestation	1 month
Sucking	28 weeks gestation	4 months
Moro	30 weeks gestation	5 months
ATNR	35 weeks gestation	6–7 months
Galant	30 weeks gestation	6 months
Stepping	Birth	2 months
Landau	3 months	15 months
Protective extension		
Forward	6 months	**Persists**
Sideways	7 months	**Persists**
Backwards	9 months	**Persists**
Tilting reaction	12 months	Persists
Parachute	7–8 months	Persists
Symmetric tonic neck	**4–6 months**	8–12 months

ATNR—Asymmetric tonic neck reflex

Developmental Milestones

First 4 weeks(Neonate)	• **Fixates on light or face in line of vision** • Dolls eye movement of eye on turning head • Turns head from side to side
1 month	• **Lifts head momentarily in prone position** • **Alerts to sound** • **Follows dangling object from midline through 90°** • **Vocalizes**
2 months	• **Head sustains in plane of body on ventral suspension** • **Social smile** • Stares momentarily at spot where object disappeared
3 months	• **Neck holding** • Brings hands together in midline • **Recognizes mother** • Anticipates feed • Coos • **Follows dangling object from midline through a range of 180°**
4 months	• Asymmetric tonic neck reflex gone • **Grasps objects with both hands** • Palmar grasp gone • Stares at own hand • Excited at sight of food • Laugh loud • **Binocular vision well established** • **Mouthing of objects**

Developmental Milestones *(Contd.)*

5 months	• Roll over
	• Foot play voluntary grasp(no release)
	• **Smiles at image in mirror**
6 months	• **Sits with support**
	• Unidextrous reach
	• **Stranger anxiety**
	• Monosyllables
	• **Transfers objects from one hand to other**
7 months	• Inhibits to no
	• Follows one step command with gesture
	• **Babbles**
	• **Enjoys mirror image**
	• **Grasps objects**
	• **Sits and leans forward on hand**
	• **Prefers mother**
	• **Pivots**
8 months	• **Sits without support**
	• **Crawls**
	• Bangs 2 cubes
	• Uncovers toy after seeing it hidden
	• **Changes position from prone to supine**
9 months	• **Stands with support**
	• **Pincer grasp develops**
	• **Waves bye bye**
	• **Bisyllables**like **baba, mama**
10 months	• Points to objects
	• **Plays peek-a-boo or pat-a-cake**
	• Responds to sound of name
	• **"Cruises" or walks holding to the furniture**
12 months	• **Stands without support**
	• **Creeps**
	• **Pincer grasp matures**
	• **Turns pages of books**
	• Comes when called
	• **Plays simple ball game**
	• Pretends to drink from cup
	• 1-2 words with meaning
	• **Uses pronouns**
15 months	• **Walks alone**
	• Creeps upstairs
	• Imitates scribbling
	• Tower of 2 blocks
	• Hugs parents
	• Indicates some desires or needs by pointing
	• **Jargon (non-verbal communication)**
	• **4–6 words vocabulary**
17 months	• Pretends play with doll
	• Uses stick to reach toy
18 months	• Runs
	• Explore drawers
	• Scribbles
	• **Tower of 3 blocks**
	• **Copies parents in task**
	• Feeds self
	• Seeks help when in trouble

Developmental Milestones *(Contd.)*

	• **May complain when wet or soiled**
	• Kisses parent with pucker
	• **10–15 words vocabulary**
	• Names pictures
	• Identifies one or more parts of bodies
2 years	• Jumps
	• Opens doors
	• Vertical and circular stroke
	• **Folds paper once imitatively**
	• **Tower of 6 blocks**
	• Asks for food, drink, toilet
	• Pulls people to show toy
	• Helps to undress
	• **Handles spoon well without spilling**
	• **Makes sentences/phrases of 2-3 words**
	• Uses pronouns
	• 100 words vocabulary
30 months	• **Walks upstairs with alternate steps**
	• **Tower of 9 blocks**
	• **Refers to self by "I"**
3 years	• **Rides tricycle**
	• **Stands momentarily on one foot**
	• **Copies circle**
	• Imitates cross
	• **Handedness develops**
	• Shares toys
	• **Helps in dressing (unbuttoning clothes, puts on shoes)**
	• Washes hand
	• Asks questions
	• **Knows full name and gender**
	• Counts 3 objects correctly
	• **Identifies color**
	• Vocabulary of 250 words
4 years	• **Walks downstairs with alternate steps**
	• **Hops on one foot**
	• Throws ball overhead
	• **Uses scissors to cut pictures**
	• **Copies cross and square**
	• Bridge with blocks
	• Plays cooperatively in a group
	• Goes to toilet alone
	• **Story telling**
	• Singing and poem reciting
5 years	• **Skips**
	• Ties shoe laces
	• Name heavier of two weights
	• **Copies triangle**
	• Dresses and undresses
	• Helps in household tasks
	• Asks meaning of words
	• Names 4 colors
6-7 years	• **Reads a sentence**

Dentition

Sequence of Teeth Eruption

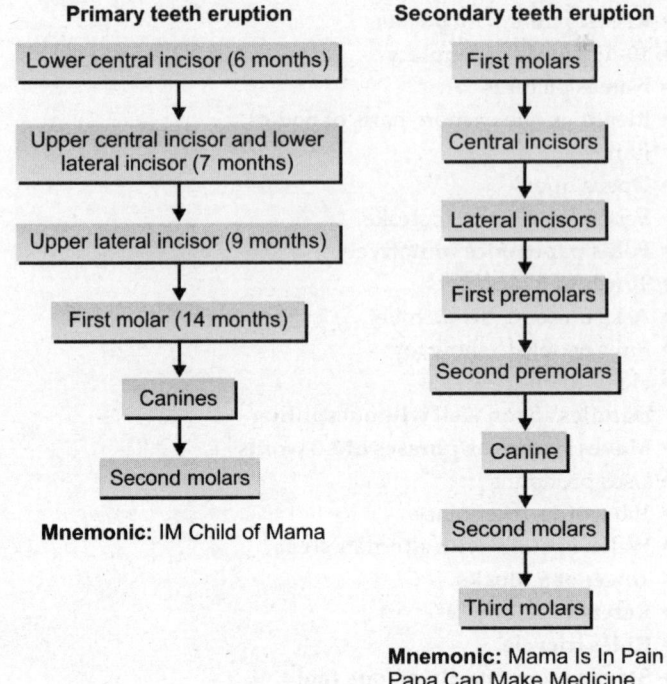

Primary teeth eruption

Lower central incisor (6 months)
↓
Upper central incisor and lower lateral incisor (7 months)
↓
Upper lateral incisor (9 months)
↓
First molar (14 months)
↓
Canines
↓
Second molars

Mnemonic: IM Child of Mama

Secondary teeth eruption

First molars
↓
Central incisors
↓
Lateral incisors
↓
First premolars
↓
Second premolars
↓
Canine
↓
Second molars
↓
Third molars

Mnemonic: Mama Is In Pain
Papa Can Make Medicine

Fig. 3

Delayed Eruption

- Delay of eruption till 12 months is considered normal if the child has no other symptoms.
- Causes of delayed eruption

Local causes	Systemic causes
• Supernumerary teeth	• P—Progeria
• Cysts	• I—Incontinentia pigmenti
• Tumours	• C—Cleidocranial dysplasia
• Overretained primary teeth	• H—Hypothyroidism, Hypopitutarism
• Ankylosed primary teeth	• D—Vitamin D deficiency Rickets, Down's syndrome
• Impaction	• A—Albright osteodystrophy
Mnemonic for systemic causes : PICHDA	

- Advanced dentition is seen in **precocious puberty** and **hyperthyroidism**.

Bone Development

- The earliest ossification center to develop in a fetus is of **calcaneus**; however other centers are also seen at birth are distal end of femur, proximal end of tibia, head of humerus, talus and cuboid.
- In a baby of **one year 2 carpal centers** are present followed by an increase in one center each year:

Age	Carpal centers
1 year	2
2 years	3
3 years	4
4 years	5
5 years	6
6 years	7

- In a baby of 3 years epiphysis of metacarpals and phalanx can be seen. Distal ulnar epiphysis is seen at an age of 8–9 years in girls and 10–12 years in boys (skeletal maturation is advanced in girls).

ADOLESCENCE

- It is a period of rapid physical, emotional, cognitive and social growth which ranges from **10 years to 19 years**. Puberty is the biologic process in which a child becomes an adult and is often described as onset of adolescence.
- Boys become more impatient, **aggressive** and irritable with rising level of testosterone. 2/3rd boys may have increased estradiol level as compared to testosterone, which leads to **physiological pubertal gynaecomastia**. Most of the times only one breast is involved and a transient tenderness can be seen. Treatment is usually not required; however in case of severe enlargement danazole can be used.
- Estradiol stimulates growth hormone secretion which subsequently increases IGF–1. **Growth hormone** and IGF 1 leads to increase in **muscle mass**.

Growth in Puberty

At puberty sensitivity of pituitary to GnRH increases.

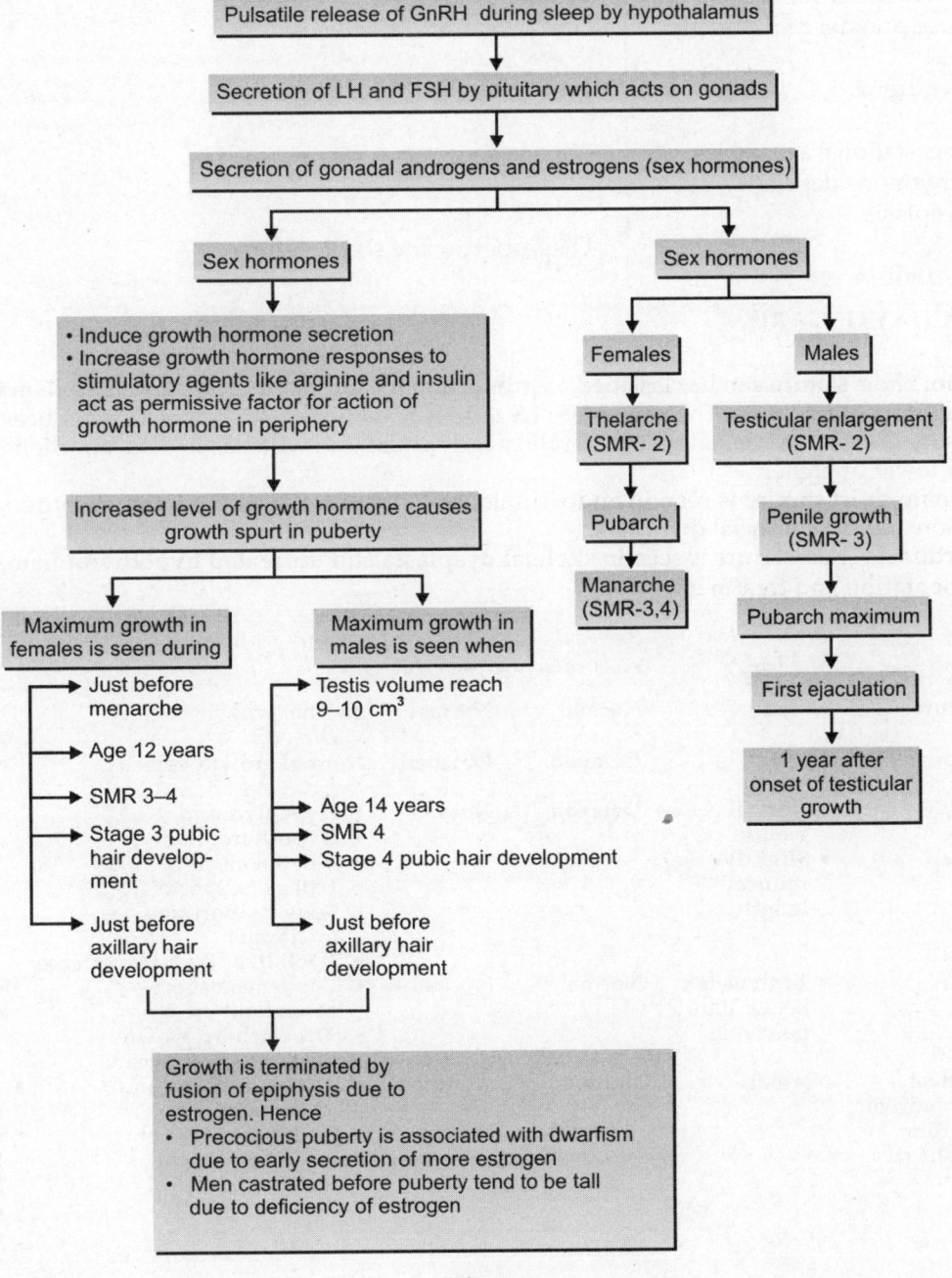

Fig. 4

DISORDERS IN GROWTH AND DEVELOPMENT

Short Stature

- Short stature is defined as:
  - ❖ Child's height below **3rd percentile.**

  Or

  - ❖ Child's height more than **2 standard deviations below the median height** corresponding to age.
- **Most common cause** is **familial short stature and constitutional growth delay**, both of which account for approximately 50% of cases. Other causes of short stature are endocrinological disorders (**hypothyroidism**, pseudohypoparathyroidism, Cushing syndrome and accelerated and delayed puberty), psychosocial dwarfism (**maternal deprivation dwarfism/Kasper Hauser syndrome**/hyperphagic syndrome), SGA babies, IUGR, skeletal dysplasia (**achondroplasia** and **rickets**) and genetic disorders (Turner syndrome, Down syndrome).

C – Constitutional, Chronic diseases **H** – Hyperphagic short stature **A** – Accelerated and delayed puberty **T** – Trisomy 21 **T** – Turner syndrome **I** – IUGR **S** – Small for gestational age babies **G** – Growth hormone deficiency	Proportionate short stature
A – Achondroplasia **R** – Rickets **H** – Hypothyroidism	Disproportionate short stature

Mnemonic: CHATTISGARH

- **Classification:** Short stature can be classified as proportionate and disproportionate based on the upper segment (US) to lower segment (LS) ratio. The values **US: LS ratio is 1.7 at birth** which gradually reduces to **1 by 10 years of age**. Proportionate short stature have a US:LS ratio nearly equal to 1; whereas in disproportionate short stature the ratio is either lower or higher.
  - ❖ Proportionate short stature is seen in endocrinological disorders, IUGR, genetic disorders, chronic diseases, malnutrition and psychosocial dwarfism.
  - ❖ Disproportionate short stature is seen in **skeletal dysplasia** and **untreated hypothyroidism**.
- **Clinical presentation and treatment**

Cause	Birth weight and length	Skeletal maturation	Timing of puberty	Other features	Treatment
Familial short stature	Normal	Normal	Normal	Normal growth velocity	**Not required/ Assurance**
Constitutional growth delay	Normal	**Delayed**	**Delayed**	**Normal growth velocity**	Not required/ Assurance
Growth hormone deficiency	• **Normal weight** • **Slightly reduced length**	Delayed	Normal	• Hypoglycemia • **Hypothyroidism** • Micropenis • Truncal adiposity • **Body proportions are normal** • "Doll like" facial appearance	Subcutaneous recombinant GH
IUGR	• Birth weight below 10th percentile	Normal	Normal	• 20% remain short throughout life • 80% catch-up growth during the first 3 years	Subcutaneous recombinant GH
Psychosocial dwarfism /**Kasper Hauser Syndrome** /**Maternal deprivation dwarfism**/Hyperphagic short stature	Normal	Normal	Normal	• Bizarre drinking and eating habits • Bladder and bowel incontinence • Social withdrawal • Delayed speech	• Foster home placement • Change in psycological environment at home • GH secretion is decreased but **GH therapy is not beneficial**

Enuresis

- It is characterized by repeated bed and cloth wetting due to voluntary or involuntary discharge of urine.
- Diagnosis is made when bed/cloth wetting occurs at least **2 times a week** for not less than **3 months**.
- **Early strict toilet training** should be discouraged as it can lead to **encopresis**.

Classification

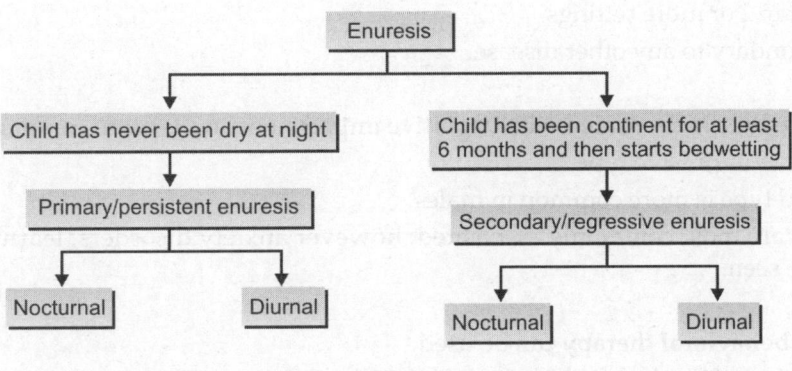

Fig. 5

- **Primary nocturnal enuresis (Night wetting)**
  - ❖ This is the **most common type of enuresis** and is **more common in boys.**
  - ❖ Cause is related to maturational delay of sleep and arousal mechanism and delay in development of increased bladder capacity.
- **Diurnal enuresis (Day time wetting)**
  - ❖ This is **more common in girls**.
  - ❖ It is seen in timid and shy children and associated with ADHD.
- **Secondary enuresis is caused by a stressful event like birth of a sibling** and loss or discord within family.

Treatment

- Treatment is not required in children **below 6 months of age**.
- First line of treatment is non-pharmacological i.e. **motivational and alarm therapy**. It is the **most effective treatment** with least chances of recurrences.
- Pharmacological therapy is initiated if motivational and alarm therapy fails. **Imipramine** alters sleep arousal mechanism. It is rarely used because causes cardiac conduction disturbances. **Oxybutynin** reduces uninhibited bladder contraction. It is useful in children with **diurnal enuresis. Desmopressin (orally or intranasally)** is preferred for special occasions like staying out at night.

Thumb Sucking

- Thumb sucking is considered normal in children till **4–5 years**. Like various other behaviors, thumb sucking is **self-soothing**. Persistence of thumb sucking in to adolescence is more common in females and is a **sign of insecurity**.
- Continuation of thumb sucking post 5 years can result in **dental misalignment** like flaring of the maxillary incisor teeth, open bite and posterior cross bite.
- To lessen the effects of misalignment it should be discontinued before **8 years**.
- Treatment
  - ❖ For children till 4–5 years parents should be advised to ignore as the habit drops spontaneously by **4 years**.
  - ❖ For children more than 5 years praising the child for other behaviors and **simple reinforcement** like giving a chocolate for not sucking thumb for a period of time is first line approach. Application of **noxious agents** to thumb is a second line treatment.

Attention Deficit Hyperactivity Disorder

- ADHD is most common neurobehavioral disorder of childhood.

- It is characterized by **inattention** and **increased distractibility, impulsivity** and decreased self-control, **motor hyperactivity** and **motor restlessness**, inefficient planning and organizing of tasks, emotional liability, low self-esteem and a**cademic underperformance.**
- The various risk factors are maternal drug use, smoking and alcohol use and genetic preponderance.
- The current **DSM IV** criteria for diagnosis is
  ❖ Behavior must begin before the age of 7 year.
  ❖ It must be present for at least 6 months.
  ❖ It must be present in 2 or more settings.
  ❖ It must not be secondary to any other disease.
- **Classification**
  ❖ ADHD, inattentive type is associated with cognitive impairment and is more common in females
  ❖ ADHD, hyperactive-impulsive type
  ❖ ADHD, combined type is more common in males.
- Language disorders are most commonly associated; however anxiety disorders, learning disabilities and mood disorders can also be seen.
- **Treatment**
  ❖ Psychosocial and **behavioral therapy** can be used.
  ❖ **Psychostimulant medications** are **most effective** treatment. The drugs used are **methylphenidate, amphetamine and dextroamphetamine preparations like Dexedrine and Adderall.** Other medications like noradrenergic reuptake inhibitor (**Atomoxetine),** tricyclic antidepressants (Imipramine, Nortriptyline) and alpha agonist (clonidine) can also be used.

Pervasive Developmental Disorders

The Diagnostic and Statistical Manual of Mental Disorders IV (DSM IV) classifies pervasive developmental disorders in to autistic spectrum disorders (autistic disorder, Asperger disorder and pervasive developmental disorder not otherwise specified), Rett syndrome and childhood disintegrative disorder.

Autistic Spectrum Disorders

Social deficits are the earliest manifestation of autistic spectrum disorder followed by **speech delay** and **language disorder** (echolalia or parroting). By **3rd year of life** other symptoms like **delayed communication**, narrow repetitive interest and insistence on sameness, stereotypic behaviors like hand flapping due to **impaired imagination** and interest in solitary play are also seen. Diagnosis can be done by screening tools like **Modified Checklist for Autism in Toddlers (M-CHAT)**, which is a questionnaire completed by parents.

- **Autistic disorder:** Autistic disorder is the most severe and most common form of pervasive developmental disorder. It is **four times more common in males** than females. In 90% cases cause cannot be identified and are called as essential. In 10% cases autism may be associated with chromosomal disorders (Fragile X syndrome, Angelman syndrome, Down syndrome), Moebius syndrome, CHARGE syndrome, tuberous sclerosis, intrauterine infections (rubella, CMV) and intrauterine drug exposure (alcohol, thalidomide, valproate)
- Apart from the symptoms mentioned above these children also have deficit in **joint attention** and **intellect**, seizures and lack of imitation. Brain overgrowth can be seen in these patients till the age of 14 months.
- **Asperger disorder:** The age of onset is delayed in these patients. These children usually are unable to express feelings and have clumsy motor skills; however other symptoms like speech and language deficit and narrow repetitive interest are not seen. These children use very pedantic language and are called as **"little professors"**.
- **Pervasive developmental disorders not otherwise specified:** These children usually have some symptoms of autism specific disorders but the severity is lesser.

Rett Syndrome

Rett syndrome is usually seen in **females**. These children develop normally till 6–18 months of age followed by **rapid regression in language and hand skills, repetitive hand movements, decreased rate of head growth (microcephaly)**, ataxia, breathing dysfunction, bruxism, scoliosis, and profound **mental retardation**. Diagnosis is confirmed by DNA analysis for methyl CpG-binding protein 2 (MECP 2).

Childhood Disintegrative Disorder

This is the least common type of pervasive developmental disorder. This is characterized by significant loss of acquired skills up to 10 years of age in language, social interaction, bladder and bowel control, play and motor skills. Loss of at least two skills is required for diagnosis.

BREATH HOLDING SPELLS

- Breath holding spells are usually seen in children of **6 months to 5 years of age**. Familial predisposition can be seen in some cases.
- The predisposing factors are frustration, anger, fear or severe pain which leads to crying and holding the breath in expiration resulting in **pallor** and **cyanosis**. Based on the predisposing factor and etiopathogenesis it can be classified as cyanotic spell and pallid spell.
- Cyanotic spell is usually caused in response to frustration and anger precipitated by scolding or refusal to fulfill any desire. These patients can develop loss of consciousness and **seizures** due to cerebral hypoxia; however **antiepileptics are not indicated**. The cause is attributed to excessive centrally mediated sympathetic activity.
- Pallid spell is usually caused in response to a painful stimuli precipitated by fall or injury. The cause is attributed to excessive centrally mediated parasympathetic activity. Hence **atropine** can be given for treatment of refractory cases.
- Treatment consists of counseling and reassuring the parents, as this is a benign disorder. They should be told to **pinch the child and not respond to the unreasonable wishes** at the onset of the episode. Oral iron therapy has been effective in some cases.

MULTIPLE CHOICE QUESTIONS

1. **A 10-year-old child is always restless inattentive to study and always wants to play outside. Parents are extremely distressed, what would you advise?**
   [AIIMS 08]
   a. It's a normal behavior
   b. Behavior therapy
   c. It's a serious illness requires medical treatment
   d. Needs change in environment

2. **A 6-year-old child has an IQ 50. Which of the following tasks the child can do:**
   [AIIMS May 07; Nov. 06, AI 07]
   a. Draw a triangle   b. Recognize colors
   c. Ride a bicycle   d. Read a sentence

3. **Reflex which is not present in child at birth is:**
   [AIIMS May 07]
   a. Moro's reflex
   b. Symmetric tonic neck reflex
   c. Crossed extensor reflex
   d. Asymmetric tonic neck reflex

4. **A 3-year-old boy with normal developmental milestones with delayed speech and difficulty in communication and concentration. He is not making friends. Most probable diagnosis is:**
   [AIIMS May 07, AI 07]
   a. Autism
   b. ADHD
   c. Mental retardation
   d. Specific learning disability

5. **Persistence of Moro's reflex is abnormal beyond the age of:**
   [AIIMS May 07]
   a. 3rd month   b. 4th month
   c. 5th month   d. 6th month

6. **A 9-year-old child disturbs other people, is destructive, interferes when people are talking, does not follow instructions and cannot wait for his turn while playing a game. He is likely to be suffering from:**
   [AIIMS Nov. 05]
   a. Emotional disorders
   b. Behavioural problems
   c. No disorder
   d. Attention deficit hyperactive disorder

7. **A 14-year-old boy has difficulty in expressing himself in writing and makes frequent spelling mistakes, does not follow instruction and cannot wait for his turn while playing game. He is likely to be suffering from:**
   [AIIMS Nov. 05]
   a. Mental retardation
   b. Lack of interest in studies
   c. Specific learning disability
   d. Examination anxiety

8. **A female child has recently learned to eat with spoon without spilling; to dress and undress herself with supervision: and to understand that she is a girl. These skills are FIRST mastered between the ages of:**
   [AIIMS Nov. 05]
   a. 2 and 3 years   b. 3 and 4 years
   c. 4 and 5 years   d. 5 and 6 years

9. A normally developing 10-month-old child should be able to do all of the following except:

[AIIMS Nov. 05; AI 06]

a. Stand alone
b. Play peek a boo
c. Pick up a pellet with thumb and index finger
d. Build a tower of 3-4 cubes

10. A 13-year-old boy has bilateral gynaecomastia. His height is 148 cm, weight 58 kg; the sexual maturity rating is stage 2. The gynaecomastia is most likely due to: [AIIMS Nov. 04]

a. Prolactinoma
b. Testicular tumor
c. Pubertal gynaecomastia
d. Chronic liver disease

11. Short stature is seen in: [AIIMS June 04]

a. Maternal deprivation syndrome
b. Hypothyroidism
c. Bulimia
d. Paternal smoking
e. IUGR

12. A two-year-old girl child is brought to the out patient with features of hand wringing stereotype movements, impaired language and communication development, breath holding spells, poor social skills and deceleration of head growth after 6 months of age. The most likely diagnosis is:

[AIIMS Nov. 03]

a. Asperger's syndrome b. Rett's syndrome
c. Fragile-X syndrome   d. Colarad syndrome

13. A 9-year-old child is restless. He is hyperactive and his teacher complaints that he doesnot listen to the teachings. Disturbs other students, he also shows less interest in playing. The likely diagnosis is:

[AIIMS May 02]

a. Cerebral palsy
b. Attention deficit hyperactive disorder
c. Delirium
d. Mania

14. A 6-year-old child has history of birth asphyxia, does not communicate well, has slow mental and physical growth, does not mix with people, has limited interests, gets widely agitated if disturbed, diagnosis is: [AIIMS Nov. 01]

a. Hyperkinetic child
b. Autistic disorder
c. Attention deficit disorder
d. Schizophrenia

15. A child climbs with alternate steps, builds a tower of 8-9 cubes, tells "I" but not his name and cannot say his age and sex the probable age is:

[AIIMS May 01]

a. 36 months   b. 24 months
c. 30 months   d. 48 months

16. Developmental examination should be further evaluated in child of 12 weeks if the child:

[AIIMS June 00; AI 02]

a. Does not vocalize
b. Does not babble
c. Does not change bright red ring from one hand to other even if given in hand
d. Does not hold head at 90°

17. A baby on examination shows unilateral moro's reflex with positive palmar grasp reflex. The site of lesion is: [AIIMS Nov. 99]

a. C1 - C4   b. C5 - C6
c. Cg - T1   d. C1 - C2

18. Meaning of baby has 15th percentile of head circumference (HC) is: [AIIMS Nov. 99]

a. 15% of children will have HC more than that
b. 15% of HC, the child is having
c. 15% of children will have HC less than that
d. 15% of children will have HC same as that

19. A mother comes with her 3-year-old female child with complain of that child is not eating anything. Her weight is 11 kg (50th percentile) and height is 88 cm (75th percentile). What should be done next:

[AIIMS Nov. 99]

a. Vitamin rich tonic to be given
b. Forceful eating
c. Nothing should be done actively and assure the patients
d. Complete investigation for UTI

20. A 4-year-old child can perform one of the following:

[AIIMS Dec. 98]

a. Can hop on single leg for 1.5 feet
b. Can skip without falling to either side
c. Can stand on one feet for 20 seconds
d. Can walk down the stairs with alternating steps holding on to the iron rail

21. Palmomental reflex is seen in lesions of:

[AIIMS Dec. 98]

a. Frontal lobe
b. Parietal lobe
c. Temporal lobe
d. Occipital lobe

22. True regarding breath holding spells is all except:

[AIIMS June 97)]

a. Antiepileptic treatment is necessary
b. Atropine is sometimes used
c. Attack of cyanosis can occur
d. Occurs between 6 months to 5 years

23. From 4–12 years child grows at the rate of 6 cm/year. Infant body weight is tripled by age of: [AIIMS 96]

a. 5 months   b. 11 months
c. 2 years   d. 18 months

24. **Which about development is not true?**
    [AIIMS May 95]
    a. Pincer grasp at 3 months
    b. Sitting at 6 months
    c. Social smile at 3 months
    d. 2-year-old can use pleurals

25. **Short stature, secondary to growth hormone deficiency is associated with:**   [AIIMS Dec. 1995]
    a. Normal body proportion
    b. Low birth weight
    c. Normal epiphyseal development
    d. Height age equal to skeletal age

26. **A 3-year-old child is expected to have all except:**
    [AIIMS Dec. 94]
    a. Speak in sentences
    b. Copy a circle
    c. Hobble 5 steps
    d. Climb upstairs and downstairs

27. **A six week old infant cannot:**   [AIIMS 92]
    a. Grasp dangling objects
    b. Fix gaze
    c. Lift and hold head
    d. Turn head towards sound

28. **Increase in muscle mass at adolescence is probably caused by:**   [AIIMS 81, PGI 83]
    a. Thyroid hormone.
    b. Adrenal hormone
    c. Growth hormone
    d. None of the above

29. **To avoid displacement of permanent teeth, finger sucking should be terminated by:**
    [PGI 79, AIIMS 78, 81]
    a. 8 years
    b. 5 years
    c. 3 years
    d. 2 years

30. **A child is below the third percentile for height. His growth velocity is normal, but chronological age more than skeletal age. The most likely diagnosis is:**
    [AI 11, 06]
    a. Constitutional delay in growth
    b. Genetic short stature
    c. Primordial dwarfism
    d. Hypopituitarism

31. **Which of the following is not true about autistic specific disorder?**   [AI 10]
    a. Impaired communication
    b. Impaired imagination
    c. Language developmental delay
    d. Vision problem

32. **Lowest recurrence in nocturnal enuresis is seen with:**   [AI 08]
    a. Bed alarms
    b. Desmopressin
    c. Imipramine
    d. Oxybutinin

33. **The most common cause of short stature is:**
    [AI 07, 08]
    a. Constitutional
    b. Systemic diseases
    c. Hypothyroidism
    d. Growth hormone deficiency

34. **Moro reflex disappears at:**   [AI 07; PGI June 98]
    a. 5 months
    b. 3 months
    c. 7 months
    d. 6 months

35. **All of the following reflexes are present at birth except:**   [AI 07; PGI June 98]
    a. Rooting reflex
    b. Symmetrical tonic neck reflex
    c. Asymmetrical neck reflex
    d. Crossed extensor reflex

36. **Which of the following appears 1st in child?** [AI 07]
    a. Creeping
    b. Crawling
    c. Mirror play
    d. Pincer grasp

37. **A child has started mouthing objects, shows likes and dislikes has and not yet developed stanger anxiety. The age of child is:**   [AI 07]
    a. 3 months
    b. 5 months
    c. 7 months
    d. 9 months

38. **The following are characteristics of autism except:**
    [AI 06]
    a. Onset after 6 years of age
    b. Repetitive behavior
    c. Delayed language development
    d. Severe deficit in social interaction

39. **The following are characteristic of autism except:**
    [AI 06]
    a. Onset after 6 years of age
    b. Repetitive behavior
    c. Delayed language development
    d. Severe deficit in social interaction

40. **WHO defines adolescent age between:**   [AI 05]
    a. 10–19 years
    b. 10–14 years
    c. 10–25 years
    d. 9–14 years

41. **A two-month-old child is able to:**   [AI 04]
    a. Show a positive parachute protective reflex
    b. Hold head steady in seated position
    c. Lift head and chest off a flat surface with extended elbows
    d. Sustain head level with the body when placed in ventral suspension

42. **All of the following are essential features of attention deficit hyperactive disease (ADHD) except:**   [AI 04]
    a. Lack of concentration b. Impulsivity
    c. Mental retardation   d. Hyperactivity

43. **What is the order of puberty:**   [AI 2K]
    a. Thelarchy - pubarchy - menarchy
    b. Puberchy - thelarchy - menarchy
    c. Puberchy - menarchy - thelarchy
    d. Adrenarchy - thelarchy–pubarchy

44. **Height of a children in 2–10 years of age is increased by:**   [AI 97]
    a. 2 cm/year   b. 4 cm/year
    c. 6 cm/year   d. 10 cm/year

45. **Peak growth velocity in adolescent girl is indicated:**   [AI 98]
    a. Breast enlargement
    b. Axillary hair
    c. Public hair
    d. Just before commencement of menarche

46. **Peak growth velocity in adolescent girls is seen just after:**   [AI 96]
    a. Appearance of pubic and axillary hair
    b. Breast enlargement
    c. Onset of menstruation
    d. Enlargement of external genitalia

47. **Maximum growth spurt is seen in girls at the time of:**   [AI 96]
    a. Pubarche   b. Thelarche
    c. Menarche   d. Adrenarche

48. **A 3-month-old baby will have:**   [PGI Nov. 09]
    a. Pincer grasp   b. Head control
    c. Sitting with support   d. Transfer objects
    e. Speak tow word sentences

49. **A boy can grasp a rattle and recently he became able to transfer objects, hand to hand. He can do:**   [PGI Dec. 08]
    a. Babble   b. Say 'mama' or 'dada'
    c. Sit without support   d. Stand with support
    e. Able to walk

50. **Drugs used in ADHD are:**   [PGI Dec. 08]
    a. Atomoxetine   b. Methylphenidate
    c. Dextro-amphetamine d. Quetiapine

51. **10-month-old child cannot do:**   [PGI Dec. 05; June 04]
    a. Change cube from one hand to another
    b. Can build a tower of 6 cubes
    c. Recognizes mother
    d. Can talk a sentence of 4 to 5 words
    e. Pincer grasp

52. **A 3-month-old can do:**   [PGI June 05; Dec. 01]
    a. Social smile
    b. Can sit without support
    c. Transfer objects from right to left
    d. Hold his neck
    e. Can change position from prone to supine

53. **Which of the following is true about eruption of teeth?**   [PGI Dec. 05]
    a. Premolar appear in primary dentition
    b. Incisors appear first in secondary dentition
    c. 3rd molar is last to develop
    d. Hypothyroidism delays dentition
    e. Canines is last to appear in primary dentition

54. **Infantile autism is characterized by:**   [PGI Dec. 04]
    a. Impaired vision
    b. Impaired neurobehavioural development
    c. Impaired folate level
    d. A socio economic hazard
    e. Parenting

55. **2-year-old child can do:**   [PGI Dec. 04]
    a. Ride tricycles
    b. Climb up and down stairs with one each time
    c. Knows sex and age
    d. Handles spoon well
    e. Can read story with picture

56. **True about head circumference measurement:**   [PGI Dec. 04]
    a. Measured in supraorbital ridge
    b. Measures hydrocephalus/microcephaly
    c. Serial measurement is useful
    d. Helps in measurement of neurological development
    e. Pediatric intelligence

57. **True about dentition:**   [PGI June 04]
    a. Hypothyroidism causes delayed dentition
    b. Premolar is not seen in primary dentition
    c. 3rd molar is the last to appear in secondary dentition
    d. Canine is the first in primary dentition
    e. Incisor is the first in secondary dentition

58. **An 18-month-old infant can do all except:**   [PGI Dec. 03]
    a. Climbing upstairs
    b. Can follow mother's activities
    c. Can turn 2-3 pages at a time
    d. Can say two or three words
    e. Can make tower of 8 cubes

59. **A baby can follow an object with 180°, can hold neck, but can't sit without support. The age of the baby is:**   [PGI June 03]
    a. 1 month   b. 3 months
    c. 5 months   d. 6 months
    e. 9 months

60. **Which of the following cannot be done by 3-year-old child?**   [PGI Dec. 02]
    a. Draw a triangle
    b. Draw a circle
    c. Arrange 9 cubes
    d. Go up and down stains
    e. Stand on one foot for 5 second

61. **Persistent Moro's reflex at 6–7 months indicates:**   [PGI 02, DPG 09]
    a. Normal child
    b. Brain damage
    c. Hungry child
    d. Irritable child

62. Persistent Moro's reflex at 6–7 months indicates:
[PGI 02, DPG 09]
a. Normal child   b. Brain damage
c. Hungry child   d. Irritable child

63. An 8 week infant can do all of the following except
[PGI Dec. 01]
a. Head control
b. Lift its head up to horizontal line in ventral suspension
c. Follows red object up to 180
d. Social smile
e. Turns head towards sound

64. Infantile proportion in adult is seen in:
[PGI Dec. 01]
a. Morquio's disease
b. Achondroplasia
c. Hypothyroidism
d. Malnutrition
e. Constitutional dwarfism

65. Treatment for breath holding spells in a child is:
[PGI Dec. 01]
a. Give extra care and love to the child
b. Inflicting painful stimulus at the beginning of the attack
c. Do not give attention to the child
d. Fulfill the wishes of the child to prevent the attack
e. Low dose barbiturates

66. A neonate is able to:
[PGI Dec. 00]
a. Fix his gaze at an object 8 to 12 inches apart
b. Focus on bright object
c. Lift his head and chest on elbow
d. Roll from side to side

67. First sign of puberty in girls: [PGI Dec. 99, AI 08]
a. Puberchy   b. Thelarchy
c. Growth spurt   d. Menarche

68. All of the following reflexes are present at birth except :
[AI 07; PGI June 98]
a. Rooting reflex
b. Symmetrical tonic neck reflex

c. Asymmetrical neck reflex
d. Crossed extensor reflex

69. Pincer grasp is attained at months: [PGI June 98]
a. 4   b. 10
c. 12   d. 18

70. Child of 9 months, which reflex is abnormal:
[PGI June 98]
a. Asymmetric neck reflex
b. Parachute reflex
c. Righting reflex
d. None

71. Atypical moro's reflex is seen in A/E: [PGI Dec. 97]
a. Clavicle   b. Sternomastoid tumor
c. Shoulder dislocation   d. Brachial plexus injury

72. Anthropometric assessment, which does not show much change in 1-4 years: [PGI Dec. 96]
a. Mid arm circumference
b. Skin fold thickness
c. Chest circumference : Head circumference
d. Height

73. Order of development of secondary sexual characteristic in male: [PGI 96]
a. Testicular development – Pubic hair – axillary hair – beard
b. Pubic hair – Testicular development – axillary hair-beard
c. Testicular development – beard – pubic hair – axillary hair
d. Axillary hair – beard – pubic hair – testicular development

74. The height of a child is double the birth height at the age of: [PGI 95]
a. 1 year   b. 2 year
c. 4 year   d. 6 year
e. 8 year

75. Which of the above diagnostic criteria are suggestive on inattention (attention deficit) on child?
a. 1 and 2 only   b. 1 and 3 only
c. 2 and 4 only   d. 1, 2, 3 and 4 only

QUESTIONS OF OTHER EXAMINATIONS

1. Which of the following is thet first sign of puberty in girls?   [Ref: MHCET 10]
a. Pubarche   b. Thelarche
c. Menarche   d. Growth spurt

2. The following is usually first sign of puberty in girls: [UPSC 10]
a. Onset of menstruation
b. Appearance of pubic hair
c. Change of voice
d. Increase in breast size

3. Child begins to sit with support, able to transfer objects from one hand to another hand and speak monosyllabic babbles at the age of: [MHCET 10]
a. 3 months   b. 6 months
c. 9 months   d. 12 months

4. Early strict toilet training can result in: [Manipal 09]
a. Nocturnal enuresis
b. Encopresis
c. Night terror
d. Temper tantrums

5. The milestones achieved at 13 months in children are all except: [DPG 09]
   a. Index finger approach
   b. Walking
   c. Casting
   d. Single words

6. The first epiphyseal center appears in: [DPG 08]
   a. Femur   b. Cuboid
   c. Os calcis   d. Clavicle

7. Best treatment for enuresis is: [DPG 08]
   a. Oxybutinin   b. Desmopressin
   c. Bed alarm   d. Imipramine

8. A child plays a simple ball game at: [Manipal 08]
   a. 52 weeks   b. 36 weeks
   c. 12 weeks   d. 48 weeks

9. A boy draws triangle but not diamond shape age is: [APPG 08]
   a. 3 years   b. 4 years
   c. 5 years   d. 6 years

10. At the end of 1 year of age, the number of carpal bones seen in the skiagram of the hand is: [COMED 08]
    a. Nil   b. 1
    c. 2   d. 3

11. Child changes a rattle from one hand to another at the age of: [COMED 07]
    a. 3 months   b. 6 months
    c. 9 months   d. 1 year

12. Which of the following activities cannot be performed by a 7 months old infant?   [UPSC 07]
    a. Pivot   b. Cruise
    c. Transfer objects   d. Enjoy mirror

13. An infant can sit with leaning forward on his hands. He bounces actively when made to stand. He laughs aloud and becomes concerned when the mother moves away. What is the most likely age? [UPSC 07]
    a. 12 weeks   b. 16 weeks
    c. 22 weeks   d. 28 weeks

14. 90% of the brain growth is achieved by the: [COMED 07, Kerala 04]
    a. 2nd year   b. 3rd year
    c. 5th year   d. 15th year

15. Birth weight of a child doubles at five months of age while the birth length doubles at the age of: [UPSC 07]
    a. 1 year   b. 2 years
    c. 3 years   d. 4 years

16. Which of the following are first incisors to erupt in an infant?   [UPSC 07]
    a. Lower central
    b. Lower lateral
    c. Upper central
    d. Upper lateral

17. A child draws circle at: [Manipal 06]
    a. 12 months   b. 24 months
    c. 30 months   d. 36 months

18. In a child one should be worried if: [KCET 06]
    a. Stammering occurs at 3 years
    b. Lack of toilet control at 2.5 years
    c. Teeth do not erupt by 11 months
    d. Social smile absent by 10 weeks

19. At which one of the following age period a child can remove front opening garment?   [COMED 06]
    a. 24 months   b. 36 months
    c. 48 months   d. 60 months

20. Postnatally when is the growth velocity maximum?   [UPSC 06]
    a. In the first year of life
    b. In the second year of life
    c. In the seventh year of life
    d. In adolescence

21. In a healthy child, the head and chest circumference equal each other around the age of: [KCET 06]
    a. 3-6 months   b. 6-9 months
    c. 9-12 months   d. 12-15 months

22. A normal healthy child has a height of 100 cm and weighs 16 kg. What is the most likely age?   [UPSC 06]
    a. 3 years   b. 4 years
    c. 5 years   d. 6 years

23. Upper segment to lower segment ratio in 3 year age child is: [Manipal 06]
    a. 1.2   b. 1.3
    c. 1.4   d. 1.6

24. Which one of the following is the correct order of events at puberty in a girl?   [UPSC 06]
    a. Thelarche-puberche- menarche-growth spurt
    b. Puberche-thelarche-growth spurt-menarche
    c. Menarche-growth spurt-thelarche-puberche
    d. Thelarche-puberche-growth spurt-menarche

25. A two month old child is most likely to: [SGPGI 05]
    a. Show a positive parachute protective reflex
    b. Hold head steady in a seated position
    c. Lift head and chest off a flat surface with extended elbows
    d. Sustain head level with the body when placed in ventral suspension

26. At what age does an infant discriminate strangers: [COMED 05]
    a. 4 weeks   b. 8 weeks
    c. 12 weeks   d. 20 weeks

27. The age by which most of the babies know their gender is: [COMED 05]
    a. 1 year   b. 2 years
    c. 3 years   d. 4 years

28. **A child can ride a tricycle, copy a circle and knows age and sex by the age of:** [J and K 05]
    a. 30 months   b. 42 months
    c. 36 months   d. 48 months

29. **Weight gain in the second year of life is:** [CMC 05]
    a. 1 kg   b. 2 kg
    c. 3 kg   d. 4 kg
    e. 5 kg

30. **Growth spurt occurs:** [SGPGI 05]
    a. Just before appearance of axillary hair
    b. Just before menarche
    c. After 16 years
    d. Before thelarche

31. **A 40 weeks old infant can do all of the following except:** [JIPMER 03]
    a. Waves bye bye
    b. Transfers objects from one hand to another
    c. Sits with support
    d. Makes a tower of 3-4 cubes

32. **Increase in height in the first year is by:** [DNB 2001]
    a. 40%   b. 50%
    c. 60%   d. 75%

33. **Handedness develops at:** [TN 01]
    a. 12 months   b. 18 months
    c. 24 months   d. 36 months

34. **A normal infant sits briefly leaning forward on her hands, reaches for and grasps a cube and transfer it from hand to hand. She babbles but cannot wave bye-bye nor she can grasp objects with the finger and thumb. Her age is:** [UPSC 2000]
    a. 4 months   b. 7 months
    c. 10 months   d. 12 months

35. **A child knows sex and name by the age of 3 years. A three old child can do which of the following except:** [Kerala 2000]
    a. Ride a tricycle
    b. Build a tower of ten cubes
    c. Knows his age and sex
    d. Use scissors to cut pictures

36. **A normal infant sits briefly leaning forward on her hands, reaches for and grasps a cube and transfer it from hand to hand. She babbles but cannot wave bye-bye nor can she grasp objects with finger and thumb. Her age is:** [UPSC 2000]
    a. 4 months   b. 7 months
    c. 10 months   d. 14 months

37. **Gender from external genitalia of fetus becomes clearly distinguished by:** [Orissa 2000]
    a. 10 weeks   b. 16 weeks
    c. 12 weeks   d. 20 weeks

38. **By .... years all milk teeth are erupted:** [AMC 2000]
    a. 1.5   b. 2
    c. 2.5   d. 3

39. **Fetal growth is maximally affected by:** [UP 2000]
    a. Insulin   b. Growth hormone
    c. Cortisol   d. Thyroxine

40. **Which of the following childhood disorder improves with increase in age?** [MP 2000]
    a. Conduct disorder   b. Emotional problems
    c. Temper tantrum   d. Sleep disorder

41. **A newborn has a head circumference of 35 cm at birth. His optimal head circumference will be 43 cm at** [UPSC 99]
    a. 4 months of age   b. 6 months of age
    c. 8 months of age   d. 12 months of age

42. **An 18-month-old baby presents with recurrent episodes of excessive crying followed by cyanosis, unconsciousness and occasional seizures since 9 months of age. The most likely diagnosis is:** [UPSC 98]
    a. Epilepsy   b. Anoxic spells
    c. Breath holding spells   d. Vasovagal attack

43. **The upper segment: lower segment ratio at 2 years of age in a normal child is:** [KCET 96]
    a. 1.8:1   b. 1.5:1
    c. 1.25:1   d. 1.12:1

44. **Vocabulary of 1.5 year old child is:** [AMU 95]
    a. 1-10 words   b. 10-20 words
    c. 20-30 words   d. 30-40 words

45. **The maximum age for growth of lymphoid tissue:** [JIPMER 95]
    a. 3-4 years   b. 5-7 years
    c. 7-11 years   d. 11-14 years

46. **Sitting height is equal to:** [Assam 95]
    a. Head circumference
    b. Chest circumference
    c. Upper segment
    d. Crown-heel length

47. **Peak Stage in height growth corresponds to .... stage of pubic hair:** [JIPMER 95]
    a. I   b. II
    c. III   d. IV

48. **Persistent Moro's reflex at 6–7 months indicates:** [PGI 02, DPG 09]
    a. Normal child   b. Brain damage
    c. Hungry child   d. Irritable child

49. **Cretinism is:** [UP 08]
    a. Disproportionate dwarfism
    b. Short stature with long trunk
    c. Short stature with short trunk
    d. Long stature with long trunk

50. **Which of the following nasal spray is very effective in control of enuresis?** [KCET 99]
    a. Pitressin
    b. Desmopressin
    c. Lipressin
    d. None of the above

51. **The behavior therapy fails in the management of enuresis. The pharmacological drug of choice for this case is:** [UP 07]
    a. Phenytoin
    b. Diazepam
    c. Imipramine
    d. Alprax

52. **Which is incorrect about thumb sucking?** [JIPMER 91]
    a. Can lead to malocclusion
    b. It is a source of pleasure
    c. It is a sign of insecurity
    d. Must be treated vigorously in the first year

53. **Which of the following is not true regarding thumb sucking?** [UP 07, 05]
    a. Feels insecurity
    b. Pleasurable sensation
    c. Leads to dental problems
    d. Child less than 4 years of age

ANSWERS

1. (b) Behaviour therapy (Ref: Ghai 7th E/P38)
- The symptom of inattentiveness, restlessness and urge to play outside is diagnostic of ADHD.
- Treatment consists of **behaviour therapy** and psychostimulant medications.

2. (b) Recognize colours (Ref: Nelson 19th E/P39)
- A 6-year-old child with IQ of 50 will have a mental development equal to 3 years.

The mentioned milestones in the options can be seen at the following ages:
- Draw a triangle – 5 years
- **Recognize colors – 3 years**
- Read a sentence – 6-7 years.

3. (b) Symmetric tonic neck reflex (Ref: Ghai 7th E/P114, Nelson 19th E/P1979)
- Symmetric tonic neck reflex only develops by 4–6 months of age and hence is not present at birth.

4. (a) Autism (Ref: Rudolph 22nd E/P352–53)
- Development of symptoms like delayed speech and difficulty in communication and concentration at 3 years of age is diagnostic of autism.

5. (d) 6 months (Ref: Ghai 7th E/P114)
- Moro reflex develops at 28 weeks of gestation and disappears by **3–6 months of age. Persistence beyond 6 months of age is considered pathological.**

6. (d) Attention deficit hyperactive disorder (Ref: Ghai 7th E/P38)

7. (c) Specific learning disability (Ref: Nelson 19th E/P110–11, Ghai 7th E/P39)

Specific learning disability (Dyslexia):
- This is the most common form of learning disability. It can be acquired both genetically as well as sporadically. The abnormalities in DCD2 gene has been implicated in the familial or genetic form.
- There is abnormality in the tempro-occipital regions of the left hemisphere.
- The child has difficulty in spelling and reading because of improper word decoding and recognition.
- Treatment in young children aims at remediation of the reading difficulty. In older children accommodation is more preferred by using computer for spelling check and giving extra time for solving questions.

8. (a) 2 and 3 years (Ref: Nelson 19th E/P39, CPDT 19th E/P73)
- Baby can **feed with spoon without spilling** at 2 years of age.
- Baby helps in **dressing (unbuttoning clothes, puts on shoes)** and **Knows full name and gender** by 3 years of age.
- Hence the best answer is between 2 and 3 years.

9. (d) Build a tower of 3-4 cubes (Ref: Nelson 19th E/P34, CPDT 19th E/P73)

A child can develop the mentioned milestones in the options by following age:
- Stand alone – 12 months
- Play peek a boo – 10 months
- Pick up a pellet with thumb and index finger — Pincer grasp develops by 9 months
- Builds a tower of 3–4 cubes – 18 months
- Hence the best answer is 'd' i.e. built a tower of 3–4 cubes.

10. (c) Pubertal gynaecomastia (Ref: Nelson 19th E/P1931)

Pubertal gynaecomastia:
- 2/3rd boys may have increased estradiol level as compared to testosterone, which leads to **physiological pubertal gynaecomastia**.
- Most of the times only one breast is involved and a transient tenderness can be seen.
- Treatment is usually not required; however in case of severe enlargement danazole can be used.

11. (a), (b) and **(e)** Maternal deprivation syndrome, Hypothyroidism and IUGR (Ref: Ghai 7th E/P18)

Causes of short stature:

Mnemonic: **CHATTISGARH**
C — Constitutional, Chronic diseases
H — Hypothyroidism
A — Accelerated and delayed puberty
T — Trisomy 21
T — Turner syndrome
I — IUGR
S — Small for gestational age babies
G — Growth hormone deficiency
A — Achondroplasia
R — Rickets
H — Hyperphagic short stature

12. (b) Rett's syndrome (Ref: Rudolph 22nd E/P353)

Rett's syndrome:

- Rett syndrome is usually seen in **females**.
- These children develop normally till 6–18 months of age followed by **rapid regression in language and hand skills, repetitive hand movements** and **decreased rate of head growth**.
- Diagnosis is confirmed by DNA analysis for methyl CpG-binding protein 2 (MECP 2).

13. (b) Attention deficit hyperactive disorder (Ref: Ghai 7th E/P38)

- The symptoms of restlessness, hyperactivity, inobidience and disturbing other students are consistent with attention deficit hyperactivity disorder.

14. (b) Autistic disorder (Ref: Rudolph 22nd E/P353)

15. (a) 30 months (Ref: Nelson 19th E/P39)

A child can develop the mentioned milestones in the question by the following age:

- **Walks upstairs with alternate steps, builds tower of 9 blocks and refers to self by "I"** by 30 months of age.
- Baby can **say his age and sex** at 3 years of age.
- Hence the most probable age of child is 30 months.

16. (a) Does not vocalize (Ref: CPDT 19th E/P73)

- Baby vocalizes at the age of 1–2 months and hence if the baby does not vocalize by 12 weeks or 3 months evaluation is warranted.

17. (b) $C_5 - C_6$ (Ref: Nelson 19th E/P565)

18. (c) 15% of children will have HC less than that (Ref: Ghai 7th E/P7)

"Percentile curves represent frequency distribution curves. For example, 25th percentile of height in a population would mean that height of 75% of individuals is above and 25% are below this value."

19. (c) Nothing should be done actively and assure the patients (Ref: Ghai 7th E/P6)

- The normal range of variation of height and weight for a child lies in between 3rd and 97th percentile.
- The normal range of target height for a male is ±8.5 cm and for female is ±7 cm. The normal range for a 3 year old female child is 95 ± 7 cm i.e. it lies in between 88 and 102 cm. Hence the height is normal.
- Thus the height and weight of the female child is appropriate for her age and nothing should be advised.

20. (d) Can walk down the stairs with alternating steps holding on to the iron rail (Ref: Nelson 19th E/P39, CPDT 19th E/P74)

Milestones of a 4 year old child:

- **Walks downstairs with alternate steps**
- **Hops on one foot**
- Throws ball overhead
- **Uses scissors to cut pictures**
- **Copies cross and square**
- Plays cooperatively in a group
- Goes to toilet alone
- Story telling

21. (a) Frontal lobe (Ref: Henry Neurological evaluation of infants and children/P63)

Palmomental reflex:

- Palmomental reflex is elicited by scratching the thenar part of hand, which leads to ipsilateral elevation and retraction of angle of mouth.
- It is normally present in infancy and older people.
- Pathological presence is associated with lesion of pyramidal tract in the opposite frontal lobe.

22. (a) Antiepileptic treatment is necessary (Ref: Nelson 19th E/P2010)

- Though seizures can be seen in breath holding spells, antiepileptic treatment is not required.
- Atropine can be used for treatment of pallid spells as excessive central parasympathetic activity is seen.
- Holding of breath leads to pallor and cyanosis.
- Mostly it is seen in between 6 months to 5 years of age.

23. (b) 11 months (Ref: Ghai 7th E/P6)

- Birth weight of a child approximately
  - Doubles by 6 months
  - Triples by 1 year
  - Quadruples by 2 years

24. (a) Pincer grasp at 3 months (Ref: Nelson 19th E/P34)

- Pincer grasp develops at 9 months and matures at 12 months.

25. (a) Normal body proportion (Ref: Rudolph 22nd E/P2017)

Cause	Birth weight and length	Skeletal maturation	Timing of puberty	Other features	Treatment
Growth hormone deficiency	• **Normal weight** • **Slightly reduced length**	Delayed	Normal	• Hypoglycemia • Hypothyroidism • Micropenis • Truncal adiposity • Body proportions **are normal** • "Doll like" facial appearance	Subcutaneous recombinant GH

26. (c) Hobble 5 steps (Ref: Nelson 19th E/P39)

- A child starts hopping by 4 years of age.

27. (a) Grasp dangling objects (Ref: Ghai 7th E/P28)

The mentioned milestones can be achieved by following age:

- Grasp dangling objects — 4 months
- Fix gaze — 1 month

- Lift and hold head — 1 months
- Turns towards sound — 1 month

28. (c) Growth hormone (Ref: Rudolph 22nd E/P2075)

29. (a) 8 years (Ref: Ghai 7th E/38)
- Continuation of thumb sucking post 5 years can result in **dental misalignment** like flaring of the maxillary incisor teeth, open bite and posterior cross bite. To lessen the effects of misalignment it should be discontinued before **8 years.**

30. (a) Constitutional growth delay (Ref: Ghai 7th E/P19)

Cause	Birth weight and length	Skeletal maturation	Timing of puberty	Other features	Treatment
Familial/Genetic short stature	Normal	Normal	Normal	Normal	Not required /Assurance
Constitutional growth delay	Normal	Delayed	Delayed	Normal growth velocity	Not required /Assurance

- Height of child below 3rd percentile is diagnostic of short stature; however the velocity of growth is normal.
- This is possible in familial short stature and constitutional growth delay.
- The child also has delayed skeletal age.
- As shown in the table constitutional short stature is associated with a delayed skeletal maturation, the best answer is option (a).

31. (d) Vision problem (Ref: Rudolph 22nd E/P353)
The findings of autistic specific disorders are:
- **Social deficits** are the earliest manifestation
- **Speech delay**
- **Language disorder** (echolalia or parroting).
- **Delayedcommunication**
- Narrow repetitive interest and insistence on sameness
- Stereotypic behaviors like hand flapping due to **impaired imagination**
- Interest in solitary play

32. (a) Bed alarms (Ref: Nelson 19th E/P74)
- First line of treatment of nocturnal enuresis is non-pharmacological i.e. **motivational and alarm therapy**. It is the **most effective treatment** with least chances of recurrences.

33. (a) Constitutional (Ref: Ghai 7th E/P19, 20, Rudolph 22nd E/P2016–17)
- **Most common cause of short stature is familial short stature and constitutional growth delay, both of which account for approximately 50% of cases.**

34. (d) 6 months of age (Ref: Ghai 7th E/P114)
- Moro reflex develops at 28 weeks of gestation and disappears by **3–6 months of age**.

35. (b) Symmetrical tonic neck reflex (Ref: Nelson 19th E/P1979, Ghai 7th E/P114)

Reflex	Emerges	Disappears
Crossed extensor	28 weeks of gestation	1–2 months
Grasp	28 weeks of gestation	2–3 month
Rooting	32 weeks of gestation	1 month
Sucking	28 weeks gestation	4 months
Moro	30 weeks gestation	5 months
ATNR	35 weeks gestation	6–7 months
Galant	30 weeks gestation	6 months
Stepping	Birth	2 months
Landau	3 months	15 months
Protective extension		
Forward	6 months	**Persists**
Sideways	7 months	**Persists**
Backwards	9 months	**Persists**
Tilting reaction	12 months	Persists
Parachute	7–8 months	Persists
Symmetric tonic neck	**4–6 months**	8–12 months

36. (c) Mirror play (Ref: Nelson 19th E/P 34)
The mentioned milestones can be seen at the following age:
- **Mirror play — 7 months**
- Creeping — 12 months
- Crawling — 8 months
- Pincer grasp — Develops at 9 months and matures at 12 months

37. (b) 5 months (Ref: CPDT 19th E/P73)
- Mouthing of objects starts at 4 months and stranger anxiety develops at 6 months.
- Hence among the given options 5 months is the best option.

38. (a) Onset after 6 years of age (Ref: Ghai 7th E/P40)
- Autism develops before 3 years of age and can be diagnosed as early as 18 months.

39. (a) Onset after 6 years of age (Ref: Rudolph 22nd E/P353)
- The symptoms of autism usually develop by 3 years of age.

40. (a) 10-19 years (Ref: Ghai 7th E/P42)

Various Stages of Growth and Development

Prenatal period	
Embryo	**From day of fertilization(generally 14th day post ovulation) to 9 weeks**
Fetus	9 weeks to birth
Perinatal period	**22 weeks of gestation to 7 days after birth**
Postnatal period	
Newborn	**First 4 weeks after birth**
Infancy	**First year**
Toddler	1–3 years
Preschool child	3–6 years
School age child	6–12 years
Adolescence	
Early	**10–13 years**
Middle	14–16 years
Late	17–**19 years**

41. (b) Hold head steady in seated position (Ref: Nelson 19th E/P34, CPDT 19th E/P73)

Milestones of a 2 month old child:
- **Holds head steady while sitting**
- Head sustains in plane of body on ventral suspension
- Social smile

42. (c) Mental retardation (Ref: Ghai 7th E/P38)

Findings in ADHD:
- **Inattention** and **increased distractibility**
- **Impulsivity**
- Decreased self-control
- **Motor hyperactivity** and **motor restlessness**
- Inefficient planning and organizing of tasks
- Emotional liability
- Low self-esteem
- **Academic underperformance.**

43. (a) Thelarchy - pubarchy–menarchy (Ref: Ghai 7th E/P498)

44. (c) 6 cm/year (Ref: Ghai 7th E/P6)

45. (d) Just before commencement of menarche (Ref: IAP 4th E/P100)

"The height velocity (maximum body growth–9-10 cm/year) is at Tanner stages II and III of mammary gland development. It is at this level of sexual maturity in girls the **menarche** is attained."

46. (a) Appearance of pubic and axillary hair (Ref: IAP 4th E/P100)

47. (c) Menarche (Ref: IAP 4th E/P100)

48. (b) Head control (Ref: Nelson 19th E/P39)

The milestones mentioned in the options develop by the following age:
- Pincer grasp – 9 months
- **Head control – 3 months**
- Sitting with support – 6 months
- Transfer objects – 7 months
- Speak two word sentences – 12 months

49. (a) Babble (Ref: Nelson 19th E/P34)
- The milestones mentioned in the question can develop by following age:
  - ❖ Grasp a rattle – 7 months
  - ❖ Transfer objects from one hand to other – 7 months
- Hence the age of baby is 7 months.
- The milestones mentioned in the options can be achieved by:
  - ❖ Babble – 7 months
  - ❖ Say mama or dada – 9 months
  - ❖ Sit without support – 8 months
  - ❖ Stand with support – 9 months
  - ❖ Able to walk – 15 months
- The 7 month old baby can babble.

50. (d) a, b and c i.e. Atomoxetine, Methylphenidate and Dextroamphetamine. (Ref: Ghai 7th E/P38, Nelson 19th E/P109)
- The first line drugs used for ADHD are **methylphenidate, amphetamine and dextroamphetamine preparations like Dexedrine and Adderral.**
- Other medications like noradrenergic reuptake inhibitor (**Atomoxetine),** tricyclic antidepressants (Imipramine, Nortriptyline) and alpha agonist (clonidine) can also be used.

51. (b) and **(d)** Can build a tower of 6 cubes and Can talk a sentence of 4 to 5 words (Ref: Nelson 19th E/P34, CPDT 19th E/P73)

The milestones mentioned in the options can develop by following age:
- Change cube from one hand to other – 6 months
- Can build a tower of 6 cubes – 2 years
- Recognizes mother – 3 months
- Can talk a sentence of 4-5 words

52. (a) and **(d)** Social smile and hold his neck (Ref: Nelson 19th E/P34, CPDT 19th E/P73)

The milestones mentioned in the options can develop by the following age:
- **Social smile – 2 months**
- Can sit without support – 8 months
- Transfer objects from right to left – 6 months
- **Hold his neck – 3 months**
- Can change position from prone to supine – 8 months

53. (c) and **(d)** 3rd molar is last to develop and Hypothyroidism delays dentition (Ref: Nelson 19th E/P36, 1204–06)

Sequence of Teeth Eruption:

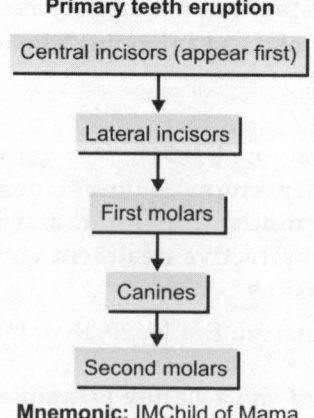

Primary teeth eruption

Central incisors (appear first) → Lateral incisors → First molars → Canines → Second molars

Mnemonic: IMChild of Mama

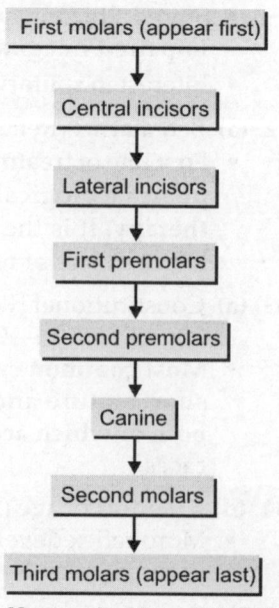

Secondary teeth eruption

First molars (appear first) → Central incisors → Lateral incisors → First premolars → Second premolars → Canine → Second molars → Third molars (appear last)

Mnemonic: Mama Is In Pain Papa Can Make Medicine

Causes of delayed eruption:
- **Hypothyroidism**
- Hypopitutarism
- Cleidocranial dysplasia
- Rickets
- Down's syndrome
- Albright osteodystrophy
- Progeria
- Incontinentia pigmenti

54. **(b)** and **(c)** (Ref: Rudolph 22nd E/P353)

55. **(b)** and **(d)** Climb up and down stairs with one each time, Handles spoon well (Ref: Nelson 19th E/P39, CPDT 19th E/P74)

The milestones mentioned in the options can be achieved by the following age:
- Ride tricycle — 3 years
- **Climb up and down stairs with one each time — 2 years**
- Knows age and sex — 3 years
- **Handles spoon well — 2 years**
- Can read a story with picture — 4 years

56. All (Ref: Nelson 19th E/P1975, Ghai 7th E/P5)
Head circumference:
- Head circumference measurement is an important part of neurological examination in the infants. It is important to add to the diagnosis of **neurological dysfunction** and **microcephaly**. A head circumference of 2 SD below the mean for age and sex is diagnostic of microcephaly. A rapid increase in head circum-ference suggests a tumor or **hydrocephalus**.
- It is **measured in every visit** and a growth chart of head is prepared. A plastic tape is used to measure the greatest circumference through the **occipital protuberance** and **supraorbital ridge**.
- The head circumference grows by 0.5 cm in first 2 weeks, 0.75 cm in 3rd week and thereafter 1 cm/week till birth. At birth the head circumference is 35 cm and by 1 year it increases to 45 cm.

57. **(a), (b)** and **(c)** (Ref: Nelson 19th E/P36, 1204–06)

58. **(a)** and **(e)** Climbing upstairs and Can make towers of 8 cubes (Ref: Nelson 19th E/P39, CPDT 19th E/P74)
The milestones mentioned in the options can be achieved by following age:
- **Climbing upstairs with alternate steps – 30 months**
- Can follow mothers activity – 18 months
- Can turn 2–3 pages at a time – 12 months
- Can say 2–3 words – 18 months
- **Can make tower of 8 cubes – 30 months**

59. **(d)** 6 months (Ref: Nelson 19th E/P34, CPDT 19th E/P73)
The milestones mentioned in the question can achieved by the following age:
- Follow an object with 180° – 3 months
- Neck holding – 3 months
- **Sit with support – 6 months**

60. **(a)** Draw a triangle (Ref: Nelson 19th E/P39)
The milestones in the options can develop by the following age:
- **Draw a triangle – 5 years**
- Draw a circle – 3 years
- Arrange 9 cubes – 30 months
- Go up and down stairs – 30 years
- Stand on one foot for 5 seconds – 3 years

61. **(b)** Brain damage (Ref: Gerald neonatal neurology/P 14)
- Moro reflex develops at 28 weeks of gestation and disappears by **3–6 months of age. Persistence beyond 6 months of age is considered pathological** and may indicate **hypoxic ischemic encephalopathy**.

62. **(b)** Brain damage (Ref: Gerald neonatal neurology/P 14)
- Moro reflex develops at 28 weeks of gestation and disappears by **3–6 months of age. Persistence beyond 6 months of age is considered pathological** and may indicate **hypoxic ischemic encephalopathy**.

63. **(a)** and **(c)** Head control and Follows red object up to 180 (Ref: Nelson 19th E/P39)
The milestones mentioned in the options can develop by the following age:
- **Head control – 3 months**
- Lift its head up to horizontal line in ventral suspension – 2 months
- **Follows red object up to 180 – 3 months**
- Social smile – 2 months
- Turns head towards sound – 1 month

64. **(b)** and **(c)** Achondroplasia and Hypothyroidism (Ref: IAP 4th E/P912–14)
- Infantile proportion means an upper segment to lower segment ratio of more than 1 or upper-segment > lower segment. This can be seen in conditions like skeletal dysplasia (**achondroplasia and rickets**) and untreated **hypothyroidism**.

65. **(b)** Inflicting painful stimulus at the beginning of the attack (Ref: Ghai 7th E/P37)

"During the episode they (parents) should **pinch the child at the onset of the spell** and **should not exhibit undue concern or excessively cuddle the child** as this reinforces the 'gain' in attention."

66. **(a)** Focus on bright object (Ref: Ghai 7th E/P30)
Milestones of a neonate:
- **Fixates on light or face in line of vision**, dolls eye movement of eye on turning head
- Turns head from side to side
- Reflexes seen are Moro's, stepping and placing; and grasp

67. (b) Thelarchy (Ref: Ghai 7th E/P498)
- Order of sexual maturity in females is thelarche followed by pubearche followed by menarche.

68. (b) Symmetrical tonic neck reflex (Ref: Nelson 19th E/P1979, Ghai 7th E/P114)

Reflex	Emerges	Disappears
Crossed extensor	28 weeks of gestation	1–2 months
Grasp	28 weeks of gestation	2–3 month
Rooting	32 weeks of gestation	1 month
Sucking	28 weeks gestation	4 months
Moro	30 weeks gestation	5 months
ATNR	35 weeks gestation	6–7 months
Galant	30 weeks gestation	6 months
Stepping	Birth	2 months
Landau	3 months	15 months
Protective extension		
Forward	6 months	**Persists**
Sideways	7 months	**Persists**
Backwards	9 months	**Persists**
Tilting reaction	12 months	Persists
Parachute	7–8 months	Persists
Symmetric tonic neck	**4–6 months**	8–12 months

69. (b) 10 (Ref: Nelson 19th E/P34)
- Pincer grasp develops at 9 months and matures at 12 months.

70. (a) Asymmetric neck reflex (Ref: Ghai 7th E/P114, Nelson 19th E/P1979)

71. (b) Sternomastoid tumor (Ref: Gerald neonatal neurology/P 14)

Moro reflex:
- When the child is held in a supine position and the head is allowed to fall, there is abduction of arm followed by adduction and closing of fists.
- It develops at 28 weeks of gestation and disappears by **3–6 months of age. Persistence beyond 6 months of age is considered pathological** and may indicate **hypoxic ischemic encephalopathy**.
- Absent moro reflex can be seen with **brachial palsy (C5-C6 lesion), fracture of humers, fracture of clavicle and shoulder dislocation.**

72. (a) Mid arm circumference (Ref: Achar's pediatrics 3rd E/P54)

"**Measurements of arm circumference**, taken at the middle of upper arm with the arm hanging relaxed at the side have been found to **remain more or less constant**, ranging between 16 and 17 cm in **two to five year old well-nourished child.**"

73. (a) Testicular development — Pubic hair — axillary hair — beard (Ref: Ghai 7th E/P498)
- Order of sexual maturity in males is testicular develoment → Pubarch → Penile growth → axillary hair →Facial hair.

74. (c) 4 years (Ref: Ghai 7th E/P6)
Height of a child approximately
- **Doubles by 4 years**
- **Triples by 12 years**

75. (c) 2 and 4 only (Ref: Ghai 7th E/P38)

QUESTIONS OF OTHER EXAMINATIONS

1. (b) Thelarche (Ref: Nelson 19th E/P1862)

2. (d) Increase in breast size (Ref: Nelson 19th E/P1862)

3. (b) 6 months (Ref: Nelson 19th E/P34)
The milestones mentioned in the question can develop by following age:
- Sit with support — 6 months
- Transfer objects from one hand to another — 6 months
- Babbles — 7 months

4. (b) Encopresis (Ref: Ahuja psychiatry 4th E/P158)

5. (c) Casting (Ref: Nelson 19th E/P34)

6. (c) Os calcis (Ref: IAP 4th E/105)

7. (c) Bed alarm (Ref: Nelson 19th E/P74)

8. (d) 48 weeks (Ref: Nelson 19th E/P39)
- A child plays a simple game at 1 year of age or 48 weeks.

9. (c) 5 years (Ref: Nelson 19th E/P39)
- A child can draw a triangle by 5 years of age.

10. (c) 2 (Ref: IAP 4th E/105)

"Two carpal centers are present at one year of age."

11. (b) 6 months (Ref: Ghai 7th E/P28)

12. (b) Cruise (Ref: Nelson 19th E/P34)
- A child starts cruising at 10 months.

13. (d) 28 weeks (Ref: Nelson 19th E/P34)
The milestones mentioned in the question can develop by the following age:
- Sits and leans forward on hand – 7 months
- Laughs loud – 4 months
- Prefers mother – 7 months

14. (a) 2nd year (Ref: Ghai 7th E/P4)
- The head size of baby at birth is 65–70% of the adult size.
- It reaches 90% of adult size by 2 years of age.

15. (d) 4 years (Ref: Ghai 7th E/P6)

16. (a) Lower central (Ref: Rudolph 22nd E/P1351)

17. (d) 36 months (Ref: Nelson 19th E/P39)

A child can draw:

- Circle at 3 years of age
- Cross and square at 4 year of age
- Triangle at 5 year of age

18. (d) Social smile absent by 10 weeks (Ref: Nelson 19th E/P34)

- Social smile develops by 8 weeks and hence if absent by 10 weeks, one should be worries.

19. (b) 36 months (Ref: Nelson 19th E/P39)

20. (a) In the first year of life (Ghai 7th E/P3)

"In the early postnatal period the velocity of growth is high, especially in the first few months. A second phase of accelerated growth occurs during puberty."

21. (c) 9-12 months (Ref: Ghai 7th E/P6)

22. (b) 4 years (Ref: Ghai 7th E/P6)

Age	Weight(Kg)	Height(cm)
Birth	3	50
6 months	6	—
1 year	9	75
2 years	12	89
3 years	14	95
4 years	16	101
12 years	39	149

23. (b) 1.3 (Ref: IAP 4th E/P35)

Ages	Upper segment to lower segment ratio
Newborn	1.8
3-4 years	1.3
9 years	1
18 years	0.9

24. (d) Thelarche-puberche-growth spurt-menarche (Ref: Nelson 19th E/P1862)

25. (d) Sustain head level with the body when placed in ventral suspension (Ref: Nelson 19th E/P34)

26. (d) 20 weeks (Ref: Ghai 7th E/P30)

- A baby develops stranger anxiety by 6 months or 24 weeks of age.

27. (c) 3 years (Ref: Nelson 19th E/P39)

28. (c) 36 months (Ref: Nelson 19th E/P39)

29. (c) 3 kg (Ref: Ghai 7th E/P6)

30. (a) and **(b)** Just before appearance of axillary hair and just before menarche (Ref: Nelson 19th E/P55, CPDT 19th E/P111)

31. (d) Makes a tower of 3-4 cubes (Ref: Nelson 19th E/P34)

- A child can make tower of 3 blocks by 18 months or 72 weeks of age.

32. (b) 50% (Ref: Ghai 7th E/P6)

- Length at birth is 50 cm and height at 1 year is 75 cm. Hence the growth is 25 cm.
- In percentage it can be expressed as $25/50 \times 100 = 50\%$.

33. (d) 36 months (Ref: Nelson 19th E/P34)

34. (b) 7 months

- The milestones mentioned in the question can be achieved by the following age
  - ❖ Sits with support — 6 months
  - ❖ Transfers cube from one hand to another — 6 months
  - ❖ Babbles — 7 months
  - ❖ Wave bye-bye — 9 months
  - ❖ Grasp object with finger — 9 months
- Hence the age of baby is 7 months

35. (d) Use scissors to cut pictures (Ref: Nelson 19th E/P39)

36. (b) 7 months (Ref: Nelson 19th E/P34)

- The milestones mentioned in the question can develop by the following age:
  - ❖ Sits with leaning forward on hand – 7 months
  - ❖ Transfer cube from hand to hand – 6 months
  - ❖ Babbles – 7 months
- Hence the child is 7 months old.

37. (c) 12 weeks (Ref: Nelson 19th E/P27)

"By 12 wk, the gender of the external genitals becomes clearly distinguishable."

38. (d) 3 years (Rudolph 22nd E/P1351)

"The primary dentition is comprised of 20 teeth, which begin to erupt at approximately 6 months of age and usually complete their eruption before the age of three years."

39. (a) Insulin (Ref: Tucker Maternal, Fetal and Neonatal physiology/P441)

- Fetal growth depends on various hormonal growth factors like
  - ❖ Insulin
  - ❖ IGF
  - ❖ Human placental lactogen (Hpl)
  - ❖ Epithelial growth factor
  - ❖ Platelet derived growth factor
  - ❖ Transforming growth factor beta
  - ❖ Leptin
- Glucocorticoids, thyroid hormones, growth hormone and sex steroid are required for growth after birth and not for fetal growth.

40. (c) Temper tantrum (Ref: Ghai 7th E/P37).

41. (b) 6 months (Ref: Ghai 7thE/P6)

42. (c) Breath holding spells (Ref: Ghai 7th E/P37)

43. (b) 1.5 (Ref: IAP 4th E/P35)

Ages	Upper segment to lower segment ratio
Newborn	1.8
3-4 years	1.3
9 years	1
18 years	0.9

- The ratio is 1.8 at birth and 1.3 at 3–4 years. Hence at 2 years it will be between 1.3 and 1.8.

44. (b) 10–20 words (Ref: Nelson 19th E/P39, CPDT 19th E/P74)

45. (b) 5–7 years (Ref: Ghai 7th E/P6)

46. (c) Upper segment (Mukherjee Growth and development/P24)

The length of the fetus is usually indicated as crown rump length and crown heel length:
- Crown-rump length (CRL) = Sitting height (upper segment)
- Crown-heel length (CHL) = Standing height

47. (c) and (d) III and IV (Ref: Nelson 19th E/P55)

48. (b) Brain damage (Ref: Gerald neonatal neurology/P 14)
- Moro reflex develops at 28 weeks of gestation and disappears by **3-6 months of age. Persistence beyond 6 months of age is considered pathological** and may indicate **hypoxic ischemic encephalopathy**.

49. (a) i.e. Disproportionate dwarfism (Ref: IAP 4th E/P914)

50. (b) Desmopressin (Ref: Nelson 19th E/P75)
- Pharmacological therapy is initiated if motivational and alarm therapy fails.

- **Imipramine** alters sleep arousal mechanism. It is rarely used because causes cardiac conduction disturbances.
- **Oxybutinin** reduces uninhibited bladder contraction. It is useful in children with **diurnal enuresis**.
- **Desmopressin** (orally or **intranasally**) is preferred for special occasions like staying out at night.

51. (c) Imipramine (Ref: Nelson 19th E/P75)
- Pharmacological therapy is initiated if motivational and alarm therapy fails.
- **Imipramine** alters sleep arousal mechanism. It is rarely used because causes cardiac conduction disturbances.
- **Oxybutinin** reduces uninhibited bladder contraction. It is useful in children with **diurnal enuresis**.
- **Desmopressin (orally or intranasally)** is preferred for special occasions like staying out at night.

52. (d) Must be treated vigorously in the first year of life (Ref: Ghai 7th E/P38)
- Thumb sucking is considered normal in children till **4–5 years**. Hence treatment should be started after this age and not at one year of age.
- Like various other behaviors, thumb sucking is **self-soothing**.
- Continuation of thumb sucking post 5 years can result in **dental misalignment** like flaring of the maxillary incisor teeth, open bite and posterior cross bite. To lessen the effects of misalignment it should be discontinued before **8 years**.

53. none (Ref: Ghai 7th E/P38, Rudolph 22nd E/P343)

2

The Fetus and Neonatal Infant

CARE OF NEWBORN

Physical Examination of the Newborn Infant

- The first examination of a newborn should be done as soon as possible after delivery to detect abnormalities and do the needful. There are various findings which are benign in the newborn and do not require special attention.

Benign findings	Cause
Mucoid vaginal discharge	Due to passage of female sex hormones from mother to baby
Vaginal bleeding	Due to withdrawal of the female sex hormones in the baby after birth
Hymenal tags	—
Mongolian blue spots — Usually disappears in the first few years but rarely may persist	Due to pigmentation of skin specially over ❖ Sacral area ❖ Buttocks ❖ Back ❖ Legs ❖ Posterior thighs ❖ Shoulder
Erythema toxicum • **Papules or pustules with erythema** seen most commonly on **second day and disappear** spontaneously	Unknown
Harlequin colour change: • When baby is placed on the side body is dissected longitudinally in to a pale upper half and deep red dependent half • Most common in low birth weight infants • Seen just after birth and **disappears** within minutes	**Imbalance in autonomic vascular regulatory mechanism**
Transient neonatal pustularmelanosis • Lesions are **present at birth** and **disappear** within 3 months	Dermatosis of unknown cause located usually on ❖ Anterior neck ❖ Forehead ❖ Lower back
Salmon patch (Nevus simplex) • **Pink macules most commonly seen on glabella, eyelids, nuchal area and upper lip.** • Lesions in the face usually **disappears** but may persist in other locations	—
Milia • Yellow pinhead sized papule on the face, gingivae and midline of palate.	Due to retention of sebum

- Can occur at any age and usually **disapper in first few weeks**

Nonretractable prepuce	—
Subconjunctival haemorrhage	Seen in babies born by vaginal delivery following vertex presentation
Prominent xiphisternum	—
Sneezing and nose block	Due to irritation by meconium, amniotic fluid or blood.
Tongue tie	Thin frenulum under the tongue
Hiccups after feed	Due to irritation of diaphragm by distended stomach
Physiological jaundice—Occurs on 2nd-3rd day of life and disappears within 7–10 days	Increased bilirubin turnover and decreased capacity of liver to excrete it
Caput succadeneum—Seen at birth and disappears in 2–3 days	❖ Edema of scalp due to local pressure and trauma during labour ❖ Crosses suture line
Cephalhematoma—Usually develops in 12–24 hours and disappear in 3–6 weeks	❖ Subperiosteal haemorrhage due to trauma during labour ❖ Does not cross suture line

Sebaceous hyperplasia
- Located most commonly on face
- Usually disappear in first 2 weeks

Palpable organs on examination of abdomen
- Liver
- Spleen
- Kidney

Delivery Room Resuscitation

- Most of the newborns successfully pass the phase of transition from intrauterine to extrauterine life. However some may require resuscitative support to sustain life. The most common cause for which baby needs resuscitation is **asphyxia.**

Steps of Resuscitation

- **Provide warmth:**
  - ❖ Infant should be received in a warm blanket and placed in preheated radiant warmer.
  - ❖ Newborn babies are at risk of hypothermia because of large surface area as compared to body weight and limited heat generating mechanisms like shivering and non shivering.

Non shivering thermogenesis	*Shivering thermogenesis*
❖ Most important	❖ Less important
❖ Increased activity	
❖ Sympathetic stimulation causes	
1. Vasoconstriction	
2. Nor epinephrine induced beta oxidation of brown fats	

  - ❖ The clinical features of hypothermia are poor weight gain, **hypoglycemia,** oliguria, azotemia, generalised bleeding, bradycardia and hypotension, tachypnea and distress, **hypoxia, apnea** and poor reflexes.
  - ❖ The baby is kept warm by keeping in incubator or radiant warmer. The mechanism of heat transfer is by **convection.**
- **Opening of airway:**
  - ❖ Infant is placed with the neck in mild extension that makes the airway more patent.
  - ❖ A bulb syringe or suction catheter is used to clear the airway of secretions.
- **Stimulation:**
  - ❖ If the baby does not breathe spontaneously or have decreased respiratory efforts then **tactile stimulation by flicking the soles or rubbing the back** can be done. The normal respiratory rate in a new born is **30-40 breaths/ minute.**

❖ After this the further management depends on the respiratory effort and heart rate of baby.

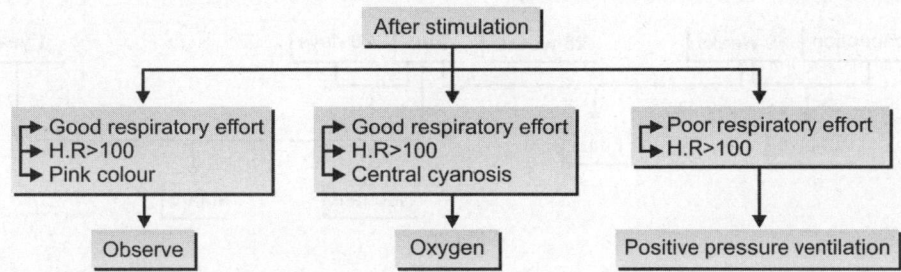

Note: Normal average heart rate of a new born infant is 120-140 beats/minute.

Fig. 1

- **Circulation:**
  - ❖ Usually ventilator support stabilises most of the infants, however if hypoxia still persists it leads to bradycardia and decreased myocardial contractility, which may decrease the blood supply to organs and further worsen the hypoxic state. Hence chest compression is done to augment the cardiac output.
  - ❖ The current resuscitation protocols recommend for chest compression is heart rate **below 60 bits per minute** despite adequate ventilation with oxygen for 30 seconds.

Assessment of Newborn

Apgar Score

The Apgar scoring system provides a quick method to assess the condition of new born baby.

Sign	0	1	2
Heart rate	Absent	<100/min	>100/min
Respiration	Absent	Weak cry	Good strong cry
Muscle tone	Limp	Some flexion	Active movements
Reflex irritability	No response	Grimace	Cough or sneeze
Colour	Blue or pale	Body pink, extremities blue	Completely pink

Inference of scoring

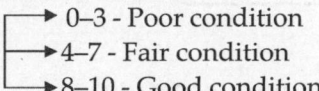 0–3 - Poor condition

4–7 - Fair condition

8–10 - Good condition

Morgan's Neonatal Neurobehavioural Examination

This consists of three parts i.e. tone and motor patterns, primitive reflexes and **behavioural responses.** The behavioural responses can be graded in to six states:

- State 1 — Deep sleep, No eye movement, Regular breathing
- State 2 — Light sleep, eyes shut, some movement
- State 3 — Dozing, eyes opening and closing
- State 4 — Awake, eyes open, minimal movement
- State 5 — Wide awake, vigorous movements
- **State 6 — Crying**

INFANTS AT RISK

Small for Gestational Age and Preterm Infant

- The fetal period ranges from **9 weeks** post conception till **birth**. Then the newborn is called **neonate** in the **first 28 days** of his life and early **neonate** in first **7 days.**

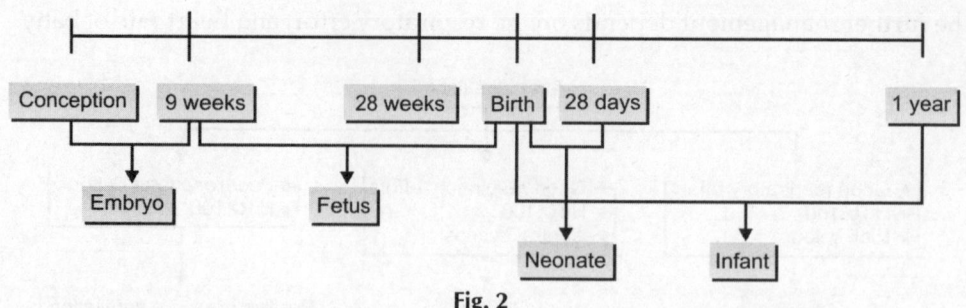

Fig. 2

- Neonatal period is crucial for the survival of baby which is reflected by the fact that almost half of the under-five child deaths occur during this period. The major causes of neonatal death are diseases associated with preterm birth, low birth weight and congenital anomalies.
- Classification of neonates as per birth weight:

Low birth weight babies	Very low birth weight babies	Extremely low birth weight babies
Weight less than **2.5 kg**	Weight less than **1.5 kg**	Weight less than 1 kg

- Classification of neonates as per duration of gestational period:

Preterm neonate	Term neonate	Post term neonate
Neonate born `before 37 weeks' (less than 259 days) of gestation	Neonate born between 37 and < 42 (259–293 days) weeks of gestation	Neonate born at gestational age of 42 weeks (294 days) or more

- Classification of neonates as per birth weight and gestational age group:

Small for date babies (Microsomia)	Appropriate for date babies	Large for date babies (Macrosomia)
Babies with birth weight of **less than 10th percentile or 2 SD** of their gestational age	Babies with birth weight between 10th- 90th percentile for their period of gestation	Babies with birth weight more than 90th percentile of their gestational age

- Preterm neonate and small for date baby (SFDB)/ Intra uterine growth retardation(IUGR):

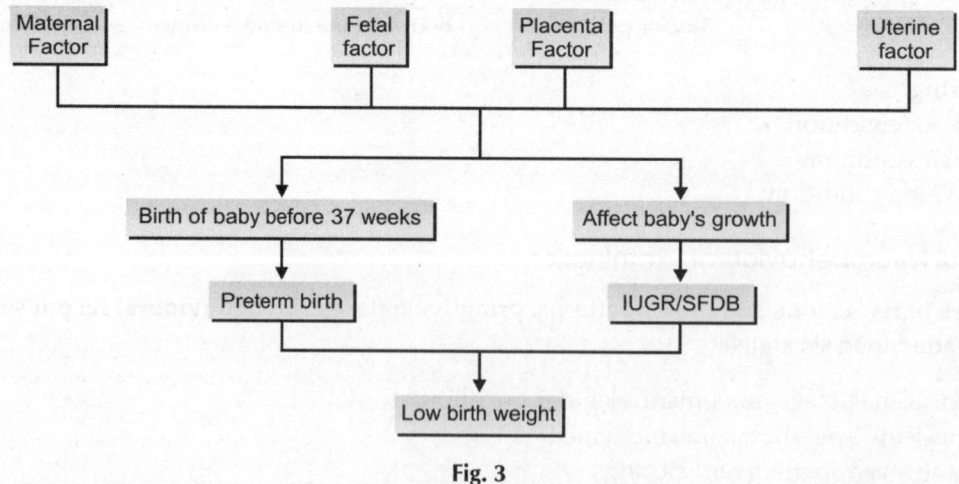

Fig. 3

- The factors associated with prematurity and IUGR/SFDB are almost similar and most of the times they are coexisting conditions.
- Most common cause of low birth weight in developed countries is **preterm birth** whereas in developing countries is **IUGR.**

Preterm Neonate

The characteristic features of preterm neonate are:
- Absence of deep sole creases.
- Size of breast nodule less than 5 mm.

- Poor elastic recoil of ear cartilage.
- Presence of lanugo hair (Lanugo hair is present on fetus and usually sheds in two periods 1. At 28 weeks and 2. At term).
- Males — Testes are located at external ring(undescended testis) and scrotum has few rugosities.
  Females — Labia majora are widely separated exposing labia minora and clitoris.

IUGR

- **Pathophysiology**

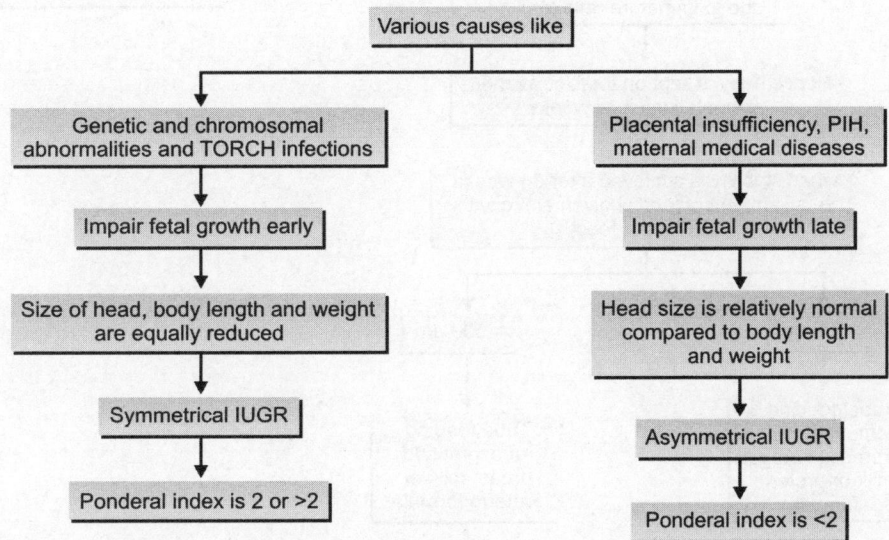

Note: Ponderal index is a measure of fetal growth. P.I = Weight (gm) $\times$ 100/Length (cm)^3

Fig. 4

- **Causes of IUGR:**

> **R — Renal disorders**
> E — Elevated blood pressure
> T — Toxemia
> A — Abruptio placentae
> R — Rubella infection
> D — Drugs of antimetabolite group and **propranolol**
> **A — Alcohol**
> T — Trisomies
> **I — Insulin deficiency in fetus**
> O — Oxygen deficiency
> **N — Nicotine**
>
> Mnemonic: **RETARDATION**

Management of Preterm and SFGD/IUGR Baby

- Apart from the routine care and procedures special attention and care is required to:
  - ❖ Maintain patent airway.
  - ❖ Prevent aspiration of gastric contents.
  - ❖ Controll temperature of baby - It can be done by isolettes (incubators) or radiant warmers.
  - ❖ Maintain adequate oxygen supply to reduce the risk of injury from hypoxia and circulatory insufficiency.

❖ **Special feeding requirements**—To breastfeed the baby a strong sucking reflex is required along with coordination of swallowing, epiglottal and uvular closure of larynx and nasal passages and normal esophageal motility, which develops at 34 week of gestation.

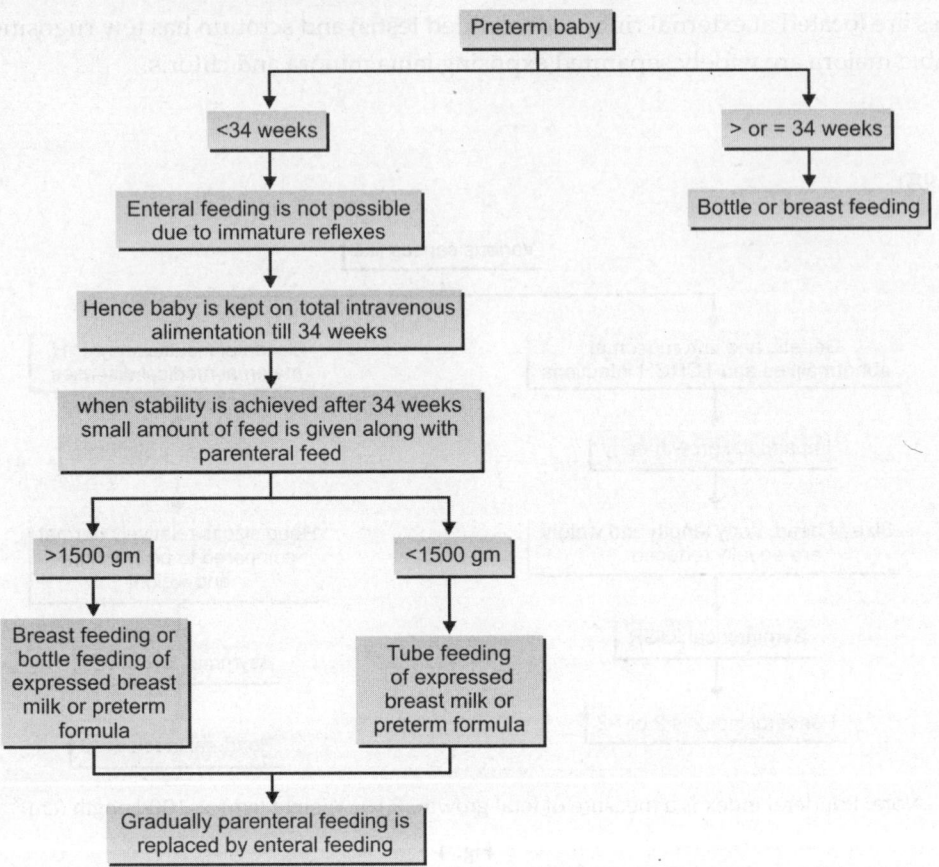

Note : Trophic feeding refers to the practice of giving very small amount of enteral nourishment to VLBW preterm infants to stimulate development of immature gastrointestinal tract.

Fig. 5

Complications

Low birth weight and premature infants lack maturity and coordination of certain body systems that manifest as various derangements.

- Metabolic derangements like hypoglycemia, hyperglycemia and hypocalcemia can be seen.
  - ❖ **Hypoglycemia** is seen due to low hepatic glycogen stores.
  - ❖ **Hyperglycemia** is seen due to immature glucose utilising mechanisms.
  - ❖ **Hypocalcemia** — Early onset is usually asymptomatic but late onset hypocalcemia presents as neonatal tetany and seizures.
- **Jaundice** can be seen as the preterm has larger RBC volume for body weight and immature hepatic enzymes and hepatic excretory capacity.
- Hematological abnormalities like **polycythemia** and **anemia** (Due to rapid destruction of fetal RBCs) can be seen.
- Immature organ systems can lead to various disorders.
  - ❖ **Intraventricular haemorrhage** can be seen due to fragile blood vessels.
  - ❖ **Retinopathy of prematurity** develops because of high oxygen saturation used during resuscitation.
  - ❖ **Osteopenia of prematurity** is caused by low levels of calcium, vitamin D and phosphorous.
  - ❖ **Respiratory distress syndrome** can be associated due to lack of surfactant.
- **Hypothermia** is seen due to **higher surface area to body weight ratio, low subcutaneous fat** and low glycogen store.

Infant of Diabetic Mother

Infants of diabetic mothers (IDM) are at increased risk for fetal, neonatal and long-term comorbidities like **congenital anomalies, macrosomia, hypoglycemia, hypomagnesemia, hypocalcemia, hyperbilirubinemia, respiratory distress,** polycythemia and cardiomyopathy.

- **Congenital anomalies:**
  - ❖ Congenital heart defects (CHD) are commonly associated with IDM. **Ventricular septal defect** is the **most common CHD** associated. Other CHDs are atrial septal defect and TGA.
  - ❖ Neural tube defects like spinal agenesis associated with **caudal regression** is found **exclusively** in IDM.
  - ❖ Gastrointestinal atresia, gastroschisis, intestinal malrotation, renal and urinary tract malformation and small left colon syndrome may be associated.
- **Macrosomia:**
  - ❖ It is defined as birth weight above the 90th percentile for gestational age, or more than 4 kg.
  - ❖ Excessive amount of glucose forms glycogen and fat which are responsible for increased body fat, muscle mass and organomegaly especially of the heart and liver.
  - ❖ It leads to various complications like **shoulder dystocia** (because of fat deposition in intrascapular area and abdomen) and birth injury.
- **Hypoglycemia:**
  - ❖ Hypoglycemia is defined as blood glucose level of less than **40 mg/dL** in neonates. It usually develops within the **first 24 hours after birth.**
  - ❖ It can cause injury to brain and neurodevelopmental complications.

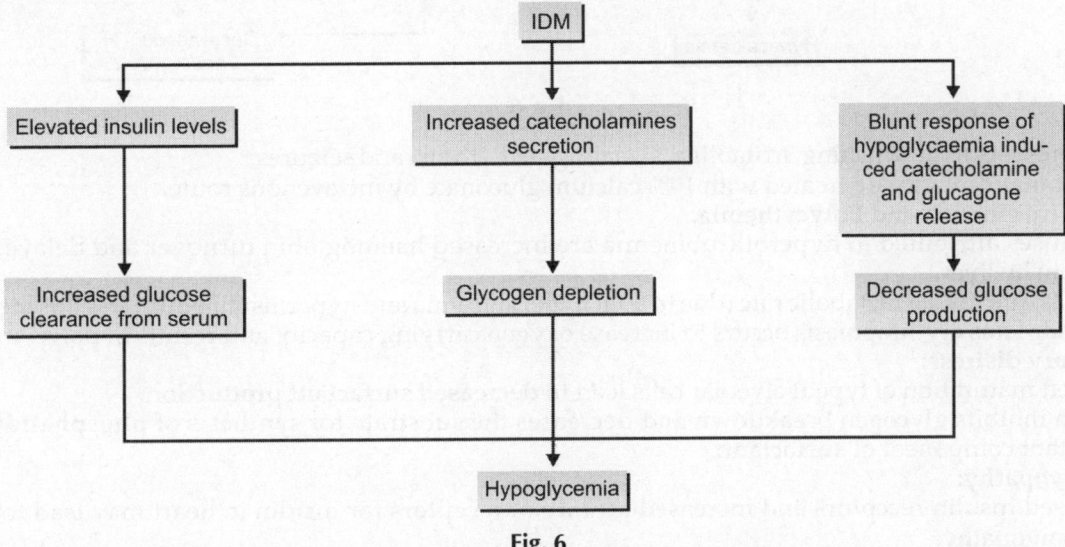

Fig. 6

- ❖ Baby presents with jitteriness, tachypnea, lethargy, poor feeding and seizures.
- ❖ Management depends on the symptoms of baby and blood glucose level.

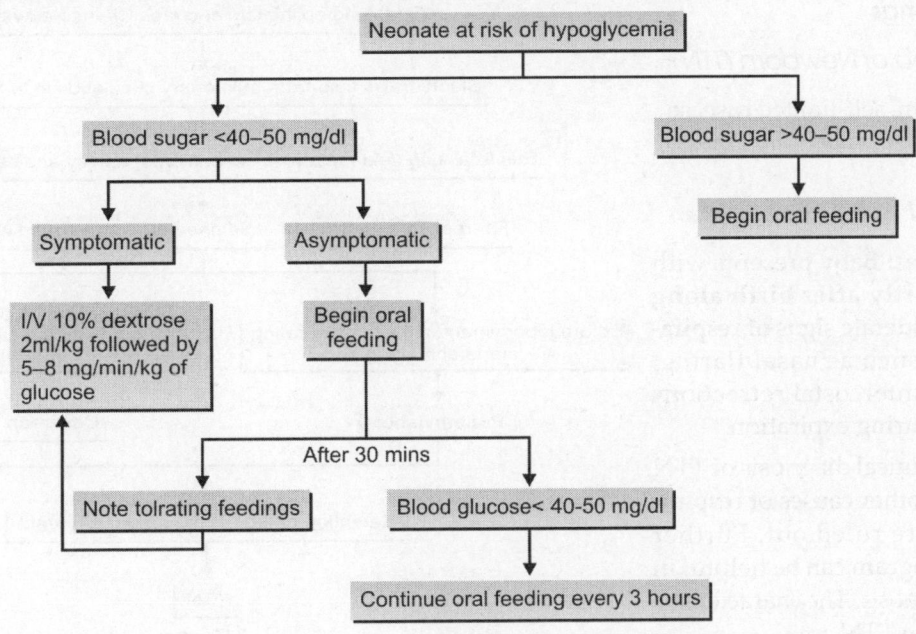

Fig. 7

- **Hypocalcemia and hypomagnesemia:**
  ❖ It is usually seen 48–72 hours after birth.

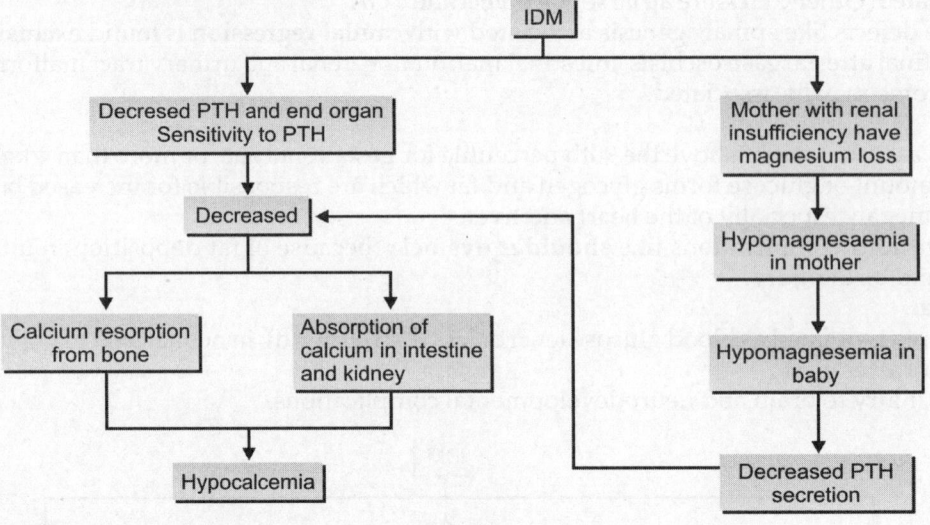

Fig. 8

❖ Baby presents with twitching, irritability, sweating, arrhythmia and seizures.
❖ Symptomatic infants are treated with 10% calcium gluconate by intravenous route.
- **Hyperbilirubinemia and Polycythemia:**
  ❖ The causes attributed to hyperbilirubinemia are increased haemoglobin turnover and delayed clearance of bilirubin by liver.
  ❖ IDM have increased metabolic rate (due to fetal hyperglycemia and hyperinsulinemia) and this increases oxygen demand. Thus erythropoiesis occurs to increase oxygen carrying capacity and results in polycythemia.
- **Respiratory distress:**
  ❖ Delayed maturation of type II alveolar cells lead to **decreased surfactant production.**
  ❖ Insulin inhibits glycogen breakdown and decreases the substrate for synthesis of **phosphatidylglycerol,** an important component of **surfactant.**
- **Cardiomyopathy:**
  ❖ Increased insulin receptors and increased affinity of receptors for insulin in heart may lead to hypertrophic cardiomyopathy.

SPECIFIC NEONATAL CONDITIONS

Abnormalities of Lungs

Transient Tachypnea of Newborn (TTN)

It is usually a benign, self-limited disease that resolves within **2–4 days.**

Pathogenesis of TTN

- **Clinical features:** Baby presents with **tachypnea shortly after birth along with mild to moderate signs of respiratory distress,** such as nasal flaring, subcostal and intercostal retractions and grunting during expiration.
- **Diagnosis:** A clinical diagnosis of TTN is arrived after other causes of respiratory distress are ruled out. Further chest roentgenogram can be helpful in differential diagnosis. The characteristic X-ray findings in TTN are:

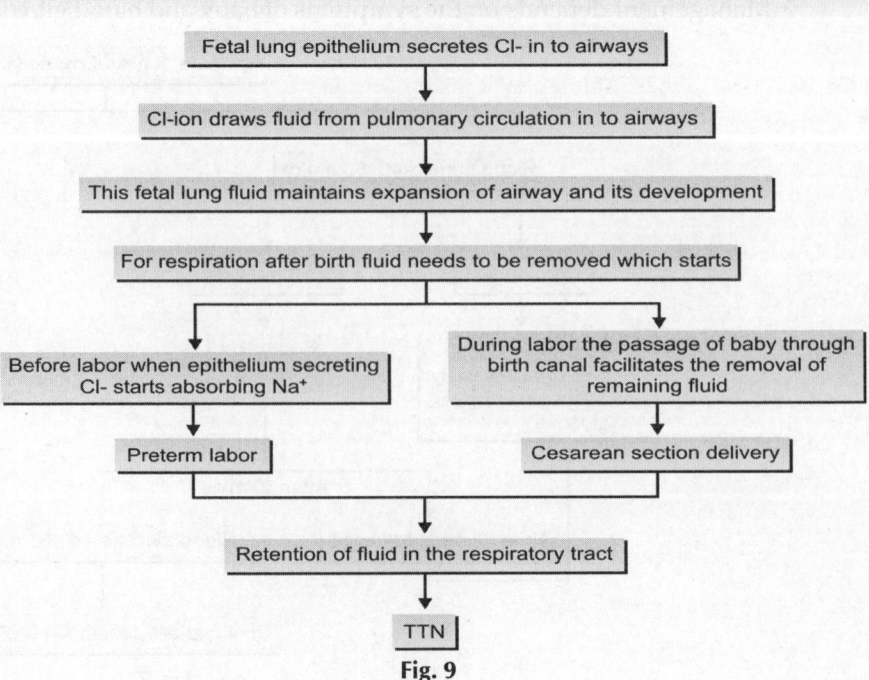

Fig. 9

  ❖ Prominent pulmonary vascular markings
  ❖ **Widened interlobar fissures due to fluid**
  ❖ **Hyperinflation with flattening of diaphragm**
  ❖ Presence of pleural effusion
  ❖ Enlarged cardiac silhouette
 • **Treatment:** Oxygen and supportive care is usually sufficient.

Meconium Aspiration Syndrome (MAS)

 • Meconium can be found in fetal intestine usually at 14 – 16 weeks of gestation. It is a black-green colour odourless substance which is composed of **water, squamous cells, vernix, lanugo, blood, amniotic fluid and intestinal secretions containing bile.**
 • Most commonly it is associated with postterm infants as passage of meconium in utero is rare before 32 weeks of gestation.

Pathogenesis of MAS

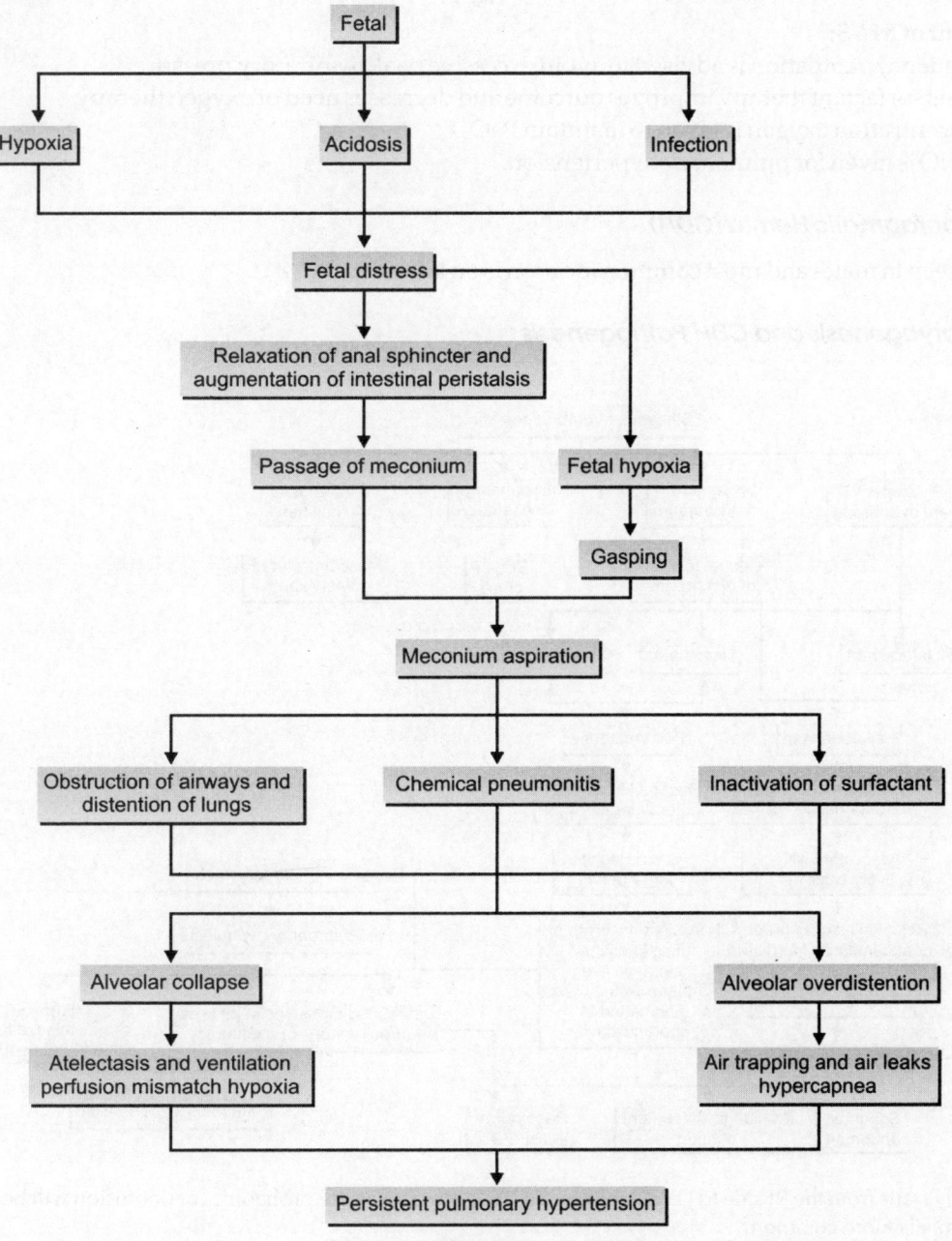

Fig. 10

- **Prevention of MAS:**
  - ❖ **Antenatal prevention:** Fetal monitoring should be done to assess the fetal well-being. Elective caesarean section has no protective effect on MAS.
  - ❖ **Postnatal prevention:** The routine intrapartum oropharyngeal and naso-pharyngeal suctioning does not prevent MAS or its complications. The current practice of effective prevention depends if the baby is vigorous or not. A vigorous baby has a strong spontaneous respira-tory effort, good muscle tone and heart rate of 100 beats / min or more.

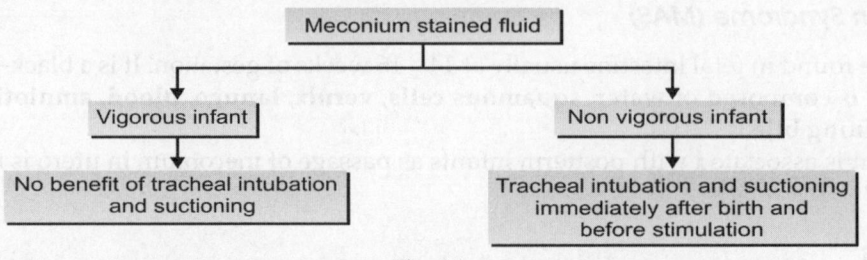

Fig. 11

- **Management of MAS:**
  - ❖ High frequency ventilation is advised to avoid excessive peak inspiratory pressure.
  - ❖ Exogenous surfactant therapy improves outcome and decreases need of oxygen therapy.
  - ❖ High concentration oxygen is given to maintain PaO_2.
  - ❖ Inhaled NO is given for pulmonary hypertension.

Congenital Diaphragmatic Hernia (CDH)

Most commonly seen in males and most common location is on left side.

Diaphragm Embryogenesis and CDH Pathogenesis

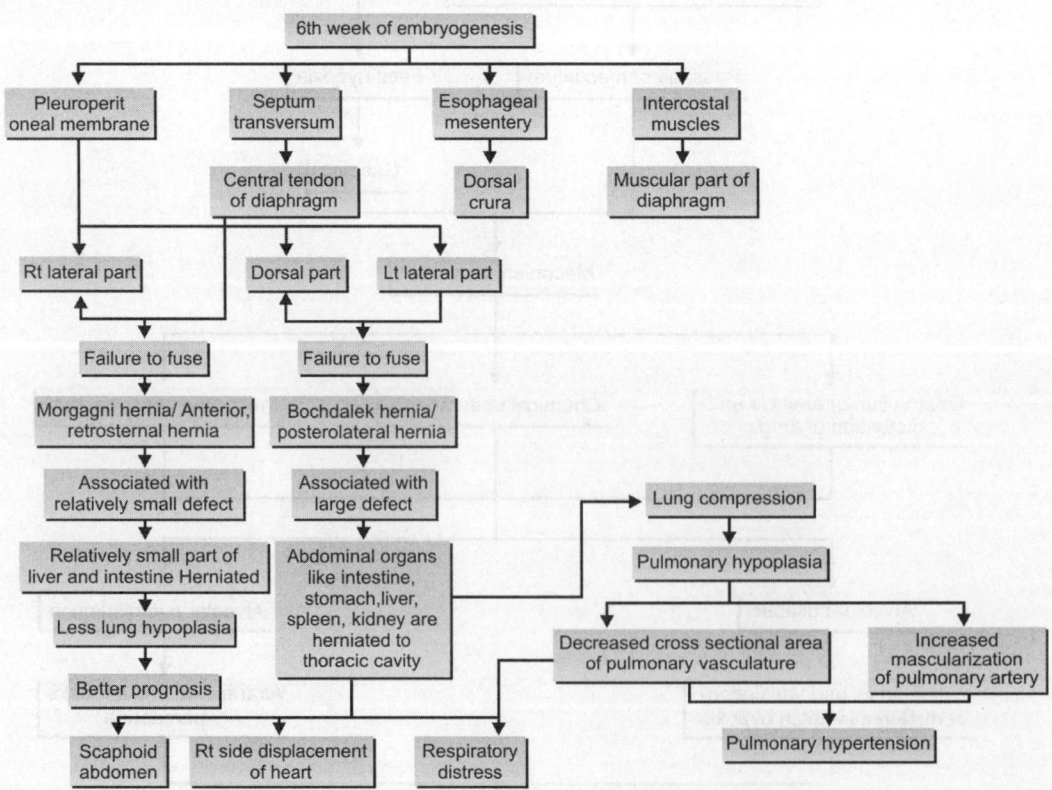

Note: Fusion usually starts from the Rt side to Lt side, hence if it stops at any time the probability of nonfusion will be maximum in Lt side. Thus morgagni hernia is more common.

Fig. 12

- **Management of CDH:** The baby presents with significant respiratory symptoms in the delivery room. The two major issues that are to be tackled are respiratory distress and pulmonary hypertension.

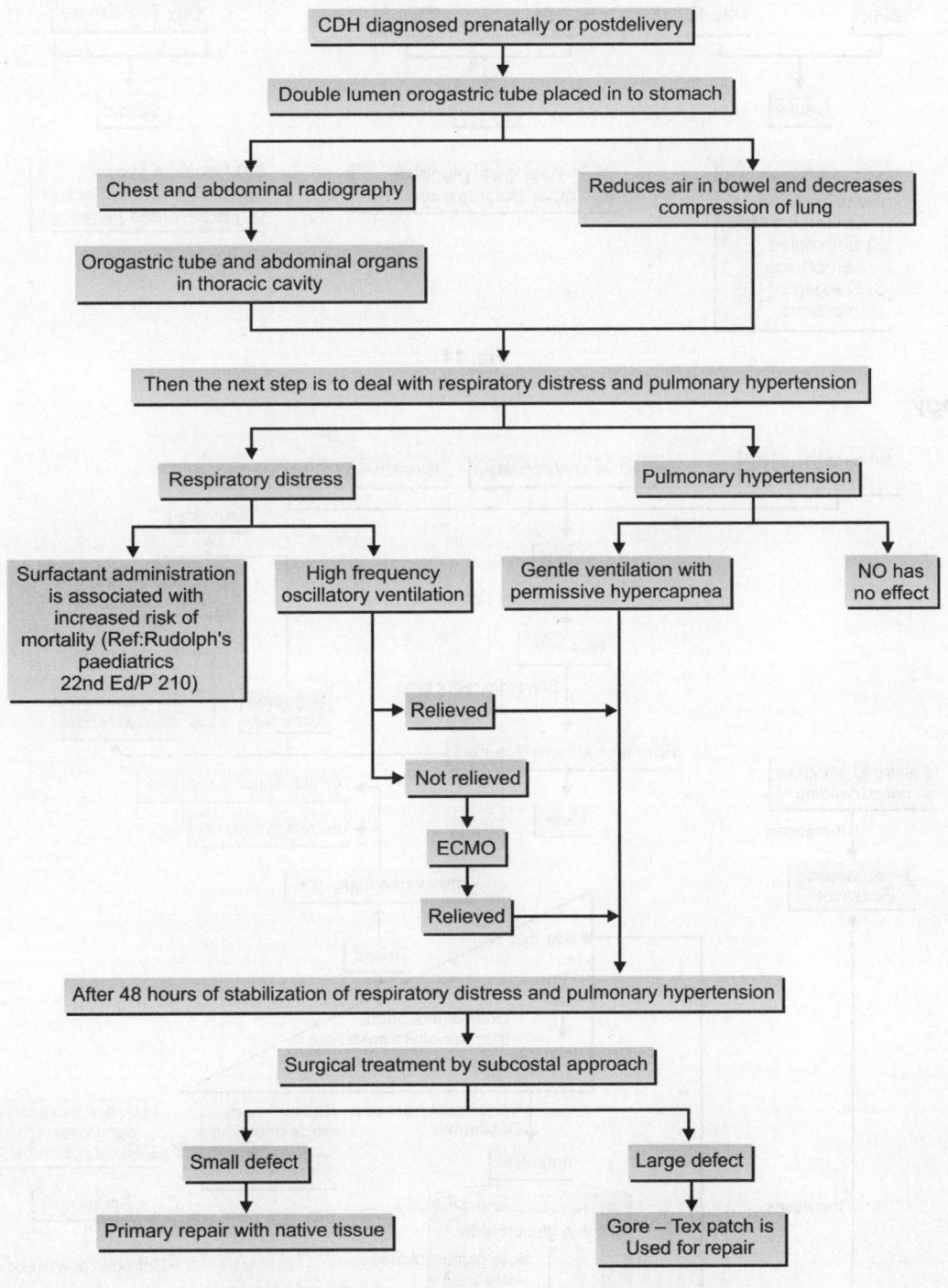

Note: ECMO - Extracorporeal Membrane Oxygenation

Fig. 13

Haematological Abnormalities

Jaundice and Hyperbilirubinemia

- Jaundice is a condition in which bilirubin excess due to overproduction or faulty elimination leads to its deposition in skin and sclera and imparting yellow colour.
- The day of presentation of neonatal jaundice is crucial as it has strong correlation with the cause.

Causes of Jaundice

Birth
Day 1
Day 2
Day 3
Day 7 and more
Cause
Cause
Cause
1) Erythroblastosis fetalis- Most common cause
2) Concealed hemorhage
3) Congenital infections
1) Physiological jaundice
2) Crigler-Najjar syndrome
1) Bacterial sepsis
2) Urinary tract infection
3) Breast feed jaundice

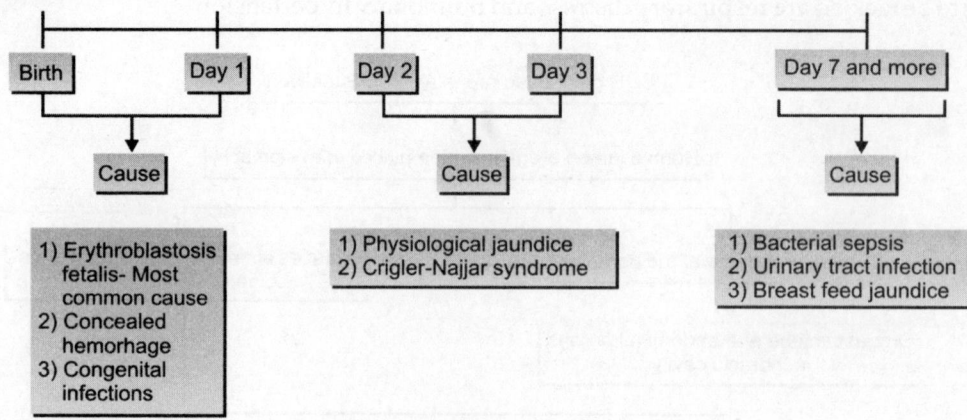

Fig. 14

Pathophysiology

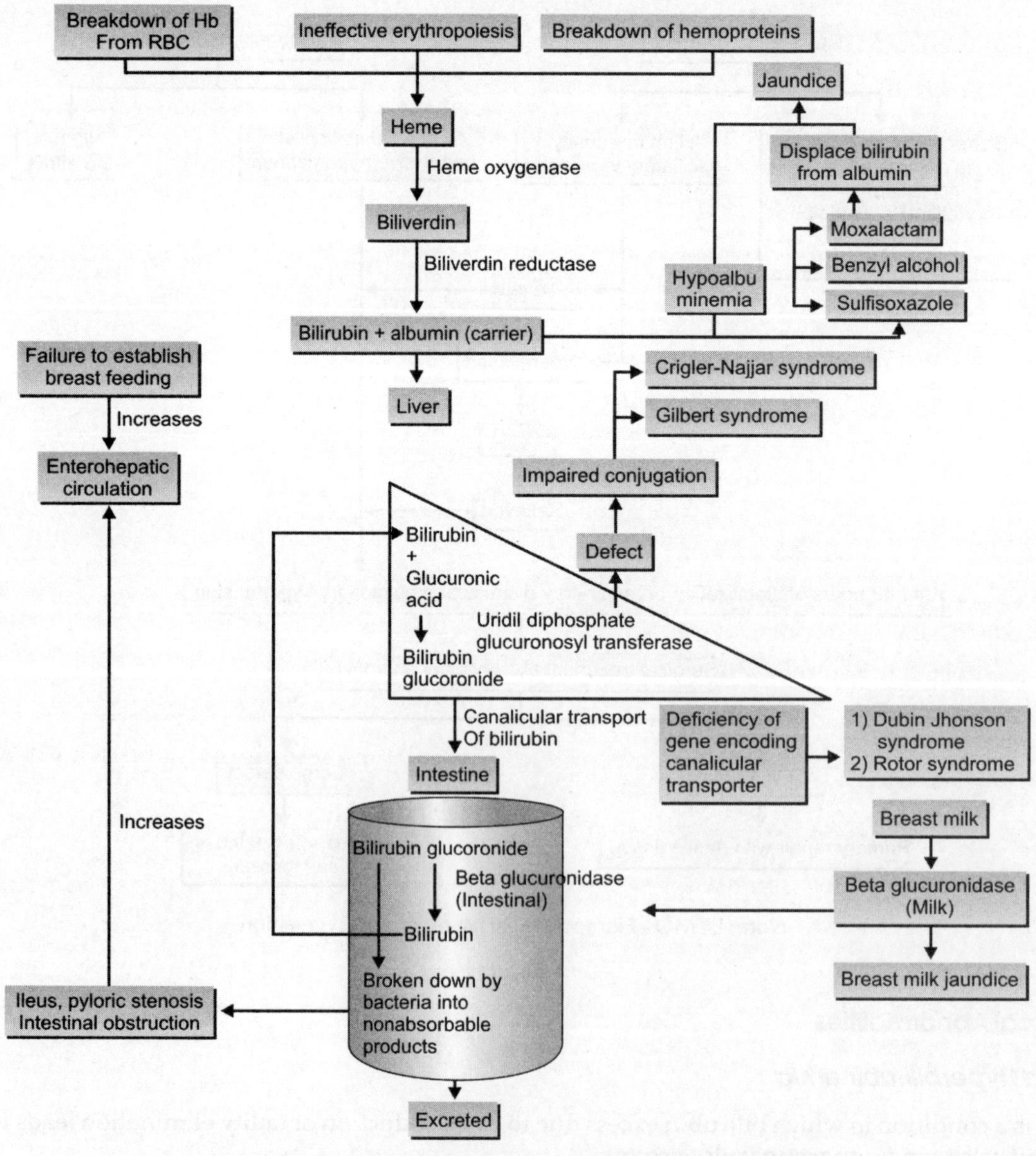

Breakdown of Hb From RBC
Ineffective erythropoiesis
Breakdown of hemoproteins
Jaundice
Heme
Heme oxygenase
Displace bilirubin from albumin
Biliverdin
Moxalactam
Biliverdin reductase
Hypoalbu minemia
Benzyl alcohol
Sulfisoxazole
Bilirubin + albumin (carrier)
Failure to establish breast feeding
Crigler-Najjar syndrome
Increases
Liver
Gilbert syndrome
Enterohepatic circulation
Impaired conjugation
Bilirubin + Glucuronic acid
Defect
Uridil diphosphate glucuronosyl transferase
Bilirubin glucoronide
Canalicular transport Of bilirubin
Deficiency of gene encoding canalicular transporter
1) Dubin Jhonson syndrome
2) Rotor syndrome
Intestine
Increases
Breast milk
Bilirubin glucoronide
Beta glucuronidase (Intestinal)
Beta glucuronidase (Milk)
Bilirubin
Broken down by bacteria into nonabsorbable products
Breast milk jaundice
Ileus, pyloric stenosis Intestinal obstruction
Excreted

Note: Each gram of hemoglobin produces 34–35 mg of bilirubin.

Fig. 15

Classification

Jaundice can be caused by rise in conjugated (direct) and/or unconjugated (indirect) bilirubin. Hence for the diagnosis the **most specific investigation** is estimation of **direct, indirect and total bilirubin level.**

Causes of unconjugated hyperbilirubinemia	*Causes of conjugated hyperbilirubinemia*
C — **Crigler-Najjar Syndrome**	Cute — **Choledochal cyst, Cystic fibrosis**
H — **Hemolysis, Hypothyroidism**	D — **Dubin Johnson syndrome**
I — Infections like malaria	A — **Atresia of bile ducts**
M — Breast **Milk jaundice**	U — **UTI**
P — **Physiological jaundice**	G — Galactosemia
I — Infant of diabetic mother	H — Hereditary fructose intolerance, **Hepatitis**
N — Neonatal intracranial hemorrhage	T — Total Parenteral nutrition, Tyrosinemia
G — **Gilbert syndrome**	E — Enzyme deficiency e.g. α_1 antitrypsin
R — **Rotor syndrome**	
Mnemonic: **CHIMPING**	Mnemonic: **Cute DAUGHTER**

Note: Hemolysis can be caused by disorders like G6PD deficiency, hereditary spherocytosis, sickle cell disease and thalassemia.

Physiological Jaundice

- In newborn increased bilirubin production due to breakdown of fetal RBCs and decreased excretion due to the limited conjugating ability of newborn's liver and increased enterohepatic circulation leads to **unconjugated hyperbilirubinemia** and **jaundice.**
- Jaundice becomes visible on **2nd to 3rd day** when **indirect bilirubin** rises at a rate of **<5 mg/dL/24 hr** and peaks on 4th to 5th day at arate of 5 - 6 mg/dL.
- **No treatment** is required as the bilirubin level is below cut-off level for phototherapy.
- Bilirubin level usually comes down to adult level by **10th to 14th day** and persistence of jaundice beyond this point suggests other causes of jaundice like haemolysis, hereditary glucuronyl transferase deficiency, breast milk jaundice, hypothyroidism and intestinal obstruction.

Breast Milk Jaundice

- It develops more gradually and presents typically in the **7th day.** The maximum level of total bilirubin can go as high as 10-30 mg/dl in the 2nd and 3rd week.
- Its cause is attributed to presence of beta - glucuronidase which unconjugates the bilirubin and increases enterohepatic circulation, which ultimately leads to **unconjugated hyperbilirubinemia.**
- If serum bilirubin is mildly elevated, breast feeding should be stopped briefly for **1–2 days.**
- Phototherapy can be used for more severe elevation in bilirubin levels.

Crigler-Najjar Syndrome

Crigler-Najjar syndrome type I	*Criggler-Najjar syndrome II*
• Caused due to complete absence of glucuronyl transferase.	• Caused due to partial absence of glucuronyl transferase.
• **Autosomal recessive** inheritance.	• **Autosomal dominant** inheritance.
• Severe **unconjugated hyperbilirubinemia.**	• Mild **unconjugated hyperbilirubinemia.** (Usually less than 10 mg/DL)
• **Kernicterus** is a **frequent complication.**	• **Kernicterus is less likely.**
• Standard hepatic biochemical tests and liver histology are normal.	• Standard hepatic biochemical tests and liver histology are normal.
• **Phototherapy** is the mainstay of treatment.	• Cytochrome p-450 inducing compounds like **phenobarbital can** improve glucunoridation by inducing hypertrophy of hepatic endoplasmic reticulum but long term treatment is not recommended.
• Liver transplantation can be curative.	

Gibert Syndrome

- Gilbert syndrome inherited as **autosomal dominant and recessive** disorder, is characterised by **defect of bilirubin uptake** as well as **conjugation (decreased activity of glucunoryl transferase).** It is more common in **males.**
- It is charcterisd by mild **unconjugated hyperbilirubinemia** and serum bilirubin level is usually less than 5 mg/dL. Standard **hepatic biochemical tests and liver histology are normal.**
- Jaundice is precipitated by stress, fatigue, alcohol, starvation, illness and relieved by calorie intake and enzyme inducers. Glucunoridation of most drugs is normal except **irinotecan,** which is glucunoridated by bilirubin-UDP-glucunoryl transferase.
- It is the most benign type and does not require any treatment.

Dubin - Jhonson Syndrome

- Dubin-Jhonson syndrome is an **autosomal recessive** disorder caused by deficiency of gene encoding canalicular transporter protein i.e. multidrug resistance protein 2. It is characterised by mild **conjugated hyperbilirubinemia.**
- Pigmented cytoplasmic globules are found in liver. **Gall bladder is not visualised** on oral cholecystography. Total urinary coporphyrin is usually normal and consists mainly of isomer I.
- When BSP (Bromosulphalein), a synthetic dye used for liver function test is injected, there is a rise in serum BSP concentration after 90 mins due to **reflux of conjugated BSP from hepatocytes** in to circulation.
- The liver function tests are normal and do not require any treatment.

Rotor Syndrome

- Rotor syndrome is an **autosomal recessive** disorder caused by defective uptake and excretion of bilirubin. It is characterised by **conjugated hyperbilirubinemia.**
- **Gall bladder is visualised** on oral cholecystography.
- There is **no reflux of BSP** from hepatocytes.
- Total urinary coporphyrin is elevated.
- The **liver function tests are normal** and do not require any treatment.

Bilirubin Toxicity and Kernicterus

- **Unconjugated bilirubin is toxic to nervous system** and its toxic symptom in newborn period due to accumulation in basal ganglia and brain stem nuclei is called as acute bilirubin encephalopathy.
- Acute bilirubin encephalopathy is characterised by poor suck, lethargy, hypotonia followed by hypertonia, opisthotonus, retrocolis, fever and loss of Moro reflex.
- Kernicterus is the term used for severe form of bilirubin toxicity which leads to permanent neurologic damage. The infant may develop delayed motor skills, movement disorder (**cheroathetosis**, ballismus, tremor), **upward gaze,** paralytic palsies, intellectual deficits and **sensorineural hearing loss.**
- Toxicity of bilirubin can be exaggerated by various factors

Hypoalbuminemia	Bilirubin binds to albumin and hypoalbuminemia causes increased free bilirubin in the blood, which can precipitate toxicity.
Drugs like Moxalactam, sulfisoxazole, benzyl alcohol	These drugs interefere with bilirubin - albumin binding and thereby increasing free bilirubin.
Acidosis	Decrease in blood Ph makes free bilirubin lipophilic and enhances it tissue uptake and toxicity.
Sepsis	Bilirubin can access to vulnerable areas of brain.
Prematurity	Premature infants have hypoalbuminemia as well as risk of acidosis, both of which can increase bilirubin toxicity.

Treatment of Hyperbilirubinemia

- The standard treatment for hyperbilirubinemia is phototherapy and, if unsuccessful, exchange transfusion is done.

- **Phototherapy:**
  - ❖ Before starting phototherapy, **eyes of the baby should be covered** to prevent retinal damage.
  - ❖ Phototherapy is used in hyperbilirubinemia because bilirubin absorbs blue light mainly at wavelength of 450 nm and causes various photochemical reactions:
    1. **Photoisomerisation** of toxic unconjugated 4Z, 15Z- bilirubin to unconjugated 4Z, 15E- bilirubin which can be excreted in bile without conjugation.
    2. Bilirubin is converted to water soluble **lumirubin** which is excreted by kidneys.
  - ❖ It can be discontinued once serum total bilirubin drops below **14 mg/dL.**
  - ❖ **Bronze baby syndrome** is a complication of phototherapy characterised by grayish - brown skin discolouration due to photo - induced modification of porphyrins. Other complications like erythematous macular rash, **dehydration, loose stools** and hypothermia can be seen.
- **Exchange transfusion:**
  - ❖ A complete exchange transfusion involves removing and replacing twice the infant's blood volume.
  - ❖ Complete exchange transfusion is performed if phototherapy has failed to reduce bilirubin level to safe range.
  - ❖ The appearance of clinical signs suggesting kernicterus at any level of serum bilirubin is an indication for exchange transfusion.
- **Phototherapy versus exchange transfusion:** The treatment of choice is based on the age, serum bilirubin level and maturity of the baby.
  - ❖ Indication for phototherapy and exchange transfusion in term babies:

Age	Phototherapy	Exchange transfusion
<24 hours	12	19
24-48 hours	15	22
48-72 hours	17.5	24
72-96 hours	20	25
>96 hours	21	25

Total serum bilirubin in mg/dL

  - ❖ Premature infants are at high risk for bilirubin toxicity and hence need special attention. They are managed on the basis of their birth weight, serum bilirubin level and overall condition:

| Birth weight | Healthy baby | | Sick baby | |
	Photo therapy	Exchange transfusion	Phototherapy	Exchange transfusion
<1000 gm	**5 – 7**	**11 – 13**	**4 – 6**	**10 – 12**
1001 – 1500 gm	7 – 10	13 – 15	6 – 8	11 – 13
1501 – 2000 gm	10 – 12	15 – 18	8 – 10	13 – 15
2001 – 2500 gm	12 – 15	18 – 20	10 – 12	15 – 18

Total serum bilirubin in mg/dL

DISORDERS SPECIFICALLY RELATED TO PRETERM BIRTH

Respiratory Distress Syndrome (RDS)/Hyaline Membrane Disease (HMD)

Respiratory distress is characterised by **failure to initiate respiration after birth.** Though RDS is a common disorder of **premature infants(< 34 weeks),** various other predisposing factors like **meconium aspiration,** male sex, caesarean section delivery, **infant of diabetic mother,** second born twin, **premature rupture of membranes,** asphyxia and cold stress are related to it. In the **first 24 hours after birth** prematurity is the most common cause; however in term neonates **meconium aspiration syndrome** is the most common cause of respiratory distress.

Pathophysiology of RDS/HMD

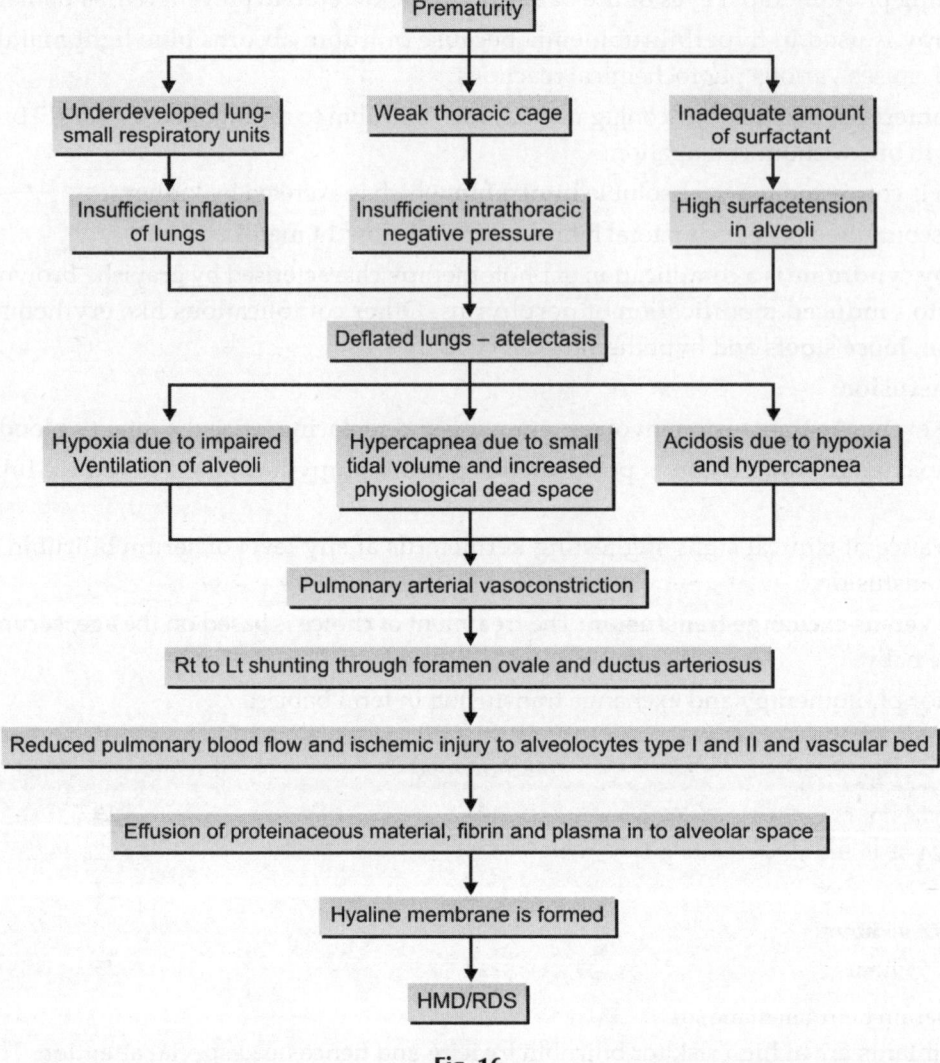

Fig. 16

- **Clinical presentation:** The baby develops respiratory distress **within first 6 hours of birth** associated with **tachypnea (RR>60/min),** prominent grunting, **intercostal and subcostal retractions, acidosis,** nasal flaring and cyanosis.
- **Diagnosis:**
  - ❖ Chest X-ray shows **reticulogranular pattern** of increased density of lung parenchyma due to miliary atelectasis and interstitial edema. Other findings are **air bronchogram, ground glass appearance** of lung and decreased lung volume.
  - ❖ There is a reduction in the **fractional residual capacity (FRC).**
  - ❖ **Tests to predict RDS/HMD:**
    - ❑ **Lecithin/Sphingomyelin ratio** of **more than 2.0** indicates lung maturity.
    - ❑ **Foam stability or shake test** — Amniotic fluid is mixed with absolute alcohol, shaken for 15 seconds and allowed to settle. If bubbles are present it indicates presence of **phosphatidylglycerol** and **phosphatidyl choline,** components of surfactant.
    - ❑ The latest test for lung maturity is **lamellar body (lamellated phospholipids carrying surfactant) count.** A lamellar body count of > 60,000 particles/μl indicates fetal lung maturity.
    - ❑ A **surfactant albumin ratio** of > 55 mg/gm indicates fetal lung maturity.
    - ❑ **Amniotic fluid tests for fetal maturity** — Optic absorbance at 650 nm indicates AF turbidity and a value of **>0.1** indicates mature fetus. **Amniotic fluid creatinine level of ≥ 2 mg/dl** indicates adequate muscle mass development and corresponds to fetal age of >37 weeks.

- **Assessment of RDS severity:** Severity of RDS can be assessed by Downe's score and Silverman's score.
  - ❖ **Downe's score:**

Signs	0	1	2
Respiratory rate	<60	60-80	>80 or apneic episodes
Cyanosis	None	With air	With 40% oxygen
Grunting	None	Audible with stethoscope	Audible without stethoscope
Retractions	None	Mild	Moderate to severe
Air entry	Good		Barely audible

  - ❖ **Inference of scores:**
    - → 1–3 - Mild RDS
    - → 4–7 - Moderate RDS
    - → 7–10 - Severe RDS

  - ❖ **Silverman's score:**

Signs	0	1	2
Thoraco abdominal movement in respiration	Significant	Thoracic lag	See-Saw
Nasal flaring	Nil	Mild	Severe
Lower intercostal retraction	Nil	Mild	Severe
Xiphoid retraction	Nil	Mild	Severe
Grunting	Nil	Audible with stethoscope	Audible without stethoscope

  Inference of scores:
  - → 1–3 - Mild RDS
  - → 4–7 - Moderate RDS
  - → 7–10 - Severe RDS

- **Management:**
  - ❖ **Prevention**
    - ❑ All foetuses between 24–36 weeks of gestation at risk of preterm delivery should be considered for antenatal corticosteroid treatment, which consists of:
      1. **2 doses of 12mg of betamethasone I.M 24 hours apart or**
      2. **4 doses of dexamethasone given I.M 12 hours apart.**

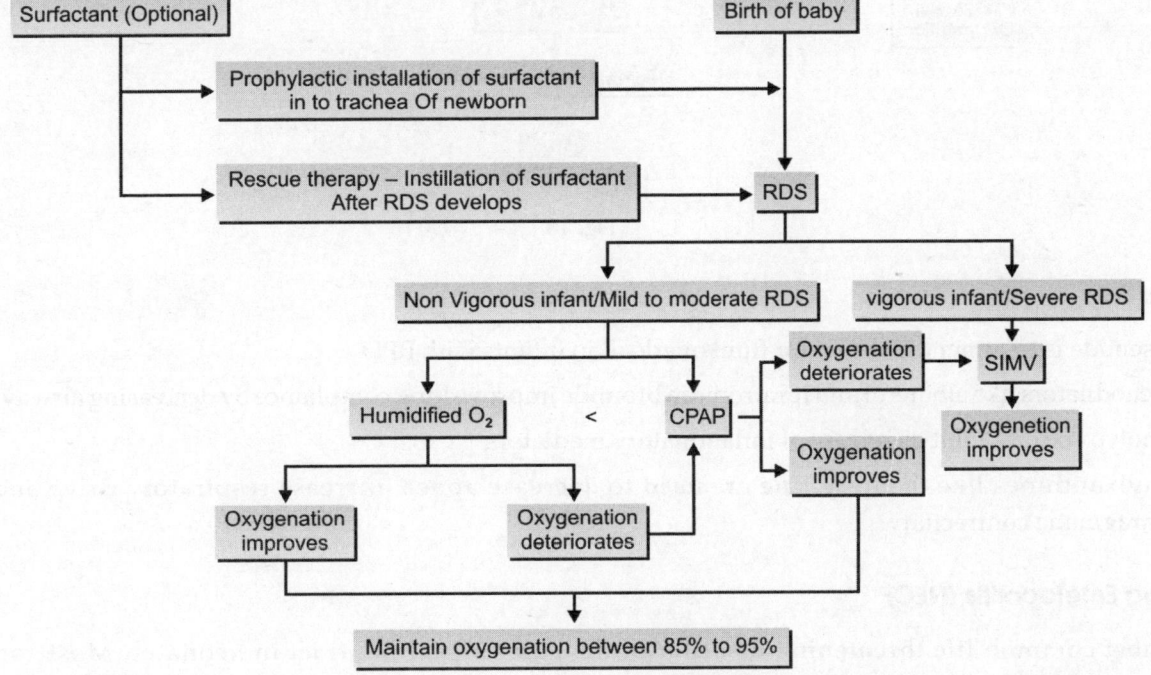

CPAP : Continuous Positive Airway Pressure, SIMV — synchronized intermittent mandatory ventilation

Fig. 17

❖ Prenatal corticosteroids administration also decreases other prematurity associated complications like **intraventricular haemorrhage,** PDA, pneumothorax and necrotising enterocolitis.

❖ **Prenatal betamethasone is more preferred than dexamethasone,** as the latter may be associated with periventricular leukomalacia and an increased incidence of RDS, IVH and death as compare to betamethasone.

❖ Contraindications to use of corticosteroids are chorioamnionitis and eclampsia.

• **Treatment:** The primary pathology towards which treatment is directed is inadequate pulmonary exchange of oxygen and carbondioxide.

Bronchopulmonary Dysplasia

Bronchopulmonary dysplasia (BPD) is a syndrome of **severe lung injury in preterm infants** usually caused by mechanical ventilation and supplemental oxygen. It occurs most frequently following preterm birth between **23–28 weeks.**

Pathophysiology of BPD

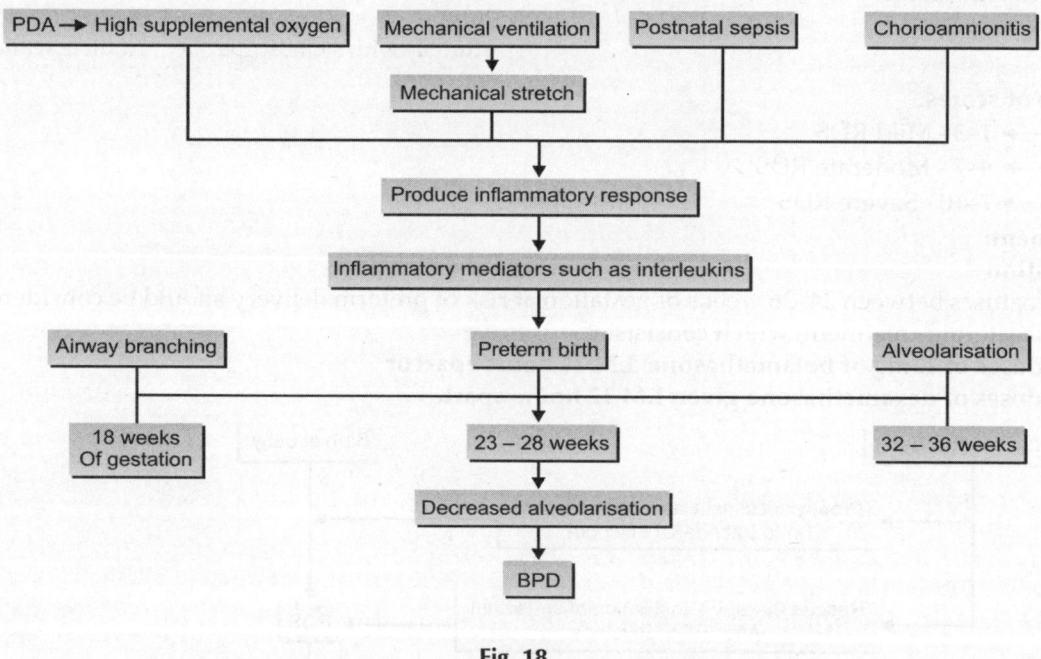

Fig. 18.

Treatment

• Furosemide is treatment of choice for fluid overload in infants with BPD.

• Bronchodilators like albuterol and ipratropium bromide improve lung compliance by decreasing airway resistance.

• Cromolyn sodium inhibits release of inflammatory mediators.

• Methylxanthines like **theophylline** are used to decrease apnea, increase respiratory drive and improve diaphragmatic contractility.

Necrotising Enterocolitis (NEC)

It is the most common life threatening disorder of the gastrointestinal tract in neonates. Most commonly it is seen in premature infants. It is characterised by inflammation and necrosis of bowel which may lead to perforation.

Pathogenesis

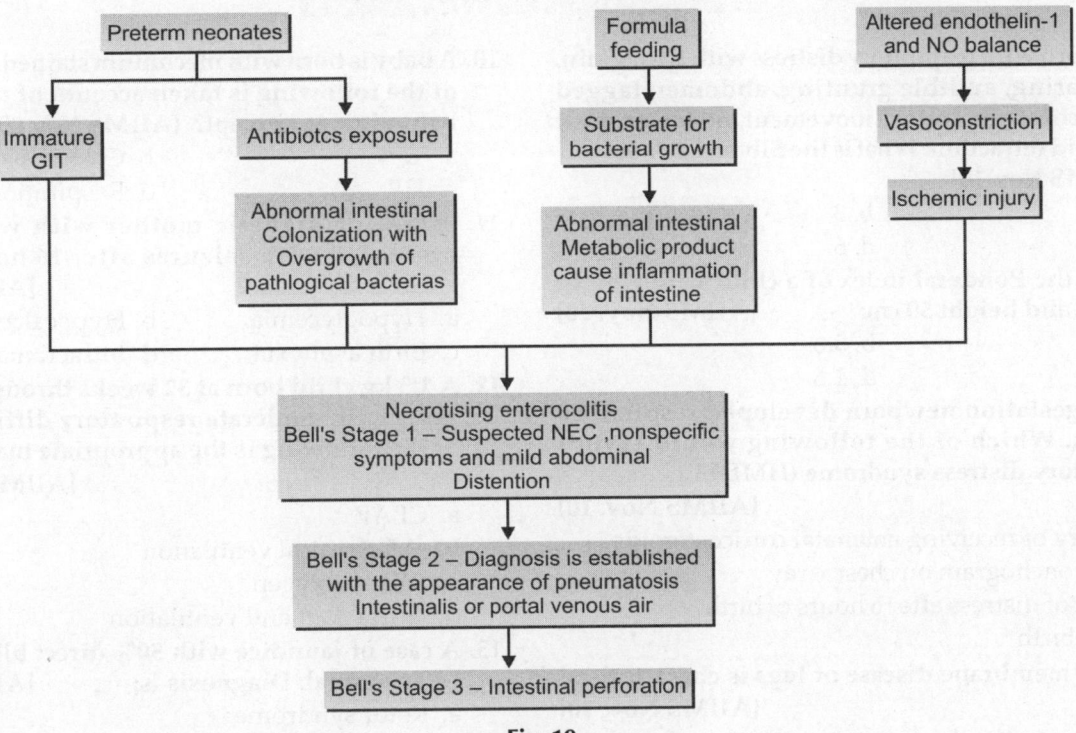

Fig. 19

- **Management:** It depends on the stage at which the neonate presents.

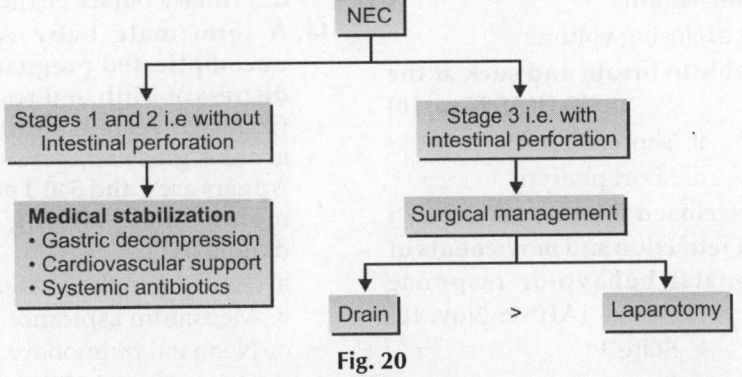

Fig. 20

Drain versus Laparotomy
(Rudolph 22nd E/P248-49)
"Outcome of infants receiving drain versus laparotomy vary depending on center and surgeon. Questions and controversy remain, however, given the small number of infants in the 1000–1500 weight group (N = 10 drain, N = 17 laparotomy), **lower survival** in infants eligible but not randomized who received **laparotomy** (15%) and the need for outcome."
(Nelson 18th E/P756)
"The role of peritoneal drainage in lieu of laparotomy in a patient with perforation   secondary to NEC remains to be determined. **Peritoneal drainage** may be helpful in patients in extremis with peritonitis who are **too unstable to undergo surgery.** Peritoneal drainage tends to be more successful in patients with **isolated intestinal perforation.** In isolated patients with **intestinal perforation treated by drainage, no further surgical procedure is needed."**

The controversy of drain versus laparotomy continues but as per information available till date drain is superior to laparotomy and first preferred procedure also.
- **Prevention of NEC:** It is an important area in the process of research; however currently the useful preventive strategies can be antenatal and postnatal.
  ❖ Antenatal use of corticosteroids is associated with decreased risk.
  ❖ Post natal intervention which are beneficial are restricted fluid administration, use of human milk and **probiotics** administration.

MULTIPLE CHOICE QUESTIONS

1. A newborn with respiratory distress with RR 86/min, nasal flaring, audible grunting, abdomen lagged behind chest respiratory movement, no lower chest or xiphoid retraction. What is the Silverman's score: [AIIMS Nov. 10]
   a. 1   b. 3
   c. 5   d. 6

2. What is the Ponderal index of a child with weight 2000 gm and height 50 cm: [AIIMS Nov. 10]
   a. 1.6   b. 3.6
   c. 2.2   d. 2.6

3. A term gestation newborn developed respiratory distress. Which of the following would favour Respiratory distress syndrome (HMD)? [AIIMS Nov. 10]
   a. History of receiving antenatal corticosteroids
   b. Air bronchogram on chest x-ray
   c. Onset of distress after 6 hours of birth
   d. Term birth

4. Hyaline membrane disease of lugs is characterised by: [AIIMS Nov. 10]
   a. FRC is smaller than closing volume
   b. FRC is greater than closing volume
   c. FRC is equal to closing volume
   d. FRC is independent of closing volume

5. Newborn babies are able to breath and suck at the same time due to: [AIIMS Nov. 10]
   a. Wide short tongue   b. Short soft palate
   c. High larynx   d. Short pharynx

6. A newborn with eyes closed 6 hours after birth lustily crying, no chest retraction and movements of all four limbs. Neonatal behaviour response grading: [AIIMS Nov. 10]
   a. State 1   b. State 3
   c. State 5   d. State 6

7. Which of the following is least likely cause of neonatal mortality in India? [AIIMS Nov. 10]
   a. Severe infections
   b. Congenital malformations
   c. Prematurity
   d. Birth asphyxia

8. Peripheral smear of neonate with ABO incompatibility will show? [AIIMS Nov. 10]
   a. Microspherocytes   b. Elliptocytes
   c. Fragmented RBCs   d. Polychromasia

9. Fetal alcohol syndrome is characterised by all except: [AIIMS Nov. 09]
   a. Microcephaly
   b. Low intelligence
   c. Large proportionate body
   d. Septal defects of heart

10. A baby is born with meconium stained liquor. Which of the following is taken account of in terming the baby vigorous except? [AIIMS Nov. 09]
    a. Tone   b. Colour
    c. HR   d. Respiration

11. Infant of diabetic mother with weight 3.8 kg presented with seizures after 16 hours of birth. What is the cause? [AIIMS Nov. 09]
    a. Hypoglycemia   b. Hypocalcemia
    c. Birth asphyxia   d. Intracranial hemorrhage

12. A 1.5 kg child born at 32 weeks through LSCS, presents with moderate respiratory difficulty. Which of the following is the appropriate management? [AIIMS Nov. 09, 10]
    a. CPAP
    b. Mechanical ventilation
    c. Warm oxygen
    d. Surfactant and ventilation

13. A case of jaundice with 50% direct bilirubin, other LFTs normal. Diagnosis is: [AIIMS May 09]
    a. Rotor syndrome
    b. Gilbert syndrome
    c. Glucuronyl transferase deficiency
    d. Primary biliary cirrhosis

14. A term male baby weighing 3.5 kg, born of uncomplicated pregnancy, developed respiratory distress at birth, not responding to surfactant, echo finding revealed nothing abnormal. X-ray showed ground glass appearance and culture is negative. Apgars are 4 and 5 at 1 and 5 minutes. History of one month fmale sibling died before. What is the diagnosis? [AIIMS Nov. 08]
    a. Total anomalous pulmonary vein connection
    b. Meconium aspiration syndrome
    c. Neonatal pulmonary alveolar proteinosis
    d. Disseminated HSV infection

15. 2 days after birth, child developed respiratory distress and had scaphoid abdomen. Breath sounds were decreased on the left side. After bag and mask ventilation, ET tube was put and the maximal cardiac impulse shifted to the right side. What should be the next step in management? [AIIMS June 08]
    a. Confirm the position of endotracheal tube
    b. Emergency surgery
    c. Nasogastric tube insertion
    d. Chest X-ray

16. A child presented with respiratory distress was brought to emergency with bag and mask ventilation. Now child is intubated. Chest X-ray shows right-sided deviation of mediastinum with scaphoid abdomen. His pulse rate is increased. What is the next step? [AIIMS Nov. 07]

a. Endotracheal intubation
b. Put a nasogastric tube
c. Surgery
d. End tidal CO_2 to confirm intubation

17. **A term neonate with unconjugated hyperbilirubinemia of 18 mg/dl on 20 days. All are common causes except:** [AIIMS May 07]
    a. Breast milk jaundice
    b. Congenital cholangiopathy
    c. G 6PD deficiency
    d. Hypothyroidism

18. **All the following can occur in a neonate for heat production except:** [AIIMS Nov. 06]
    a. Shivering
    b. Breakdown of brown fat with adrenaline secretion
    c. Universal flexion like a fetus
    d. Cutaneous vasoconstriction

19. **All of the following are the complications in the new born of a diabetic mother except:** [AIIMS May 06]
    a. Hyperbilirubinemia   b. Hyperglycemia
    c. Hypocalcemia   d. Hypomagnesemia

20. **Administration of glucose solution is prescribed for all of the following situations except:** [AIIMS May 06]
    a. Neonates
    b. Child of a diabetic mother
    c. History of unconsciousness
    d. History of hypoglycemia

21. **Which mechanism in phototherapy is chiefly responsible for reduction in serum bilirubin?** [AIIMS May 05]
    a. Photo-oxidation
    b. Photo-isomerization
    c. Structural isomerization
    d. Conjugation

22. **Characteristics radiological feature of transient tachypnea of newborn is:** [AIIMS May 05]
    a. Reticulogranular appearance
    b. Low volume lungs
    c. Prominent horizontal fissure
    d. Air bronchogram

23. **A 5-year-old child is rushed to casualty reportedly electrocuted while playing in a park. The child is apneic and is ventilated with bag and mask. There are bums on each hand. What will be the next step in the management :** [AIIMS Nov. 05, 04]
    a. Check pulses   b. Start chest compressions
    c. Intubate   d. Check oxygen saturation

24. **Bag and mask ventilation is contraindicated in:** [AIIMS May 04; June 99]
    a. Cleft lip
    b. Meconium aspiration

c. Diaphragmatic hernia
d. Multicentric bronchogenic cyst

25. **Asphyxial injury in a term baby is characterized by all except:** [AIIMS Nov. 03]
    a. Seizures
    b. Differential hypotonia (lower limbs>upper limbs)
    c. Altered sensorium
    d. Difficulty in clearing oral secretions

26. **A new born baby has been referred to the casualty as a case of congenital diaphragmatic hernia. The first clinical intervention is to:** [AIIMS May 03]
    a. Insert a central venous pressure line
    b. Bag and mask ventilation
    c. Insert a nasogastric tube
    d. Ventilate with high frequency ventilator

27. **All of the following groups of newborns are at an increased risk of hypoglycemia except:** [AIIMS Nov. 02]
    a. Birth asphyxia
    b. Respiratory distress syndrome
    c. Maternal diabetes
    d. Post-term infant

28. **A full term baby, exclusively breast fed, at the end of 1 week was passing golden yellow stools and was found to have adequate hydration with normal systemic examination. The weight of the baby was just same as it was at birth. The pediatrician should now advise:** [AIIMS May 02]
    a. Give oral solution with breast feeding
    b. Start top feeding
    c. Investigate for lactic acidosis
    d. Reassure the mother that nothing is abnormal

29. **Transient tachypnea of new born (TTN) is commonly seen in which of the following situations:** [AIIMS May 02]
    a. Term delivery requiring forceps
    b. Term requiring ventouse
    c. Elective cesarean section
    d. Normal vaginal delivery

30. **A child has bilirubin of 4 mg. Conjugated bilirubin and alkaline phosphatase are normal, bile salts and bile in urine are absent. However urobilinogen in urine is raised. What is the likely diagnosis?** [AIIMS Nov. 01]
    a. Obstructive jaundice   b. Rotor's syndrome
    c. Biliary cholestasis   d. Hemolytic jaundice

31. **A 6 months old child having severe dehydration comes to the casualty with weak pulse and unrecordable BP Repeated attempt in gaining IV access has failed. The next best step is:** [AIIMS May 01]
    a. Try again
    b. Jugular vein catheterization
    c. Intraosseous IV fluids
    d. Venesection

32. **Retinopathy of prematurity is commonly pre-disposed by:** [AIIMS June 00]
    a. Less gestation age   b. Low birth weight
    c. O2 toxicity   d. Carbohydrate excess

33. **A full term, 80 hrs old newborn baby develops jaundice. What should be minimum level of serum bilirubin to start phototherapy:** [AIIMS June 99]
    a. 20 mg%   b. 12.5 mg%
    c. 18 mg%   d. 15 mg%

34. **All are true about Gilbert's syndrome except:** [AIIMS Dec. 97]
    a. Mild conjugated hyperbilirubinemia
    b. Autosomal dominant
    c. Normal liver histology
    d. Almost normal liver function tests

35. **Which is not a component of APGAR score?** [AIIMS June 97]
    a. Colour of body
    b. Muscle tone
    c. Heart rate/minutes
    d. Respiratory rate per minute

36. **One gm of Hb liberates mg of bilirubin:** [AIIMS June 97]
    a. 40   b. 34
    c. 15   d. 55

37. **Full term small for date babies are predisposed to:** [AIIMS May 95]
    a. Hypercalcemia
    b. CNS infections
    c. Hypoglycemia
    d. PDA

38. **In asymmetrical IUGR which organ is not affected:** [AIIMS 94]
    a. Subcutaneous fat   b. Muscle
    c. Liver   d. Brain

39. **For a term small for date baby true is:** [AIIMS May 93]
    a. No nipple nodule
    b. No palmar plantar crease
    c. Weight less than 10th percentile
    d. Hyperbilirubinemia

40. **Unconjugated bilirubin is increased in all except:** [AIIMS May 93]
    a. Crigler-Najjar syndrome
    b. Dubin Johnson syndrome
    c. Gilbert syndrome
    d. Hemolytic anemia

41. **IUGR is caused by all except:** [AIIMS 91]
    a. Diabetes   b. Alcohol
    c. Smoking   d. Chronic renal failure

42. **Intrauterine growth retardation can be caused by all except:** [AIIMS 87]
    a. Nicotine   b. Alcohol
    c. Propranolol   d. Phenothiazine

43. **Risk of kernicterus is increased by all except:** [AIIMS 84]
    a. Low level of serum albumin
    b. Prematurity
    c. Acidosis
    d. High levels of serum albumin

44. **A premature infant is more likely than a full term infant to:** [AIIMS 80, PGI 85]
    a. Suffer from jaundice of hepatic origin
    b. Maintain normal body temperature in a cold environment
    c. Excrete urine with a uniform specific gravity
    d. Suffer from anemia

45. **Infants receiving phototherapy:** [AIIMS 80, PGI 83]
    a. Have increased insensible water loss
    b. Generally develop a bronze discolouration of skin
    c. Should have their eyes patched during therapy
    d. Often become constipated

46. **A hymenal tag in a newborn is best treated by:** [AIIMS 80, PGI 82]
    a. Steroids   b. Surgery
    c. Leaving it alone   d. None of the above

47. **A neonate weighing 1500 grams is delivered at 33 weeks. Which of the following would be most appropriate method of nutrition for baby?** [AI 11]
    a. IV fluids and oral feeding
    b. Nasogastric feeding/alternate oral feeding
    c. Total parenteral nutrition
    d. IV fluids and assessment/follow up

48. **Most common fetal response to acute hypoxia is:** [AI 09]
    a. Tachycardia
    b. Bradycardia
    c. Cardiac arrest tachypnea
    d. Ventricular arrhythmia

49. **Probiotics have been found beneficial for use in:** [All India 2008]
    A. Necrotizing enterocolitis
    B. Neonatal sepsis
    C. Candidiasis
    D. Intestinal perforation

50. **A child presented with severe respiratory distress two days after birth. On examination he was observed to have a scaphoid abdomen and decreased breath sounds on the left side. He was managed by prompt endotracheal intubation. After ET tube placement the maximal cardiac impulse shifted further to the right side. What should be the next step in management?** [AI 08]

a. Confirm the position of endotracheal tube by chest X-ray
b. Remove tube and reattempt intubation
c. Nasogastric tube insertion and decompress the bowel
d. Chest X-ray to confirm diagnosis

51. **A neonate having congenital diaphragmatic hernia developed respiratory distress. Breath sounds were decreased on the left side. After bag and mask ventilation, ET tube was put and the maximal cardiac impulse shifted to the right side. What should be the next step in management?**   **[AI 08]**
    a. Confirm the position of endotracheal tube by X-ray chest
    b. Emergency surgery
    c. Nasogastric tube insertion
    d. Chest X-ray

52. **A very low birth weight preterm baby is on ventilator for respiratory distress. Baby presents with clinical features of necrotizing enterocolitis with perforation. What is the appropriate management?**   **[AI 08]**
    a. Conservative management
    b. Immediate laparotomy
    c. Extra corporeal membrane oxygenation with surgery after stabilization
    d. Peritoneal drainage

53. **A nonventilated preterm baby in incubator is under observation. Which is the best way to monitor the baby's breathing and detect apnea?**   **[AI 07]**
    a. Infrared throraric movement study
    b. Capnography
    c. Nasal digital temperature monitoring
    d. Impedence technique

54. **All of the following are features of prematurity in a neonate, except:**   **[AI 06]**
    a. No creases on sole   b. Abundant lanugo
    c. Thick ear cartilage   d. Empty scrotum

55. **Which of the following is the principal mode of heat exchange in an infant incubator?**   **[AI 06]**
    a. Radiation   b. Evaporation
    c. Convection   d. Conduction

56. **Which of the following malformation in a newborn is specific for maternal insulin dependent diabetes mellitus?**   **[AI 06]**
    a. Transposition of great arteries
    b. Caudal regression
    c. Holoprosencephaly
    d. Meningomyelocele

57. **In unconjugated hyperbilirubinemia, the risk of kernicterus increases with the use of:**   **[AI 05]**
    a. Ceftriaxone   b. Phenobarbitone
    c. Ampicillin   d. Sulfonamide

58. **All of the following therapies may be required in a 1 hour old infant with severe birth asphyxia except:**   **[AI 05]**
    a. Glucose   b. Dexamethasone
    c. Calcium gluconate   d. Normal saline

59. **The appropriate approach to a neonate presenting with vaginal bleeding on day 4 of life is:**   **[AI 05]**
    a. Administration of vitamin K
    b. Investigation for bleeding disorder
    c. No specific therapy
    d. Administration of 10 ml/kg of fresh frozen plasma over 4 hours

60. **With reference to RDS, all of the following statements are true except:**   **[AI 02], [PGI Dec. 99]**
    a. Usually occurs in infants born before 34 weeks of gestation
    b. Is more common in babies born to diabetic mothers
    c. Leads to cyanosis
    d. Is treated by administering 100% oxygen

61. **Full term, small-for-date babies are at high-risk of:**   **[AI 00]**
    a. Hypoglycemia
    b. Intraventricular hemorrhage
    c. Bronchopulmonary dysplasia
    d. Hyperthermia

62. **What should be measured in a newborn who presents with hyperbilirubinemia?**   **[AI 00]**
    a. Total and direct bilirubin
    b. Total bilirubin only
    c. Direct bilirubin only
    d. Conjugated bilirubin only

63. **True statement about IUGR is:**   **[AI 99]**
    a. Hepatomegaly is due to fatty infiltration
    b. Head circumference is 3 cm more than chest circumference
    c. Hyaline membrane disease is a common cause of death
    d. Hypothermia does not occur due to good shivering mechanism

64. **Unconjugated hyperbilirubinemia in neonate is seen in all except:**   **[AI 98]**
    a. Physiological jaundice
    b. Dubin Johnson syndrome
    c. Hypothyroidism
    d. Hemolytic anemia

65. **Meconium aspiration is done for 3 times but no breathing occurs. Next step in resuscitation would be:**   **[AI 97]**
    a. Chest compression
    b. O$_2$ inhalation
    c. Bag and mask ventilation
    d. Trikling of sole

66. **Vomiting on the first day of baby's life may be caused by all of the following except:**   [AI 97]
    a. Pyloric stenosis
    b. Esophageal atresia
    c. Aerophagy
    d. Amniotic gastritis

67. **All of the following are causes of bronchopulmonary dysplasia except:**   [AI 96]
    a. Oxygen toxicity
    b. Theophylline use
    c. Traumatic damage to lungs
    d. Pulmonary oedema due to capillary leakage

68. **Defective hepatic conjugation is seen in all the following except:**   [AI 96]
    a. Neonatal jaundice
    b. Gilbert syndrome
    c. Crigler-Najjar syndrome
    d. Novobiocin therapy

69. **Jaundice at birth or within 24 hours of birth is commonly due to:**   [AI 95]
    a. Erythroblastosis
    b. Congenital hyperbilirubinemia
    c. Biliary atresia
    d. Physiological

70. **A 3hours old neonate with apnea is on bag and mask ventilation for last 30 seconds, now showing spontaneous breathing with heart rate 110/min. The next step should be:**   [AI 92]
    a. Discontinue ventilation
    b. Continue ventilation
    c. Give chest compression
    d. ET intubation

71. **Neonatal jaundice first time appears in 2nd week not a cause:**   [AI 92]
    a. Galactosemia
    b. Rh incompatibility
    c. Hypothyroidism
    d. Breast milk jaundice

72. **Hyaline membrane seen in lung is composed of:**   [AI 88]
    a. Globulin
    b. Fibrin
    c. Mucoprotein
    d. Polysaccharide

73. **Macrosomia is seen in:**   [PGI Nov. 09]
    a. GDM
    b. Maternal obesity
    c. Maternal hypothyroidism
    d. Hyperbilirubinemia
    e. Fetal goiter

74. **MCV (fl) in infant of one month of age is:**   [PGI Nov. 09]
    a. 76 – 80
    b. 80 – 100
    c. 90 –110
    d. 101 – 125
    e. 125 – 135

75. **Drugs that can be used in kernicterus:**   [PGI June 06; Dec. 02; PGI June 09]
    a. Barbiturates
    b. Benzodiazepines
    c. Phenytoin
    d. Chlorpromazine
    e. Carbamazepine

76. **Low birth weight is defined as:**   [PGI Dec. 08]
    a. Weight < 2.5 kg
    b. Weight < 2.0 kg
    c. Weight < 1.5 kg
    d. Weight < 10 percentile for their gestational age
    e. Weight < 2.5 SD for their gestational age

77. **Common sites for Mongolian spots are:**   [PGI Dec. 08]
    a. Face
    b. Neck
    c. Lumbosacral area
    d. Leg
    e. Thigh

78. **Skin changes in newborn that disappear spontaneously:**   [PGI Dec. 08]
    a. Harlequins skin change
    b. Mongolian spots
    c. Erythema toxicum
    d. Lymphoma
    e. Milia

79. **Neonatal apnea is seen in all except:**   [PGI Nov. 08]
    a. Prematurity
    b. Hyperglycemia
    c. Hypoglycemia
    d. Hypercalcemia
    e. Hyperthermia

80. **A child presented in the casualty with fever, unconscious and papilloedema. What next to be done:**   [PGI Nov. 08]
    a. Intubation
    b. Oxygenation
    c. CT scan
    d. Lumber puncture

81. **Unconjugated hyperbilirubinemia is seen in:**   [PGI Dec. 07]
    a. Physiological jaundice
    b. Breast milk jaundice
    c. Gilbert syndrome
    d. Biliary atresia
    e. Rotor syndrome

82. **Loss of pulmonary surfactant in premature infant:**   [PGI Dec. 2007]
    a. Pulmonary edema
    b. Collapse of alveoli
    c. Decreased compliance

83. **Components of neonatal resuscitation:**   [PGI Dec. 07]
    a. Maintenance of temperature
    b. Maintenance of respiration
    c. Maintenance of circulation
    d. Chest compression

84. **Still born child is defined by:**   [PGI Dec. 07]
    a. > 20 weeks
    b. > 24 weeks
    c. > 28 weeks
    d. > 32 weeks
    e. > 1300 gm

85. **Infants of diabetic mother manifests:**   [PGI Dec. 07]
    a. Hyperglycemia
    b. Hypoglycemia
    c. Hypocalcemia
    d. Increased fetal defect
    e. Hyperbilirubinemia

86. **Conjugated hyperbilirubinemia in infancy is seen in:** [PGI Dec. 06]
    a. Gilbert syndrome
    b. Crigler-Najjar syndrome
    c. Dubin Johnson syndrome
    d. Rotor syndrome
    e. Neonatal hepatitis

87. **The different manifestations of hypothermia are:** [PGI June 06]
    a. Apnea
    b. Hypoglycemia
    c. Hyperglycemia
    d. Tachycardia
    e. Hypoxia

88. **Conjugated hyperbilirubinemia in infancy seen in:** [PGI Dec. 04]
    a. Choledochal cyst
    b. Extra hepatic biliary atresia
    c. Crigler - Najjar disease
    d. Gilbert disease

89. **A term baby developed jaundice on 3rd day up to the thigh with normal stool and urine. Mother's blood group is 'O'-ve and that of baby's 'A'+ve. The cause of jaundice is:** [PGI Dec. 04; Dec. 02]
    a. Rh incompatibility
    b. Physiological jaundice
    c. Extrahepatic biliary atresia
    d. Sepsis
    e. Glucose-6 phosphate dehydrogenase deficiency

90. **A 3 kg term baby delivered by cesarian section develops respiratory distress soon after birth. The liquor was meconium stained. Breathing rate is 90/minute. Correct statements :** [PGI Dec. 04]
    a. Transient tachypnea of newborn
    b. Meconium aspiration syndrome
    c. Reticulonodular shadows in X-ray chest
    d. Surfactant production
    e. Oral feeding started early

91. **Respiratory distress in newborn is defined when:** [PGI June 04]
    a. Respiration rate >60/min
    b. Intercostal recession
    c. Aspiration > 20 ml
    d. Hypoxemia
    e. Reticulonodular shadow in CXR

92. **A 4 kg baby born to a diabetic mother found i.e. lethargic which of the following is to be done:** [PGI Dec. 03]
    a. Reasses the baby again after 2 hours
    b. Give 10% dextrose IV
    c. Start oral feeding
    d. Give injection insulin

93. **A women delivered a baby of 2.2 kg weight her LMP is not known. To know the maturity of baby, following are used:** [PG June 03]
    a. Sole crease
    b. Ear cartilage
    c. Breast nodule
    d. Anterior fontanelle
    e. Weight of the baby

94. **Infants of diabetic mother have the followings:** [PGI June 03]
    a. Macrosomia
    b. Neural tube defect
    c. Hyperglycemia
    d. Hypocalcemia

95. **True about physiological jaundice:** [PGI June 03]
    a. Jaundice appears within first 24 hours
    b. Jaundice disappear in 3rd week
    c. Sudden rise of bilirubin
    d. Breast feeding should be stopped

96. **Hypothermia in neonate is characterized by :** [PGI Dec. 02]
    a. Hyperactivity
    b. Hypoglycemia
    c. Apnea
    d. Increased urinary output

97. **Normal finding in term neonate:** [PGI Dec. 02, Dec. 98]
    a. Erythema toxicum
    b. Epstein's pearl
    c. Bilateral cryptorchidism
    d. Subconjunctival hemorrhages
    e. Erythema nodosum

98. **Which of the following is true about Gilbert's syndrome:** [PGI June 02]
    a. Increased liver transaminases
    b. Unconjugated hyperbilirubinemia
    c. Bleeding tendency
    d. Presence of autoantibodies
    e. Increased toxicity of irinotecan

99. **A Newborn weighing 1000 g is born at gestational age of 30 weeks with respiratory distress after 2–3 hours of birth. What are the diagnostic possibilities:** [PGI June 01]
    a. Diaphragmatic hernia
    b. Cong. bronchopulmonary cysts
    c. Bronchopulmonary dysplasia
    d. HMD
    e. Pulmonary hemorrhage

100. **Which of the following are signs of neonatal respiratory distress syndrome?** [PGI June 01]
    a. Intercostal retraction
    b. RR > 60/min
    c. Absence of cyanosis
    d. PH < 7.2
    e. A linear streak on CXR

101. **True about physiological jaundice in neonate:** [PGI Dec. 00]
    a. Occurs in first 6 hours of delivery
    b. Unconjugated hyperbilirubinemia
    c. Neurological sequelaare common
    d. Best treated by phototherapy
    e. Starts on 2nd day of life

102. **Newborn with APGAR score of 2 at 1 min. and 6 at 5 min. has respiratory distress and mediastinal shift diagnosis is :** [PGI Dec. 00]
    a. Congenital adenomatoid lung disease
    b. Pneumothorax
    c. Diaphragmatic hernia
    d. Transient tachypnea of newborn
    e. HMD

103. **Small for date baby is:** [PGI June 00]
    a. < 10 percentile for the gestational age
    b. < 50 percentile for gestational age
    c. < 2000 gm
    d. < 2500 gm

104. **Bronze baby syndrome is due to:** [PGI Dec. 98]
    a. Phototherapy
    b. Wilson disease
    c. Chloramphenicol toxicity
    d. Hemochromatosis

105. **Hypoxic ischemic encephalopathy true is:** [PGI Dec. 98]
    a. Lower limbs affected more than upper limbs
    b. Proximal muscles>distal muscles
    c. Seizure
    d. Trunk involved

106. **Small for gestational age infant is having:** [PGI Dec. 97]
    a. Undescended testis   b. Wrinkled sole
    c. Lanugo sole   d. Breast nodule

107. **Granulomatous appearance of lung with air bronchogram in neonates represents:** [PGI Dec. 97]
    a. Aspiration pneumonia
    b. Hyaline membrane disease
    c. Staph pneumonia
    d. ARDS

108. **True about Crigler-Najjar syndrome type II is:** [PGI Dec. 97]
    a. Diglucuronide deficiency
    b. Recessive trait
    c. Kernicterus is seen
    d. Phenobarbitone not useful

109. **Respiratory distress syndrome in infants is seen in:** [PGI 89]
    a. Babies of diabetics
    b. Premature rupture of membrane
    c. More than 2500 gm
    d. Less than 37 weeks

110. **Meconium contains all except:** [PGI 88]
    a. Lanugo   b. Bacterial flora
    c. Epithelial debris   d. Bilirubin

111. **At birth the normal heart rate is:** [PGI 81, Bihar 91]
    a. 60–80   b. 80–110
    c. 70–120   d. 110–150

112. **The clinical sign of hyaline membrane disease generally first appears:** [PGI 81, AMU 88]
    a. In the first six hours of life
    b. Between 12 and 24 hours of life
    c. Between 36 and 48 hours of life
    d. After 48 hours of life

QUESTIONS OF OTHER EXAMINATIONS

1. **In neonate jaundice appears for the first time in the second week. The following is not a cause:** [DPG 10]
    a. Galactosemia   b. Rh incompatibility
    c. Hypothyroidism   d. Breast milk jaundice

2. **The late features of kernicterus includes all of the following except:** [DPG 09]
    a. Hypotonia
    b. Sensorineural hearing loss
    c. Choreoathetosis
    d. Upward gaze palsy

3. **Most common newborn rash which presents at 24-48 hours of life is?** [UPSC 09]
    a. Erythematous papularpustular lesions
    b. Milia
    c. Transient pustularmelanosis
    d. Hemangioma

4. **Which of the following is an abnormal finding in a neonate?** [DPG 09]
    a. Glycosuria   b. Bacteruria
    c. WBCs in urine   d. Hyperbilirubinemia

5. **In a newborn, what is the normal respiratory rate?** [UPSC 08]
    a. 10–20 breaths/min   b. 30–40 breaths/min
    c. 40–60 breaths/min   d. 60–80 breaths/min

6. **A newborn presented with jaundice. Most diagnostic investigation of choice is:** [UP 08]
    a. Total and direct bilirubin
    b. Conjugated bilirubin
    c. Serum bilirubin
    d. Uroporphyrin levels

7. **Fetal lung maturity assessed by all except:** [UP 08]
    a. Measurement of α fetoprotein
    b. Lecithin : sphingomyelin ratio

c. Measurement of amniotic fluid creatinine

d. Phosphatidyl choline concentration in amniotic fluid

8. **The following factors contribute to hypothermia in preterm babies except:** [UPSC 08]

a. Decreased subcutaneous fat and brown fat

b. Large surface area in relation to body weight

c. Less oxygen consumption

d. Increased muscular activity

9. **Not seen in small for date babies:** [APPG 08]

a. Hypoglycemia   b. Polycythemia

c. Intracranial bleed   d. Hypocalcemia

10. **The blood sugar in a neonate shortly after birth reaches the lowest level of 30 mg/dl at the age of:** [DPG 08]

a. 1 hour   b. 3 hours

c. 6 hours   d. 8 hours

11. **All of the following statements about prenatal steroids are true except:** [UPSC 08]

a. They cause 50% reduction in respiratory distress syndrome and intraventricular hemorrhage

b. These are advocated to mothers at risk of preterm delivery at 24-34 weeks of gestation

c. These can be safely administered to mothers with hypertension or diabetes

d. These can be given even in presence of chorio-amnionitis clinically

12. **The dose of betamethasone in prenatal period to prevent respiratory distress syndrome is:** [UP 07]

a. 6 mg   b. 12 mg every 24 hours

c. 6 mg every 12 hours   d. 4 mg stat

13. **A 32 week old premature infant, 900 gm weight on the third day. The serum bilirubin is 13 mg%. The treatment of choice is:** [UP 07]

a. Exchange transfusion

b. Phototherapy

c. Wait and watch

d. Pharmacologic therapy

14. **Which of the following medical disorder leads to delayed fetal lung maturity?** [UPSC 07]

a. Heart disease   b. Diabetes

c. Thalassemia major   d. Epilepsy

15. **Failure to initiate and maintain spontaneous respiration following birth is clinically k/a:** [COMED 07]

a. Birth asphyxia

b. RDS—Respiratory distress syndrome

c. Respiratory failure

d. Pulmonary edema

16. **All of the following factors affect APGAR score except:** [COMED 07]

a. Prematurity

b. Mental retardation

c. Neurological condition of the newborn

d. Mode of delivery

17. **Autosomal dominant familial nonhemolytic hyper-bilirubinemia occurs in all except:** [UP 07]

a. Crigler-Najjar syndrome

b. Dubin Johnson syndrome

c. Gilbert syndrome

d. Cryoglobulinemia

18. **A 50 hour old full term breast fed newborn boy weighing 3100 gm presents with clinically evidence jaundice. Physical examination is otherwise normal. The total bilirubin is 11 mg/dl with a direct bilirubin of 4 mg/dl. What would be the correct statement?** [UPSC 07]

a. Continue breast feeds and review after 48 hours

b. Stop breast feeds and review after 24 hours

c. Continue breast feeds and start blue light phototherapy

d. Arrange for a double volume exchange transfusion

19. **A 26-year-old third gravida mother delivered a male baby weighing 4.2 kg at 37 weeks of gestation through an emergency caesarean section for obstructed labour. The child developed respiratory distress one hour after birth. He was kept nil per orally and given intravenous fluids. He maintained oxygen saturation on room air. No antibiotics were given. Chest radiograph revealed fluid in interlobar fissure. Respiratory distress settled by 24 hours of life. What is the most likely diagnosis?** [UPSC 06]

a. Transient tachypnea of newborn

b. Meconium aspiration syndrome

c. Persistent fetal circulation

d. Hyaline membrane disease

20. **Meconium aspiration is done 3 times but no breathing occurs. Next step in resuscitation would be:** [MHCET 05]

a. Chest compression

b. O_2 inhalation

c. Bag and mask ventilation

d. Tickling of sole

21. **Microsomia is defined as:** [MHCET 05]

a. Birth weight below 90th percentile

b. Birth weight below 10th percentile

c. Birth weight below 20th percentile

d. Birth weight below 50th percentile

22. **Very low birth weight babies are:** [SGPGI 05]

a. < 2500 gm of birth weight

b. < 1500 gm of birth weight

c. < 1000 gm of birth weight

d. Between 2500-3000 gm of birth weight

23. **Hyperbilirubinemia in a child can be due to:** [MHCET 05]

a. Breast milk jaundice

b. Cystic fibrosis

c. Fanconi's syndrome

d. Alpha 1 antitrypsin deficiency

24. **The newborn heart rate is about:** [TN 04]
   a. 120-160/min
   b. 160-180/min
   c. 180-200/min
   d. 200-220/min

25. **Early neonatal period is:** [Kerala 03]
   a. 1 day
   b. 7 days
   c. 28 days
   d. 14 days

26. **Bag and mask ventilation is newborn resuscitation is contraindicated in:** [UPSC 02]
   a. Diaphragmatic hernia
   b. Pulmonary hypoplasia
   c. Tracheo-esophageal fistula
   d. Laryngomalacia

27. **Hypoglycemia in late infant and child occurs if blood glucose level is:** [CUPGEE 01]
   a. 40 mg/dl
   b. 60 mg/dl
   c. 10 mg/dl
   d. 20 mg/dl

28. **Which of the following is true of hyaline membrane disease of the newborn?** [UPSC 99]
   a. Prematurity provides relative protection of the occurrence
   b. Maternal steroid exposure increase severity of disease
   c. Phosphatidyl glycerol estimation is a reliable method of diagnosis
   d. Surfactant increases the surfacetension of alveoli

29. **The foetus born during 6th month of intrauterine life will not be able to survive due to:** [ICS 98]
   a. Lack of subcutaneous tissue
   b. Lack of coordination between the respiratory and nervous system
   c. Absence or insufficient amount of surfactant
   d. Lack of sufficient capillaries

30. **The fetal length is affected if the mother has under-nutrition during the:** [UPSC 98]
   a. First trimester
   b. Second trimester
   c. Third trimester
   d. Anytime during the pregnancy

31. **A term baby was brought with complaints of breathing difficulty. He was born normally to primigravida. Mother's antenatal period and labour record was normal. On examination he was in respiratory distress. Abdomen was flat. There was no organomegaly. The most likely cause is:** [UPSC 98]
   a. Congenital heart disease with dextrocardia
   b. Respiratory distress syndrome
   c. Diaphragmatic hernia
   d. Aspiration pneumonia

32. **Jaundice in the newborn is physiological when:** [UPSC 98]
   a. The infant is visibly jaundiced in the first 24 hours of birth
   b. The total bilirubin concentration in the serum increases by 1mg/dl per day

c. The total bilirubin concentration is above 15 mg/dl
d. Jaundice persists for more than one week in a term infant

33. **Jaundice seen immediately after birth in:** [AP 97]
   a. Septicemia
   b. Rh incompatibility
   c. Breast milk jaundice
   d. Physiological jaundice

34. **Which of the following is true about Transient tachypnea of newborn (TTN)?** [UPSC 97]
   a. It is the commonest respiratory disorder caused by absence of surfactant
   b. In premature babies it is often fatal
   c. Onset of respiratory distress is immediately after birth and it rarely lasts beyond 48 hours
   d. It often leads to chronic lung disease

35. **Which of the following substance is toxic to neurons?** [JIPMER 95]
   a. Unconjugated bilirubin
   b. Bile salts
   c. Hemoglobin
   d. Melanin

36. **In a child cessation of breathing for 20 sec with bradycardia is:** [AMU 95]
   a. Apnea
   b. Dyspnea
   c. Cheyne stokes respiration
   d. None

37. **Foetal maturity is assessed by:** [Kerala 94]
   a. L/S ratio
   b. Bilirubin content of amniotic fluid
   c. Ultrasound
   d. Amniocentesis

38. **Most common cause of respiratory distress after birth in first 24 hours is:** [JIPMER 95]
   a. Neonatal sepsis
   b. Meconium aspiration
   c. Bacterial pneumonia
   d. Air embolism

39. **Harlequin skin change in the newborn is seen in:** [JIPMER 93]
   a. Autonomic dysfunction
   b. Icthyosis
   c. Septicemia
   d. Polycythemia

40. **The following is of serious pathological significance in infants:** [KCET 89]
   a. Loss of weight
   b. Palpable left kidney
   c. Palpable spleen
   d. Deviation of trachea from midlines

41. **Neonatal period extends up to:** [JIPMER 81, UPSC 84]
   a. 21 days of life
   b. 30 days of life
   c. 28 days of life
   d. 35 days of life

42. **At birth the normal heart rate is:** [PGI 81, Bihar 91]
   a. 60–80
   b. 80–110
   c. 70–120
   d. 110–150

43. **Cephalhematoma usually disappears within:** [JIPMER 80, UPSC 82]
   a. 3–5 months
   b. 2–5 weeks
   c. 3–5 weeks
   d. 5–7 weeks

ANSWERS

MULTIPLE CHOICE QUESTIONS

1. (c) 5 (Ref: Kulkarni Manual of neonatology/P267)
Silverman's score:

Signs	0	1	2
Thoraco abdominal movement in respiration	Significant	Thoracic lag	See-Saw
Nasal flaring	Nil	Mild	Severe
Lower intercostal retraction	Nil	Mild	Severe
Xiphoid retraction	Nil	Mild	Severe
Grunting	Nil	Audible with stethoscope	Audible without stethoacope

- Putting the values for the signs in the question
  - ❖ Nasal flaring — 2
  - ❖ Audible grunting — 2
  - ❖ Abdomen lagging — 1
  - ❖ Intercostal retraction absent — 0
  - ❖ Xiphoid retraction absent — 0
- Hence the Silverman's score is 5 and the child is having moderate RDS.

2. (a) 1.6 (Ref: Ghai 7th E/P109)
- Ponderal index is a measure of fetal growth.
- P.I = Weight (gm) × 100/Length (cm)^3
- Putting the values in the formula
  P.I = 2000 × 100/50^3 = 1.6

3. (b) Air bronchogram on chest X-ray (Ref: Ghai 7th E/P143, Nelson 19th E/P577)
- Chest X-ray in RDS shows reticulogranular pattern of increased density of lung parenchyma due to miliary atelectasis and interstitial edema. Other findings are **air bronchogram,** ground glass appearance of lung and decreased lung volume.
- Antenatal corticosteroids are given to decrease the incidence of RDS.
- Onset of distress in RDS is usually seen in the first 6 hours of life.
- RDS is usually associated with preterm birth.

4. (a) FRC is smaller than closing volume (Ref: Lynn Pediatric respiratory medicine 2nd E/P379)

"A reduction in functional residual capacity (FRC) and a marked decrease in lung compliance are characteristics of RDS."

5. (c) High larynx (Ref: Rudolph 22nd E/P1329)
- In infants the superior border of larynx is located at the level of first cervical vertebrae. This high location of larynx elevates epiglottis to the level of palate and facilitates nasal breathing.

- Further during breast feeding the forward thrust of tongue further elevates larynx and facilitates baby's nasal breathing while feeding.

6. (d) State 6 (Ref: Tecklin Pediatric physical therapy 3rd E/P88)
Morgan's neonatal neurobehavioural examination: This consists of three parts i.e. tone and motor patterns, primitive reflexes and behavioural responses. The behavioural responses can be graded in to six states—
- State 1 — Deep sleep, No eye movement, Regular breathing.
- State 2 — Light sleep, eyes shut, some movement.
- State 3 — Dozing, eyes opening and closing.
- State 4 — Awake, eyes open, minimal movement
- State 5 — Wide awake, vigorous movements
- **State 6 — Crying**

7. (b) Congenital malformations (Park's PSM 20th E/P485)

Causes of neonatal mortality in India	%age
Preterm birth	28
Infections	26
Birth asphyxia	23
Congenital anomalies	8
Neonatal tetanus	7
Diarrhoea	3

8. (a) Microspherocytes (Ref: Avery's disease of newborn 8th E/P1191)

Features	Rh disease	ABO disease
Incidence	Less common	More common
Pallor and jaundice	Marked	Minimal
Hydrops	Common	Rare
Hepatosplenomegaly	Marked	Minimal
Blood type		
Mother		
Baby		
Rh -ve		
Rh +ve		
O		
A or B		
Anemia	Marked	Minimal
Direct coombs test	Positive	Usually negative
Indirect coombs test	Positive	Positive
Peripheral smear	Nucleated RBCs	**Spherocytes/ Microspherocytes**

9. **(c)** Large proportionate body (Ref: Nelson 19th E/P612)
   Features of fetal alcohol syndrome:
   - **Growth retardation**
   - **Mental retardation**
   - **Microcephaly**
   - Small palpebral fissures
   - Short nose
   - Smooth philtrum
   - Thin upper lip
   - **Cardiac defects (ASD, VSD)**
   - Hypoplastic fifth finger nails

10. **(b)** Colour (Ref: Rudolph 22nd E/P 205, Ghai 7th E/P 100)

    "A vigorous infant is defined as one who has strong **spontaneous respiratory effort, good muscle tone** and **heart rate** of 100 or more beats per minute."

    Babies born with meconium stained fluid are classified in to vigorous and non-vigorous for further management. (Kindly see text for details of management of meconium aspiration syndrome)

11. **(a)** Hypoglycemia (Ref: Rudolph 22nd E/P 197, Nelson 18th E/p785)

    "Hypoglycemia develops within first 24 hours of life. Infants can be asymptomatic or present with non-specific symptoms like jitterness, irritability, tachypnea, lethargy, hypotonia, poor feed and frank seizure activity."

    Rudolph 22nd E/P 197

    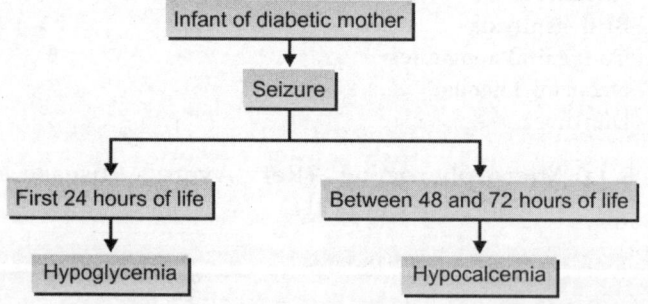

12. **(a)** CPAP (Ref: Rudolph 22nd E/P 238, Ghai 7th E/P 144)

    - "Recent studies suggest that prophylactic nasal CPAP applied immediately after birth may reduce the need for surfactant treatment and mechanical ventilation without any negative effect on mortality."
    - "Mild to moderate RDS can be managed with CPAP. Preterm baby developing severe RDS often require mechanical ventilation in the form of SIMV."
    - Though all other modalities may be required for management of RDS the first thing that is needed to be done is to put baby on CPAP and then depending on the further course of disease a decision on surfactant therapy or mechanical ventilation can be taken.

13. **(a)** Rotor syndrome (Ref: Ghai 7th E/P149, Nelson 19th E/P1321)
    - This is a case of conjugated hyperbilirubinemia with normal LFTs.
    - Gilbert syndrome and glucuronyl transferase deficiency cause unconjugated hyperbilirubinemia.
    - Primary biliary cirrhosis causes conjugated hyperbilirubinemia with deranged LFTs.
    - Rotor syndrome causes conjugated bilirubinemia with normal LFTs and hence is the answer of choice.

14. **(c)** Neonatal pulmonary alveolar proteinosis (Ref: Nelson 19th E/P1453–54)
    Pulmonary alveolar proteinosis (PAP):
    - PAP is characterised by accumulation of surfactant in the alveoli because of increased production or decreased clearance.
    - Congenital PAP is characterised by early onset, grave prognosis and **positive family history.** The baby presents with **severe respiratory distress after birth.** It can be caused by inherited deficiency of surfactant protein B. Other factors that may play a role are abnormalities in production of GM-CSF, IL 4 and surfactant protein D.
    - In older children the symptoms of respiratory distress develop gradually. Males are more commonly affected than female.
    - Gold standard for diagnosis is histopathological examination of lung biopsy. BAL fluid can be examined for surfactant in adults.
    - Recurrent BAL is done to remove the accumulated surfactant.

15. **(a)** Confirm position of endotracheal tube (Ref: Rudolph 22nd E/P 210, Nelson 18th E/P 747,48)
    - Respiratory distress, scaphoid abdomen and decreased breath sounds on the left side are sufficient to make a diagnosis of congenital diaphragmatic hernia.
    - If we look at the flow chart in the text, invariably the first thing to be done is to put a double lumen nasogastric tube. But in this case the baby was intubated and then the cardiac impulse shifed to right side, which indicates overinflation of intestine. The only thing that could have done this is faulty intubation of endotracheal tube in to esophagus. Hence the best next thing to do is to check the position of endotracheal tube.

    Kindly see text for details of management of congenital diaphragmatic hernia.

16. (b) Put a nasogastric tube (Ref: Rudolph 22nd E/P 210, Nelson 18th E/P 747, 48)

- This is also a case of congenital diaphragmatic hernia but here there is no right shift after intubation. Hence intubation was successful and the next best thing to be done is insertion of a double lumen nasogastric tube and decompression of bowel.

Rudolph 22nd E/P 210

"When CDH has been diagnosed prenatally or as soon as the diagnosis is suspected, a **double lumen nasogastric tube** should be placed in to the infant's stomach in the delivery room to reduce air in the bowel and decrease compression of lungs."

17. (b) Congenital cholangiopathy (Ref: Nelson 18th E/P 757)

Causes of unconjugated hype rbilirubinemia: (Table 1)

Causes of Conjugated hyperbilirubinemia: Rudolph 22nd E/P 1498

1. Billiary atresia
2. Choledochal cyst
3. Alagille syndrome
4. Hypopituitarism
5. DubinJhonson syndrome
6. Rotor syndrome
7. Cystic fibrosis
8. Metabolic diseases like
   - Tyrosinemia
   - Galactosemia
   - Hereditary fructose intolerance
   - Mitochondrial enzyme defect
9. Idiopathic neonatal hepatitis
10. Alpha-1-Antitrypsin deficiency
11. Sepsis

18. (c) Universal flexion like a fetus (Ref: Rudolph 22nd E/P171)

Rudolph 22nd E/P171

"Heat production postnatally is the result of shivering and nonshivering thermogenesis. In general non-shivering thermogenesis is thought to be more important than shivering thermogenesis in newborn. Although under usual circumstances nonshivering thermogenesis may be the primary means by which heat is generated in the newborn, at least some capacity for shivering may exist."

As per text the other mechanisms of heat production are :

- Vasoconstrition
- Norepinephrine induced beta oxidation of brown fats

19. (b) Hyperglycemia (Ref: Rudolph 22nd E/P195,96,97, Ghai 7th E/P 156)

- Hypoglycemia and not hyperglycemia is a complication in infant of diabetic mother. For details of complications kindly see text.

20. (c) History of unconsciousness (Ref: Nelson 19th E/P280)

- Neonates have limited glycogen store and hence are at risk of hypoglycemia.
- Child of diabetic mother develop hypoglycemia after birth and require glucose administration.
- If patient with history of hypoglycemia develop symptoms of hypoglycemia or found unconscious then glucose should be administered.

21. (b) Photoisomerisation (Ref: Nelson 18th E/P 762) Kindly see text for details.

22. (c) Prominent horizontal fissure (Ref : Rudolph 22ndE/P 202, Ghai 7thE/P 146)

X-ray feature of TTN:

"Chest X ray may show hyperexpanded lung fields, prominent vascular markings and prominent interlobal fissures."

Table 1

Increase load of bilirubin	Decrease in the activity of glucunoryl	Competetive block glucunoryl transferase	Decresed bilirubin uptake by liver cells
1. **Hemolytic anemia**	1. Genetic deficiency — e.g. Criggler-Najjar syndrome I, II, Gilbert syndrome	1. Drugs that require glucuronic acid for conjugation	1. Genetic defect—e.g. Gilbert syndrome
2. Polycythemia	2. **Thyroid deficiency**		2. Prematurity
3. Shortened Rbc lif—e.g. **Physiological jaundice**	3. Hypoxia		
4. Increased enterohepatic circulation— e.g. **Breast milk jaundice, Physiological jaundice**			
5. Infection			

23. (a) Check pulses (Ref: Ghai 7th E/P98)
- The patient is ventilated with bag and mask and hence the first two steps of resuscitation i.e. air way and breathing has been taken care of.
- The best next step is to assess the circulation by checking the pulse and if inadequate, chest compressions should be started.

24. (c) Diaphragmatic hernia (Ref: Rudolph 22nd E/P 210, Ghai 7thE/P 153)

"Bag and mask ventilation should be avoided in babies with congenital diaphragmatic hernia."

- Bag and mask ventilation will allow substantial amount of air to enter the esophagus and subsequently it will inflate the intestine. In CDH this will lead to further compression of lungs and worsening of condition. Hence bag and mask ventilation is not indicated in CDH.

25. (c) Altered sensorium
Clinical presentation of asphyxia: (Table 2)

26. (c) Insert a nasogastric tube (Ref: Rudolph 22nd E/P 210, Nelson 18th E/P 747, 48)

27. (d) Post term infant (Ref: Rudolph 22ndE/P212)
Causes of neonatal hypoglycaemia:

Decreased substrate availability	Increased utilization	Hyperinsulinemia	Miscelleneous
• IUGR	• Perinatal asphyxia	• **IDM**	• Sepsis
• Prematurity	• Hypothermia	• Beckwith-widemann syndrome	• Congenital heart disease
• Glycogen storage disease		• Erythroblastosis fetalis	• CNS abnormalities
• Inborn errors e.g. fructose intolerance		• Exchange transfusion	
		• Islet cell dysplasia	
		• Maternal β agonist to colytics	
		• Improperly placed umbilical artery catheter	

28. (d) Reassure the mother that nothing is abnormal (Ref: Ghai 7thE/P6, Nelson 18th E/P760)

"During the first few days after birth, the newborn loses extracellular fluid equivalent to about 10% of the body weight. Most infants regain their weight by the age of 10 days."

- Thus the inability of child to gain weight till 6th day is not a concern.

"Breast-feeding jaundice occurs in first week of life in breast feed infants who normally have higher bilirubin levels than formula fed infants. Giving supplements of glucose to breast fed infants is associated with higher bilirubin levels, in part because of reduced intake of higher caloric density of breast milk."

- Thus the baby passing golden yellow stool on 6th day is having breast — feeding jaundice. The treatment consists of frequent breast feeding and **discouraging 5% dextrose or water.**

29. (c) Elective caesarean section (Ref: Rudolph 22nd E/P 201)

"TTN of newborn is associated with caesarean section delivery."

For details of cause of TTN kindly see flowchart in text.

30. (d) Hemolytic jaundice (Ref: Nelson 18th E/P 757, Rudolph 22nd E/P 1498)
- It is a case of unconjugated hyperbilirubinemia as conjugated bilirubin and LFT is normal.
- From the given options unconjugated hyperbilirubinemia is seen only in haemolytic jaundice.

31. (c) Intraosseus IV fluids (Ref: Rudolph 22nd E/P405)

"The bone marrow cavity is effectively a non-collapsible vascular space, even in the setting of shock or cardiac arrest. Therefore, intraosseus access is the initial vascular access site of choice in patients with life threatening problems such as cardiopulmonary arrest or decompensated shock."

- In this case the patient is having severe dehydration and unrecordable BP with failure in gaining IV access.

Table 2

CNS	CVS	Pulmonary	Renal	GIT	Metabolic
• Hypoxic-ischemic encephalopathy	• Myocardial ischemia	• Pulmonary hypertension	• RenalAcute tubular or cortical necrosis	• Gastrointestinal	• Inappropriate secretion of anti-diuretic hormone
• Infarction	• Poor contractility	• Pulmonary hemorrhage	• AdrenalAdrenal hemorrhage	• Perforation or ulceration with hemorrhage and necrosis	• Hyponatremia
• Intracranial hemorrhage	• Tricuspid insufficiency	• Respiratory distress syndrome			• Hypoglycemia
• **Seizures**	• Hypotension				• Hypocalcemia, myoglobinuria Subcutaneous fat necrosis
• Cerebral edema					
• **Hypotonia**					
• **Hypertonia**					

- Hence **intraosseus route is the best way of management, which medical personnel can access in less than a minute time.**

32. **(c)** Oxygen toxicity (Ref: Ghai 7thE/P645, Rudolph 22nd E/P2313)

"Retinopathy of prematurity is seen in preterm babies due to early exposure to oxygen and other environmental factors by a premature, under-developed retinal vascular system."

- Risk factors associated with retinopathy of prematurity:
  - ❖ Prematurity, specially birth before 32 weeks.
  - ❖ Birth weight less than 1500 gm.
  - ❖ Supplemental oxygen therapy — Most significant causative factor.
  - ❖ Hypoxemia.
  - ❖ Hypercarbia.
  - ❖ Septicemia.

Also know:

"Threshold" disea se is a developing retinopathy that requires ablative laser treatment of the vascular zone of retina to check further progression.

33. **(a)** 20mg% (Ref: Nelson 19th E/P597)

Indication for phototherapy in term babies:

Age	Phototherapy	Exchange transfusion
<24 hours	12	19
24-48 hours	15	22
48-72 hours	17.5	24
72-96 hours	**20**	25
>96 hours	21	25

34. **(a)** Mild conjugated hyperbilirubinemia (Ref: Rudolph 22nd E/P1509-10)

35. **(d)** Respiratory rate per minute (Ref: Ghai 7th E/P107)

Apgar score:

Sign	0	1	2
Heart rate	Absent	<100/min	>100/min
Respiration	Absent	Weak cry	Good strong cry
Muscle tone	Limp	Some flexion	Active movements
Reflex irritability	No response	Grimace	Cough or sneeze
Colour	Blue or pale	Body pink, extremities blue	Completely pink

36. **(b)** 34 (Ref: Tucker Maternal, fetal and neonatal physiology/P647)

37. **(c)** Hypoglycemia (Ref: Ghai 7th E/P129–30)

Metabolic derangements like hypoglycemia, hyperglycemia and hypocalcemia can be seen in small for date babies.

- ❖ Hypoglycemia is seen due to low hepatic glycogen stores.

- ❖ Hyperglycemia is seen due to immature glucose utilising mechanisms.
- ❖ Hypocalcemia — Early onset is usually asymptomatic but late onset hypocalcemia presents as neonatal tetany and seizures.

38. **(d)** Brain (Ref: Ghai 7th E/P129)
- In asymmetrical IUGR growth of brain is usually not restricted.

39. **(c)** Weight less than 10th percentile (Ref: Ghai 7th E/P109)

Small for date babies	Appropriate for date babies	Large for date babies
• Babies with birth weight of **less than 10th percentile or 2 SD** of their gestational age.	• Babies with birth weight between 10th-90th percentile for their period of gestation.	• Babies with birth weight more than 90th percentile of their gestational age.

- Other findings are seen in a preterm baby and not in a term baby.

40. **(b)** Dubin Johnson syndrome (Ref: Ghai 7th E/P149, Nelson 19th E/P1321)

41. **(a)** Diabetes (Ref: Nelson 19th E/P551)

Causes of IUGR:

R — **Renal disorders**
E — Elevated blood pressure
T — Toxemia
A — Abruptio placentae
R — Rubella infection
D — Drugs of antimetabolite group and **propranolol**
A — **Alcohol**
T — Trisomies
I — **Insulin deficiency in fetus**
O — Oxygen deficiency
N — **Nicotine**

Mnemonic: **RETARDATION**

42. **(d)** Phenothiazine (Ref: Nelson 19th E/P551)

43. **(d)** High levels of serum albumin (Ref: Nelson 19th E/P596)

Factors increasing risk of kernicterus:

Hypoalbuminemia	Bilirubin binds to albumin and hypoalbuminemia causes increased free bilirubin in the blood, which can precipitate toxicity
Drugs like Moxalactam Sulfisoxazole Benzyl alcohol	These drugs interefere with bilirubin-albumin binding and thereby increasing free bilirubin
Acidosis	Decrease in blood Ph makes free bilirubin lipophilic and enhances it tissue uptake and toxicity
Sepsis	Bilirubin can access to vulnerable areas of brain
Prematurity	Premature infants have hyppoalbuminemia as well as risk of acidosis, both of which can increase bilirubin toxicity

44. (a) and **(d)** Suffer from jaundice of hepatic origin and anemia (Ref: Ghai 7th E/P129–30)

Low birth weight and premature infants lack maturity and coordination of certain body systems that manifest as various derangements.

- Metabolic derangements like hypoglycemia, hyperglycemia and hypocalcemia can be seen.
  - ❖ Hypoglycemia is seen due to low hepatic glycogen stores.
  - ❖ Hyperglycemia is seen due to immature glucose utilising mechanisms.
  - ❖ Hypocalcemia — Early onset is usually asympto-matic but late onset hypocalcemia presents as neonatal tetany and seizures.
- **Jaundice** can be seen as the preterm has **larger RBC volume** for body weight and immature hepatic enzymes and hepatic excretory capacity.
- Hematological abnormalities like polycythemia and anemia (Due to rapid destruction of fetal RBCs) can be seen.
- Immature organ systems can lead to various disorders.
  - ❖ Intraventricular haemorrhage can be seen due to fragile blood vessels.
  - ❖ Retinopathy of prematurity develops because of high oxygen saturation used during resuscitation.

- ❖ Osteopenia of prematurity is caused by low levels of calcium, vitamin D and phosphorous.
- ❖ Respiratory distress syndrome can be associated due to lack of surfactant.
- Hypothermia is seen due to higher surface area to body weight ratio, low subcutaneous fat and low glycogen store.

45. (a), (b) and **(c).** Have increased insensible water loss, Generally develop a bronze discolouration of skin, Should have their eyes patched during therapy (Ref: Ghai 7th E/P173)

46. (c) Leave it alone (Ref: Ghai 6th E/P146)

47. (c) Total prenteral nutrition (Ref: Nelson 19th E/P554) To breastfeed the baby a strong sucking reflex is required along with coordination of swallowing, epiglottal and uvular closure of larynx and nasal passages and normal esophageal motility, which develops at 34 week of gestation [See Flowchart 1].

48. (b) Bradycardia (Ref: Rudolph 22nd E/P156)

"If uterine contractions are occurring, a fall in fetal heart rate after the onset of a contraction with a gradual return to baseline after the contraction has ceased suggests decreased fetal oxygenation."

Flowchart 1

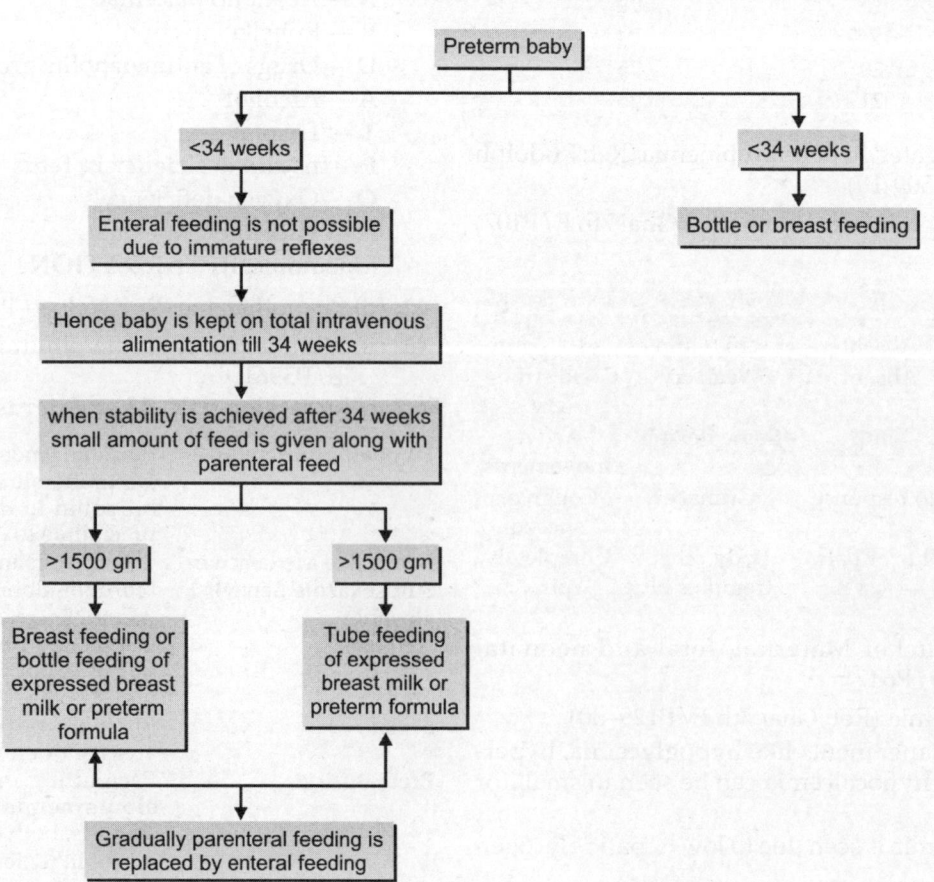

49. (a) Necrotising enterocolitis (Ref: Rudolph 22nd E/P249)

Prevention of NEC:

"Among postnatal interventions, only restricted fluid administration, use of human milk and administration of **probiotics** demonstrated a protective effect when randomized controlled trials were analysed in meta-analysis."

50. (c) Remove tube and reattempt intubation (Ref: Rudolph 22nd E/P 210, Nelson 18th E/P 747,48)

- For management of congenital diaphragmatic hernia, If we look at the flow chart in the text, invariably the first thing to be done is to put a double lumen nasogastric tube. But in this case the baby was intubated and then the cardiac impulse shifted to right side, which indicates overinflation of intestine. The only thing that could have done this is faulty intubation of endotracheal tube in to esophagus. Hence the position of tube is to be checked (not by X-ray as it will not be able to distinguish faulty intubation)and if it is not in place the best next thing to do is to remove the tube and reattempt intubation.

51. (c) Nasogastric tube insertion (Ref: Rudolph 22nd E/P 210, Nelson 18th E/P 747,48)

- For management of congenital diaphragmatic hernia, If we look at the flow chart in the text, invariably the first thing to be done is to put a double lumen nasogastric tube. But in this case the baby was intubated and then the cardiac impulse shifed to right side, which indicates overinflation of intestine. The only thing that could have done this is faulty intubation of endotracheal tube in to esophagus. Thus the next steps are as earlier to check the position of endotracheal tube(Not by X-ray as it will not be distinguish faulty intubation) and if not in position then reattempt intubation (not in option). Then the next best thing is to put a nasogastric tube.

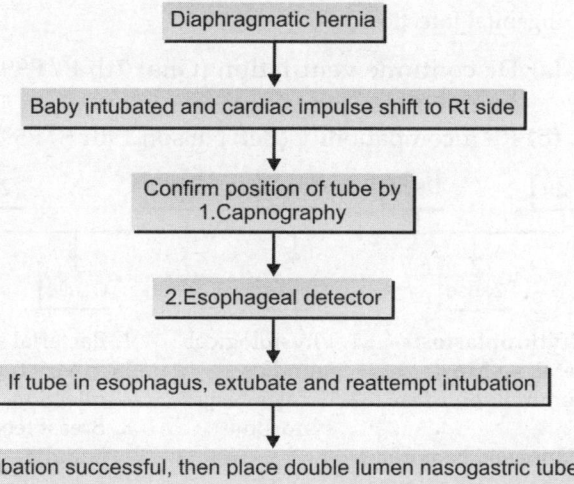

52. (d) Peritoneal drainage (Ref: Rudolph 22nd E/P2 48–49, Nelson 18th E/P756)

- **Management of necrotising enterocolitis:** It depends on the stage at which the neonate presents.

53. (d) Impedance technique (Ref: Rudolph 21st E/P1937)

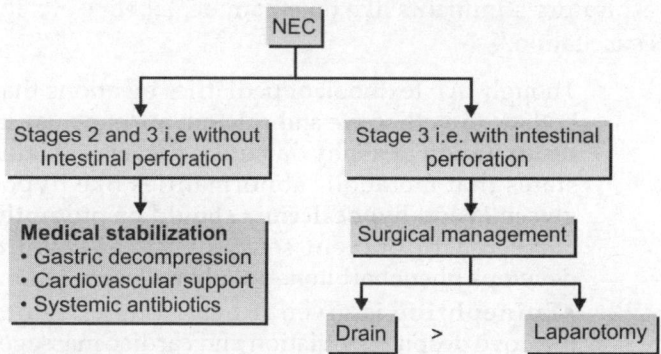

"The management of recurrent apnea depends on the etiology. Infants are typically monitored with heart rate/ impedance monitors, and it should be noted that impedance-based monitors detect chest wall motion and thus will not detect obstructive apnea unless the episode produces significant bradycardia."

54. (c) Thick ear cartilage (Ref : Ghai 7thE/P 109)

The characteristic features of **preterm neonate** are:

- Absence of **deep sole creases.**
- Size of **breast nodule** less than 5 mm.
- **Poor elastic recoil** of ear cartilage.
- Presence of **lanugo hair** (Lanugo hair is present on fetus and usually sheds in two periods 1)at 28 weeks and 2) At term).
- Males — **Testes** are located at **external ring** and scrotum has few rugosities.
- Females — Labia majora are widely separated exposing labia minora and clitoris.

55. (c) Convection (Ref: Ghai 7th E/P117)

"The mechanism of heat transfer in incubator is by **convection**."

56. (b) Caudal regression (Ref: Rudolph 22ndE/P196)

"Spinal agenesis associated with caudal regression syndrome is a congenital anomaly found exclusively in IDMs."

Kindly see text for details of congenital malformation associated with IDMs.

57. (d) Sulfonmide (Ref: Rudolph 22ndE/P 231)

"Use of agents such as sulfisoxazole and benzyl alcohol can interfere with bilirubin albumin binding and predispose an infant to bilirubin toxicity."
Sulfisoxazole is a drug that belongs to sulphonamide group.

58. (b) Dexamethasone (Ref: IAP 4th E/P53-55)

"A large majority of asphyxiated babies can be effectively revived and resuscitated by using bag and mask ventilation alone and intubation is usually not required. There is no role for dexamethasone, atropine, calcium and respiratory stimulants like nikethamide, lobeline etc. in resuscitation."

- Though IAP textbook of pediatrics mentions that both **dexamethasone** and **calcium** are of no use in resuscitation of asphyxia per se; however it later states that metabolic abnormalities like hypoglycemia and **hypocalcemia should be promptly corrected** to prevent seizures and if seizure develops phenobarbitone should be given.
  •**Epinephrine** is given if heart rate does not improve despite ventilation and cardiac massage.
- If baby is in shock plasma espanders like blood, plasma and **saline** should be given.
- **Sodium bicarbonate** is given if effective ventilation is not established by 10 minutes.
- **Calcium gluconate** and **glucose** is administered to prevent seizures.

59. (c) No specific therapy
- Due to withdrawl of the female sex hormones in the baby after birth vaginal bleeding can be seen. It is a normal condition and does not require specific treatment.

60. (d) Is treated by administering 100% oxygen (Ref: Rudolph 22nd E/P233–38, Ghai 7th E/P143)

"Baby with RDS should be kept on CPAP with a **mixture of oxygen and air** in order to maintain the arterial PaO$_2$ between 50 and 70 mm Hg."

- **100% oxygen** is not given as in a premature baby with RDS it can lead to bronchopulmonary dysplasia as well as retinopathy of prematurity.
- **RDS** occurs predominantly in **prematurely born infants.**

61. (a) Hypoglycemia (Ref: Ghai 7th E/P155)
Common causes of hypoglycemia:

Inadequate substrate	Relative hyperinsulinemia	Sickness
• Small for gestational age	• Infant of diabetic mother	• Hypothermia
• Preterm babies	• Large for date babies	• Sepsis
• Low birth weight babies	• Rh isoimmuniza-tion	• Asphyxia

- Preterm and LBW infants are at high risk for Intraventricular haemorrhage.
- Preterm infants are at high risk for bronchopulmonary dysplasia.

62. (a) Total and direct bilirubin (Ref: Nelson 22nd E/P758)

"Regardless of gestation or time of appearance of jaundice patients with significant hyperbilirubi-nemia and those with symptoms and signs require a complete diagnostic evaluation which includes determination of **direct and indirect bilirubin** fractions, haemoglobin, reticulocyte count, blood type, coombs test and peripheral blood smear."

63. (b) Head circumference is 3 cm more than chest circumference (Ref: Ghai 7th E/P6)
- The head circumference is usually 3 cm more than chest circumference at birth.
- In case of symmetric IUGR the difference will remain same and in asymmetric IUGR as growth of body is retarded more as compared to head, the difference will be increased.

64. (b) Dubin Johnson syndrome ((Ref: Ghai 7th E/P149, Nelson 19th E/P1321)

65. (d) Trikling of sole (Ref: Ghai 7th E/P98–99)
- The first step of resuscitation i.e. clearing of airway has been done and the next step should be to stimulate breathing by fickling the soles or rubbing the back.

66. (a) Pyloric stenosis (Ref: Nelson 19th E/P1229)
- Vomiting in neonates with pyloric stenosis is typically seen in **3rd week** of life.

67. (b) Theophylline use (Ref: Ghai 7th E/P146)
68. (d) Novobiocin therapy (Nelson 19th E/P1320–21)
69. (a) Erythroblastosis (Ref: Nelson 19th E/P593)
Causes of jaundice:

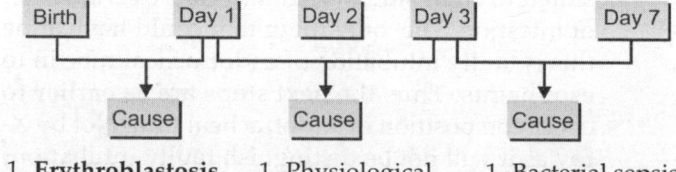

1. **Erythroblastosis fetalis—Most comm on cause**
2. Concealed hemorrhage
3. Congenital infections

1. Physiological jaundice
2. Crigler — Najjar syndrome

1. Bacterial sepsis
2. Urinary tract infection
3. Breast feed jaundice

70. (a) Discontinue ventilation (Ghai 7th E/P99) (See Flowchart 2)
71. (b) Rh incompatibility (Ref: Nelson 19th E/P593)

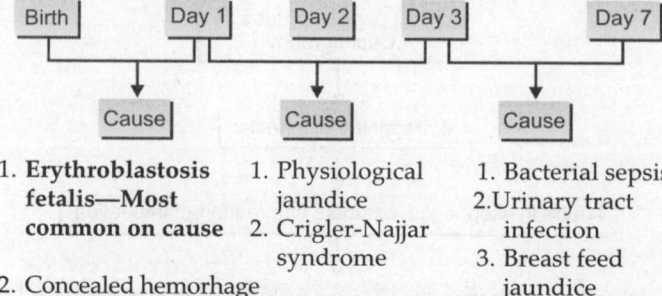

1. **Erythroblastosis fetalis—Most common on cause**
2. Concealed hemorrhage
3. Congenital infections

1. Physiological jaundice
2. Crigler-Najjar syndrome

1. Bacterial sepsis
2. Urinary tract infection
3. Breast feed jaundice

Flowchart 2

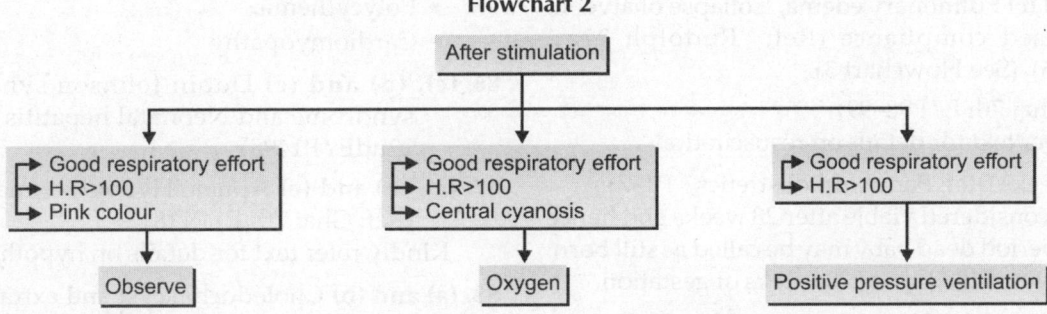

72. **(b)** Fibrin (Ref: Ghai 7th E/P143)
    - Effusion of proteinaceous material, **fibrin** and plasma in to alveolar space because of alveolocytes damage leads to hyaline membrane formation.

73. **(a)** and **(b)** GDM and Maternal obesity (Ref: Nelson 18th E/P 710)
    - "The oversized infants are usually born at term, but preterm infants with weights high for gestational age also have a significant higher mortality than do infants of the same size born at term; maternal diabetes and obesity are predisposing factors."

74. **(c)** 90 – 110 (Ref: Ghai 7th E/P 298)
    - Mean PCV of 1 month infant is 104
    - Range of PCV of 1 month infant is 85–104
    - Thus the best possible answer is 90–110.

75. **(a)** Barbiturates (Ref : Rudolph 22nd E/P 1510)

"In Crigler-Najjar syndrome type II hyperbilirubi-nemia of less than 10 mg/Dl is usually observed and this is typically responsive to cytochrome P450 inducing compounds such as **phenobarbital**."

    - Phenobarbital belongs to the barbiturate group of drugs.

76. **(a)** Weight < 2.5 kg (RefGhai 7th E/P128)

Low birth weight babies	Very low birth weight babies	Extremely low birth weight babies
• Weight less than 2.5 kg	• Weight less than 1.5 kg	• Weight less than 1 kg

77. **(c), (d)** and **(e)** Lumbosacral area, Leg and Thigh (Ref: Nelson 19th E/P2162)
    Mongolian blue spots are caused due to pigmentation of skin especially over:
    - Sacral area
    - Buttocks
    - Back
    - Legs
    - Posterior thighs
    - Shoulder.

78. **(a), (b), (c)** and **(e)** Harlequins colour change, Mongolian spots, Erythema toxicum and Milia (Ref: Nelson 19th E/P2161–64)

Transient skin changes of newborn:
- Mongolian spots
- Milia
- Harlequins colour change
- Erythema toxicum
- Stroke bite
- Neonatal pustular melanosis.

79. **(b), (d)** and **(e)** Hyperglycemia, Hypercalcemia and hyperthermia (Ref: Ghai 7th E/P146, Nelson 19th E/P573)

Causes of neonatal apnea:
- Prematurity
- Metabolic abnormalities like hypocalcemia, hypoglycemia, hypothermia, hypo and hypernatremia and hyperammonemia
- Sepsis
- Respiratory distress
- Anemia
- Polycythemia

80. **(a)** Intubation

81. **(a), (b)** and **(c)** Physiological jaundice, Breast milk jaundice and Gilbert syndrome (Ref: Fleischer Emergency textbook of Pediatrics/P 360)

Causes of unconjugated hyperbilirubinemia	Causes of conjugated hyperbilirubinemia
C—Crigler-Najjar Syndrome	Cute—Choledochal cyst, Cystic fibrosis
H—Hemolysis, Hypothyroidism	D—Dubin Johnson syndrome
I—Infections like malaria	A—Atresia of bile ducts
M—Breast Milk jaundice	U—UTI
P—Physiological jaundice	G—Galactosemia
I—Infant of diabetic mother	H—Hereditary fructose intolerance, Hepatitis
N—Neonatal intracranial hemorrhage	T—Total Parenteral nutrition, Tyrosinemia
G—Gilbert syndrome	E—Enzyme deficiency e.g. α_1 antitrypsin
	R—Rotor syndrome
Mnemonic: **CHIMPING**	Mnemonic: Cute **DAUGHTER**

Note: Hemolysis can be caused by disorders like G6PD deficiency, hereditary spherocytosis, sickle cell disease and thalassemia.

82. **(a), (b) and (c)** Pulmonary edema, Collapse of alveoli, decreased compliance (Ref: Rudolph 22nd E/P236) (See Flowchart 3)

83. **All** (Ref: Ghai 7th E/P98–99)
    Kindly refer text for details on resuscitation.

84. **(c)** > 28 weeks (Ref: Padubidri obstretics/ P157)
    • A baby is considered viable after 28 weeks and hence after this period dead baby may be called as still born. Baby is around 1000 gm at 28 weeks of gestation.

85. **(b), (c), (d) and (e)** Hypoglycemia, Hypocalcemia, Increased fetal defect and Hyperbilirubinemia (Ref: Nelson 19th E/P614)
    Infants of diabetic mothers (IDM) are at increased risk for fetal, neonatal and long-term comorbidities:
    • **Congenital anomalies**
    • Macrosomia
    • **Hypoglycemia**
    • Hypomagnesemia
    • **Hypocalcemia**
    • **Hyperbilirubinemia**
    • **Respiratory distress**

    • Polycythemia
    • Cardiomyopathy

86. **(c), (d) and (e)** Dubin Johnson syndrome, Rotor syndrome and Neonatal hepatitis (Ref: Rudolph 22ndE/P1498)

87. **(a), (b) and (e)** Apnea, Hypoglycemia and Hypoxia (Ref: Ghai 7th E/P118)
    Kindly refer text for details on hypothermia.

88. **(a) and (b)** Choledochal cyst and extrahepatic biliary atresia (Ref: Rudolph 22ndE/P1498)

89. **(b)** Physiological jaundice (Ref: Ghai 7th E/P147)
    • In newborn increased bilirubin production due to breakdown of fetal RBCs and decreased excretion due to the limited conjugating ability of newborn's liver and increased enterohepatic circulation leads to **unconjugated hyperbilirubinemia** and jaundice.
    • Jaundice becomes visible on **2nd to 3rd** day when **indirect bilirubin** rises at a rate of <5 mg/dL/24 hr and peaks on 4th to 5th day at a rate of 5–6 mg/dL.

90. **(b)** Meconium aspiration syndrome (Ref: Rudolph 22nd E/P204–5)

Flowchart 3

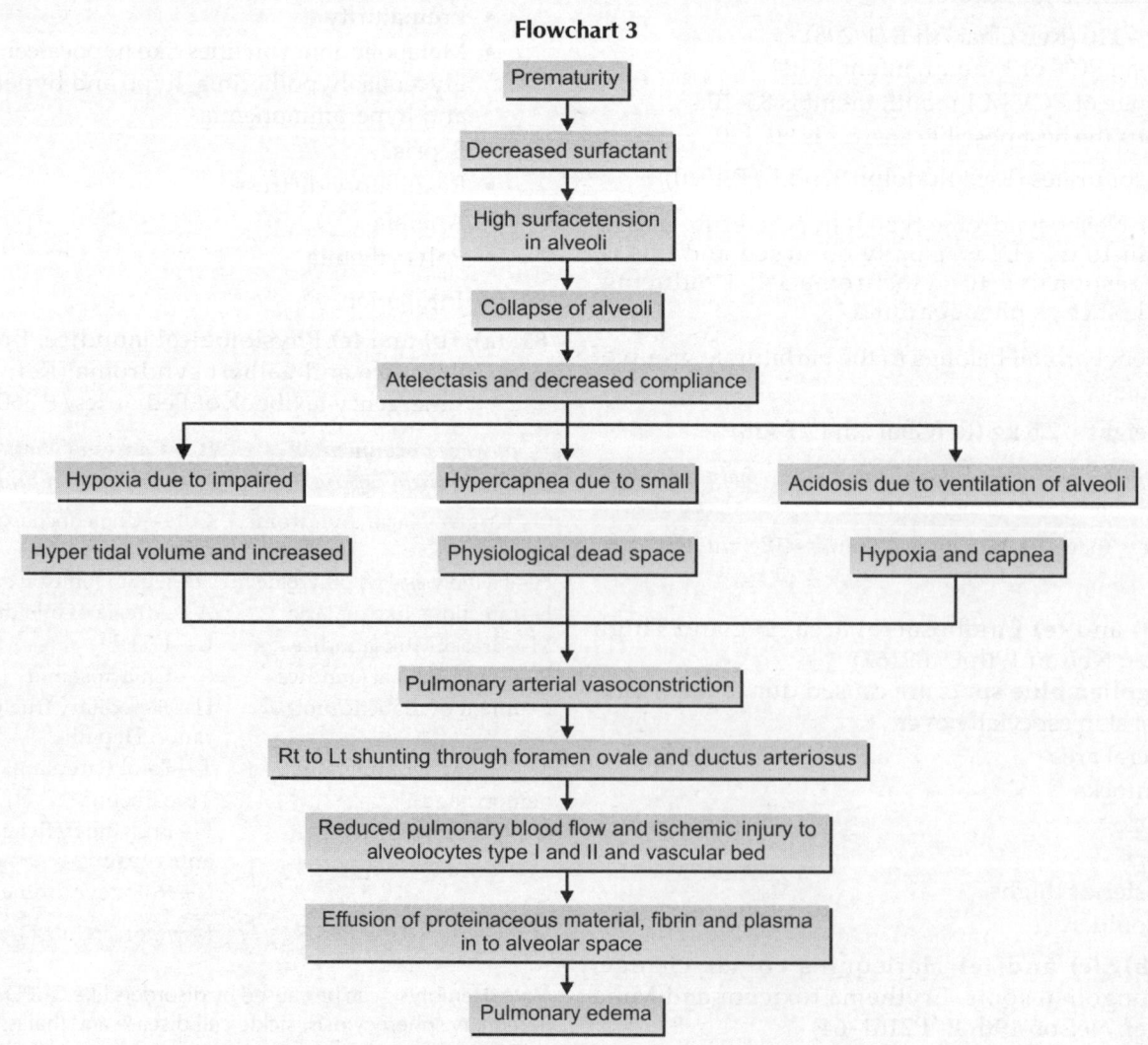

- First of all presence of **meconium stained fluid** points towards meconium aspiration syndrome.
- The other points consolidating the diagnosis are:
  ❖ MAS is characterised by respiratory distress, **tachypnea (baby in question has RR 90/min),** retractions and cyanosis.
  ❖ Most commonly it is associated with near **term,** term and postterm infants as passage of meconium in utero is rare before 32 weeks of gestation.

Also know:
- Radiological features of MAS do not always correlate with the severity of the disease. The radiological findings are:
  ❖ Overinflation with flattened diaphragm
  ❖ Patchy infiltrates
  ❖ Pneumomediastinum ⎱ Both are complication of
                  MAS and can be seen
  ❖ Pneumothorax ⎰ even on initial radiograph

91. (a) and (b) Respiratory rate>60/min and intercostal recession (Ref: Ghai 7th E/P142)

Findings in respiratory distress:
- Tachypnea — RR > 60/min
- Prominent grunting
- Intercostal and subcostal retractions
- Nasal flaring
- Cyanosis
- Acidosis

92. (a) Give 10% dextrose IV (Ref: Rudolph 22nd E/P213)
- The baby in the question is lethargic i.e. symptomatic.
- So according to flowchart he should be given 10% dextrose IV (See Flowchart 4)

93. (a), (b) and (c) Sole creases, Ear cartilage and Breast nodules (Ref: Ghai 7th E/P109)
The characteristic features of **preterm neonate** are:
- Absence of **deep sole creases.**

- Size of **breast nodule** less than 5mm.
- **Poor elastic recoil** of ear cartilage.
- Presence of **lanugo hair** (Lanugo hair is present on fetus and usually sheds in two periods 1)At 28 weeks and 2) At term).
- Males — **Testes** are located at **external ring** and scrotum has few rugosities.
- Females — Labia majora are widely separated exposing labia minora and clitoris.

Absence of these features will confirm the maturity of the baby.

94. (a), (b) and (d) Macrosomia, Neural tube defect and Hypocalcemia (Ref: Rudolph 22nd E/P195–7)
- Infants of diabetic mother at risk for developing:
  ❖ Hypoglycemia
  ❖ Hypocalcemia
  ❖ Hypomagnesemia
  ❖ Hyperbilirubinemia
  ❖ Polycythemia
  ❖ Cardiomyopathy
  ❖ Respiratory distress
  ❖ Congenital anomalies like
    ❑ Congenital heart defects (CHD):
      1. **Ventricular septal defect** is the **most common CHD** associated.
      2. Other CHD are atrial septal defect, TGA.
    ❑ Spinal agenesis associated with **caudal regression** is found **exclusively** in IDM.
    ❑ **Neural tube defects.**
    ❑ Gastrointestinal atresia, gastroschisis, intestinal malrotation, renal and urinary tract malformation and small left colon syndrome may be associated.

Flowchart 4

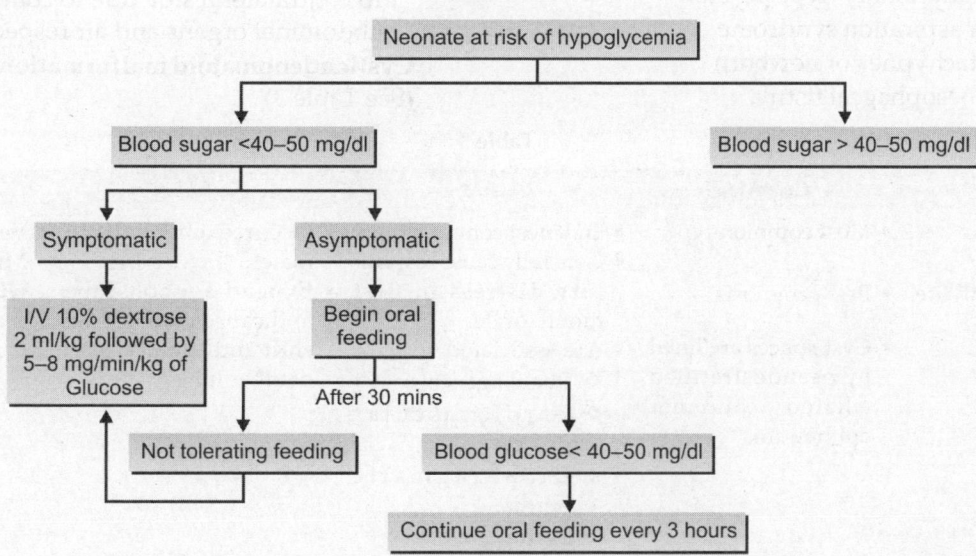

95. None (Ref: Ghai 7th E/P147–49)
    - Jaundice appears on 2nd to 3rd day of life and disappears on 2nd week.
    - **Indirect bilirubin** rises at a rate of **<5 mg/dL/24 hr** and peaks on 4th to 5th day at a **rate of 5–6 mg/dL.**
    - Breast feeding should never be stopped.

96. **(b)** and **(c)** Hypoglycemia and Apnea (Ref: Ghai 7th E/P118)
    Kindly refer text for details on hypothermia.

97. **(a), (b)** and **(d)** Erythema toxicum, Ebstein Pearls and subconjunctival haemorrhage (Ref: Ghai 7th E/P 112–13)
    Kindly refer text for all the normal findings in a newborn.

98. **(b)** and **(e)** Unconjugated hyperbilirubinemia and Increased toxicity of irinotecan (Ref: Rudolph 22nd E/P1509–10)
    Gibert syndrome:
    - Gilbert syndrome inherited as **autosomal dominant** and recessive disorder is characterised by defect of bilirubin uptake as well as conjugation (decreased activity of glucunoryl transferase). It is more common in **males.**
    - Gilbert syndrome is charcterised by **mild-unconjugated hyperbilirubinemia** and serum bilirubin level is usually less than 5mg/dL. Standard **hepatic biochemical tests and liver histology are normal.**
    - Irinitecan is metabolised by **glucunoryl transferase** in phase II and its absence can lead to toxicity.

99. **(a), (d)** and **(e)** Diaphragmatic hernia, HMD and Pulmonary haemorrhage (Ref: Ghai 7th E/P142, Nelson 18th E/P752)
    Pulmonary causes of Respiratory distress in a baby:
    - **Pulmonary haemorrhage**
    - Pneumonia
    - Persistent pulmonary hypertension
    - Meconium aspiration syndrome
    - Transient tachypnea of newborn
    - Tracheo – oesophageal fistula
    - RDS/HMD
    - Diaphragmatic hernia
    - Lobar emphysema
    - Bilateral choanal atresia
    - Vascular rings

100. **(a), (b)** and **(d)** Intercostal retraction, RR>60/min and ph<7.2 Ref: (Ref: Ghai 7th E/P142)
    Clinical features oF respiratory distress:
    - Respiratory distress within first 6 hours of birth
    - **Tachypnea — RR > 60/min**
    - Prominent grunting
    - **Intercostal and subcostal retractions**
    - Nasal flaring
    - Cyanosis
    - **Acidosis.**

101. **(b)** and **(e)** Unconjugated hyperbilirubinemia and Starts on 2nd day of life (Ref: Nelson 18th E/P758, Ghai 7th E/P147)
    - In newborn increased bilirubin production due to breakdown of fetal RBCS and decreased excretion due to the limited conjugating ability of newborn's liver and increased enterohepatic circulation leads increase in **unconjugated bilirubin level** and jaundice.
    - Jaundice becomes visible on **2nd to 3rd day** when indirect bilirubin rises at a rate of < 5 mg/dL/24 hr and peaks on 4th to 5th day at a rate of 5–6 mg/dL.
    - **No treatment is required** as the bilirubin level is below cut-off level for phototherapy.
    - If jaundice appears in the first 24 - 36 hours then other causes should be searched for

102. **(a), (b)** and **(c)** Congenital adenomatoid lung disease, Pneumothorax and Diaphragmatic hernia (Ref: Rudolph 22nd E/P1931, Ghai 7th E/P142)
    - Congenital adenomatoid lung, diaphragmatic hernia and pneumothorax cause mediastinal shift to contralateral side due to compression by cysts, abdominal organs and air respectively.

    Cystic adenomatoid malformation of lung (CCAM):
    (See Table 3)

Table 3

CCAM 0	CCAM1	CCAM 2	CCAM 3	CCAM 4
• Also called acinar dysplasia. • Incompatible with life.	• Most common type. • Best prognosis. • Cyst spaces are lined by pseudostratified ciliated columnar epithelium.	• 2nd most common type. • Generally cause **respiratory distress** in first month of lfe. • Are associated with: ❖ Renal agenesis. ❖ Cardiovascular defects. ❖ Diaphragmatic hernia. ❖ Syringomyelia.	• Occur exclusively in males. • Expand a whole lobe and cause mediastinal shift and compression of other lung.	• Very rare. • Multiloculated, thin walled cysts are present.

103. (a) <10% for gestational age (Ref: Ghai 7th E/P129)

Small for date babies	Appropriate for date babies	Large for date babies
• Babies with birth weight of less than 10th percentile of their gestational age.	• Babies with birth weight between 10th-90th percentile for their period of gestation.	• Babies with birth weight more than 90th percentile of their gestational age.

104. (a) Phototherapy (Ref: Nelson 19th E/P598)
- **Bronze baby syndrome** is a complication of phototherapy characterised by grayish - brown skin discolouration due to photo - induced modification of porphyrins.

105. (c) Seizure (Ghai 7th E/P141)

Stages of hypoxic ischemic encephalopathy:

Stage 1	Stage 2	Stage 3
Hyperalert and Irritable	Lethargic	Comatose
Normal muscle tone	Mild hypotonia	Flaccid
Mydriasis	Miosis	Anisocoria
No seizures	Sezuires are common	Seizures are less common

106. (a) and **(d)** Undescended testis and Breast nodule (Ref: Ghai 7th E/P109)

If the cause of SGA baby is prematurity, than it can have features like:
- Absence of **deep sole creases.**
- Size of **breast nodule** less than 5mm.
- **Poor elastic recoil** of ear cartilage.
- Presence of **lanugo hair** (Lanugo hair is present on fetus and usually sheds in two periods: 1. At 28 weeks and 2. At term).
- Males — **Testes** are located at **external ring (undescended testis)** and scrotum has few rugosities.
  Females — Labia majora are widely separated exposing labia minora and clitoris.

107. (b) Hyaline membrane disease (Ref: Ghai 7th E/P143)

108. (a) Diglucuronide deficiency (Ref: Nelson 19th E/P1320)

Crigler-Najjar syndrome II:
- Caused due to partial absence of **glucuronyl transferase.**
- Predominantly **autosomal dominant** inheritance.
- Mild **unconjugated hyperbilirubinemia.** (Usually less than 10 mg/DL).
- **Kernicterus is less likely.**
- Standard hepatic biochemical tests and liver histology are normal.
- Cytochrome p-450 inducing compounds like **phenobarbital** can improve glucunoridation by inducing hypertrophy of hepatic endoplasmic reticulum but long term treatment is not recommended.

109. (a) and **(b)** Babies of diabetics and Premature rupture of membranes (Ref: Ghai 7th E/P143)
- RDS is the most common cause of respiratory failure in early days of a neonate.
- Though it is a common disorder of **premature infants (< 34 weeks),** various other predisposing factors like male sex, caesarean section delivery, **infant of diabetic mother, premature rupture of membranes,** second born twin, asphyxia and cold stress are related to it.

110. (b) Bacterial flora (Ref: Ghai 7th E/P144–45)
- Meconium can be found in fetal intestine usually at 14–16 weeks of gestation.
- It is a black — green colour odourless substance which is composed of **water, squamous cells, vernix, lanugo, blood, amniotic fluid and intestinal secretions containing bile.**

111. (d) 110–150 (Ref: Nelson 19th E/P1482)

112. (a) In the first six hours of life (Ref: Ghai 7th E/P143)
- The baby develops respiratory distress **within first 6 hours of birth** associated with **tachypnea (RR > 60/min),** prominent grunting, **intercostal and subcostal retractions, acidosis,** nasal flaring and cyanosis.

QUESTIONS OF OTHER EXAMINATIONS

1. (b) Rh incompatibility (Ref: Nelson 19th E/P593)

2. (a) Hypotonia (Ref: Nelson 19th E/P596)
- Kernicterus is the term used for severe form of bilirubin toxicity which leads to permanent neurologic damage.
- The infant may develop delayed motor skills, movement disorder (**cheroathetosis,** ballismus, tremor), **upward gaze,** paralytic palsies, intellectual deficits and **sensorineural hearing loss.**

3. (a) Erythematous popular pustular lesions (Ref: Nelson 19th E/P2162)
- **Erythema toxicum — Papules or pustules with erythema** seen most commonly on **second day and disappear** spontaneously.
- **Milia** —Yellow pinhead sized papule on the face, gingivae and midline of palate. Can occur at any age and usually **disapper in first few weeks.**
- **Transient neonatal pustularmelanosis** — Lesions are **present at birth** and **disappear** within 3 months.

4. (b) Bacteruria (Ref: Nelson 19th E/P1733)

5. (b) 30–40 breaths/min (Ref: Ghai 7th E/P180)

6. (a) Total and direct bilirubin (Ref: Ghai 7th E/P147–48)

7. (a) Measurement of α fetoprotein (Ref: Burton Interpretation of diagnostic tests 8th E/P876)

8. (d) Increased muscular activity (Ref: Ghai 7th E/P115)

9. (c) Intracranial bleed (Ghai 7th E/P129–30)

10. (b) 3 hours (Ref: Nelson 19th E/P508)

11. (d) These can be given even in presence of chorio-amnionitis clinically (Ref: Nelson 19th E/P577)

12. (b) 12 mg every 24 hours (Ghai 7th E/P144)
- All foetuses between 24 and 36 weeks of gestation at risk of preterm delivery should be considered for antenatal corticosteroid treatment, which consists of:
  1. 2 doses of 12 mg of betamethasone I.M 24 hours apart or
  2. 4 doses of dexamethasone given I.M 12 hours apart.

13. (a) Exchange transfusion (Ref: Nelson 19th E/P597)
Indication for phototherapy and exchange transfusion in preterm babies:

Birth weight	Healthy baby		Sick baby	
	Photo therapy	Exchange transfusion	Photo therapy	Exchange transfusion
<1000 gm	5–7	**11–13**	4–6	10-12
1001–1500 gm	7–10	13–15	6–8	11–13
1501–2000 gm	10–12	15–18	8–10	13–15
2001–2500 gm	12–15	18–20	10–12	15–18

14. (b) Diabetes (Ref: Nelson 19th E/P613–14)
Respiratory distress in infants of diabetic mother:
- Delayed maturation of type II alveolar cells lead to **decreased surfactant production.**
- Insulin inhibits glycogen breakdown and **decreases the substrate for synthesis of phosphatidyl-glycerol, an important component of surfactant.**

15. (b) RDS — Respiratory distress syndrome (Ref: Ghai 7th E/P142–43)

16. (d) Mode of delivery (Ghai 7th E/P144)

17. (b) Dubin Johnson syndrome (Ref: Ghai 7th E/P149)

18. (b) Stop breast feeds and review after 24 hours (Ref: Nelson 19th E/P596)

"If nursing is discontinued, the serum bilirubin level falls rapidly, usually reaching normal levels within a few days. Cessation of breast-feeding for 1-2 days and substitution of formula for breast milk results in a rapid decline in serum bilirubin, after which nursing can be resumed without a return of the hyperbilirubinemia to its previously high levels."

19. (a) Transient tachypnea of newborn (Ref: Ghai 7th E/P146)
- TTN is usually a benign, self-limited disease that resolves within **2–4 days.**
- The characteristic X-ray findings in TTN are:
  ❖ Prominent pulmonary vascular markings
  ❖ **Widened interlobar fissures due to fluid**
  ❖ Hyperinflation with flattening of diaphragm
  ❖ Presence of pleural effusion
  ❖ Enlarged cardiac silhouette

20. (d) Tickling of sole (Ref: Ghai 7th E/P99)

21. (b) Birth below 10th percentile (Ref: IAP 4th E/P47)

Small for date babies	Appropriate for date babies	Large for date babies
• Babies with birth weight of less than 10th percentile or 2 SD of their gestational age	• Babies with birth weight between 10th-90th percentile for their period of gestation	• Babies with birth weight more than 90th percentile of their gestational age

22. (b) < 1500 gm of birth weight (Ref: IAP 4th E/P47)

Low birth weight babies	Very Low birth weight babies	Extremely low birth weight babies
• Weight less than 2.5 kg	• Weight less than 1.5 kg	• Weight less than 1 kg

23. (a), (b) and **(d).** Breast milk jaundice, Cystic fibrosis and Alpha 1 antitrypsin deficiency (Ref: Ghai 7th E/P147)

24. (a) 120–160/min (Ref: Nelson 19th E/P1482)

"The heart rate of newborn infants is rapid and subject to wide fluctuations. The **average rate ranges from 120 to 140 beats/min** and may increase to 170+ beats/min during crying and activity or drop to 70–90 beats/min during sleep."

25. (b) 7 days (Ref: Ghai 7th E/P96)

26. (a) Diaphragmatic hernia (Ref: Ghai 7th E/P153)

27. (a) 40 mg/dl (Ref: Ghai 7th E/P155)

28. (c) Phosphatidyl glycerol estimation is a reliable method of diagnosis (Ref: Ghai 7th E/P144)
- **Foam stability or shake test** — Amniotic fluid is mixed with absolute alcohol, shaken for 15 seconds and allowed to settle. If bubbles are present it indicates sufficient surfactant (dipalmitoyl-phosphatidylcholine, phosphatidylglycerol, proteins and cholesterol) indicating lung maturity.

29. (c) Absence or insufficient amount of surfactant (Ref: Ghai 7th E/P143)

30. (a) Anytime during pregnancy

"Maternal nutritional status both before and during pregnancy is associated with fetal growth patterns."

31. **(c)** Diaphragmatic hernia (Ref: Rudolph 22nd E/P 210, Nelson 18th E/P 747, 48)

32. **(b)** The total bilirubin concentration in the serum increases by 1mg/dl per day (Ref: Ghai 7th E/P147)
   - Jaundice becomes visible on **2nd to 3rd day** when **indirect bilirubin** rises at a rate of **<5 mg/dL/24 hr** and peaks on 4th to 5th day at a rate of 5–6 mg/dL.

33. **(b)** Rh incompatibility (Ref: Nelson 19th E/P593)

34. **(c)** Onset of respiratory distress is immediately after birth and it rarely lasts beyond 48 hours (Ref: Ghai 7th E/P146)
   - TTN is usually a benign, self-limited disease that resolves within **2–4 days.**
   - Baby presents with **tachypnea shortly after birth along with mild to moderate signs of respiratory distress,** such as nasal flaring, subcostal and intercostal retractions and grunting during expiration.

35. **(a)** Unconjugated bilirubin (Ref: Nelson 19th E/P596)

36. **(a)** Apnea (Ref: Ghai 7th E/P146)
   - Apnea is defined as cessation of breathing for 20 seconds or more, or less than 20 seconds along with bradycardia or cyanosis.

37. **(a)** L/S ratio (Ref: Ghai 7th E/P144)
   - Tests to predict RDS/HMD:
     ❖ **Lecithin/Sphingomyelin ratio** of **more than 2.0** indicates lung maturity.
     ❖ Foam stability or shake test — Amniotic fluid is mixed with absolute alcohol, shaken for 15 seconds and allowed to settle. If bubbles are present it indicates sufficient surfactant (dipalmitoylphosphatidylcholine, **phosphatidylglycerol,** proteins and cholesterol) indicating lung maturity.

38. **(b)** Meconium aspiration (Ref: IAP 4th E/P567)
   - In the **first 24 hours after birth** prematurity is the most common cause; however in term neonates meconium aspiration syndrome is the most common cause of respiratory distress.

39. **(a)** Autonomic dysfunction (Ref: Nelson 19th E/P2162)
   Harlequin colour change:
   - When baby is placed on the side body is dissected longitudinally in to a pale upper half and deep red dependent half.
   - Most commonly seen in low birth weight infants; however disappears within minutes.
   - It is caused by **imbalance in autonomic vascular regulatory mechanism.**

40. **(d)** Deviation of trachea from midline (Ref: Nelson 19th E/P526, Leonard Imaging of the newborn infant and young child 5th E/P5))

   "**Abdomen:** The **liver** is usually palpable, sometimes as much as 2 cm below the rib margin. Less commonly, the tip of the **spleen** may be felt. The approximate size and location of each **kidney** can usually be determined on deep palpation."

   - In young infant the trachea is more mobile and flexible and hence normal deviation of the trachea to the right on expiration can be seen in chest X-rays.
   - The newborn may lose 10% of weight in the first week of life; however it is regained in following weeks. However any weight loss after this period indicates serious disorder.

41. **(c)** 28 days of life (Ref: Ghai 7th E/P96)

42. **(d)** 110–150 (Ref: Nelson 19th E/P1482)

43. **(c)** 3–5 weeks (Ref: Ghai 7th E/P112)

3

Nutrition

Nutrition is the basic need to support growth and development in early phase of life and sustain various functions in the later phase. The macronutrients (carbohydrates, fats and proteins) provide energy as well as build the body, whereas the micronutrients (vitamins and minerals) facilitate various metabolic processes. Breast milk contains all the macro and micronutrients in sufficient amount and hence serves as the best feed for the baby.

FEEDING OF INFANTS

Breast Feeding

Breast milk is the **best food for both preterm and term neonates.** It contains all the essential micronutrients (vitamins and minerals) and macronutrients (10% proteins, **40% carbohydrates** and 50% fats) required for the growth of baby. Breast feeding is initiated within **1 hour** after normal delivery and **4 hours** after caesarean section. Exclusive breast feeding is recommended till **6 months** of age. Complimentary feeding should be started at 6 months of age and breast feeding should be continued till 2 years of age. Maximum breast milk output is seen at **5–6 months.**

Signs of Good Attachment during Breast Feeding

- Baby's mouth should be wide open
- Only the upper areola should be visible
- Baby's chin should touch the breast
- Baby's lower lip should be everted

Maturation of Human Milk

Time	Milk type	Constituents
Premature delivery	Premature milk	Contains more proteins, iron, sodium, Ig and calories but **less lactose**
3-4 days post delivery	Colostrum	Rich in **protein,** antibodies and vitamin A, D, E and K
4th day- 2nd week	Transitional milk	Rich in fat and sugar but less protein and antibodies
2nd week onwards	Mature milk	Less viscous but contains all nutrients for normal growth

Change in breast milk during the course of breast feeding:

Fore milk	Hind milk
Milk secreted at the beginning of feeding. It is rich in <ul><li>Water — Quenches thirst of baby</li><li>**Protein**</li><li>Sugar</li><li>Vitamin</li><li>Minerals</li></ul>	Milk secreted at the end phase of feeding It is rich in <ul><li>**Fat content** — Satisfies hunger of baby and provides energy</li></ul>

Components of Breast Milk and Cow Milk

Contents	Cow milk (gm/l)	Human milk (gm/l)
Proteins	More i.e. 33	Less i.e. 11
	60% whey	18% whey
	40% casein	82% protein
Carbohydrates e.g. Lactose	**Less i.e. 50**	**More i.e. 70**
Fats (Linoleic acid)	More i.e. 3.5	Less i.e. 1
Minerals	More i.e.	Less i.e.
Calcium	1400	350
Phosphorous	900	150
Iron	1	0.15
Sodium	25	6.5
Chloride	29	12

Benefits of Human Milk

- Decreased gastrointestinal disturbances like diarrhea can be seen because of various antimicrobial factors. Moreover mother's milk is **free of contaminating bacteria.**
- **Epidermal growth factor** present in breast milk enhances the maturation of intestinal cells. Hence there is decreased incidence of allergy to cow milk, **evening colic,** "spitting up", occult malena and atopic eczema.
- Breast milk has components of both active and passive immunity:
  - ❖ It has high concentration of secretory **Ig A** antibodies that prevents microorganisms from adhering to intestinal mucosa.
  - ❖ Macrophages in human milk **may** synthesize **lysozyme, complement and lactoferrin.** Lactoferrin has an inhibitory effect on growth of E.coli.
  - ❖ Bile stimulated lipase in human milk kills Giardia Lamblia and Entamoeba Histolytica.
  - ❖ **Decreased incidence of infections** like respiratory infections, otitis media, bacteremia and meningitis is seen because of various viral and bacterial **Ig G antibodies;** and various substances like interferon that inhibits the growth of viruses.
  - ❖ **Para amino benzoic acid (PABA)** provides protection against **malaria.**
  - ❖ α-**Lactalbumin** in human milk has **immunostimulatory, antibacterial** and antitumor effect.
- High level of essential polyunsaturated fatty acids like linoleic acidand α-linolenic-acid whose derivatives like arachidonic, eicosapentaenoic and **docosahexaenoic (DHA) acid** are required for brain development are present.
- Breast milk has **more lactose** than any other milk which is required for growth of brain, **growth of lactobacillus** in intestine (**lactose inhibits growth of harmful bacteria in intestine by secreting lactic acid which keeps intestinal pH low or acidic)** and **absorption of calcium.**
- **Decreased sodium concentration** in human milk has a protective effect on infant's kidney. **Calcium is better absorbed** because Calcium/phosphorous ratio is high in human milk.
- Breast milk has ample amount of vitamins like Vitamin A and Vitamin C, micronutrients like copper, selenium and cobalt; however is **deficient in vitamin K** (can lead to hemorrhagic disease of newborn), **iron, fluoride** and **vitamin D.** Though iron is limited in human milk, the baby has sufficient stores for 6 months and hence should be supplemented with iron **after 6 months of age.**
- Breast fed babies are **less prone to develop allergic disorders and chronic disorders** like diabetes, heart disease and lymphoma in future.It **protects babies** from tendency to **obesity.**

Expressed Breast Milk

In the absence of mother, expressed breast milk can be given to the baby. The expressed breast milk can be stored at **room temperature for 6-8 hours, refrigerator for 24 hours** and freezer at −20°C for 3 months.

MALNUTRITION

The clinical features of malnutrition depend on the type of macro or micronutrient deficiency.

Macronutrient Deficiency

Protein energy Malnutrition

PEM is a serious, lethal disease affecting children mostly in low income countries. It is a result of inadequate intake of proteins and calories or faulty digestion and absorption of proteins. The clinical presentation of PEM can be discussed as two different entities called as marasmus and kwashiorkor.

- **Marasmus and kwashiorkor:**

Marasmus	*Kwashiorkor*

• Prolonged starvation leads to selective depletion of somatic compartment (skeletal muscle) proteins to provide energy.
• Body fat is depleted to provide energy as well as low leptin levels stimulate the release of cortisol which leads to lipolysis.
• Severe muscle wasting and minimal subcutaneous fat leads to manifestations like
  ❖ **Monkey facies** — Buccal pad fat loss that creates wrinkled appearance.
  ❖ **Baggy pants appearance** — Loose skin of buttocks hanging down.
• Visceral compartment **(liver)** is spared, hence serum albumin level is normal and there is no edema.
• The child appears to be alert.
• Appetite is good.
	• Protein deprivation is relatively more than calorie deficiency. In Ghanaian language 'Ga' means a **child displaced from mother's breast.**
	• There is selective loss of protein from visceral compartment **(liver)** and hence leads to hypoalbuminemia.
	• Decreased serum albumin leads to **generalized edema** which masks the severe weight loss. The **letter 'K'** is added to PEM grade to indicate **presence of edema.**
	• Relative sparing of subcutaneous fat and muscle mass gives sugar baby appearance.
	• Skin pigmentation called as **flaky paint appearance** or enamel spots is seen.
	• Alternate bands of hypopigmentation and normally **pigmented hair** are called as **flag sign.**
	• Affected child is **apathic, irritable and cries intermittently.**
	• Appetite is decreased.

- **Complications of Protein energy malnutrition:** These complications are the usual cause of death in severe malnutrition.

Mnemonic: HIDE

❖ H — Hypoglycemia , Hypothermia, Heart failure
❖ I — Infections and sepsis due to compromised immune system
  1. **Cell mediated immunity** is compromised. The thymus is reduced in size and T8>T4 cell production is reduced.
  2. **Humoral immunity** — Immunoglobulin production by B cells is **normal or increased.** However **secretory Ig A production is reduced** which can compromise the mucosal immunity.
  3. **Complement production** is usually decreased (C3 > C4)
  4. **Phagocytic activity** of polymorphnuclearcells is impaired.
❖ D — Dehydration,
Deficiency of micronutrients and vitamins
  1. Iron - Microcytic hypochromic anemia
  2. Vitamin A - Xeropthalmia, Night blindness, **Bitot spots**, Keratomalacia, Growth failure
  3. Vitamin B12 - Megaloblastic anemia
  4. Vitamin C - Scurvy
  5. Vitamin D - Rickets
❖ E — Electrolyte imbalance
  1. Hyponatremia
  2. **Hypokalemia**
  3. Hypomagnesemia

- **Diagnosis:** Malnutrition can be assessed by several age dependent factors and independent factors.
  - ❖ Age dependent factors like height and weight are best indicators of growth and malnutrition.

Factors	*Indicator*	*Type of malnutrition*
Low height for age	**Stunting**	**Chronic**
Low weight for height	**Wasting**	**Acute**
Low weight for age	**Underweight**	**Acute and chronic**

❖ Age independent factors like MAC, bangle test, skin fold thickness and various ratios can also be used.

MAC	Bangle test	Skin fold thickness	Ratios
❖ Normal value is 16–17 cm in age group of 1–5 years ❖ 12.5 – 3.5 — Borderline malnutrition ❖ <12.5 — Severe malnutrition	In cases of malnutrition a bangle of 4 cm diameter passes above elbow.	A skin fold thickness in triceps above 10 mm is normal and below 6 mm indicates malnutrition.	❖ Kanawati index ❖ Dugdale's index ❖ Quaker arm circumference ❖ Jeliffe's ratio

- **Severity of malnutrition:**
  - ❖ WHO classification

    WHO classification is based on weight for height, height for age and presence of edema.

Factors	Moderate malnutrition	Severe malnutrition
Symmetrical edema	No	Yes
Weight for height	SD is between –2 to –3	SD is less than –3
Height for age	SD is between – 2 to –3	SD is less than –3

  - ❖ IAP classification

    IAP classification is based on weight for age values.

Grade of malnutrition	Weight for age value (%)
Normal	>80
Grade I or mild	71–80
Grade II or moderate	61–70
Grade III or severe	**51–60**
Grade IV or very severe	<50

  - ❖ **Gomez classification:** Gomez classification is based on comparison of weight of malnourished child to a normal child of same age, which is 50th percentile of Boston standards. This classification holds good for hospitalised children as the cut off values were obtained from weight of admitted children.

$$\text{Weight for age (\%)} = \frac{\text{Weight of the child}}{\text{Weight of normal child of same age}} \times 100$$

Grade of malnutrition	Weight for age
Normal child	90–110 %
1st degree, Mild	**75–89 %**
2nd degree, Moderate	60–74 %
3rd degree, Severe	**<60 %**

- **Treatment:** Patient is managed in 3 different stages.
  - ❖ First stage — During first 24–48 hours dehydration and infections are dealt with adequate rehydration therapy and good antibiotic coverage respectively.
  - ❖ Second stage — Then for next 7–10 days along with antibiotic therapy, patient is put on a diet of 75 cal/Kg required to maintain the protein and energy need.
  - ❖ Third stage — This stage is aimed at restoring the patient's protein and fat content of the body by providing a diet of up to **150 Kcal/kg/24 hours.**

MICRONUTRIENT DEFICIENCY

Vitamin A Deficiency

- **Different forms of Vitamin A:**
  - ❖ Alcohol form — All-trans-retinol (Vitamin A)
  - ❖ Storage form (in liver)-Retinyl palmitate
  - ❖ Aldehyde form **(for vision)-11-cis-retinal**

- **Sources of Vitamin A:**

Preformed Vitamin A	Provitamin A caretinoids
• Richest source is **shark oil and cod liver oil.**	• Richest source is green leafy vegetables. • **All — trans β-carotene** is the most effective precursor of vitamin A.

- **Functions of vitamin A and manifestations of its deficiency**

Functions of vitamin A	Manifestations of deficiency
11-cis-retinal form of vitamin A is required for night vision.	Night blindness
Immunomodulatory	Leukopenia and infections like measles
All — trans- retinoic acid promotes nuclear transcription and controls epithelial cell differentiation, division and death.	❖ Dry scaly hyperkeratotic skin patches called as **phrynoderma or toad skin** ❖ Diarrhea due to intestinal mucosa damage ❖ Keratinization and opacification of cornea known as **xeropthalmia.** ❖ Infection and weakening of cornea know as **Keratomalacia** ❖ Keratinization of conjunctiva leads to plaque formation called as **Bitot spots.**
Bone development	Bone overgrowth leads to compressive optic nerve palsy
Fetal development	❖ Mental retardation ❖ Hydrocephalus ❖ Poor growth

- **Recommended daily allowance of Vitamin A:**

Infants	300–400 μg
Children	400–600 μg
Adolescent	700 μg

- **Prevention of xeropthalmia:**
  - ❖ Short term action refers to administration of large doses of vitamin A to subjects susceptible to its efficiency.

Vitamin A Prophylaxis

Age group	Oral dose of Vitamin A	Timing
Newborn	50000 IU	At birth
Infants	**100000 IU**	Once every 4–6 months
Children> 1 year of age	200000 IU	Once every 4–6 months
Women of child bearing age	300000 IU	Within 1 month of giving birth
Pregnant or lactating women	5000 IU or 20000 IU	Daily or weekly

- ❖ Medium term action refers to fortification of certain foods with vitamin A like adding of vitamin A to dalda.
- ❖ Long term action refers to action on factors leading to ocular diseases.
  1. Increasing awareness among people to consume food rich in vitamin A like green leafy vegetables.
  2. Encouraging breast feeding for as long as possible.
  3. Taking care of factors that can lead to vitamin A deficiency like prevention (safe water supply and maintenance of sanitary latrines) and treatment of diarrhea, immunization against measles.

Vitamin C Deficiency

- Human beings are unable to synthesize vitamin C as they lack the enzyme gulonolactone oxidase. Hence to meet the demand body needs exogenous vitamin C which is readily available in **breast milk,** certain vegetables and citrus foods.
- Richest source of vitamin C in fruits is amla (600 mg/100 gm) and in vegetables is cabbage (124 mg/100 gm).
- Functions of vitamin C and manifestation of its deficiency

  Deficiency of vitamin C leads to Scurvy, which usually manifests clinically in infants and young children in the age group of 6 – 24 months. Although Scurvy is rarely seen in present time, earlier it was most commonly seen in babies fed exclusively with **cow's milk.** The requirement of vitamin C is increased during infectious and diarrheal diseases.

Function of Vitamin C	*Manifestation of deficiency*
Hydroxylation of lysine and proline in collagen formation.	Weakening of collagen in various parts of body. • **Blood vessels** — Fragility of blood vessels present as purpura, ecchymosis, perifollicular hemorrhages, gum bleeding, subperiosteal bleeding and epistaxis. • Bones and cartilage — **Osteoblasts cannot form osteoid** as collagen is an important part of osteoid. This leads to **epiphyseal separation, rosary at the costochondral junction,** depression of the sternum and arthralgia. The pain results in **pseudoparalysis** i.e. decreased movement at joints and the characteristic **frog like** position, in which baby lies is legs flexed at knees and hips partially flexed and externally rotated. • **Gums** — Bluish purple, spongy swellings in the mucosa over upper incisors. • **Muscle** — Weakness and degeneration of skeletal muscle and cardiac muscle hypertrophy
Conversion of dopamine to norepinephrine and tryptophan to serotonin.	Decreased norepinephrine and serotonin may produce irritability and other psychological manifestations.
Non heme iron absorption and transfer of iron from transferrin to ferritin.	Iron deficiency anemia.
Formation of tetrahydrofolic acid which plays an important role in hematopoetic system	Megaloblastic anemia.

- **Diagnosis of vitamin C deficiency:**
  - ❖ Leucocyte concentration of vitamin C is the best indicator of body stores, which is estimated by **buffy coat preparation,** but it is a difficult test to perform.
  - ❖ Urinary vitamin C excretion after administration of a test dose is usually performed. Excretion of less than 80% of administered dose indicates deficiency of vitamin C.
  - ❖ Plasma and serum vitamin C is a poor indicator of body stores.
  - ❖ Radiological features — The typical radiological features are best seen in the knee joint.
    - ❑ **White line of Fraenkel** — Zone of well calcified cartilage at the metaphysis.
    - ❑ **Pelkan Spur** — Lateral prolongation of white line.
    - ❑ **Wimsberger sign** — Epiphyseal centres of ossification surrounded by a white line.
    - ❑ Metaphyseal rarefaction zone seen as a triangular defect in the lateral part.
    - ❑ Ground glass appearance of the bone.
    - ❑ **Epiphyseal separation.**

Vitamin D Deficiency

The important sources of vitamin D are cutaneous synthesis mediated by sunlight and food of animal origin. **Halibut liver** oil is the richest source of vitamin D. Deficiency of vitamin D causes **rickets** in children and **osteomalacia** in adults.

Steps of Vitamin D Synthesis and Mechanism of Deficiency

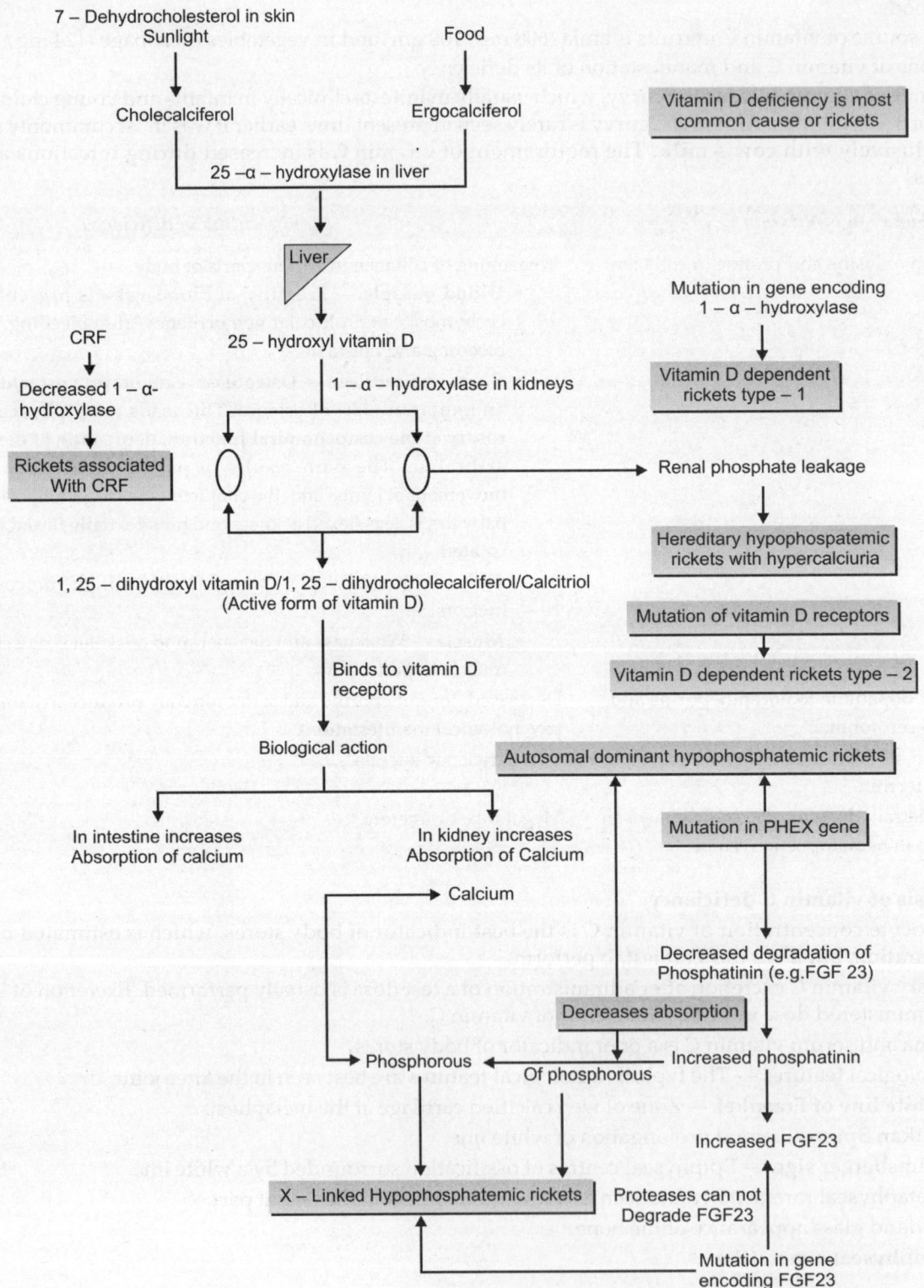

7 – Dehydrocholesterol in skin
Sunlight

Food

Cholecalciferol

Ergocalciferol

Vitamin D deficiency is most common cause or rickets

25 –α – hydroxylase in liver

Liver

Mutation in gene encoding 1 – α – hydroxylase

CRF

25 – hydroxyl vitamin D

Decreased 1 – α- hydroxylase

1 – α – hydroxylase in kidneys

Vitamin D dependent rickets type – 1

Rickets associated With CRF

Renal phosphate leakage

Hereditary hypophospatemic rickets with hypercalciuria

1, 25 – dihydroxyl vitamin D/1, 25 – dihydrocholecalciferol/Calcitriol (Active form of vitamin D)

Mutation of vitamin D receptors

Vitamin D dependent rickets type – 2

Binds to vitamin D receptors

Autosomal dominant hypophosphatemic rickets

Biological action

Mutation in PHEX gene

In intestine increases Absorption of calcium

In kidney increases Absorption of Calcium

Calcium

Decreased degradation of Phosphatinin (e.g.FGF 23)

Decreases absorption

Phosphorous

Of phosphorous

Increased phosphatinin

Increased FGF23

X – Linked Hypophosphatemic rickets

Proteases can not Degrade FGF23

Mutation in gene encoding FGF23

Fig. 3.1

Note: **Phosphatinins** also block **1-α-hydroxylase** in kidney. **Elevated levels of phosphatinine can be seen in** McCune - Albright syndrome, epidermal nevus syndrome, neurofibromatosis and tumor-induced osteomalacia

- **Rickets:** Bone is made up of a protein matrix called as osteoid and mineral matrix composed of calcium and phosphorous. Rickets occurs due to defective mineralization of the matrix of bone at growth plates.
  - ❖ **Classical Clinical features:**
    - ❑ **Craniotabes** — Softening of the cranial bones makes the skull like a ping-pong ball. It is the **earliest presentation.** Craniotabes can also be seen in premature neonates, hypervitaminosis A, **syphilis,** hydrocephalus and **osteogenesis imperfecta.**
    - ❑ **Caput quadratum or hot cross bun sign** — This is caused due to widening of suture and thickening of bones around it.
    - ❑ **Rachitic rosary** — It is **non-tender** widening of the costochondral junction that gives a feeling of beads of a rosary on examination.
    - ❑ **Harrison groove** — It is horizontal depression along the lower anterior chest due to pulling of softened ribs by the diaphragm during inspiration.
    - ❑ **Growth plate widening** — It results in widening of wrist and ankle.
    - ❑ Increased risk of **pneumonia** and **atelectasis** due to impairment in air movement because of softening of ribs.
    - ❑ **Large anterior fontanel** and its delayed closure and frontal bossing of skull can be seen.
    - ❑ Delayed eruption of temporary teeth and **dental caries** can be seen.
    - ❑ **Growth retardation** can be seen.
    - ❑ **Bone changes** — **Tenderness and pain** in bones is the earliest presentation. **Bowlegs/ knock knees/genu valgum and windswept deformity** is caused due to bending of softened shafts of femur, tibia and fibula.
    - ❑ **Pectus carinatum** — This is caused by anterior projection of sternum.
    - ❑ **Pot belly** — Laxity of abdominal muscle leads to forward protrusion.

MNEMONIC: HELICOPTER
H — Harrison's groove, Hot cross bun sign   E — Enlarged growth plate   L — Large anterior fontanel   I — Infection of lungs   C — Craniotabes, Caries   O — Os deformity **(Bowlegs/ knock knees/genu valgum and windswept deformity)**   P — Pectus carinatum, Pot belly   T — Tenderness and pain in bone   E — Enlarged ankles and wrists   R — Retardation of growth, Rachitic rosary

  - ❖ **Different causes of rickets —**

Vitamin D Deficiency

	Nutritional vitamin D deficiency	Vitamin D - Dependent rickets type 1	Vitamin D - Dependent rickets type 2	Chronic renal failure
Clinical manifestations (Classical features are similar in all)	Prolonged laryngospasm, symptoms of hypocalcemia.	Metabolic acidosis, aminociduria.	**Alopecia,** epidermal cysts.	Secondary hyperparathyroidism, metabolic acidosis.
Causes	Breast fed infants without adequate sun exposure (Breast milk is a poor source of vitamin D)	**Autosomal recessive** disease caused by mutation in the gene encoding **1-α-hydroxylase.**	**Autosomal recessive** disease caused by mutation in gene encoding vitamin D receptor.	Can be complication of different diseases like diabetes mellitus and hypertension.
Treatment	• 600,000 IU (15 mg) of vitamin D is given once or daily for 10 days **or** • 2000–5000 **IU**/day for 4–6 weeks	**Calcitriol**	High doses of vitamin D and oral calcium.	Calcitriol, Dietary phosphorous restriction, use of oral phosphorous chelaters (As CRF is associated with hyperphosphatemia due to inability of kidney to excrete phosphorous, and calcitriol will also increase serum phosphorous level).

Deficiency of minerals (Calcium and phosphorous)

	Calcium deficiency	X-Linked Hypophosphatemic rickets	Autosomal dominant Hypophosphatemic rickets	Hereditary hypophosphatemic rickets with hypercalciuria	Fanconi syndrome
Clinical manifestations (Classical features are similar in all)	It occurs later than nutritional deficiency rickets.	Abnormalities predominantly in lower extremities, delayed dentition and tooth abscesses.	—	Kidney stones, bone pains	Polyuria, polydipsia and metabolic acidosis.
Causes	Calcium depleted diet, malabsorption syndromes.	**PHEX gene mutation** causes increased phosphatinine, which decreases absorption of phosphorous.	Mutation in gene encoding **FGF23** leads to decreased breakdown by proteases and **increased FGF23 (phosphatinine).**	Renal phosphate leak	Cystinosis, Wilson's disease, Lowe syndrome, tyrosinemia and heavy metal exposure.
Treatment	Dietary calcium supplementation .	**Oral phosphorous and calcitriol.**	**Oral phosphorous and calcitriol.**	**Oral phosphorous.**	Treatment of the etiology, **calcitriol, phosphorous and bicarbonate.**

❖ **Diagnosis of rickets:**

Rickets is usually diagnosed by classic radiographic findings supported by classical clinical features and laboratory parameters.

❑ **Radiological findings:**

Rickets is associated with defective mineralization of bone i.e. decreased calcium deposition in the bones which gives rise to various radiological signs.

Radiological Sign	Cause
Loss of normal zone of provisional calcification is the **earliest sign.**	Decreased osteoid matrix formation due to decreased calcium deposition.
Fraying of metaphysis	Edge of metaphysis loses its sharp border.
Cupping and splaying of metaphysis	Effect of weight on the softened metaphysis.
Widening of growth plate	Lack of metaphyseal calcification.

❑ **Differential diagnosis:**

The physiological processes involved in regulation of body calcium and phosphorous levels are mediated by three hormones vitamin D, parathyroid hormone and calcitonin. The understanding of physiological process is important to understand the changes in different disorders.

Hormone	Effect on serum calcium	Effect on serum phosphorous
Vitamin D (Calcitriol)	Intestine ⎤ Increases kidney ⎦ absorption ↑ Serum calcium	Intestine ⎤ Increases kidney ⎦ absorption ↑ Serum phosphorous
PTH	Bones — Increases resorption and serum calcium Kidney — Increases absorption Intestine — Increases absorption ↑ Serum calcium	Kidney — Decreases absorption ↓ Serum phosphorous
Calcitonin	Bones — Decreases resorption and serum calcium Kidney — Increases excretion ↑ Serum calcium	No role

In different types of rickets and disorders mimicking it, the laboratory parameters vary because of their difference in cause

Type of rickets	Ca	PO$_4$	ALP	PTH	HCO$_3$	Urine Ca	Urine PO$_4$
Vitamin D deficiency	Decreased	Decreased	Increased	Increased	Normal	Decreased	Increased
Vitamin D dependent	Normal or decreased	Normal or decreased	Increased	Increased	Increased	Decreased	Increased
Hypophosphatemic	Normal	Decreased	Increased	Normal	Normal	Decreased	Increased
Hyperparathyroidism	Increased	Decreased	Increased	Increased	Normal	Decreased	Increased
Distal RTA	Decreased	Normal	Increased	Increased	Normal	Increased	Normal

Note: Normal levels of serum Ca = 9–10 mg/dl, PO$_4$ = 3–4.5 mg/dl, ALP = 30–120 IU/5–15 KA, PTH = 10–55 units, HCO$_3$ = 22–28 units

MULTIPLE CHOICE QUESTIONS

1. **True about cow's milk are all except:**
   [AIIMS May 10, 07]
   a. Cow's milk contains 80% whey protein not casein
   b. Cow milk has less carbohydrate than mothers milk
   c. Has more K4 and Na+ than infant formula feeds
   d. Has more protein than breast milk

2. **Best indicator for nutritional status for a child is:**
   [AIIMS May 10, AIIMS Nov. 06]
   a. Mid arm circumference
   b. Head circumference
   c. Rate of increase of height and weight
   d. Chest circumference

3. **Which vitamin deficiency can result in Neonatal Seizures?**   **[AIIMS Nov. 09]**
   a. Thiamine   b. Pyridoxine
   c. Cyanocobalamin   d. Vitamin-C

4. **All are true about scurvy except:**   **[AIIMS May 09]**
   a. Skeletal changes in adult occur with clinical deficiency of vit C
   b. Defective proximal calcification is the central cause for bone change
   c. Cartilaginous overgrowth results in widening of epiphyseal plate
   d. Bowing of legs.

5. **Rickets in infant present as all except:**
   [AIIMS May 07]
   a. Craniotabes   b. Widened fontanel
   c. Rachitic Rosary   d. Bow legs

6. **Common to both acute and chronic malnutrition is:**
   [AIMS May 07]
   a. Weight for age   b. Weight for height
   c. Height for age   d. BMI

7. **The important fatty acid present in breast milk which is important for growth is:** **[AIIMS Nov. 06]**
   a. Docosahexaenoic acid b. Palmitic acid
   c. Linoleic acid   d. Linolenic acid

8. **Deficit in weight for height in a 3 years old child indicates:**   **[AIIMS Nov. 05]**
   a. Acute malnutrition
   b. Chronic malnutrition
   c. Concomitant acute and chronic
   d. Under weight

9. **Deficit in weight for height in a 3 years old child indicates:**   (AIIMS Nov. 05)
   a. Acute malnutrition
   b. Chronic malnutrition
   c. Concomitant acute and chronic
   d. Under weight

10. **The vitamin A supplement administered in "Prevention of nutritional blindness in children program" contain:**   **[AI 03, AIIMS Nov. 05]**
    a. 25,000 lU/ml   b. 1 Lakh IU/ml
    c. 3 Lakh IU/ml   d. 5 Lakh lU/ml

11. **All of the following conditions are observed in Marasmus, except:**   **[AIIMS May 05, DPG 09]**
    a. Hepatomegaly
    b. Muscle wasting
    c. Low insulin levels
    d. Extreme weakness

12. **A 2-year-old boy has vitamin D resistant rickets. His investigations revealed serum Calcium- 9 mg/dl, Phosphate-2.4 mg/dl, alkaline phosphatase-1041IU, normal intact parathyroid hormone and bicarbonate 22 mEq/L. Which of the following is the most probable diagnosis?**   **[AIIMS May 04; Nov. 02]**
    a. Distal renal tubular acidosis
    b. Hypophosphatemic rickets
    c. Vitamin D dependent rickets
    d. Hypoparathyroidism

13. **All of the following are seen in Rickets except:**
    [AIIMS May 03]
    a. Bow legs   b. Gunstock deformity
    c. Pot belly   d. Craniotabes

14. **All of the following are characteristic features of kwashiorkor except:** [AIIMS May 03]
    a. High blood osmolarity
    b. Hypoalbuminemia
    c. Edema
    d. Fatty liver

15. **A 2 years child with vitD resistant rickets was evaluated. His lab investigation reveals:** [AIIMS May 02]

    Serum calcium — 9 mg/dl
    Serum phosphate — 2.4 mg/dl
    Serum alkaline phosphate — 1041 IU
    Parathormone level — 59 units
    The likely diagnosis is:
    a. Distal renal tubular acidosis
    b. Vit. D dependent rickets
    c. Hypophosphatemic rickets
    d. Hyperparathyroidism

16. **Basanti a 7 year old girl, presents with recent onset of genu valgum and difficulty in walking. On X-ray examination there is metaphyseal widening and osteoporosis. Investigations showed a serum calcium of 9 mg/dl. Serum phosphorus of 2.5mg/dl and alkaline phosphatase of 30Ka units, the possible cause is :** [AIIMS Nov. 00]
    a. Nutritional rickets
    b. Hypophosphatemic rickets
    c. Azotemic renal dystrophy
    d. Primary Hyperparathyroidism
    d. Calcitonin

17. **A child is suffering from severe PEM. Calories to be given per kg of body weight to regain weight:** [AIIMS June 99]
    a. 200 Kcal   b. 150 Kcal
    c. 400 Kcal   d. 100 Kcal

18. **Most common cause of genu valgum in children is:** [AIIMS 98]
    a. Osteoarthritis   b. Rickets
    c. Paget disease   d. Rheumatoid arthritis

19. **Wind swept deformity is seen in:** [AIIMS 98]
    a. Scurvy   b. Rickets
    c. Achondroplasia   d. Osteoporosis

20. **Daily dose of vitamin A in a 6–12 months old child is:** [AIMS June 97]
    a. 500 microgram   b. 200 microgram
    c. 300 microgram   d. 700 microgram

21. **Earliest manifestation of rickets is:** [AIIMS June 97]
    a. Craniotabes   b. Rachitic rosary
    c. Harrison groove   d. Pigeon chest

22. **Which is deficient in exclusively breast fed baby:** [AIIMS Feb. 97]
    a. Vitamin B   b. Vitamin A
    c. Vitamin C   d. Proteins

23. **Percentage of lactose in human milk is:** [AIIMS June 97]
    a. 7.2 gm   b. 4.5 gm
    c. 8.0 gm   d. 6.7 gm

24. **Which of the following will occur in an exclusively breast fed baby?** [AIIMS Sep. 96]
    a. Jaundice   b. Scurvy
    c. Tetany   d. Eczema

25. **Exclusive breastfeeding may be associated with all of the following except:** [AI 98, AIIMS 96]
    a. Hemolysis due to vitamin K deficiency
    b. Evening colic
    c. Golden colour stool
    d. Prolongation of physiological jaundice

26. **A 2-year-old child has a weight of 6.4 kg and has vitamin A deficiency. What is the grade of malnutrition in this child:** [AIIMS 87]
    a. First degree   b. Second degree
    c. Third degree   d. Fourth degree

27. **All of the following are features of vitamin D intoxication except:** [PGI 79, AIIMS 86]
    a. Nausea and vomiting
    b. Muscular weakness
    c. Anorexia
    d. Oliguria
    e. Metastatic calcification

28. **The most important factor to overcome protein energy malnutrition in children less than 3 years is:** [AIIMS 83]
    a. Supply of subsidised food from ration shop
    b. Early supplementation of solids in infants
    c. Immunization to child
    d. Treatment of anemia and pneumonia in infant and toddlers

29. **Primary metabolic bone disorder in scurvy is:** [AI 10]
    a. Decreased mineralisation.
    b. Decreased osteoid matrix formation.
    c. Increased bone resorption.
    d. Decreased bone mass with normal mineralisation and osteoid formation.

30. **Deficient mineralisation in epiphyseal growth cartilage is seen in:** [AI 09]
    a. Rickets   b. Osteomalacia
    c. Scurvy   d. Hyperparathyroidism

31. **All of the following nutritional assessment methods indicate inadequate nutrition except:** [AI 09]
    a. Hb<11.5 gm/dl during 3rd trimester of pregnancy
    b. Increased 1–4 year mortality rate
    c. Birth weight<2500 gm
    d. Decreased weight for height

32. **The following statement about Gomez classification is false:** [AI 08]
    a. Based on height retardation
    b. Based on 50th percentile Boston standards
    c. Between 75 and 89% implies in malnutrition
    d. This classification has prognostic value for hospitalization children

33. **Compared with Cow's milk, mother's milk has more:** [AI 07]
    a. Lactose   b. Vitamin D
    c. Proteins   d. Fats

34. **Which of the following is the best indicator of long term nutritional status?** [AI 07]
    a. Mid arm circumference
    b. Height for age
    c. Weight for age
    d. Weight for height

35. **The protective effects of breast milk are known to be associated with:** [AI 05]
    a. IgM antibodies   b. Lysozyme
    c. Mast cells   d. IgA antibodies

36. **The protective effects of breast milk are known to be associated with:** [AI 05, DPG 09]
    a. Ig M antibodies   b. Lysozyme
    c. Mast cells   d. Ig A antibodies

37. **A 10-year-old boy has a fracture of femur. Biochemical evaluation revealed Hb 11.5 gm/dl and ESR 18 mm 1st hr. Serum calcium 12.8 mg/dL, serum phosphorus 2.3 mg/dL, alkaline phosphate 28 Ka units and blood urea 32 mg/dL. Which of the following is the most probable diagnosis in his case:** [AI 04]
    a. Nutritional rickets
    b. Renal rickets
    c. Hyperparathyroidism
    d. Skeletal dysplasia

38. **The current recommendation for breast feeding is that:** [AI 04]
    a. Exclusive breast feeding should be continued till 6 month of age followed by supplementation with additional foods.
    b. Exclusive breast feeding should be continued till 4 month of age followed by supplementation with additional foods.
    c. Colostorum is the most suitable food for a newborn baby but it is best avoided in first two days.
    d. The baby should be allowed to breast feed till one year of age.

39. **Elemental iron and folic acid content of pediatric iron folic acid tablet supplied under RCH program:** [AI 03]
    a. 20 mg iron and 100 microgram folic acid
    b. 40 mg iron and 100 microgram folic acid
    c. 40 mg iron and 50 microgram folic acid
    d. 60 mg iron and 100 microgram folic acid

40. **The vitamin A supplement administered in "Prevention of nutritional blindness in children program" contain:** [AI 03, AIIMS Nov. 05]
    a. 25,000 IU/ml   b. 1 Lakh IU/ml
    c. 3 Lakh IU/ml   d. 5 Lakh IU/ml

41. **Kwashiorkor is characterized by all of the following features except:** [AI 99]
    a. Edema
    b. Patchy depigmentation of hair
    c. Fatty liver
    d. Fatty infiltration of pancreas

42. **Caloric supplementation required for a severely malnourished child (per kg-body weight) is:** [AI 99]
    a. 100 cal/kg   b. 125 cal/kg
    c. 150 cal/kg   d. 175 cal/kg

43. **Exclusive breast feeding may be associated with the following except:** [AI 98]
    a. Hemolysis due to vit K deficiency
    b. Evening colic
    c. Golden colour stool
    d. Prolongation of physiological jaundice

44. **Exclusive breast feeding is at least till:** [AI 98]
    a. 4 months   b. 6 months
    c. 8 months   d. 10 months

45. **A child with alopecia, hyperpigmentation psoriatic dermatitis in genitals and mouth and hypogonadism is likely to be suffering from:** [AI 98]
    a. Cu deficiency   b. Iron deficiency
    c. Zn deficiency   d. Mg deficiency

46. **Exclusive breastfeeding may be associated with all of the following except:** [AI 98, AIIMS 96]
    a. Hemolysis due to vitamin K deficiency
    b. Evening colic
    c. Golden colour stool
    d. Prolongation of physiological jaundice

47. **The amount of calories required in a 1 year of age are:** [AI 96]
    a. 900 Kcal/day   b. 1000 Kcal/day
    c. 1200 Kcal/day   d. 1400 Kcal/day

48. **All are seen in marasmus except:** [AI 95]
    a. Hepatomegaly   b. Muscle wasting
    c. Voracious appetite d. Weight loss

49. **Flaky paint appearance of the skin is seen in:** [AI 95]
    a. Dermatitis   b. Pellagara
    c. Marasmus   d. Kwashiorkor

50. **In Kwashiorkor which immunoglobulin is most affected:** [AI 94]
    a. Ig D   b. Ig A
    c. Ig E   d. Ig M

51. **Kwashiorkor is diagnosed in growth retarded children along with:**   [AI 91]
    a. Edema and mental changes
    b. Hypopigmentation and anemia
    c. Edema and hypopigmentation
    d. Hepatomegaly and anemia

52. **Kwashiorkor is characterised by all except:**   [AI 89]
    a. Dermatitis   b. Edema
    c. Flag sign   d. Alertness

53. **Anti-infective vitamin is:**   [PGI 87, 88, AI 89]
    a. Vitamin B6   b. Vitamin A
    c. Vitamin D   d. Vitamin C

54. **True about breast feeding:**   [PGI Nov. 09]
    a. Best for both preterm and term
    b. 50% energy from protein
    c. Promote lactobacillus growth in bowel
    d. Predispose to necrotising Enterocolitis
    e. Decrease allergic disorders

55. **Manifestations of vitamin c deficiency are:**
                                              [PGI Dec. 08]
    a. Pseudoparalysis   b. Sabre tibia
    c. Epistaxis   d. Craniotabes
    e. Costochondral junction becomes dome shaped

56. **In breast fed infant less chance of enteric infection is due to:**   [PGI Dec. 08]
    a. Alkaline pH of stool
    b. Breast milk nutrients have beneficial effect on immune system
    c. Ig G in breast milk
    d. Bacteroides and clostridium in gut
    e. Sterile nature of breast milk

57. **Benefits of breast milk are:**   [PGI June 08]
    a. Better nutrition   b. Less infection
    c. More diarrhea   d. Less allergy
    e. High sodium contents

58. **Pseudoparalysis in an infant is suggestive of:**
                                              [PGI 06]
    a. Acute rheumatic fever
    b. Vitamin B6 deficiency
    c. Vitamin E deficiency
    d. Vitamin C deficiency

59. **Hypervitaminosis of which of the following will cause bony abnormalities:**   [PGI Dec. 06]
    a. Vit A   b. Vit D
    c. Vit C   d. Vlt E
    e. Vit K

60. **In rickets seen:**   [PGI Dec. 06]
    a. ↑ ALP   b. ↓ALP
    c. Hypo PO_4 in blood   d. Hyper PO_4 in blood
    e. Hyperphosphaturia

61. **Acute complications of PEM:**   [PGI June 05, 06]
    a. Hypothermia   b. Hypoglycemia
    c. Hypokalemia   d. Hypermagnesemia
    e. Eosinophilia

62. **Acute malnutrition is manifested by:** [PGI June 05]
    a. Weight for age   b. Weight for height
    c. Age for height   d. Broca's index
    e. Ponderal index

63. **True about vit. D deficiency rickets:**   [PGI Dec. 04]
    a. Vit. D3 given at a dose of 50-150 mg/day
    b. X-ray knee joint is diagnostic
    c. Rachitic rosary is tender
    d. Increased chances of respiratory tract infection
    e. Hyponatremia

64. **Vitamin A deficiency is characterized by:**
                                              [PGI Dec. 04]
    a. Bitot spot   b. Xerophthalmia
    c. Night blindness   d. Tranta's spot

65. **Zinc deficiency causes:**   [PGI Dec. 03]
    a. Sexual infantilism
    b. Loss of libido
    c. Poor weight gain
    d. Poor wound healing

66. **True about nutritional rickets:**   [PGI Dec. 03]
    a. Craniotabes   b. Multiple fractures
    c. Widening of wrists d. Phosphate in serum
    e. Growth retardation

67. **Vitamin D deficiency rickets is characterised by:**
                                              [PGI June 03]
    a. Increased forehead sweating
    b. Characteristically decreased calcium
    c. Anterior fontanel is widened
    d. Increased alkaline phosphatase

68. **About scurvy true A/E:**   [PGI June 2000]
    a. Subperiosteal hematoma with tenderness
    b. Separation of epiphysis
    c. Increased alkaline phosphatase
    d. Gingival bleeding
    e. Growth retardation

69. **Wimsberger sign is present in:**   [PGI 2000]
    a. Rickets   b. Scurvy
    c. Secondary syphilis d. Tuberculosis

70. **Following are radiological features of scurvy except:**
    [PGI Dec. 99]
    a. Bony thickening
    b. Metaphyseal widening
    c. Metaphyseal calcification
    d. Epiphyseal separation

71. Grade III malnutrition according to IAP is:

[PGI June 99]

    a. 50%   b. 51–60%
    c. 61–80%   d. 81–100%

72. Splaying and cupping of metaphysis is seen in:

[PGI June 99]

    a. Rickets   b. Scurvy
    c. Chondrodystrophy   d. Syphilis

73. Seen in rickets all except: [PGI June 98]
    a. Cupping of metaphysis
    b. Defective mineralisation
    c. Epiphyseal dysgenesis
    d. Defective osteoid formation

74. Breast milk storage in a refrigerator is up to:

[PGI Dec. 98, UP 08]

    a. 4 hours   b. 8 hours
    c. 12 hours   d. 24 hours

75. Craniotabes is seen in the following except:

[PGI Dec. 97]

    a. Rickets
    b. Syphilis
    c. Osteogenesis imperfecta
    d. Thalassemia

76. True about serology of rickets is: [PGI June 97]

    Alk PO$_4$ Serum PO$_4$
    a. ↓   ↓
    b. ↑   ↑
    c. ↑   ↓
    d. ↓   ↑

77. Rachitic rosary are seen in all except: [PGI Dec. 97]
    a. Rickets   b. Scurvy
    c. Chondrodystrophy   d. Syphilis

78. A six month old infant fed totally on cow's milk has been brought with bleeding spots, anemia, fever and generalised tenderness. On examination there was swelling in both the lower extremities and the blood count was normal. The most likely diagnosis is: [PGI 96]
    a. Arthritis   b. Poliomyelitis
    c. Osteomyelitis   d. Scurvy

79. All of the following statements are true regarding vitamin A deficiency except: [PGI 96]
    a. Growth retardation is common
    b. Frequent infections can occur
    c. Hydrocephalus is infrequent
    d. Anterior segment of the eye is initially involved

80. Deficiency of vitamin c in infant is best estimated by vitamin c level in: [PGI 95]
    a. Plasma
    b. Urinary excretion
    c. Buffy coat estimation
    d. Adrenal cortical vitamin C estimation

81. The normal calorie requirement for a 5 year old child is: [PGI 93]
    a. 800 calories   b. 1000 calories
    c. 1500 calories   d. 2000 calories

82. Phrynoderma is due to deficiency of:

[Kerala 90, KCET 89, PGI 90]

    a. Vitamin D   b. Niacin
    c. Vitamin A   d. Essential fatty acids

83. Breast milk at room temperature stored for:

[PGI 88]

    a. 4 hrs   b. 8 hrs
    c. 12 hrs   d. 24 hrs

84. Anti-infective vitamin is: [PGI 87, 88, AI 89]
    a. Vitamin B6   b. Vitamin A
    c. Vitamin D   d. Vitamin C

QUESTIONS OF OTHER EXAMINATIONS

85. In Kwashiorkor the letter K is post-fixed to denote:

[MHCET 10]

    a. Weight for height
    b. Skin changes
    c. Edema
    d. Muscle wasting

86. After premature delivery, mother's milk is low in:

[MHCET 10]

    a. Lactose   b. Fat
    c. Protein   d. Sodium

87. Calorie requirement per day of a child weighing 15 kg would be: [MHCET 10]
    a. 1150 kcal   b. 1250 kcal
    c. 1450 kcal   d. 1550 kcal

88. Which of the following is not the correct sign of good attachment of a baby to the breast?   [UPSC 09]
    a. Baby's mouth wide open
    b. Lower areola more visible
    c. Baby's lower lip everted
    d. Baby's chin touching the breast.

89. Which of the following is not a sign of active rickets?

[COMED 09]

    a. Prominent fontanel   b. Hot cross bun sign
    c. Saddle nose   d. Caries teeth

90. All of the following conditions are observed in Marasmus, except: [AIIMS May 05, DPG 09]
    a. Hepatomegaly   b. Muscle wasting
    c. Low insulin levels   d. Extreme weakness

91. **The protective effects of breast milk are known to be associated with:**   [AI 05, DPG 09]
    a. Ig M antibodies   b. Lysozyme
    c. Mast cells   d. Ig A antibodies

92. **With reference to malnourished child, the follow-ing statements are correct except:**   [UPSC 09]
    a. Skin and mucosa are not effective barriers to infection
    b. There is impairment of chemotaxis associated with defective candidicidal, bactericidal capacities of polymorphs
    c. There is impairment of cell mediated immunity and delayed hypersensitivity
    d. There is impairment of humoral response to immunizing agents and reduces number of B cells

93. **Mostly death in PEM is due to all except:**   [DPG 09]
    a. Hypothermia   b. CCF
    c. Worm infestation   d. Electrolyte imbalance

94. **The skin changes seen in protein energy malnutri-tion can be due to deficiency of all of the following nutrients except:**   [DPG 09]
    a. Zinc   b. Tryptophan
    c. Essential fatty acids   d. Pyridoxine

95. **Deficiency of which element can lead to syndrome of growth failure, anemia and hypogonadism:**   [COMED 09]
    a. Calcium   b. Copper
    c. Zinc   d. Magnesium

96. **Abnormalities of copper metabolism are implica-ted in the pathogenesis of all the following except:**   [UPSC 09]
    a. Wilson's disease
    b. Menke's kinky hair syndrome
    c. Indian childhood cirrhosis
    d. Keshan disease

97. **When can a severely malnourished child be safely discharged from the hospital?**   [UPSC 08]
    a. The child attains height for age
    b. The child reaches his ideal weight for height
    c. The child loses edema and starts gaining weight
    d. The child attains weight for his age

98. **Hind milk is richer in:**   [COMED 07]
    a. Carbohydrate   b. Protein
    c. Fat   d. Minerals

99. **Para amino benzoic acid of breast milk prevents the infection of:**   [UP 07]
    a. *Plasmodium vivax*   b. *Klebsiella pneumonia*
    c. Giardia   d. *E. coli*

100. **One of the following is false regarding complica-tions of protein energy malnutrition:**   [COMED 07]
    a. Hyperglycemia   b. Hyperthermia
    c. Septic shock   d. Electrolyte imbalance

101. **Which one of the following vitamin deficiencies causes corneal vascularisation, poor growth and photophobia:**   [UPSC 07]
    a. Riboflavin   b. Pyridoxine
    c. Niacin   d. Thiamine

102. **Breast milk is maximum at:**   [APPG 04]
    a. 1–2 months   b. 3–4 months
    c. 5–6 months   d. 7–8 months

103. **Rett's syndrome occurs due to deficiency of:**   [Kerala 04]
    a. Niacin   b. Biotin
    c. Carotene   d. Vitamin D

104. **Child with frog like position and resistance to move the limbs:**   [CMC 2001]
    a. Scurvy   b. Rickets
    c. Trauma   d. Congenital dislocations

105. **Pseudoparalysis is seen in:**   [CMC 2001]
    a. Scurvy   b. Rickets
    c. Polio   d. Osteomalacia

106. **Kwashiorkor in GhanianGa language means:**   [Kerala 2000]
    a. Condition seen in 2nd child
    b. Condition seen in displaced child
    c. Condition seen in cousin
    d. Condition seen in step child
    e. Condition seen in 3rd child

107. **Breast milk storage in a refrigerator is up to:**   [PGI Dec. 98, UP 08]
    a. 4 hours   b. 8 hours
    c. 12 hours   d. 24 hours

108. **The following are radiographic features of rickets except:**   [KCET 96]
    a. Increased in width of growth plate
    b. Decreased bone density
    c. Rachitic rosary
    d. Subperiosteal bleeding

109. **The substance that has anti infective property directly or indirectly in the milk are all except:**   [JIPMER 95]
    a. Lactoferrin   b. Lactalbumin
    c. Lysozyme   d. Nucleotides

110. **Growth retardation, taste alteration, hepatospleno-megaly, hypochromic microcytic anemia, loss of hair, hypogonadism in a boy indicate deficiency of:**   [KCET 95]
    a. Selenium   b. Copper
    c. Zinc   d. Iron

111. **Human colostrum contains more of the following nutrients than mature human milk except:**   [KCET 94]
    a. Lactose   b. Minerals
    c. Proteins   d. Vitamin A

112. One year old baby exclusively breast fed has a 1 cm hepatomegaly, severe pallor and no splenomegaly. The most important investigation is: [TN 90]
a. B 12 estimation
b. Serum iron estimation
c. Folic acid estimation
d. Fetal hemoglobin estimation

113. Phrynoderma is due to deficiency of:
[Kerala 90, KCET 89, PGI 90]
a. Vitamin D
b. Niacin
c. Vitamin A
d. Essential fatty acids

114. Costochondral junction swelling are seen in:
[JIPMER 87]
a. Scurvy
b. Rickets
c. Chondrodystrophy
d. All of the above

115. Breast feeding should begin ....hours after delivery:
a. 2   b. 4
c. 8   d. 12

116. Toad skin is seen in deficiency of vitamin:
a. A   b. B
c. D   d. Biotin

ANSWERS

MULTIPLE CHOICE QUESTIONS

1. (a) Cow's milk contains 80% whey protein not casein (Ref: Rudolph 22nd E/P99)

"Mature human milk provides a protein content of approximately 0.9g/100 ml with 60% whey and 40% casein compared with 3.3g/100 ml protein in **cow milk** with **18% whey** and **82% protein**."

Contents	Cow milk (gm/l)	Human milk (gm/l)
Proteins	More i.e. 33 60% whey 40% casein	Less i.e. 11 18% whey 82% protein
Carbohydrates **e.g. Lactose**	**Less i.e. 50**	**More i.e. 70**
Fats (Linoleic acid)	More i.e. 3.5	Less i.e. 1
Minerals	More i.e.	Less i.e.
Calcium	1400	350
Phosphorous	900	150
Iron	1	0.15
Sodium	25	6.5
Chloride	29	12

2. (a) Rate of increase of height and weight (Ref: Ghai 7th E/P6, 62)

Age dependent factors like height and weight are **best indicators of growth and malnutrition.**

Factors	Indicator	Type of malnutrition
Low height for age	Stunting	Chronic
Low weight for height	Wasting	Acute
Low weight for age	Underweight	Acute and chronic

3. (b) Pyridoxine (Ref: Nelson 19th E/P 193)
"Four clinical disturbances caused by vitamin B6 deficiency has been described in humans; convulsions in infants, peripheral neuritis, dermatitis and anemia."
- There are three forms of vitamin B6 i.e. pyridoxine, pyridoxal and pyridoxamine.
- Pyridoxal-5- phosphate (PLP) is the active form which acts as coenzyme in various reactions.
- Manifetation of pyridoxine deficiency:

Manifestations	Cause
Convulsions	As pyridoxal phosphate is coenzyme for both glutamic decarboxylase and gamma aminobutyric acid trans-aminase, pyridoxine deficiency causes decrease in GABA.
Microcytic, hypo-chromic anaemia	As aminolevulinate synthase, the first enzyme in heme synthesis requires PLP as cofactor, pyridoxine deficiency causes decreased Hb synthesis.
Cystathionuria peripheral neuritis dermatitis	Cystithionase is a vitamin B_6 dependent enzyme.
Homocystinemia	As vitamin B_6 is required for conversion of homocysteine to cystathionine.

Note: Pyridoxine at high doses causes sensory neuropathy and ataxia.

4. (b) Defective proximal calcification is the central cause of bone change (Ref: Nelson 18th E/P)

"Vitamin C deficiency results in scurvy, a condition in which formation of collagen and chondroitin sulphate is impaired. Osteoblasts cannot form osteoid and enchondral bone formation cannot take place."

- Bone is made up of a protein matrix called as **osteoid and mineral matrix composed of calcium and phosphorous.**
- Rickets occurs due to **defective mineralization (calcification)** of the matrix of bone at growth plates.
- Scurvy occurs due to **impaired osteoid formation.**

5. (d) Bow legs (Ref: Ghai 7th E/P82)
Classical features of Rickets:

MNEMONIC: HELICOPTER
H — Harrison's groove, Hot cross bun sign
E — Enlarged growth plate
L — Large anterior fontanel
I — Infection of lungs
C — Craniotabes, Caries
O — Os deformity **(Bowlegs/ knock knees/genu valgum and windswept deformity)**
P — Pectus carinatum, Pot belly
T — Tenderness and pain in bone
E — Enlarged ankles and wrists
R — Retardation of growth, Rachitic rosary

- For bowlegs to appear weight of the patient should be beard by the soft bones of leg. The given patient is an infant and hence cannot walk (Infant - Baby till 12 months, baby starts walking after 12 months). So bowlegs will not be seen in this patient.

6. (a) Weight for age (Ref: Ghai 7th E/P62)

Factors	Indicator	Type of malnutrition
Low height for age	Stunting	Chronic
Low weight for height	Wasting	Acute
Low weight for age	Underweight	Acute and chronic

7. (a) Docosahexaenoic acid (Ref: Rudolph 22nd E/P100, Park 20th E/P463)
- Breast milk has high level of essential polyunsaturated fatty acids like **linoleic acid** and α-linolenic acid whose derivatives like arachidonic acid, eicosapentaenoic and **docosahexaenoic (DHA) acid** required for brain development.

8. (a) i.e. Acute malnutrition (Ref: Ghai 7th E/P62)

Factors	Indicator	Type of malnutrition
Low height for age	Stunting	Chronic
Low weight for height	Wasting	Acute1
Lowweight for age	Underweight	Acute and chronic

9. (a) Acute malnutrition (Ref: Ghai 7th E/P62)

Factors	Indicator	Type of malnutrition
Low height for age	Stunting	Chronic
Low weight for height	Wasting	Acute
Low weight for age	Underweight	Acute and chronic

10. (b) 1 Lakh IU/ml (Ref: Park's PSM 20th E/P532)
Vitamin A prophylaxis:

Age group	Oral dose of Vitamin A	Timing
Newborn	50000 IU	At birth
Infants	100000 IU	Once every 4 – 6 months
Children > 1 year of age	200000 IU	Once every 4 – 6 months

11. (a) Hepatomegaly (Ghai 7th E/P67)
Marasmus:
- Prolonged starvation leads to selective depletion of somatic compartment (skeletal muscle) proteins to provide energy.
- Body fat is depleted to provide energy as well as low leptin levels stimulate the release of cortisol which leads to lipolysis. Severe **muscle wasting** and minimal subcutaneous fat is seen which gives the characteristic appearance.
  - ❖ Monkey facies — Buccal pad fat loss that creates wrinkled appearance.
  - ❖ Baggy pants appearance — Loose skin of buttocks hanging down.
- Visceral compartment **(liver)** is spared, hence serum albumin level is normal and there is **no edema.**

- The child appears to be alert.
- Appetite is **good.**

12. (b) Hypophosphatemic rickets (Ghai 7th E/P83, Nelson 19th E/P2345)
Laboratory parameters in different types of rickets: (See Table 1)
- Now comparing the values in question we find that serum:
  - ❖ Ca — Normal
  - ❖ PO_4 — Decreased
  - ❖ ALP — Increased
  - ❖ PTH — Normal
- Thus the patient is having hypophosphatemic rickets.

13. (b) Gunstock deformity (Ref: Ghai 7th E/P82)
Clinical presentation of rickets:

MNEMONIC: HELICOPTER
H — Harrison's groove
E — Enlarged growth plate
L — Large anterior fontanel
I — Increased risk of pulmonary infections
C — Craniotabes
O — Os deformity **(Bowlegs/knock knees/genu valgum and windswept deformity)**
P — Pectus carinatum, Pot belly
T — Tenderness and pain in bone
E — Enlarged ankles and wrists
R — Retardation of growth, Rachitic rosary

14. (a) High blood osmolarity (Ref: Ghai 7th E/P67)
15. (c) Hypophosphatemic rickets (Ghai 7th E P83, Nelson 19th E/P2345)
16. (c) Hypophosphatemic rickets (Ghai 7th E/P83, Nelson 19th E/P2345)
17. (b) 150 Kcal (Ref: Ghai 7th E/P73)
- Gain of weight is the aim of treatment in the third phase, in which 150Kcal/Kg/24 hour is provided to the patient.
18. (b) Rickets (Ref: Ghai 7th E/P82)
19. (b) Rickets (Ref: Ghai 7th E/P82)

Table 1

Type of rickets	Ca	PO₄	ALP	PTH	HCO₃	Urine Ca	Urine PO₄
Vitamin D deficiency	Decreased	Decreased	Increased	Increased	Normal	Decreased	Increased
Vitamin D dependent	Normal or decreased	Normal or decreased	Increased	Increased	Increased	Decreased	Increased
Hypophosphatemic	Normal	Decreased	Increased	Normal	Normal	Decreased	Increased
Hyperparathyroidism	Increased	Decreased	Increased	Increased	Normal	Decreased	Increased
Distal RTA	Decreased	Normal	Increased	Increased	Normal	Increased	Normal

Note: Normal levels of serum Ca = 9–10 mg/dl, PO_4 = 3–4.5 mg/dl, ALP = 30–120 IU/5–15 KA, PTH = 10–55 units

20. (c) 300 microgram (Ref: Ghai 7th E/P79)

Daily recommended allowance of vitamin A:

Infants	300 – 400 μg
Children	400 – 600 μg
Adolescent	700 μg

21. (a) Craniotabes (Ref: Ghai 7th E/P82)

22. (a) Vitamin B (Ref: Riordan's Breast feeding and lactation/P108)

"A mother eating a vegan diet (i.e. without milk or dietary products) may produce milk deficient in vitamin B12."

23. (a) 7.2 gm (Ref: Duggan's nutrition in pediatrics 4th E/P344)

Contents	Cow milk (gm/l)	Human milk (gm/l)
Proteins	More i.e. 33	Less i.e. 11
	60% whey	18% whey
	40% casein	82% protein
Carbohydrates e.g. Lactose	**Less i.e. 50**	**More i.e. 70**
Fats (Linoleic acid)	More i.e. 3.5	Less i.e. 1
Minerals	More i.e.	Less i.e.
Calcium	1400	350
Phosphorous	900	150
Iron	1	0.15
Sodium	25	6.5
Chloride	29	12

- Amount of lactose in human milk is around 70 gm/L or 7 gm/100 ml.

24. (a) Jaundice (Ref: Ghai 7th E/P147)

"The **increased frequency of jaundice in breastfed babies** is not related to characteristics of breast milk but rather to inadequate breast feeding."

25. (b) Evening colic (Ref: Nelson 19th E/P158)

26. (c) Third degree (Ref: Ghai 7th E/P64)
- The appropriate age for a 2 year old child is 12 kg.
- In the given child the weight is 6.4 kg. The degree of malnutrition can be found by comparing the weight i.e. as per Gomez classification.
- Now weight for age = 6.4 × 100 = 53.3%.
- Gomez classification of malnutrition:

Grade of malnutrition	Weight for age
Normal child	90-110 %
1st degree, Mild	75-89 %
2nd degree, Moderate	60-74 %
3rd degree, Severe	**< 60 %**

27. (d) Oliguria (Ref: Nelson 19th E/P189)

Hypervitaminosis D:
- Hypotonia and **muscle weakness.**

- GIT symptoms like **nausea, vomiting, anorexia** and constipation.
- Generalised symptoms like irritability, pallor and polydipsia.
- Metabolic disorders like hypercalcemia and hypercalciuria.
- CVS disorders like aortic valvular stenosis and hypertension.
- Retinopathy, and clouding of the cornea and conjunctiva.
- Renal damage associated with proteinuria and **polyuria.**
- Long bones reveal **metastatic calcification** and generalized osteopetrosis.

28. (c) Immunization to child (Ref: Ghai 7th E/P77)

Prevention of malnutrition:
- Exclusive breastfeeding for first 6 months.
- Introduction of complimentary feed at 6 months of age.
- Vaccination.
- Discouragement of feeding restriction in fevers and diarrhoea.
- Adequate gape in between pregnancies.

29. (b) Decreased osteoid matrix formation (Ref: Ghai 7th E/P91)
- Vitamin C is critical for hydroxylation of lysine and proline which are required in collagen formation.
- **Osteoblasts cannot form osteoid** in scurvy as collagen is an important part of osteoid.

Note: Defective mineralisation is a feature of rickets.

30. (a) Rickets (Ref: Ghai 7th E/P82)

31. (a) Hb<11.5 gm/dl during 3rd trimester of pregnancy (Ref: Park 20th E/P565)

Indicators of nutritional status:

Phenomenon	Indicator
Maternal nutrition Infant and preschool child nutrition	**Birth weight**
	- Proportion of being breast fed and on weaning foods, by age in months
	- **Mortality rate in children of 1-4 years age**
	- If age is known
	❖ Height for age
	❖ Weight for age
	- If age is not known
	❖ **Weight for height**
	❖ Arm circumference
	❖ Clinical signs and syndromes
School child nutrition	- Height for age and weight for height at 7 years or school admission
	- Clinical signs

32. (a) Based on the height retardation (Ref: Park 20th E/P554)

Gomez classification

- Gomez classification is based on comparison of weight of malnourished child to a normal child of same age, which is 50th percentile of Boston standards. This classification holds good for hospitalised children as the cut off values were obtained from weight of admitted children.

- Weight for age (%)

$$= \frac{\text{Weight of the child}}{\text{Weight of normal child of same age}} \times 100$$

- **Classification:**

Grade of malnutrition	Weight for age
Normal child	90–110 %
1st degree, Mild	75–89 %
2nd degree, Moderate	60–74 %
3rd degree, Severe	< 60 %

33. (a) Lactose (Ref: Rudolph 22nd E/P99)

Contents	Cow milk (gm/l)	Human milk (gm/l)
Proteins	More i.e. 33	Less i.e. 11
	60% whey	18% whey
	40% casein	82% protein
Carbohydrates e.g. Lactose	**Less i.e. 50**	**More i.e. 70**
Fats (Linoleic acid)	More i.e. 3.5	Less i.e. 1
Minerals	More i.e.	Less i.e.
Calcium	1400	350
Phosphorous	900	150
Iron	1	0.15
Sodium	25	6.5
Chloride	29	12

34. (b) Height for age (Ref: Ghai 7th E/P62)

Factors	Indicator	Type of malnutrition
Low height for age	Stunting	Chronic
Low weight for height	Wasting	Acute
Low weight for age	Underweight	Acute and chronic

35. (d) IgA antibodies (Ref: Nelson 19th E/P158)

- "Human milk contains bacterial and viral antibodies including relatively high concentrations of **secretory Ig A** that prevents microorganisms from adhering to the intestinal mucosa."

- About option 'b' Lysozyme Nelson states that "Macrophages in human milk **may synthesize** lactoferrin, lysozyme and complement."

- Thus option b is not wrong but if we have to choose among options b and d then d is a more correct answer as its beneficial role is well established.

36. (d) Ig A antibodies (Ref: Nelson 19th E/P158)

- Breast milk has high concentration of **Ig A** that prevents microorganisms from adhering to intestinal mucosa.

- Macrophages in human milk **may synthesize lysozyme, complement and Lactoferrin.** Lactoferrin has an inhibitory effect on growth of E.coli.

- Bile stimulated lipase in human milk kills Giardia Lamblia and Entamoeba Histolytica.

- **Decreased incidence of infections** like respiratory infections, otitis media, bacteremia and meningitis is seen because of various viral and bacterial **Ig G antibodies;** and various substances that inhibit the growth of viruses.

- Though more than one option is correct, the best answer is Ig A as its effect is more established and important for the baby.

37. (c) Hyperparathyroidism (Nelson 19th E/P1895)

- Serum calcium level is increased and ALP level is also increased which can be seen with hyperparathyroidism.

- All other options will lead to decreased calcium levels.

38. (a) Exclusive breast feeding should be continued till 6 month of age followed by supplementation with additional foods (Ref: Ghai 7th E/P60).

- Breast feeding is initiated within **1 hour** after normal delivery and **4 hours** after caesarean section.

- Exclusive breast feeding is recommended till **6 months** of age.

39. (a) 20 mg iron and 100 microgram folic acid (Ref: Nutrition in children in developing countries/P498)

- Recommendation of dosage by National nutritional anemia control programme — In preschool children i.e. 1–5 years of age a pediatric tablet containing 20 mg of iron and 100 mcg of folic acid is given daily for 100 days in a year.

40. (b) 1 Lakh IU/ml (Ref: Park's PSM 20th E/P532)

Vitamin A prophylaxis:

Age group	Oral dose of Vitamin A	Timing
Newborn	50000 IU	At birth
Infants	100000 IU	Once every 4–6 months
Children > 1 year of age	200000 IU	Once every 4–6 months

41. (d) Fatty infiltration of Pancreas (Ref: Ghai 7th E/P67)

Kwashiorkor:

- Protein deprivation is relatively more than calorie deficiency.

- There is selective loss of protein from visceral compartment **(liver)** and hence leads to hypoalbuminemia.

- Decreased serum albumin leads to **generalized edema** which masks the severe weight loss.
- Relative sparing of subcutaneous fat and muscle mass gives sugar baby appearance.
- Skin pigmentation called as **flaky paint appearance** or enamel spots is seen.
- Alternate bands of hypopigmentation and normally **pigmented hair** are called as **flag sign.**
- Affected child is **apathic, irritable and cries intermittently.**
- Appetite is decreased.

42. (c) 150 cal/kg (Ghai 7th E/P73)

Treatment of malnutrition: Patient is managed in 3 different stages—

- **First stage** — During first 24–48 hours dehydration and infections are dealt with adequate rehydration therapy and good antibiotic coverage respectively.
- **Second stage** — Then for next 7–10 days along with antibiotic therapy, patient is put on a diet of 75 cal/Kg required to maintain the protein and energy need.
- **Third stage** — This stage is aimed at restoring the patient's protein and fat content of the body by providing a diet of up to 150 Kcal/kg/24 hours.

43. (b) Evening colic (Ref: Nelson 19th E/P158)

- **Decreased incidence of allergy** and/or intolerance to cow milk is seen, as epidermal growth factor present in breast milk enhances the maturation of intestinal cells. There is **decreased incidence of evening colic,** "spitting up", occult malena and atopic eczema.

44. (b) 6 months (Ref: Ghai 7th E/P60)

45. (c) Zn deficiency (Ref: Harrison 18th E/CHAPTER 74, TABLE 74–2)

Manifestations of zinc deficiency:

- **Growth retardation**
- Decreased taste and smell
- Alopecia
- Dermatitis
- Diarrhea
- **Immune dysfunction**
- Failure to thrive
- **Gonadal atrophy**
- Congenital malformations
- **Poor wound healing**
- Hepatosplenomegaly

Also know:

Mineral deficiency	Presentation
Selenium	• Cardiomyopathy • Heart failure • Striated muscle degeneration
Molybdenum	• Severe neurologic abnormalities

Fluoride	• Dental caries
Chromium	• Impaired glucose tolerance
Copper	• Anemia
	• Growth retardation
	• Defective keratinization
	• Pigmentation of hair
	• Hypothermia
	• Degenerative changes in aortic elastin
	• Osteopenia
	• Mental deterioration

46. (b) Evening colic (Ref: Nelson 19th E/P158)

47. (c) 1200 Kcal/day (Ref: Park 20th E/P552)

Recommended daily allowance in children:

Age group	KiloCalories required per day
0–6 months	108/kg
6–12 months	98/kg
1–3 years	**1240**
4–6 years	1690
7–9 years	1950

48. (a) Hepatomegaly (Ref: Ghai 7th E/P67)

Marasmus:

- Prolonged starvation leads to selective depletion of somatic compartment (skeletal muscle) proteins to provide energy.
- Body fat is depleted to provide energy as well as low leptin levels stimulate the release of cortisol which leads to lipolysis.
- Severe **muscle wasting** and minimal subcutaneous fat gives appearance of monkey facies and baggie pants.
  - ❖ **Monkey facies** — Buccal pad fat loss that creates wrinkled appearance.
  - ❖ **Baggy pants appearance** — Loose skin of buttocks hanging down.
- Visceral compartment **(liver)** is spared, hence serum albumin level is normal and there is **no edema.**
- The child appears to be alert.
- Appetite is **good.**

49. (d) Kwashiorkor (Ghai 7th E/P67)

50. (b) Ig A (Ref: Duggan Nutrition in Pediatrics 4th E/P131)

Effect of malnutrition on immune system:

- Cell mediated immunity is compromised. The thymus is reduced in size and T8 > T4 cell production is reduced.
- **Humoral immunity** — Immunoglobulin production by B cells is normal or increased. However **secretory Ig A production is reduced** which can compromise the mucosal immunity.
- Complement production is usually decreased (C3 > C4).
- Phagocytic activity of polymorphnuclear cells is impaired.

51. **(a)** Edema and mental changes (Ref: Ghai 7th E/P67)
Kwashiorkor:
- Protein deprivation is relatively more than calorie deficiency.
- There is selective loss of protein from visceral compartment **(liver)** and hence leads to hypo-albuminemia.
- Decreased serum albumin leads to **generalized edema** which masks the severe weight loss.
- Relative sparing of subcutaneous fat and muscle mass gives sugar baby appearance.
- Skin pigmentation called as **flaky paint appearance** or enamel spots is seen.
- Alternate bands of hypopigmentation and normally **pigmented hair** are called as **flag sign.**
- Affected child is **apathic, irritable and cry intermittently (mental changes).**

52. **(d)** Alertness (Ghai 7th E/P67)

53. **(b)** Vitamin A (Ghai 7th E/P79)
- Vitamin A has immunomodulatory function and deficiency can lead to leukopenia and infections like measles.

54. **(a), (c)** and **(e)** Best for both preterm and term, Promote lactobacillus growth in bowel, Decrease allergic disorders (Ref: Ghai 7th E/P122–29)
- Breast milk is the best food for both preterm and term neonates.
- It contains all the essential micronutrients (vitamins and minerals) and macronutrients (10% proteins, **40% carbohydrates** and 50% fats) required for the growth of baby.
- It has **more lactose** than any other milk which is required for **growth of lactobacillus** in intestine as lactose inhibits growth of harmful bacteria in intestine by secreting lactic acid which keeps intestinal pH low.
- Baby who are on formula feed are at increased risk of necrotising Enterocolitis but breast milk is protective.
- Breast fed babies are **less prone to develop allergic and chronic disorders** like diabetes, heart disease and lymphoma in future.

55. **(a)** and **(c)** Pseudoparalysis and Epistaxis (Ref: Ghai 7th E/P91)
Weakening of collagen in various parts of body is seen in scurvy:
- **Blood vessels —** Fragility of blood vessels present as purpura, ecchymosis, perifollicular hemorrhages, gum bleeding, subperiosteal bleeding and epistaxis.
- **Bones and cartilage —** Osteoblasts cannot form osteoid as collagen is an important part of osteoid. This leads to epiphyseal separation, rosary at the costochondral junction, depression of the sternum

and arthralgia. The pain results in **pseudo-paralysis** i.e. decreased movement at joints and the characteristic position in which baby lies is legs flexed at knees and hips partially flexed and externally rotated.
- **Gums —** Bluish purple, spongy swellings in the mucosa over upper incisors.

56. **(b), (c)** and **(e)** Breast milk nutrients have beneficial effect on immune system, Ig G in breast milk and Sterile nature of breast milk (Ref: Nelson 19th E/P158)
- Lactose in breast milk forms lactic acid which is required for acidic environment to prevent growth of pathogenic organisms.
- Breast milk Macrophages in human milk **may synthesize lysozyme, complement and Lacto-ferrin.** Lactoferrin has an inhibitory effect on growth of *E.coli.* Bile stimulated lipase in human milk kills *Giardia lamblia* and *Entamoeba histolytica.*
- Mother's milk is **free of contaminating bacteria.**

57. **(a), (b)** and **(d)** Better nutrition, Less infection and Less allergy (Ref: Ghai 7th E/P122–27, Nelson 19th E/P158)
- Breast milk is the best food for both preterm and term neonates.
- **Decreased incidence of infections** like respiratory infections, otitis media, bacteremia and meningitis is seen because of various viral and bacterial antibodies; and various substances that inhibit the growth of viruses.
- Decreased gastrointestinal disturbances can be seen because of various factors.
  - ❖ Mother's milk is free of contaminating bacteria.
  - ❖ It has high concentration of **Ig A** that prevents microorganisms from adhering to intestinal mucosa.
  - ❖ Macrophages in human milk **may** synthesize **lysozyme, complement and Lactoferrin.** Lactoferrin has an inhibitory effect on growth of *E.coli.*
  - ❖ Bile stimulated lipase in human milk kills *Giardia lamblia* and *Entamoeba histolytica.*
- Breast fed babies are **less prone to develop allergic and chronic disorders** like diabetes, heart disease and lymphoma in future.
- **Decreased sodium concentration** in human milk has a protective effect on infant's kidney.

58. **(d)** Vitamin C deficiency (Ref: Ghai 7th E/P91)
- The joint pain in scurvy results in **pseudoparalysis** due to decreased movement at joints and the characteristic position in which baby lies is legs flexed at knees and hips partially flexed and externally rotated.

59. (a) and **(b)** Vit A and Vit D (Ref: Ghai 7th E/P80, Nelson 19th E/P181, 189)
Hypervitaminosis:

Vitamin A	Vitamin D
• Generalised symptoms like pruritus, lack of weight gain, irritability and anorexia • Limitation of motion, with tender swelling of the bones • Alopecia • Skin disorders like seborrheic cutaneous lesions and desquamation of the palms and soles • Fissuring of the corners of the mouth • Increased intracranial pressure • Hepatomegaly • Craniotabes • **Hyperostosis affecting several long bones**	• Hypotonia and **muscle weakness** • GIT symptoms like **nausea, vomiting,** anorexia and constipation • Generalised symptoms like irritability, pallor and **polydipsia** • Metabolic disorders like hypercalcemia and hyper-calciuria • CVS disorders like aortic valvular stenosis and hyper-tension • Retinopathy, and clouding of the cornea and conjunctiva • Renal damage associated with proteinuria and **polyuria** • **Long bones reveal meta-static calcification and gene-ralized osteopetrosis**

60. (a), (c) and **(e)** ALP, Hypo PO4 in blood and Hyper-phosphaturia (Ghai 7th E/P82) (See Table 2)

61. (a), (b) and **(c)** Hypothermia, Hypoglycemia and Hypokalemia (Ref: Ghai 7th E/P69, Nelson 19th E/P172)

Complications of Protein energy malnutrition:
- **H — Hypoglycemia , Hypothermia**
- **I —** Infections
- **D —** Dehydration,

Deficiency of micronutrients and vitamins
1. Iron - Microcytic,hypochronic anemia
2. Vitamin A - Xeropthalmia, night blindness, **bitot spots,** Keratomalacia and growth faliure
3. Vitamin B12 - Megaloblastic anemia
4. Vitamin C - Scurvy
5. Vitamin D - Rickets
- **E —** Electrolyte imbalance
  1. Hyponatremia
  2. **Hypokalemia**
  3. Hypomagnesemia

62. (b) Weight for height (Ref: Ghai 7th E/P62)

Factors	Indicator	Type of malnutrition
Low height for age	Stunting	Chronic
Low weight for height	Wasting	Acute
Low weight for age	Underweight	Acute and chronic

63. (b) and **(d)** X-ray knee joint is diagnostic , Increased chances of respiratory tract infection (Ref: Ghai 7th E/P83)
- For treatment of vitamin D deficiency rickets, **600,000 IU (15 mg)** of vitamin D is given once or daily for 10 days or **2000–5000 IU**/day for 4–6 weeks.
- X-ray along with the clinical features are mainstay of diagnosis.
- Rachitic rosary is not tender.
- Increased risk of **pneumonia** and **atelectasis** due to impairment in air movement because of softening of ribs.

64. (a), (b) and **(c)** Bitot spot, Xeropthalmia and Night blindness (Ref: Ghai 7th E/P79)
Manifestation of vitamin A deficiency:

Functions of vitamin A	Manifestations of deficiency
11-cis-retinal form of vitamin A is required for night vision	**Night blindness**
Immunomodulatory	Leukopenia and infections like measles
All-trans-retinoic acid pro-motes nuclear transcription and controls epithelial cell differentiation, division and death	• Dry scaly hyperkeratotic skin patches • Diarrhea due to intestinal mucosa damage • Keratinization and opacifi-cation of cornea known as xeropthalmia ↓ Infection and weakening of cornea **Keratomalacia** • Keratinization of conjunctiva leads to plaque formation called as **Bitot spots**
Bone development	Bone overgrowth leads to compressive optic nerve palsy
Fetal development	• Mental retardation • Hydrocephalus • Poor growth

Table 2

Type of rickets	Ca	PO$_4$	ALP	PTH	HCO$_3$	Urine Ca	Urine PO$_4$
Vitamin D deficiency	Decreased	Decreased	Increased	Increased	Normal	Decreased	Increased
Vitamin D dependent	Normal or decreased	Normal or decreased	Increased	Increased	Increased	Decreased	Increased
Hypophosphatemic	Normal	Decreased	Increased	Normal	Normal	Decreased	Increased
Hyperparathyroidism	Increased	Decreased	Increased	Increased	Normal	Decreased	Increased
Distal RTA	Decreased	Normal	Increased	Increased	Normal	Increased	Normal

(Ref: Harrison 18th E/Chapter 74, Table 74-2)

65. Manifestations of zinc deficiency:

- **Growth retardation**
- Decreased taste and smell
- Alopecia
- Dermatitis
- Diarrhea
- **Immune dysfunction**
- Failure to thrive
- **Gonadal atrophy**
- Congenital malformations
- **Poor wound healing**
- Hepatosplenomegaly

66. (a), (c), (d) and **(e)** Craniotabes, Widening of wrists, Phosphate in serum and Growth retardation (Ghai 7th E/P82)

Clinical features of rickets:

Mnemonic: HELICOPTER
H — Harrison's groove E — Enlarged growth plate L — Large anterior fontanel I — Increased risk of pulmonary infections C — Craniotabes O — Os deformity **(Bowlegs/knock knees/genu valgum and windswept deformity)** P — Pectus carinatum, Pot belly T — Tenderness and pain in bone E — Enlarged ankles and wrists R — Retardation of growth, Rachitic rosary

- In rickets serum calcium and phosphate are decreased.

67. (c) and **(d)** Anterior fontanel is widened and Increased alkaline phosphatase (Ref: Ghai 7th E/P82)

68. (c) Increased alkaline phosphatase (Ref: Ghai 7th E/P91, Nelson 19th E/P185)

Scurvy is associated with weakening of collagen in various parts of body:

- Blood vessels — Purpura, ecchymosis, perifollicular hemorrhages, **gum bleeding, subperiosteal bleeding**
- Bones and cartilage — **Osteoblasts cannot form osteoid** as collagen is an important part of osteoid. This leads to **epiphyseal separation, rosary at the costochondral junction,** depression of the sternum and arthralgia. The pain results in **pseudoparalysis** i.e. decreased movement at joints and the characteristic position in which baby lies is legs flexed at knees and hips partially flexed and externally rotated.
- Gums — Bluish purple, spongy swellings in the mucosa over upper incisors can be seen.
- Muscle — Weakness and degeneration of skeletal muscle and cardiac muscle.

69. (b) Scurvy (Ref: Sutton's Radiology 6th E/P238)

- **Wimsberger** sign seen in scurvy represents epiphyseal centres of ossification surrounded by a white line.

70. (b) Metaphyseal widening (Ref: Ghai 7th E/P91, Nelson 19th E/P185)

The typical radiological features of scurvy are best seen in the knee joint:

- **White line of Fraenkel** — Zone of well **calcified cartilage at the metaphysis.**
- **Pelkan Spur** — Lateral prolongation of white line.
- **Wimsberger sign** — Epiphyseal centres of ossifica-tion surrounded by a white line.
- Metaphyseal rarefaction zone seen as a triangular defect in the lateral part.
- Ground glass appearance of the bone.
- **Epiphyseal separation**

Note: Metaphyseal widening is a feature of rickets.

71. (b) 51-60% (Ref: Ghai 7th E/P64)

IAP Classification of malnutrition:

Grade of malnutrition	Weight for age value (%)
Normal	>80
Grade I or mild	71-80
Grade II or moderate	61-70
Grade III or severe	**51-60**
Grade IV or very severe	<50

72. (a) Rickets (Ref: Ghai 7th E/P82)

73. (c) and **(d)** Epiphyseal dysgenesis and defective osteoid formation (Ref: Ghai 7th E/P 82)

Radiological sign	Cause
Loss of normal zone of provisional calcification is the earliest sign	Decreased mineralisation of the bone
Fraying of metaphysis	Edge of metaphysis loses its sharp border
Cupping and splaying of metaphysis	Effect of weight on the softened metaphysis
Widening of growth plate	Lack of metaphyseal calcification

74. (d) 24 hours (Ref: Ghai 7th E/P127)

Storage of expressed breast milk:

Method of storage	Time of storage
Room temperature	6–8 hours
Refrigerator	24 hours
Freezer at –20 °C	3 months

75. (d) Thalassemia (Ref: Nelson 19th E/P181, 187)

Causes of craniotabes:

- Prematurity
- **Rickets**
- Hypervitaminosis A
- **Osteogenesis imperfecta**
- Hydrocephalus
- **Syphilis.**

76. (c) (Ref: Ghai 7th E/P82)

77. (d) Syphilis (Ref: http://radiopaedia.org/articles/rachitic-rosary)
- A **rachitic rosary** refers to expansion of the anterior rib ends at the costochondral junctions and is most frequently seen in rickets.
- Causes
    ❖ Rickets
    ❖ Scurvy
    ❖ Chondrodystrophy.

78. (d) Scurvy (Ref: Ghai 7th E/P91)
- Symptoms like bleeding spots, anemia, fever and generalised tenderness indicate towards scurvy.
- Further it is consolidated by the fact that the baby was exclusively fed with cow's milk.

79. (d) Anterior segment of the eye is initially involved (Ref: Ghai 7th E/P79)

80. (c) Buffy coat estimation (Ref: Nelson 19th E/P186)
- Leucocyte concentration of vitamin C is the best indicator of body stores, which is estimated by **buffy coat preparation,** but it is a difficult test to perform.
- Urinary vitamin C excretion after administration of a test dose is usually performed. Excretion of less than 80% of administered dose indicates deficiency of vitamin C.
- Plasma and serum vitamin C is a poor indicator of body stores.

81. (c) 1500 calories (Ref: Park 20th E/P552)
Recommended daily allowance in children:

Age group	KiloCalories required per day
0–6 months	108/kg
6–12 months	98/kg
1–3 years	**1240**
4–6 years	1690
7–9 years	1950

82. (d) Vitamin A (Ref: Thappa Clinical Pediatric Dermatology/P160)

"**Phrynoderma (Toad skin)** is a type of follicular hyperkeratosis typically seen in **vitamin A deficiency.** This eruption has also been seen with deficiencies of vitamin B complex, C and E, calories and essential fatty acids."

83. (b) 8 hrs (Ref: Ghai 7th E/P127)

84. (b) Vitamin A (Ghai 7th E/P79)
- Vitamin A has immunomodulatory function and deficiency can lead to leukopenia and infections like measles.

85. (c) Edema (Ref: Partha Pediatrics/P103)

86. (a) Lactose (Ref: Ghai 7th E/P125)

87. (b) 1250 kcal (Ref: Ghai 7th E/P90)

88. (b) Lower areola more visible (Ref: Ghai 7th E/P126)

Signs of good attachment during breast feeding:
- Baby's mouth should be wide open
- **Only the upper areola should be visible**
- Baby's chin should touch the breast
- Baby's lower lip should be everted.

89. (c) Saddle nose (Ref: Ghai 7th E/P82)

90. (a) Hepatomegaly (Ghai 7th E/P67)
Marasmus:
- Prolonged starvation leads to selective depletion of somatic compartment (skeletal muscle) proteins to provide energy.
- Body fat is depleted to provide energy as well as low leptin levels stimulate the release of cortisol which leads to lipolysis. Severe **muscle wasting** and minimal subcutaneous fat is seen which gives the characteristic appearance.
    ❖ Monkey facies — Buccal pad fat loss that creates wrinkled appearance.
    ❖ Baggy pants appearance — Loose skin of buttocks hanging down.
- Visceral compartment **(liver)** is spared, hence serum albumin level is normal and there is **no edema.**
- The child appears to be alert.
- Appetite is **good.**

91. (d) Ig A antibodies (Ref: Nelson 19th E/P158)
- Breast milk has high concentration of **Ig A** that prevents microorganisms from adhering to intestinal mucosa.
- Macrophages in human milk **may synthesize lysozyme, complement and Lactoferrin.** Lactoferrin has an inhibitory effect on growth of E.coli.
- Bile stimulated lipase in human milk kills Giardia Lamblia and Entamoeba Histolytica.
- **Decreased incidence of infections** like respiratory infections, otitis media, bacteremia and meningitis is seen because of various viral and bacterial **Ig G antibodies;** and various substances that inhibit the growth of viruses.
- Though more than one option is correct, the best answer is Ig A as its effect is more established and important for the baby.

92. (d) There is impairment of humoral response to immunizing agents and reduces number of B cells (Ref: Duggan Nutrition in Pediatrics 4th E/P131)
Effect of malnutrition on immune system:
- Cell mediated immunity is compromised. The thymus is reduced in size and T8>T4 cell production is reduced.
- Humoral immunity — Immunoglobulin production by B cells is normal or increased. However secretory Ig A production is reduced which can compromise the mucosal immunity.
- Complement production is usually decreased (C3 > C4).
- Phagocytic activity of polymorphnuclear cells is impaired.

93. **(c)** Worm infestation (Ref: Ghai 7th E/P68)
    Causes of death in malnutrition:
    - Hypoglycemia
    - Hypothermia
    - Electrolyte imbalance
    - Heart failure
    - Infections

94. **(d)** Pyridoxine (Ghai 7th E/P59, 92)

95. **(c)** Zinc (Ref: Ghai 7th E/P92)

96. **(d)** Keshan disease (Ref: Ghai 7th E/P93)
    Disorders associated with copper deficiency and abnormal metabolism:

Mnemonic: WILMS
• **W** — Wilson's disease • **I** — Indian childhood cirrhosis • **L** — Long bone abnormalities like cupping, flaring, periosteal elevation and fractures • **M** — Menke's steely hair syndrome, Microcytic hypochromic anemia • **S** — Seborrheic dermatitis

Note: Keshan disease is caused by selenium deficiency.

97. **(c)** The child loses edema and starts gaining weight (Ref: Ghai 7th E/P75)
    Criteria for discharge of severely malnourished child:
    - Attainment of 90% of NCHS median of weight for height and has no edema.
    - Child is alert and active and taking at least 120–130 Kcal/kg/day, with consistent weight gain on oral feeding
    - No infection
    - Complete immunization for age
    - Adequate micronutrient supplement

98. **(c)** Fat (Ghai 7th E/P125)

Fore milk	Hind milk
Milk secreted at the beginning of feeding. It is rich in: • **Water**—Quenches thirst of baby. • **Protein** • Sugar • Vitamin • Minerals	Milk secreted at the end phase of feeding. It is rich in: **Fat content**—Satisfies hunger of baby and provides energy.

99. **(a)** Plasmodium vivax (Ref: Parathasarthy pediatrics/P102)

100. **(a)** and **(b)** Hyperglycemia and hyperthermia (Ref: Ghai 7th E/P69–70)

101. **(a)** Riboflavin (Ref: Ghai 7th E/P87)

102. **(c)** 5–6 months (Ref: Ghai 19th E/P422)

103. **(a)** Niacin (Ref: Coleman The Biology of Autistic syndromes/P208)

"In **Rett syndrome,** decreased amount of **nicotinamide (vitamin B3)** have been reported."

104. **(a)** Scurvy (Ref: Ghai 7th E/P91)
    - This is a case of scurvy presenting with pseudoparalysis.

105. **(a)** Scurvy (Ref: Ghai 7th E/P120)

106. **(b)** Condition seen in displaced child (Ref: Riordan breast feeding and human lactation/811)
    - In Ghanian language Ga, 'Kwashiorkor' means the disease of displaced child, where by a baby is displaced from mother's breast and develops malnutrition.

107. **(d)** 24 hours (Ref: Ghai 7th E/P127)
    Storage of expressed breast milk:

Method of storage	Time of storage
Room temperature	6-8 hours
Refrigerator	24 hours
Freezer at –20 °C	3 months

108. **(c)** Rachitic rosary (Ref: Ghai 7th E/P82)
    - Rachitic rosary is found on clinical examination and not on X-ray.

109. **(d)** Nucleotides (Ref: Duggan Nutrition in pediatrics 4th E/P346)

110. **(c)** Zinc (Ref: Ghai 7th E/P92)

111. **(a)** Lactose (Ref: Ghai 7th E/P125)

Time	Milk type	Constituents
3-4 days post delivery	Colostrum	Rich in protein, antibodies, minerals and vitamin A, D, E and K but **less carbohydrate**
4th day – 2nd week	Transitional milk	Rich in fat and carbohydrate but protein and antibodies decrease
2nd week onwards	Mature milk	Less viscous but contains all nutrients for normal growth

112. **(b)** Serum iron estimation (Ref: Nelson 19th E/P158)
    - Iron is limited in human milk; however the baby has sufficient stores for 6 months and hence should be supplemented with iron **after 6 months of age.**
    - This baby of 1 year on exclusively breast milk has developed iron deficiency anemia. Hence serum iron should be estimated for diagnosis.

113. **(d)** Vitamin A (Ref: Thappa Clinical Pediatric Dermatology/P160)

"Phrynoderma (Toad skin) is a type of follicular hyperkeratosis typically seen in **vitamin A deficiency.** This eruption has also been seen with deficiencies of vitamin B complex, C and E, calories and essential fatty acids."

114. **(d)** All of the above (Ref: http://radiopaedia.org/articles/rachitic-rosary)

115. **(a)** 2 (Ref: Nelson 19th E/P157)

116. **(a)** A (Ref: Thappa Clinical Pediatric Dermatology/P160)

Cardiovascular System

4

CONGENITAL HEART DISEASES

Congenital heart diseases **(CHD)**are abnormalities of the heart or great vessels caused by faulty embryogenesis between 3rd and 8th week, when major cardiovascular structures form and begin to function. These are the most common cause of mortality in children with congenital malformation. Various genetic and environmental factors can be attributed to the cause of congenital heart disease. Based on the pathophysiological changes caused by the abnormalities in heart, congenital heart diseases can be broadly divided in to conditions causing abnormal connections between different chambers of heart or great vessels **(left to right shunt and right to left shunt)** and **obstructive lesions,** restricting free blood flow. **Nada's criteria** are used for the assessment of presence of heart diseases in children.

Genetic Factors

- Single gene mutation in genes can give rise to:
  - ❖ **Noonan syndrome** — Pulmonary stenosis and hypertrophic cardiomyopathy,**ASD**
  - ❖ **Apert syndrome** — Coarctation of aorta and VSD
  - ❖ **Holt-Oram syndrome** — **ASD** and VSD
  - ❖ **Ellis-Van creveld syndrome** — Single atrium, **ASD**
  - ❖ **TAR (Thrombocytopenia-Absent Radius) syndrome** — **ASD** and TOF.
  - ❖ **DiGeorge syndrome** — Cardiac outflow tract defects
  - ❖ **Alagille syndrome** — Pulmonary artery stenosis, Tetralogy of Fallot
- Chromosomal abnormalities can give rise to:
  - ❖ Cridu chat syndrome
  - ❖ **Down syndrome – ASD**
  - ❖ Trisomy 13
  - ❖ Trisomy 18

  VSD is the most common cardiac lesion seen in these conditions.

  - ❖ Turner syndrome – Bicuspid aortic valve and coarctation of aorta are commonly seen.

Environmental Factors

- Exposure to teratogenic drugs and substances like **lithium (Ebstein's anomaly),** retinoic acid, alcohol and progesterone can cause CHD.
- Maternal diseases like gestational diabetes most commonly gives rise to **transposition of great vessels**, however **sacral agenesis** is more specific.
- Viral infection of mother during pregnancy like **rubella (PDA** and pulmonary stenosis), coxscakie virus and mumps (Endocardial fibroelastosis) can cause CHD.

CHD Causing Left to Right Shunt

These lesions are also called as **acyanotic CHD** as initially they increase the pulmonary blood flow, which triggers adaptation mechanisms in the circulation by causing medial hypertrophy and vasoconstriction. Gradually the pulmonary pressure surpasses the systemic pressure and the flow changes from right to left (shunt reversal - Eisenmenger syndrome).

Pathophysiology of Acyanotic Heart Diseases

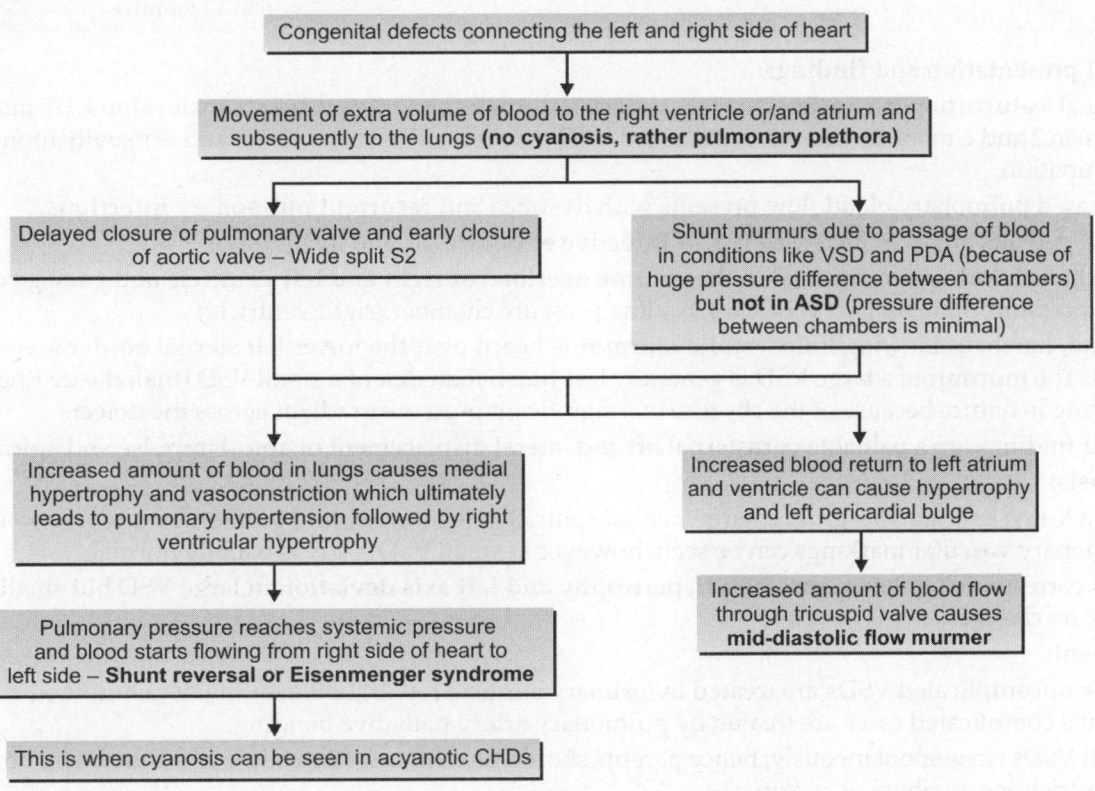

Fig. 4.1

Eisenmenger Syndrome

It is defined as an increase in the pulmonary vascular resistance by a ratio of pulmonary to systemic ratio of **more than 1.** It is **usually seen in patients with VSD** but can be associated with **ASD, PDA** or any aortopulmonary connection.

- **Clinical presentation**

  Patients become symptomatic usually after 3rd decade of life with initial mild presentations like cyanosis, fatigue and dyspnea which can progress to heart failure. The clinical findings can be a right ventricular heave, **loud single or narrow split S$_2$, loud P$_2$** and murmurs of tricuspid regurgitation and pulmonary insufficiency (early decrescendo diastolic murmur or **Ghram steel murmur**).

- **Diagnosis**
  - ❖ X-ray shows a prominent pulmonary artery, **enlarged pulmonary vessels in the hilar areas which taper down at the periphery.**
  - ❖ Echocardiographical **"W" sign** is the characteristic sign of early midsystolic closure of the pulmonary valve.
  - ❖ **Pulmonary capillary wedge pressure is usually normal.**

- **Treatment**

  The best way of treatment is to prevent it in infancy by surgical approach. However once it has developed the patient is given symptomatic (phlebotomy with volume replacement for polycythemia), medical (calcium channel blocker and prostacyclin analogue i.e. epoprosterenol) and/or surgical (combined heart-lung or bilateral lung transplantation) treatment.

Ventricular Septal Defect (VSD)

VSD is the **most common form of CHD,** which results from incomplete closure of ventricular septum. Morphologically VSDs can be classified based on their site of location.

Membranous VSD	Infundibular VSD	Muscular VSD
• This is the **most common type of VSD post infancy** involving membranous interventricular septum.	• These are located below the pulmonary valve.	• This is the most **common type of VSD at birth,** located in the muscular septum, however close spontaneously between 6 to 12 months.

- **Clinical presentation and findings:**
    - ❖ Clinical features depend on the size of the defect. If the defect is large the baby can develop **CHF** most commonly between 2 and 6 months, whereas small sized VSD may remain asymptomatic and is usually found in a routine examination.
    - ❖ Increased pulmonary blood flow presents with dyspnea and **recurrent pulmonary infections.**
    - ❖ These patients are at an increased risk of **infective endocarditis** and arrhythmia.
    - ❖ The clinical findings correspond to the **volume overload of right and left ventricle** and passage of blood from high pressure chamber (left ventricle) to a low pressure chamber (right ventricle).
    - ❖ A loud, harsh, or blowing **holosystolic murmur** is heard over the lower left sternal border accompanied by a thrill. The murmur of a large VSD is generally less harsh than that of a small VSD (maladie de Roger) and more blowing in nature because of the absence of a significant pressure gradient across the defect.
    - ❖ Other findings are a palpable parasternal lift and lateral displacement of apical impulse and apical thrust.
- **Diagnosis:**
    - ❖ **Chest X-ray:** In large VSD gross enlargement of ventricles, left atrium, and pulmonary artery as well as increased pulmonary vascular markings can be seen, however in small VSD X-ray is usually normal.
    - ❖ **ECG** corresponds to **left ventricular hypertrophy and left axis deviation** in large VSD but small VSD usually show no change.
- **Treatment:**
    - ❖ Large uncomplicated VSDs are treated by primary surgical repair, however in later childhood and premature infant's complicated cases are treated by pulmonary artery palliative banding.
    - ❖ Small VSDs close spontaneously; hence parents should be encouraged to allow children to live normal life with no restrictions on physical activity.

Atrial Septum Defect (ASD)

There are three different types of ASD, i.e. Ostium primum ASD, ostium secundum ASD and Sinus venosus defect.

Ostium primum ASD	Ostium secundum ASD	Sinus venosus defect
• Seen in 5% of cases	• **Most common type of ASD**, seen in 90% of cases.	• Seen in 5% of cases.
• Located adjacent to AV valves and are caused by abnormal endocardial cushion development.	• Located in the centre of septum and is caused by incomplete closure of hole of septum primum by septum secundum.	• Located in the superior portion of atrial septum, generally extending in to SVC.
• Associated with mitral and tricuspid valve abnormalities as they also develop from endocardial cushion.	• May be associated with **partial anomalous pulmonary venous connection** or pulmonic stenosis.	• May be associated with anomalous pulmonary venous return to right atrium.
• Clinical features — Rarely may present with CHF and arrhythmias in late teenage or early adulthood.	• Clinical features —	
• Most commonly seen with **Down's syndrome.**	❖ **Most commonly seen in females** and may be associated with **Holt Oram syndrome.**	
	❖ Usually defects less than 6mm in diameter close spontaneously, but larger defects may present as failure to thrive in younger and exercise intolerance in older children.	

- Clinical findings on examination secondary to **increased blood flow to the right side** of heart through ASD are:
- ❖ A palpable **right ventricular systolic liftor heave at the left sternal border.**
- ❖ A **fixed and widely split 2nd heart sound.**
- ❖ A **systolic pulmonic ejection click murmur** is produced by the **increased flow across the right ventricular outflow tract into the pulmonary artery, not by low-pressure flow across the ASD.**
- Chest x-ray shows:
  - ❖ **Enlarged right atrium and ventricle.**
  - ❖ Large pulmonary artery.
  - ❖ Increased pulmonary vascularity.
  - ❖ **Small aortic shadow.**

• ECG shows changes corresponding to **left axis deviation**, right ventricular hypertrophy.	• ECG shows changes corresponding to **right axis deviation** and right ventricular hypertrophy.	• Hemodynamic disturbance, clinical features, ECG, and x-ray findings are similar to those seen in secundum ASD.
• Treatment — **Surgical closure** of primary defect is highly effective but subaortic stenosis is a commonly encountered sequel.	• Treatment — **Nonsurgical closure with an umbrella like device (e.g. amplatzer)** is preferred over surgical closure. Elective closure is usually done **after the 1st year and before entry into school.Ref : Rudolph 22ⁿᵈ E/P1812.**	• Treatment — **Surgical closure by patch** and incorporating the entry of anomalous veins into the left atrium.

Note: A **patent foramen ovale (PFO)** is a common finding during infancy, which occurs due to incomplete closure of foramen ovale post birth. It is usually of no hemodynamic significance and **is not considered an ASD.**

Patent Ductus Arteriosus (PDA)

Ductus arteriosus is an essential fetal structure that normally shunts blood from the **pulmonary artery to the aorta**, which serves to bypass the deflated lungs but it closes post birth and forms **ligamentum arteriosum** due to contraction because of decreased prostaglandins and increased oxygen concentration. In the full term infants, the **physiological (functional) closure** occurs within **10 to 15 hours**, whereas the **anatomical closure** may take place only in the **3ʳᵈpostnatal week**. It is two times **more common in females** than males. PDA can be seen in both mature as well as premature infants; however the cause and management differin both cases.

Premature infants	Mature infants
• PDA is caused by **immaturity and hypoxia** (Causes vasodilation). • As time progresses due to improvement in both factors, spontaneous closure occurs in most cases. • If spontaneous closure doesn't occur then **prostaglandin inhibitor indomethacin (As prostaglandins cause vasodilation and interfere with its closure)**, 0.2 mg/kg at 12-24 hr intervals for three doses may induce pharmacologic closure by inhibiting prostaglandin synthesis.	• PDA is caused because ductus is deficient in both the mucoid endothelial and the muscular layer which is required for contraction. • **Rubella infection** in the first trimester of pregnancy is highly associated with PDA. • Because of the anatomical defect, **PDA persisting beyond 1 week in mature infants rarely close spontaneously** or with pharmacological intervention (Prostaglandin inhibitors). • PDA less than 5mm may be treated by trans- catheter coil or an umbrella like device, whereas larger ones require surgical closure by **ligation and division of ductus** by thoracoscopic approach. • Surgery should be preferably done before child attains 1 year of age.Nelson 19ᵗʰ E/P1512

Note: **Pg E1 analogues (misoprostol and alprostadil) are used to maintain patency of ductus arteriosus** in some ductus dependent CHDs. (Remember: Prostaglandin maintains Patency)

Ductus dependent pulmonary blood flow	Ductus dependent systemic blood flow
• **Pulmonary atresia with intact ventricular septum** • Tricuspid atresia • Critical pulmonary stenosis • TOF	• **Coarctation of aorta** • **Aortic arch interruption** • **Hypoplastic left heart syndrome**

- **Clinical presentation and findings:**
  - ❖ A small PDA is usually asymptomatic, but large PDA may result in **CHF** due to volume overload of right and left ventricle and left atrium. **CHF** is the **most common cause of death in adolescents**, however they may present with other frequent complications like **infective endocarditis**, pulmonary or systemic embolism and **pulmonary hemorrhage**. Infective endocarditis is more common with **smaller lesions** and hence requires early closure.
  - ❖ **Bounding peripheral arterial pulses** can be seen because of increased stroke volume (increased systolic B.P). Wide pulse pressure can be seen (**Pulse pressure = systolic B.P – Diastolic B.P**) due to passage of blood into the pulmonary artery during diastole and reflex peripheral vasodilation(decreased diastolic BP).
  - ❖ A prominent apical pulse and systolic thrill is maximally seen in the 2nd left interspace.
  - ❖ **Machinery like or thunder rolling murmur** is heard because of continuous passage of blood from aorta to pulmonary artery. The patient has other features like resting tachycardia, **CO_2 retention**, frequent apnoea and a hyperactive precordium.
  - ❖ **Differential cyanosis** can be seen when PDA is associated with severe pulmonary hypertension or reversal of shunt.
- **Diagnosis:**
  - ❖ **Chest x-ray** shows prominent pulmonary artery with increased intrapulmonary vascular markings and cardiomegaly due to dilation of left atrium and ventricle.
  - ❖ **E.C.G** corresponds to left or biventricular hypertrophy.
  - ❖ **Differential diagnosis**–PDA should be carefully distinguished from other conditions like **aorto-pulmonary window**, truncus arteriosus, VSD with aortic regurgitation and arteriovenous fistula

CHD Causing Right to Left Shunt

Right to left shunt facilitates mixing of poorly oxygenated venous blood with systemic arterial blood and causes **hypoxemia and cyanosis**. Chronic cyanosis causes **clubbing of fingers and toes** (hypertrophic osteoarthropathy) and polycythaemia.The peripheral emboli can directly access to systemic circulation and cause paradoxical **embolism of brain** resulting in **infarction and abscess**.The different lesions associated with right to left shunt and cyanosis are **TOF, tricuspid atresia**, TGA, double outlet right ventricle, TAPVC, truncus arteriosus, double ventricle, **hypoplastic left heart syndrome (Cyanosis is seen at birth)** and **Eisenmenger complex.**

Tetralogy of Fallot (TOF)

Faulty embryogenesis causing misalignment of the outlet septum relative to muscular septum causes unequal division of truncus arteriosus in to small pulmonary and large aortic components. The small pulmonary component results in right ventricular outflow obstruction and hypertrophy. This gives rise to TOF, which primarily consists of four components i.e. **right ventricular outflow tract (infundibular stenosis>pulmonary valve stenosis) obstruction, right ventricular hypertrophy, ventricular septal defect** and **dextroposition of the aorta. Pentalogy of Fallot** consists of the features of tetralogy along with **ASD**.

- **Clinical presentation**

  Though TOF is classically a cyanotic CHD, it may present without cyanosis depending on the magnitude of pulmonic stenosis and patency of PDA.

Acyanotic TOF	*Cyanotic (classical) TOF*
• Insignificant obstruction to right ventricular outflow makes the TOF quite similar to an isolated VSD, as there is no right to left shunt. Such condition is also known as **pink TOF**. • A patent PDA can direct the flow of blood from aorta to pulmonary artery. Thus even if there is significant right ventricular outflow obstruction cyanosis does not occur. Thus relaxation of ductal smooth muscle (dilatation of the ductus arteriosus)by administration of **Pg E1** provides adequate pulmonary blood flow until a surgical procedure can be performed.	• Significant obstruction to right ventricular outflow facilitates movement of deoxygenated blood through VSD to aorta and causes cyanosis.**TOF is the most common cyanotic cardiac lesion.** • **Cyanosis is not seen at birth** and rather towards the end of 1st year. • **Blue spells or hypercyanotic episodes** are caused due to acute reduction in pulmonary blood flow by various reasons like prolonged crying and fever. It is usually seen in first 2 years of life. • Dyspnoea occurs on exertion and the child acquires a **squatting position**, which increases the systemic B.P and increases blood flow to lungs through VSD. • Growth retardation may occur if oxygen saturation is chronically low.

- **Clinical findings in classical TOF:**
  - ❖ A bulge in the anterior hemithorax can be seen because of right ventricular hypertrophy; however **heart is of normal size.** Substernal right ventricular impulse can be felt.
  - ❖ **Loud and harsh ejection systolic murmur is heard at 2nd intercostal space** in left sternal border due to turbulence through the right ventricular outflow tract. **Single loud second sound** corresponding to aortic valve closure is heard. A continuous murmur may be audible if prominent collaterals are present.
  - ❖ Normal venous and arterial pressure keep the **pulse (arterial, venous) normal. JVP** is usually normal.
- **Diagnosis:**
  - ❖ Chest x-ray shows **boot or wooden shoe shaped heart (Coeur en sabot), clear hilar areas and lung fields** because of diminished pulmonary blood flow, large aorta and a right sided aortic arch.
  - ❖ **ECG** corresponds to **right ventricular hypertrophy and right axis deviation.**
- **Complications of classical TOF:**
  - ❖ Extreme polycythaemia and dehydration leads to cerebral thrombosis. It is most commonly seen in children younger than 2 year.
  - ❖ Brain abscess is less common than cerebral thrombosis and usually seen in children older than 2 year.
  - ❖ Bacterial endocarditis is frequently seen, which makes antibiotic prophylaxis compulsory before and after dental and certain surgical procedures.
  - ❖ **CHF is usually not seen in classical TOF** but may be seen in pink TOF.
  - ❖ A **right sided aortic arch** can be seen in association with TOF.
- **Treatment:**
  - ❖ **Corrective surgery** is done usually within 4-12 months of birth.
  - ❖ **Blalock-Taussig shunt (aortopulmonary shunt)** is the **most commonly done** which joins **subclavian artery** to the homolateral branch of the **pulmonary artery. Pott's shunt** joins descending aorta to pulmonary artery and **Waterson's shunt** joins ascending aorta to right pulmonary artery.
  - ❖ **Treatment of cyanotic spell:**
    The main aim in treating a cyanotic spell is to increase oxygenation by providing oxygen and increasing pulmonary blood flow.
    - ❑ Place infant on the abdomen in the knee-chest position.
    - ❑ **Morphine** is useful in terminating a **prolonged and severe attack.**
    - ❑ Beta blockers like **propranolol** are used for prophylaxis to reduce the frequency of attacks.
    - ❑ Administration of oxygen relieves dyspnea.
    - ❑ Drugs increasing systemic B.P like methoxamine or **phenylephrine**, improve right ventricular outflow, decrease the right-to-left shunt, and thus improve the symptoms.
    - ❑ Development of metabolic acidosis warrants intravenous administration of **sodium bicarbonate.**

Transposition of Great Vessels (TGV)

In a normal heart the aorta arises from left ventricle(located on **the right posterior side of pulmonary artery**), whereas pulmonary artery from right ventricle. TGV causes ventriculo-arterial discordance, i.e. aorta arises from right ventricle (located on the **right anterior side of pulmonary artery**) and pulmonary artery from left ventricle. It is most commonly seen in **infants of diabetic mother** and **male babies.**

- **Pathophysiology**
  The existence of two parallel circuits in TGA is clearly shown in the diagram. Deoxygenated blood is circulated in the systemic circuit consisting of the right side of heart, aorta and systemic circulation, whereas oxygenated blood is circulated in the pulmonary circuit of left side of heart, pulmonary artery and lungs. The only way by which these infants can survive is by mixing of oxygenated and deoxygenated blood facilitated by **VSD (associated in 50% cases), ASD and PDA.**

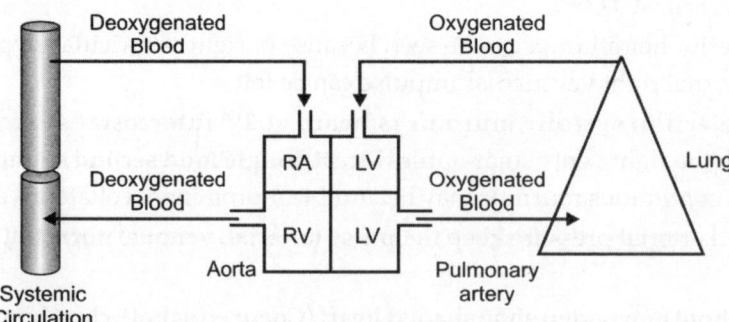

Fig. 4.2

- The clinical features and management depend on the presence or absence of VSD and pulmonary artery stenosis (PAS).

Simple or isolated TGA	TGA with VSD	TGA with VSD and PAS
• TGA is not associated with VSD or PAS. • Baby presents with **cyanosis in first few hours or days** of life as the ductus arteriosus begins to close. • Severe hypoxemia is seen, however CHF is less frequent. • A **loud second heart sound with soft systolic ejection murmur** may be seen. • Chest X-ray shows a characteristic **egg on side appearance.** • Simple TGA is a **medical emergency** and treatment should be initiated as soon as the diagnosis is made. • **Prostaglandin E1** is given to maintain the patency of ductus arteriosus. • **Rashkind balloon atrial septostomy** *is* done if patient still remains hypoxemic on Pg E1 or delay in definite surgery is anticipated. • **Jantene (arterial switch)** operation is the definite surgical procedure of choice usually done within first two weeks of life. Aorta and pulmonary artery is divided above the sinuses and re-anastomosed in their correct positions.	• TGA is associated with VSD and at times alongwith PAS. • Cyanosis is usually delayed because of mixing of oxygenated and deoxygenated blood through VSD. • **CHF is a frequent** complication and it should be repaired within first months of life. • **Digitalis and diuretics** is given till the patient is awaited for definite surgical procedure. • **Jantene (arterial switch)** operation **with closure of VSD** is the surgical procedure of choice.	• This combination of anomalies may mimic TOF and present with similar features like cyanosis, exercise intolerance and growth retardation. • Treatment usually consists of measures to increase oxygenation. • **PgE1** is given to maintain patency of ductus arteriosus. • Surgical procedures like aortopulmonary shunt (most preferred) and atrial septostomy is done to gain time for the definite procedure. • **Rastelli operation** is the definite surgical procedure.

Total Anomalous Pulmonary Venous return (TAPVC)

During embryological development of heart, failure of connection between pulmonary vein and left atrium results in faulty connection of pulmonary vein directly with right atrium or indirectly by connection with various vessels draining in to right atrium. The **pulmonary veins almost always join together** to form a common vein that connects the right side of heart.

- **Pathophysiology:** It is clear from the diagram that volume overload of right side of heart and lungs occur because of flow of both oxygenated and deoxygenated blood. Volume over load causes hypertrophy of right atrium and ventricle as well as pulmonary congestion and right sided heart failure.

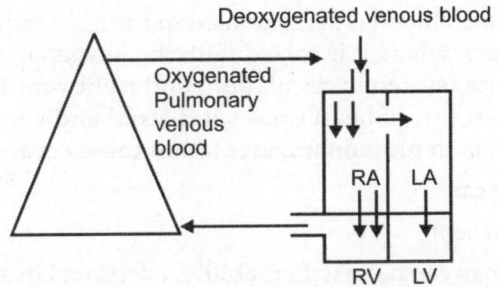

Fig. 4.3

- TAPVC can be classified in to four types depending on its direct or indirect connection by a particular vessel with right ventricle.

Supracardiac TAPVC	*Cardiac TAPVC*	*Infracardiac/ Infradiaphragmatic TAPVC*	*Mixed TAPVC*
• Pulmonary vein connects to coronary sinus or superior vena cava by a vertical vein. • It is the **most common type of TAPVC,** seen in 50% cases. • Obstruction is quite infrequent, but when present it is most commonly caused by compression of left vertical artery by left pulmonary artery anteriorly and left bronchus posteriorly.	• Pulmonary vein directly drains in to right atrium. • It is seen in 25% cases. • Obstruction is rarely seen.	• Pulmonary vein connects to the inferior vena cava by ductus arteriosus. • It is seen in 25% cases. • It is almost always associated with pulmonary vein out flow obstruction which may be caused by narrowness of the trunk, compression by oesophageal hiatus of diaphragm or a constriction in ductus venosus.	• A combination of various connections can be seen. • It is the **least common type** encountered.

- Clinical features and management depend on the presence or absence of obstruction.

TAPVC with obstruction	*TAPVC without obstruction*

• Due to severe pulmonary congestion caused by obstruction, the baby presents with very early onset dyspnoea, intense cyanosis and right sided heart failure.
 • A loud 2nd heart sound, gallop rhythm and systolic murmur of tricuspid regurgitation may be heard.
 • X-ray shows a **ground glass appearance** as seen in RDS.
 • E.C.G corresponds to **right atrium and ventricular hypertrophy**.
 • Due to its nature of presentation it is a medical emergency
   ❖ **Pg E1** is given to dilate ductus venosus and arteriosus. However **patient may worsen after Pg E1 administration** due to further shunting of blood to the right side of heart, thereby decreasing systemic circulation. In this case Pg E1 administration should be stopped immediately.
   ❖ **CPAP with oxygen and diuretics** are required until patient is prepared for cardiopulmonary bypass.
   ❖ **Surgery is the definite treatment in which, common pulmonary venous trunk is anastomosed directly to the left atrium, ASD is closed, and the connection to the systemic venous circuit is terminated.**
	• Due to absence of obstruction these babies may develop minimal cyanosis and even can be asymptomatic during infancy because of mixing of pulmonary and venous blood through foramen ovale and ASD.
	 • Heart sounds are usually normal and murmurs are not heard.
	 • X-ray shows an enlarged heart termed as **figure of eight or snowman**, which is caused by dilated left vertical vein, innominate vein, right superior vena cava along with dilated heart.
	 • E.C.G corresponds to right atrium and ventricular hypertrophy.
	 • **Surgery** is the definite treatment in which, common pulmonary venous trunk is anastomosed directly to the left atrium, ASD is closed, and the connection to the systemic venous circuit is terminated.

Tricuspid Atresia

Faulty embryogenesis leading to unequal division of the atrio-ventricular (A-V)canal causes A-V canal defect, which gives rise to a **small and atretic tricuspid valve**, a larger mitral valve, ASD, VSD and a **hypoplastic right ventricle**.

- **Pathophysiology:** The deoxygenated blood is accumulated in the right atrium and flows to the left side of heart by an **ASD and patent foramen ovale**, where it is mixed with the oxygenated blood. Further from the left ventricle mixed blood is pumped in to aorta (systemic circulation) and right ventricle (pulmonary circulation) by a VSD. Clearly volume overload of the left side of heart causes **left atrial and ventricular hypertrophy**, whereas **limited supply of blood for oxygenation in to pulmonary circulation** causes **cyanosis** at birth.

- **Clinical presentation and findings:**

  ❖ At birth Cyanosis is usually present.

  ❖ As the baby grows other findings can be easy fatigability, exertional dyspnea, and occasional hypoxic episodes as a result of compromised pulmonary blood flow.

  ❖ An **increased left ventricular impulse** differentiates it from other cyanotic CHDs (Increased right ventricular impulse).

  ❖ **Holosystolic murmur** is heard along the left sternal border. The **2nd heart sound is usually single**.

- **Diagnosis:**

  ❖ X-ray shows a small heart with a distinctive **round or apple configuration** resulting from deficiency of right ventricular and pulmonary artery segments. (Ref: Rudolph 22nd E/P1824)

  ❖ E.C.G corresponds to **left axis deviation and left ventricular hypertrophy**, which **distinguishes it from most cyanotic CHDs.**

- **Treatment:**

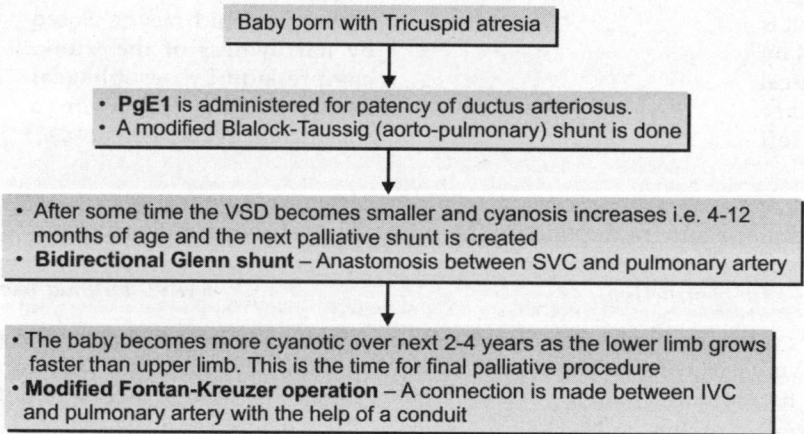

Fig. 4.4

CHDs Causing Obstructive Lesions

Based on their anatomic location obstructive lesions of aorta can be classified as transverse **aortic arch hypoplasia and/or atresia** (preductal type) and juxtaductal coarctation of aorta (post ductal type).

Juxtaductal Coarctation of Aorta

It is the **most common type** of coarctation which arises **distal to origin of left subclavian artery** near the origin of the ductus arteriosus. **Males are more commonly affected;** however in **females** it is commonly seen in association with **Turner syndrome**. It can be associated with the other form of coarctation (**aortic arch hypoplasia and/or atresia**) and various congenital abnormalities like **bicuspid aortic valve (most common),** aberrant origin of subclavian artery, VSD and PDA. When associated with left sided obstructive lesions like subaortic stenosis and parachute mitral valve (supravalvular mitral ring) it is called as **Shone complex.**

- **Clinical presentation and findings:**

  ❖ It is also called as **adult – type coarctation** as the patient may present in adulthood even with severe coarctation and are diagnosed only on routine examinations. **Most commonly it presents insidiously in the 60% of children** with no symptoms in infancy. The symptoms can be **exercise induced claudication and pain in lower limbs, headache** and **dyspnea.**

❖ However it can present in infancy with signs of lower body hypoperfusion, acidosis, and **severe heart failure** if severe coarctation is associated with transverse arch hypoplasia.

❖ The classical sign of coarctation is **radial-femoral pulse delay** i.e. femoral pulse is felt after radial (Normally femoral pulse can be felt earlier than radial). **Pulse in the upper limb is felt well than in the lower limb**.

❖ The blood pressure is **decreased in lower extremities** and **increased in the upper extremities** (Normally B.P in lower limbs is 10-20 mmHg higher than in arms).

❖ A short **systolic murmur** can be heard at the left sternal border in the **3rd and 4th intercostal** spaces, which can be transmitted to the left infrascapular area and neck. A **systolic ejection click murmur** can be heard if a bicuspid aortic valve is associated. Systolic or continuous murmurs may be heard over the left and right sides of the chest laterally and posteriorly due to formation of **collaterals** by periscapular, transverse cervical, **intercostal**, **superior and inferior epigastric artery** and internal mammary arteries.

- **Diagnosis:**
  ❖ A **"figure 3"** sign can be seen in chest X-ray because of prominence of aorta proximal to coarctation, indentation of aortic outline at coarctation and dilation of post-stenotic segment. **Notching of the inferior ribs** by large intercostal arteries can be seen.

  ❖ ECG in **older children** shows **left ventricular hypertrophy**; however **infants** with severe coarctation usually show **right ventricular hypertrophy.**

- **Complications:** If not treated on time there can be various complications like premature coronary artery disease, **heart failure**, hypertensive encephalopathy, **intracranial haemorrhage**, aortic aneurysm and **infective endocarditis or endarteritis.**

- **Treatment:**
  ❖ **Surgery** is the definite **procedure of choice**. However if infants present after closure of ductus arteriosus with rapid deterioration prostaglandin E1 should be administered to maintain the patency.

  ❖ The surgical correction can be complicated by rebound hypertension and restenosis. **Balloon angioplasty** is the **treatment of choice for restenosis,** whereas medical management for rebound hypertension is required.

HEART FAILURE

- Heart failure is the inability of the heart to meet the metabolic demands of the body. It can be caused by **CHDs** (**most common cause in infants**), RHD (most common cause in children beyond 5 years of age), infective endocarditis, myocarditis and arrhythmias.

- Infants and younger children usually present with poor feeding, respiratory distress, diaphoresis and lethargy. On general examination edema (usually seen in eyelids and sacrum but lower **limbs are spared),** **hepatomegaly** and splenomegaly is present most of the times. **JVP** is raised but **difficult to measure** in infants because of short neck. On cardiac examination precordium is prominent with displacement of apical impulse, heart tones are distant and a gallop rhythm is present.

ACQUIRED HEART DISEASES

Infective Endocarditis

- Infective endocarditis can be caused by a wide range of bacteria, viruses and fungi. However the most common causes are bacteria like **viridians streptococci (α hemolytic)** followed by staphylococcus aureus.

CPDT 19th E/P560-61"Common organisms causing IE are **viridians streptococci (30–40 % of cases)**, *Staphylococcus aureus* (25–30%) and fungal agents (about 5%)."

- IE can be caused by various factors:
  ❖ **Congenital heart diseases** — The CHDs like **VSD, aortic stenosis, TOF and PDA** are at increased risk of developing IE because of intracardiac high velocity ejection of blood causing endocardial damage.

  ❖ Rheumatic heart disease.

  ❖ **Central venous line** — In this case the most common cause is *Staphylococcus epidermidis*.

  ❖ **Open heart surgery** — This is the **most common cause of IE in infants**. The organisms responsible are usually fungus.

  ❖ **Valve replacement or valve conduit repair** — *Staphylococcus aureus* is the most common organism causing IE in this setting.

- **Clinical presentation and findings:**
  - ❖ The clinical presentation can range from mere fever and weight loss for months as seen in case of streptococcal IE to severe conditions like myocardial and cerebral abscess, mycotic aneurysms and embolic strokes in staphylococcal IE.
  - ❖ On general examination one can find various manifestations of vasculitis caused by **immune complexes**.
    - ❏ **Osler nodes** — Intradermal nodes in the pads of fingers and toes.
    - ❏ **Janeway lesions** — Erythematous lesions on palms and soles.
    - ❏ **Splinter haemorrhages** — Linear lesions beneath the nails.
    - ❏ **Roth spot** — Retinal haemorrhages.
    - ❏ **Glomerulonephritis** — It presents as microscopic hematuria.
    - ❏ **Arthralgia, myalgia, clubbing and splenomegaly.**
    - ❏ Auscultation may reveal a **new or changing murmur** which indicates towards heart failure.
- **Diagnosis:**
  - ❖ The investigation of choice for IE is a **blood culture**, however for specific diagnosis **Duke criteria** is considered as the golden standard.
  - ❖ **Duke criteria:**

Major criteria	*Minor criteria*
• Two separate positive blood culture. • Echocardiographic evidence of endocardial involvement like oscillating intracardiac mass on valves or other supporting structures.	• Predisposing conditions • Fever • Embolic vascular signs • Immune complex phenomena • Single positive blood culture • Serological evidence of infection

For diagnosis of IE there should be at least 2 major or 1 major and 3 minor or 5 minor criteria.
- **Treatment:** As soon as IE is suspected antibiotic therapy should be started. The most common regimen is **vancomycin** with or without gentamicin for 6 weeks.

Rheumatic Fever and Rheumatic Carditis

Rheumatic fever is the most common cause of acquired heart disease in children. It is more commonly encountered in developing countries because of presence of predisposing conditions like **low socioeconomic status**, overcrowding, poor nutrition and poor hygiene. It is usually seen in the age group of **5–15 years**. The onset of rheumatic fever is preceded by infection of the upper respiratory tract by **group A β haemolytic streptococci**. The antibodies against the streptococci cross react with various connective tissues of cardiac muscle, striated muscle and vascular smooth muscle in human body.

Clinical Presentation

Clinical manifestations can be divided in to 5 major and 4 minor ones as per T. Duckett Jones (**Jones criteria**) which help in establishing the diagnosis of rheumatic fever.
- **Major manifestations:**
  - ❖ **Carditis** — This is the **second most common manifestation** of rheumatic fever seen in 50% of cases and **most common cause of mortality**. Involvement of all three layers of heart can be seen i.e. endocarditis, myocarditis and pericarditis collectively known as **pancarditis**; however endocarditis is more commonly seen than the latter. Almost all the valves of the heart can be involved.
    - ❏ **Mitral valve** — It is the **most common valve involved** and most common following sequalae is **mitral insufficiency** which is characterised by high pitch apical holosystolic murmur. An apical short and **low density mid diastolic murmur (Carrey Coomb's murmur)** can be heard because of flow through an edematous mitral valve. **Mitral stenosis** on the other hand is usually seen after 5-10 years of an acute attack and is **more common in adults** than in children.
    - ❏ **Aortic valve** — It is the second most commonly involved which usually presents as aortic insufficiency and is characterised by high pitched decrescendo diastolic murmur.
    - ❏ **Pulmonary valves** are almost **never affected**.

❖ **Migratory polyarthritis** — This is the **most common and earliest manifestation** of rheumatic fever seen in almost 70% of cases. There is a typical involvement of multiple **large joints** like knees, ankles, wrists and elbows in a migratory fashion. The **pain can precede arthritis** and may be disproportionate to other findings like swelling, redness, heat and tenderness. The characteristic feature is that it responds excellently to even small doses of aspirin.

❖ **Chorea** — It is characterised by involuntary and purposeless movements associated with emotional liability, poor school performance and facial grimacing which increase with stress and disappear with sleep. When other manifestations like carditis and arthritis develop within 4 weeks after infection, **chorea** takes months to develop and is often **not associated with other features**. It is self-limiting and usually resolves by 6 weeks. **Prepubertal girls** of 8–12 years are more prone to develop chorea and it can be **aggravated by pregnancy** and intake of **OCPs**.

❖ **Erythema marginatum** — It is a characteristic macular, serpeginious and erythematous rash of migratory nature, which is seen predominantly on the trunk and extremities but **face is spared.**

❖ **Subcutaneous nodules** — **Nontender**, nonpruritic, freely movable nodules of less than 2 cm diameter are seen along the **extensor surfaces of joints**, scalp and spinal column. This is the **least common manifestation** seen in less than 1% of patients but when present **it indicates towards** severe form of disease like rheumatic **carditis**. These are nonspecific as they can also be seen with RA and SLE.

- **Minor manifestations:**
  ❖ **Arthralgia** or joint pain in the absence of polyarthritis.
  ❖ **Fever** with a temperature of at least 39°C.
  ❖ Laboratory parameters like **CRP** and **ESR** are elevated.
  ❖ **Prolonged PR interval** in ECG (1st degree heart block).
  ❖ **Leucocytosis**

Diagnosis

The diagnosis of rheumatic fever is confirmed if there are **2 major criteria or 1 major and 2 minor criteria with evidence of preceding streptococcal infection**. The evidences of infection can be increased titres of **antistreptolysin O** or other antibodies like antihyaluronidase and anti-DNAse B; and positive throat culture for Group A streptococcus.

Treatment and Prophylaxis

- Benzathine penicillin G is the drug of choice but in patients allergic to penicillin **erythromycin** can be used.
- Low dose aspirin is given for relief from arthritis and fever.
- Corticosteroids are given in case of severe carditis and heart failure.

CPDT 19th E/P555"The **steroid of choice is prednisolone**, which is given in a dose of 2 mg/kg/d for 2 weeks followed by gradual reduction **till end of 3rd week.**"

- The drug of choice for prophylaxis is **benzathine penicillin** once in 21 days at a dose of 6, 00,000 units for children up to 6 years and 1.2 million units for older ones till the age of 25–30 years.
- Other drugs that can be used for prophylaxis are **sulfadiazine, penicillin V** and **erythromycin**.

MULTIPLE CHOICE QUESTIONS

1. **Preterm baby with PDA, which is the least likely finding?** [AIIMS Nov. 10]
   a. CO₂ washout
   b. Bounding pulses
   c. Pulmonary hemorrhage
   d. Necrotising Enterocolitis

2. **What is pentalogy of Fallot:** [AIIMS May 2010, AI 07]
   a. TOF with PDA
   b. TOF with ASD
   c. TOF with COA
   d. TOF with TGA

3. **Eisenmenger syndrome is characterized by all except:** [AIIMS May 2010, AI 05]
   a. Return of left ventricle and right ventricle to normal size
   b. Pulmonary veins not distended
   c. Pruning of peripheral pulmonary arteries
   d. Dilatation of central pulmonary arteries

4. **Which of the following is not a major criteria of Jones in rheumatic fever?** [AIIMS Nov. 10]
   a. Pancarditis   b. Arthritis
   c. Chorea   d. Elevated ESR

5. **All are signs of impending Eisenmenger syndrome except:** [AIIMS May 2010]
   a. Increased flow murmur across tricuspid and pulmonary valve
   b. Single S2
   c. Increased intensity of P2
   d. Graham Steel murmur

6. **Regarding ASO titre all are seen except:** [AIIMS Nov. 09]
   a. ASO can be increased in school children
   b. May be negative in post streptococcal glomerulo-nephritis
   c. ASO titre included in major criteria in Jones criteria
   d. May not be elevated in 20% cases of carditis

7. **Essential criteria for TOF includes all except?** [AIIMS Nov. 08]
   a. Valvular stenosis   b. Infundibular stenosis
   c. Over riding of aorta   d. RVH

8. **In post ductal coarctation of the aorta, blood flow to the lower limb is maintained through which of the following arteries:** [AIIMS Nov. 07]
   a. Umblical artery and subcostal arteries
   b. Thoracic and pericardiophrenic arteries
   c. Intercostal arteries and superior epigastric artery
   d. Ant and post circumflex arteries

9. **Drug of choice for Rheumatic fever prophylaxis in penicillin allergic patient:** [AIIMS May 07]
   a. Erythromycin   b. Clindamycin
   c. Vancomycin   d. Gentamycin

10. **A premature infant is born with a patent ductus arteriosus. Its closure can be stimulated by administration of:** [AIIMS May 06]
    a. Prostaglandin analogue
    b. Estrogen
    c. Anti-estrogen compounds
    d. Prostaglandin inhibitors

11. **About carey coomb's murmur which is false:** [AIIMS Nov. 06]
    a. Delayed diastole murmur
    b. Seen in rheumatic fever
    c. Can be associated with AR
    d. Low pitched murmur

12. **Recurrent respiratory tract infections may occur in all of the following except:** [AIIMS Nov. 05]
    a. Ventricular septal defect
    b. Tetralogy of Fallot
    c. Transposition of great arteries
    d. Total anomalous venous return

13. **All of the following are true regarding Tetralogy of Fallot except:** [AIIMS May 05]
    a. Ejection systolic murmur in second intercostal space
    b. Single second heart sound

    c. Predominantly left to right shunt
    d. Normal jugular venous pressure

14. **Which of the following syndromes is best associated with congenital heart disease?** [AIIMS May 05]
    a. Lesch-Nyhan syndrome
    b. Rasmussen syndrome
    c. Holt Oram syndrome
    d. Leopard syndrome

15. **A 6 months old child with Tetralogy of Fallot develops cyanotic spell initiated by crying. Which one of the following drugs you would like to avoid?** [AIIMS Nov. 04]
    a. Sodium bicarbonate   b. Propranolol
    c. Phenylephrine   d. Isoprenaline

16. **The most appropriate management for maintaining patency of ductus arteriosus in a neonate is:** [AIIMS May 04]
    a. Prostaglandin E1   b. Oxygen
    c. Nitric oxide   d. Indomethacin

17. **Which one of the following does not produce cyanosis in the first year of life:** [AIIMS May 03]
    a. Atrial septal defect
    b. Hypoplastic left heart syndrome
    c. Truncus arteriosus
    d. Double outlet right ventricle

18. **A young female presents with history of dyspnea on exertion. On examination, she has wide, fixed split S2 with ejection systolic murmur (m/VI) in left second intercostal space. Her ECG shows left axis deviation. The most probable diagnosis is:** [AIIMS May 2003]
    a. Total anomalous pulmonary venous drainge.
    b. Tricuspid atresia
    c. Ostium primum atrial septal defect
    d. Ventricular septal defect with pulmonary arterial hypertension

19. **A 4½ years old girl always had to wear warm socks even in summer season. On physical examination, it was noticed that she had high blood pressure and her femoral pulse was weak as compared to radial and carotid pulse, a chest radiography showed remarkable notching of ribs along with their lower borders. This was due to:** [AIIMS Nov. 02]
    a. Femoral artery thrombosis
    b. Coarctation of aorta
    c. Raynaud's disease
    d. Takayasa arteritis

20. **A child with large perimembranous VSD has congestive heart failure. What may be the cause of improvement of cardiac failure in the patient?** [AIIMS Nov. 01]
    a. Aortic regurgitation
    b. Vascular changes in pulmonary circulation

c. Infective endocarditis

d. Closure of VSD spontaneously

21. A neonate has central cyanosis and short systolic murmur on the 2nd day of birth. The diagnosis is:
[AIIMS May 01]

a. Tetralogy of Fallot

b. Transposition of great vessels

c. Atrial septal defect

d. Ventricular Septal defect

22. A 29-day-old child presents with features of congestive cardiac failure and left ventricular hypertrophy. Auscultation shows a short systolic murmur. Most likely diagnosis is: [AIIMS Nov. 00]

a. Rheumatic fever

b. Tetralogy of fallot

c. Transposition of great arteries

d. Ventricular septal defect

23. A five years old child presents with left ventricular hypertrophy and central cyanosis what is the most probable diagnosis? [AIIMS Nov. 00]

a. Tricuspid atresia

b. Eisenmenger syndrome

c. Tetralogy of Fallot

d. Total anomalous pulmonary venous drainage

24. A child with VSD presents with development of cyanosis because of Eisenmenger physiology. What is the correct sequence of events which leads to this change? [AIIMS Nov. 00]

a. Left to right shunt, pulmonary hypertension, right ventricular hypertrophy, right to left shunt.

b. Left to right shunt, right ventricular hypertrophy, pulmonary hypertension, right to left shunt.

c. Pulmonary hypertension, right to left shunt right ventricular hypertrophy, left to right shunt.

d. Left to right shunt, right ventricular hypertrophy, right to left shunt, pulmonary hypertension.

25. All are true about rheumatic fever, except:
[AIIMS June 99]

a. Common in poor socioeconomic group

b. Develops after streptococcal pharyngitis

c. Communicable disease

d. Seen in 5–15 years of children

26. Tetralogy of Fallot present with one of the following: [AIIMS Dec. 98]

a. Central cyanosis with clubbing

b. Cardiomegaly

c. Left ventricular hypertrophy

d. Normal ECG and Chest X-ray

27. All of the following are characteristics features of Tricuspid Atresia except: [AIIMS Dec. 98]

a. Left Axis deviation

b. Right ventricular hypoplasia

c. Pulmonary vascularity is diminished

d. Splitting of S2

28. Infective endocarditis is not seen in one of the following conditions: [AIIMS Dec. 98]

a. PDA

b. ASD

c. TOF

d. VSD

29. Coarctation of aorta is associated with all except:
[AIIMS June 98]

a. Turner's syndrome

b. Bicuspid aortic valve

c. Pulmonary stenosis

d. Atresia of aortic arch

30. All are true regarding tricuspid atresia except:
[AIIMS Dec. 97]

a. Split S_2

b. Patent foramen ovale

c. Pulmonary oligemia in chest X-ray

d. Left axis deviation in ECG

31. True about VSD is all except: [AIIMS June 97]

a. Small hole closes spontaneously

b. Defect is usually in membranous part

c. Endocarditis is a common complication

d. Pulmonary oligemia in chest X-ray

32. NADA's criteria are used for :
[AIIMS Feb. 1997, AI 96]

a. Assessment of child for degree of dehydration

b. Assessment of child for degree of malnutrition

c. Assessment of child for presence of heart disease

d. Assessment of child for degree of mental retardation

33. True about 1 year old child with PDA is:
(AIIMS May 95)

a. Symptoms similar to pulmonary window

b. Chances of spontaneous closure high

c. Indomethacin may help in closure

d. Endocarditis is rare

34. Earliest valular lesion in case of rheumatic fever is:
(AIIMS May 94)

a. Mitral regurgitation (MR)

b. Aortic regurgitation (AR)

c. Mitral stenosis (MS)

d. Aortic stenosis (AS)

35. Commonest cause of systemic hypertension in children is: [AIIMS 89]

a. Coarctation of aorta

b. Acute glomerulonephritis

c. Nephrotic syndrome

d. Congenital adrenal hyperplasia

36. A child with tetralogy of Fallot uses which of the following positions: [DPG 10, AIIMS 87]

a. Supine

b. Prone

c. Squatting

d. Leaning forwards

37. The following is false about atrial septal defect:
[AIIMS 81]

a. Ostium secundum most common

b. Right to left shunt

c. May be associated with TAPVC

d. CCF is very rare

38. **Which condition is most commonly associated with coarctation of aorta?** [AI 11, 09, AI 08]
    a. PDA
    b. Bicuspid aortic valve
    c. Aortic stenosis
    d. VSD

39. **A ten-year-old boy presents to the pediatric emergency unit with seizures. Blood pressure in the upper extremity measured as 200/140 mm Hg. Femoral pulses were not palpable. The most likely diagnosis amongst the following is:** [AI 10]
    a. Takayasu aortoarteritis
    b. Renal parenchymal disease
    c. Grandmal seizures
    d. Coarctation of aorta

40. **A 10 year old boy is having hypertension. There is no other significant history and urine analysis, cause for his hypertension:** [AI 10]
    a. Chronic glomerulonephritis
    b. Polycystic kidney disease
    c. Reflux nephropathy
    d. Renal parenchymal disease

41. **All of the following statements about Patent Ductus Arteriosus (PDA) are true, except:** [AI 08]
    a. It is more common in males than females
    b. It is a common heart lesion in rubella
    c. Treatment is closure of defect by ligation or division of ductus
    d. Hypoxia and immaturity are important in maintaining the patency

42. **Which of the following is a minor criteria for diagnosis of Rheumatic fever (RF) according to modified Jones criteria?** [AI 07]
    a. ASO titer
    b. Past history of Rheumatic fever
    c. Fever
    d. Subcutaneous nodules

43. **What is pentalogy of Fallot?**
    [AIIMS May 2010, AI 07]
    a. TOF with PDA
    b. TOF with ASD
    c. TOF with COA
    d. TOF with TGA

44. **In which of the following conditions left atrium is not enlarged?** [AI 06]
    a. Ventricular septal defect
    b. Atrial septal defect
    c. Aortopulmonary window
    d. Patent ductus arteriosus

45. **The following features are true for tetralogy of Fallot, except:** [AI 06]
    a. Ventricular septal defect
    b. Right ventricular hypertrophy
    c. Atrial septal defect
    d. Pulmonary stenosis

46. **Blalock and Taussig shunt is done between:** [AI 06]
    a. Aorta to pulmonary artery
    b. Aorta to pulmonary vein

c. Subclavian artery to pulmonary vein
d. Subclavian vein to artery

47. **A 1 month old boy is referred for failure to thrive. On examination, he shows feature of congestive failure. The femoral pulses are feeble as compared to brachial pulses. The most likely clinical diagnosis is:** [AI 06]
    a. Congenital aortic stenosis
    b. Coarctation of aorta
    c. Patent ductus arteriosus
    d. Congenital aortoiliac disease

48. **The most common type of total anomalous pulmonary venous connection is:** [AI 05]
    a. Supracardiac
    b. Infracardiac
    c. Mixed
    d. Cardiac

49. **Eisenmenger syndrome is characterized by all except:** [AIIMS May 2010, AI 05]
    a. Return of left ventricle and right ventricle to normal size
    b. Pulmonary veins not distended
    c. Pruning of peripheral pulmonary arteries
    d. Dilatation of central pulmonary arteries

50. **In which of the following a 'Coeur en Sabot' shape of the heart is seen?** [AI 04]
    a. Tricuspid atresia
    b. Ventricular septal defect
    c. Transposition of great arteries
    d. Tetralogy of Fallot

51. **A five-day-old, full term male infant was severely cyanotic at birth. Prostaglandin E was administered initially and later ballooned atrial septostomy was done which showed improvement in oxygenation. The most likely diagnosis of this infant is:** [AI 04]
    a. Tetralogy of Fallot
    b. Transposition of great vessels
    c. Truncus arteriosus
    d. Tricuspid atresia

52. **All of the following are true about ASD except:** [AI 01]
    a. Right atrial hypertrophy
    b. Left atrial hypertrophy
    c. Right ventricular hypertrophy
    d. Pulmonary hypertension

53. **A patient presents with LVH and pulmonary complications. ECG shows left axis deviation. Most likely diagnosis is:** [AI 01]
    a. TOP
    b. Tricuspid atresia
    c. TAPVC
    d. VSD

54. **Potts shunt is:** [AI 01]
    a. Right subclavian artery to right pulmonary artery
    b. Descending aorta to left pulmonary artery
    c. Left subclavian to left pulmonary artery
    d. Ascending aorta to right pulmonary artery

55. **A patient presents with LVH and pulmonary complications. *ECG,*shows left axis deviation. Most likely diagnosis is:**   **[AI 01]**
    a. TOF   b. Tricuspid atresia
    c. TAPVC   d. VSD

56. **A neonate has recurrent attacks of abdominal pain, restless irritability and diaphoresis on feeding. Cardiac auscultation reveals a nonspecific murmur. He is believed to be at risk for MI Likely diagnosis here is:**   **[AI 01]**
    a. ASD
    b. VSD
    c. TOF
    d. Anomalous coronary artery

57. **True statement about Ductus Arteriosus is: [AI 00]**
    a. It undergoes anatomic closure within 24 hours of birth
    b. Forms the ligamentum venosum in later life
    c. It is induced to close by high levels of prosta-glandins
    d. May cause a machinery murmur by its patency

58. **Most common congenital heart diseases: [AI 99]**
    a. ASD   b. VSD
    c. PDA   d. TOF

59. **Figure of 8 configuration on chest X-ray is seen:**
                                                  [AI 99]
    a. TOF   b. ASD
    c. TAPVC   d. VSD

60. **A child presented with headache, dizziness, intermittent claudication with occasional dyspnea. The most probable diagnosis in:**   **[AI 99]**
    a. ASD   b. PDA
    c. TOP   d. Coarctation of aorta

61. **True about coarctation of aorta: [AI 99]**
    a. Most common site is distal to the origin of the left subclavian artery
    b. Most common age of presentation is at 15-20 years
    c. Upper rib notching is due to erosion by dilated collateral vessels
    d. Right ventricular hypertrophy

62. **Ribnotching of 4–9th ribs with double bulging is seen in :**   **[AI 98]**
    a. Aortic aneurysm   b. Aortic dissection
    c. Coarctation of aorta d. Diaphragmatic hernia

63. **True about ASD:**   **[AI 98]**
    a. Foramen ovale is patent
    b. Left parasternal heave is due to increased pulmonary artery flow
    c. S2 is wide and variable
    d. Systolic murmur is due to rapid flow of blood across the shunt

64. **Most common manifestation of rheumatic fever:**
                                                  [AI 98]
    a. Arthritis   b. Carditis
    c. Subcutaneous nodule d. Raised ASLO

65. **Which is going to best declare the case as that of interatrial septal defect with other cardiac abnormalities?**   **[AI 97]**
    a. Elevated pressure in left atrium
    b. Elevated pressure in right atrium
    c. Elevated PO2 in pulmonary artery
    d. Systolic murmur

66. **All of the following statements regarding total anomalous pulmonary venous connection are true except:**   **[AI 97]**
    a. The total pulmonary venous blood reaches the right atrium
    b. Always associated with a VSD
    c. The oxygen concentration of the blood in the pulmonary artery is higher than in the aorta
    d. Infracardiac type is always obstructive

67. **Total anomalous pulmonary venous connection false statement is:**   **[AI 97]**
    a. All pulmonary veins enter by a single trunk
    b. Need not always be associated with a septal defect
    c. Radiologically has figure of 8 appearance
    d. Is a cyanotic heart disease

68. **Coarctation of aorta is common in which syndrome?**
                                                  [AI 95]
    a. Down's   b. Turner's
    c. Klinefelter's   d. Noonan's

69. **Sustained severe hypertension in children is most commonly suggestive of:**   **[AI 95]**
    a. Coarctation of aorta
    b. Pheochromocytoma
    c. Renal parenchymatous disease
    d. Drug induced

70. **In patent ductus arteriosus connection is between:**
                                                  [AI 93]
    a. Aorta and coronary artery
    b. Aorta and pulmonary artery
    c. Aorta and subclavian artery
    d. Pulmonary artery and subclavian artery

71. **Congestive cardiac failure is diagnosed in an infant by:**   **[AI 88]**
    a. Basal crepts   b. Elevated JVP
    c. Pedal edema   d. Liver enlargement

72. **Which of the following statements is/are false about ostium secundum ASD?**   **[PGI June 09]**
    a. Fixed splitting of 2nd heart sound
    b. Narrow splitting of 2nd heart sound
    c. Lt axis deviation of ECG
    d. Shunt murmur prominent
    e. Rt axis deviation

73. **7 day old baby presented in the emergency department with unconscious, blue in appearance with 85 % in Oxygen saturation. The diagnosis:**
    [PGI Dec. 08]
    a. Tetralogy of Fallot   b. TGA
    c. TAPVC   d. PDA

74. **Cardiac tumor in childhood includes:** [PGI Dec. 08]
    a. Rhabdomyoma   b. Lymphoma
    c. Atrial myxoma   d. Sarcoma
    e. Fibroma

75. **A child after 4 weeks of birth acyanotic, ejection systolic murmur detected causes are:** [PGI June 08]
    a. VSD   b. PDA
    c. TOF   d. Coarctation of aorta
    e. Tricurpid stenosis

76. **True about subcutaneous nodule in Rheumatic fever:**   [PGI Dec. 07]
    a. Non tender
    b. Most common manifestation
    c. Present on extensor surfaces
    d. Associated with arthritis

77. **True about TGA:**   [PGI Dec. 07]
    a. Cyanosis at birth   b. CHF
    c. VSD   d. AS
    e. None

78. **Fallots tetralogy manifestation are:** [PGI Dec. 05]
    a. Left axis deviation
    b. Left ventricular hypertrophy
    c. VSD
    d. Blalock taussig shunt is between pulmonary artery and subclavian artery
    e. Morphine is contraindicated in cyanotic spells

79. **8 years old child presented with altered sensorium and seizure. On examination BP was 180/120. Correct statements:**   [PGI Dec. 04]
    a. Sodium nitroprusside strips
    b. Cause of hypertension is essential hypertension
    c. IV labetolol, hydralazine, and diaoxide are given
    d. Nifedipine is used
    e. Pheochromocytoma mimics the condition

80. **2 years old children presented with sudden onset of altered sensorium on examination BP was 200/100:**
    [PGI Dec. 04]
    a. Renal artery stenosis   b. Coarctation of aorta
    c. Glomerulonephritis   d. Essential hypertension
    e. Pheochromocytoma

81. **Components of Tetralogy of Fallot is/are:**
    [PGI June 04]
    a. VSD
    b. Lt. Ventricular hypertrophy
    c. Lt. Axis deviation

    d. Taussig-Blalock shunt is between pulmonary and subclavian artery
    e. Morphine is given for Cyanosis

82. **True about Rheumatic fever:**   [PGI Dec. 03]
    a. Chorea is aggravated during pregnancy
    b. Chorea and arthritis co-existing
    c. Subcutaneous nodules are tender
    d. Erythema multiforme seen

83. **True about rheumatic fever in children:**
    [PGI Dec. 03]
    a. Polyarthritis
    b. Caused by á haemolytic streptococci
    c. Erythema marginatum is most common manifestation
    d. Most common valve involved is mitral
    e. Erythema marginatum is common in face

84. **Bacterial endocarditis is most commonly caused by:**
    [PGI Dec. 03]
    a. α-Hemolytic Streptococci
    b. β-Hemolytic Streptococci
    c. *Staphylococcus aureus*
    d. Cardiobacterium
    e. *Staph-epidermidis*

85. **ASD is seen in a/e :**   [PGI June 01]
    a. Turner's syndrome
    b. Ellis-van Creveld syndrome
    c. Down's syndrome
    d. Halt-oram syndrome
    e. TAR syndrome

86. **Cyanosis is seen in :**   [PGI Dec. 01]
    a. Persistent ductus arteriosus
    b. Tricuspid atresia
    c. Ostium primum ASD
    d. Eisenmenger complex
    e. Tetralogy of Fallot

87. **ASD is seen in a/e:**   [PGI June 01]
    a. Turner's syndrome
    b. Ellis-vancreveld syndrome
    c. Down's syndrome
    d. Halt-oram syndrome
    e. TAR syndrome

88. **Eisenmenger complex is common in adult in:**
    [PGI June 00]
    a. VSD   b. ASD
    c. PDA   d. Cushion defect

89. **A 2-year-old known case of RHD presents with 3 wks history of fever, hematuria and palpitations diagnosis is:**   [PGI Dec. 99]
    a. *Streptococcal endocarditis*
    b. Collagen vascular disease
    c. Reactivation
    d. *Staphylococcal endocarditis*

90. MC cause of death in adult with PDA is:

[PGI Dec. 99]

a. CCF
b. Infective endocarditis
c. Rupture
d. Embolism

91. Congenital cyanotic heart disease with pulmonary oligemia is seen with :

[PGI Dec. 99]

a. ASD
b. VSD
c. Tricuspid atresia
d. Hypoplastic left ventricle

92. True about TGA:

[PGI 99]

a. Acyanotic heart disease
b. Cyanotic disease
c. Aorta anterior to pulmonary artery
d. VSD

93. A patient of VSD in CCF develops clubbing with no cyanosis diagnosis is:

[PGI 98]

a. Right to left shunt
b. Left to right shunt
c. Subacute bacterial endocarditis
d. Pulmonary edema

94. The most common cause of secondary hypertension in children is:

[PGI 93]

a. Renal artery stenosis
b. Renal disease
c. Systemic vasculitis
d. Adrenal tumors

95. In atrial septal defect the aorta is:

[PGI 86]

a. Small
b. Normal
c. Enlarged
d. Aneurysmal

96. Which of the following are immune complex lesions in SBE?

[PGI 86]

a. Meningitis
b. Osler nodes
c. Microscopic hematuria
d. Roth spots
e. Mycotic aneurysms

97. All of the following causes death in coarctation of Aorta except:

[PCI June 2000]

a. Infective endocarditis
b. CCF
c. Intra cranial hemorrhage
d. Anterior MI

QUESTIONS OF OTHER EXAMINATIONS

1. Which one of the following is a cyanotic congenital heart disease?

[UPSC 10]

a. Patent ductus arteriosus
b. Atrial septal defect
c. Ventricular septal defect
d. Tetralogy of Fallot

2. A child with tetralogy of Fallot uses which of the following positions?

[DPG 10, AIIMS 87]

a. Supine
b. Prone
c. Squatting
d. Leaning forwards

3. A 7-year-old child with rheumatic heart disease presents with pallor, fever and a palpable spleen. The following investigations would be needed to arrive at a diagnosis except:

[UPSC 10]

a. Electrocardiogram
b. Echocardiogram
c. Blood culture
d. Urine examination

4. An 8-month-old female child presented to emergency with a heart rate of 220/min and features of congestive heart failure. Heart rate comes down to normal after administration of intravenous adenosine. What is the most likely diagnosis?

[UPSC 10]

a. Atrial fibrillation
b. Atrial flutter
c. Paroxysmal supraventricular tachycardia
d. Ventricular tachycardia

5. A newborn infant was referred with intermittent cyanosis which improved on crying but worsened when quiet. What is the most likely diagnosis?

[UPSC 10]

a. Diaphragmatic hernia
b. Congenital heart disease (cyanotic)
c. Choanal atresia
d. Tracheal agenesis

6. A newborn baby develops cyanosis on day three of life. On auscultation, there is systolic murmur. Echocardiography reveals a cyanotic heart disease in the baby. Which one of the following drugs can be administered to prolong the life of baby pending intervention?

[UPSC 09]

a. Indomethacin
b. Ibuprofen
c. Prostaglandin E1
d. Propranolol

7. All are characteristic of Fallot except:

[DPG 09, Jipmer 86]

a. Infundibular stenosis
b. VSD
c. Overriding of aorta
d. Left ventricular hypertrophy

8. A 2-month-old infant is brought to the hospital emergency with marked respiratory distress. On examination, the infant has cyanosis and bilateral crepitation. Heart rate is 180/min, respiratory rate 56/min and the liver span 7.5 cm. The child has had repeated episodes of fever, cough and respiratory

distress since the time of birth. **Cardiovascular examination reveals grade III ejection systolic murmur in left parasternal area and the chest X-ray reveals cardiomegaly with a narrow base and plethoric lung fields. What is the most likely diagnosis?** [UPSC 09]

a. Congenital methemoglobinemia
b. Transposition of great arteries
c. Cystic fibrosis
d. Tetralogy of Fallot

9. **Umbilical cord has:** [DPGEE 08]

a. 1 vein and 2 arteries
b. 2 vein and 2 arteries
c. 1 vein and 1 artery
d. 2 veins and 1 artery

10. **The clinical features associated with coarctation of aorta in older children are the following except:** [UPSC 08]

a. Upper body hypertension
b. Prominent pulsation in neck
c. Fatiguanleness, tiredness in leg
d. Absence of flow murmurs over scapular region

11. **In which of the following differential cyanosis is found?** [UPSC 08]

a. VSD with reversal of shunt
b. PDA with reversal of shunt
c. ASD with reversal of shunt
d. Tetralogy of Fallot

12. **Ductus arteriosus closes in response to:** [UPSC 08]

a. Decrease in peripheral oxygen saturation
b. Indomethacin therapy
c. Prostaglandin E1
d. Increase in pulmonary vascular resistance

13. **Systolic murmur in TOF is due to?** [APPG 08]

a. VSD   b. Pulmonary stenosis
c. ASD   d. None

14. **A newborn presents with deepening cyanosis at birth, with congestive heart failure and normal first heart sound. X-ray reveals cardiomegaly, diagnosis is:** [UP 08]

a. Tetralogy of Fallot's
b. Ebstein anomaly
c. Transposition of great vessels
d. Ventricular septal defect

15. **Egg on side appearance is seen in:** [UP 08]

a. Fallot's tetralogy
b. Ebstein anomaly
c. Transposition of great vessels
d. Tricuspid atresia

16. **Commonest cause of heart failure in infancy is:** [COMED 08]

a. Myocarditis   b. Rheumatic fever
c. Cardiomyopathy   d. Congenital heart disease

17. **Cause of death in acute rheumatic fever is:** [UP 08]

a. Pericarditis   b. Myocarditis
c. Endocarditis   d. Streptococcal sepsis

18. **Most common type of atrial septal defect is:** [UP 07, 06]

a. Ostium primum
b. Ostium secundum
c. Endocardial cushion defect
d. Endocardial hypertrophy

19. **All of the following are acyanotic congenital heart diseases except:** [SGPGI 05]

a. VSD   b. ASD
c. PDA   d. Tetralogy of Fallot

20. **Not a feature of Fallot's tetralogy:** [MAHE 05]

a. Left ventricular hypertrophy
b. Boot shaped heart
c. VSD
d. Overriding of arch of aorta

21. **In a patient of rheumatic carditis full dose of steroid is given for:** [Kerela 04]

a. 3 Weeks   b. 6 weeks
c. 9 weeks   d. 12 weeks

22. **Children born to mothers with systemic lupus erythematosis are likely to have one of the following anomalies:** [KCET 03]

a. Atrial septal defect
b. Tetralogy of Fallot
c. Transposition of great vessels
d. Complete heart block

23. **Which of the following is most common cause of cyanotic heart diseases:** [UPSC 02]

a. Dextrocardia   b. Fallot's tetralogy
c. Atrial septal defect d. Coarctation of aorta

24. **Uncommon finding in congestive cardiac failure in newborn is:** [CMC 01]

a. Tachycardia   b. Tachypnoea
c. Hepatomegaly   d. Pedal edema

25. **Commonest cause of enlarged cardiac shadow in X-ray of a child is:** [KCET 2000]

a. PDA   b. Coarctation of aorta
c. Pericarditis   d. Rheumatic carditis

26. **The following statements are true of patent ductus arteriosus (PDA) except:** [Kerala 2000]

a. Spontaneous closure occurs in some term infants
b. Pulmonary hypertension develops
c. Bacterial endocarditis is more frequent with small PDA
d. Recurrent chest infection and congestive failure may develop
e. Anatomic existence of PDA is an indication for surgery

27. **Emergency treatment of TGV is:** [TN 99]
    a. Balloon septostomy   b. Oxygen
    c. Ventilation   d. Digoxin

28. **Infantile myocarditis and pericarditis is due to:** [TN 99]
    a. Coxscakie A   b. Coxscakie B
    c. Mumps   d. Pox virus

29. **The commonest cyanotic heart disease manifesting as congestive cardiac failure during first week of life is:** [MP 98]
    a. Pulmonary stenosis
    b. Fallot's tetralogy
    c. Tricuspid atresia
    d. Hypoplastic left heart syndrome

30. **In infective endocarditis which of the following is not immune mediated:** [Kerala 97]
    a. Roth spots   b. Osler nodes
    c. Glomerulonephritis   d. None

31. **Balloon valvotomy is successful in all of the following cases except:** [Ref: UPSC 97]
    a. Congenital pulmonary stenosis
    b. Calcified mitral stenosis
    c. Mitral stenosis in pregnancy
    d. Congenital aortic stenosis

32. **The most common anomaly seen in fetus of a mother taking lithium carbonate is:** [UP 97]
    a. Cardiac deformities
    b. Neural tube defect
    c. Limb reduction
    d. Genitourinary deformities

33. **Intracavitary electrocardiography is a diagnostic aid in:** [UPSC 96]
    a. Tricuspid regurgitation
    b. Endocardial fibroelastosis
    c. Endomyocardial fibrosis
    d. Ebstein's anomaly of tricuspid valve

34. **Steroids are given in rheumatic fever when there is:** [AMU 95]
    a. Carditis   b. Chorea
    c. Subcutanous nodules   d. All

35. **Commonest cause of systemic hypertension in children is:** [AIIMS 89]
    a. Coarctation of aorta
    b. Acute glomerulonephritis
    c. Nephrotic syndrome
    d. Congenital adrenal hyperplasia

36. **Which of the following are immune complex lesions in SBE?** [PGI 86]
    a. Meningitis
    b. Osler nodes
    c. Microscopic hematuria
    d. Roth spots
    e. Mycotic aneurysms

37. **Which of the following is not a characteristic of right sided failure?** [JIPMER 80]
    a. Pulmonary edema   b. Ascites
    c. Oliguria   d. Dependent edema

ANSWERS

1. (a) CO$_2$ washout (Ref: Richard neonatology P291)
Clinical presentation of PDA:
- Precordial murmur
- Hyperactive precordium
- **Bounding pulses**
- Resting tachycardia
- Frequent apnea
- **Carbon dioxide retention**
- **Necrotising Enterocolitis** is frequently seen in premature infants.
- **Pulmonary hemorrhage** is a frequent complication of PDA.

2. (b) TOF with ASD (Ref: Julia Fetal echocardiography/P221)
- TOF primarily consists of four components i.e. **right ventricular outflow tract (infundibulum) obstruction, right ventricular hypertrophy, ventricular septal defect** and **dextroposition of the aorta. Pentalogy of Fallot** consists of the features of tetralogy along with **ASD**.

3. (a) Return of left ventricle and right ventricle to normal size (Ref: Nelson 19th E/P1549–50)
- It is defined as an increase in the pulmonary vascular resistance by a ratio of pulmonary to systemic ratio of **more than 1.**
- X-ray shows a prominent pulmonary artery, **enlarged pulmonary vessels in the hilar areas which taper down at the periphery.**
- The best way of treatment is to prevent it in infancy by surgical approach because once the changes develop they never come back to normal.

4. (d) Elevated ESR ((Ref: CPDT 19th E/P554)
Jones criteria for diagnosis of rheumatic fever:

Major criteria	Minor criteria
• Carditis	• Fever
• Polyarthritis	• Polyarthralgia
• Sydenhams chorea	• Previous rheumatic fever or rheumatic heart disease
• Subcutaneous nodules	• Elevated ESR, CRP
• Erythema marginatum	• Leucocytosis
	• Prolonged PR interval or 1st degree AV block.

- For diagnosis of rheumatic fever any 2 major criterias or 1 major and 2 minor criterias are required along with the concrete evidence of preceding streptococcal infection. The evidences of streptococcal infection are:
  1. Increased titres of anti streptococcal antibodies like **antistreptolysin O,** antihyaluronidase or anti-DNAse B.
  2. Positive throat culture for group A streptococcus.

5. (c) Increased flow murmur across tricuspid and pulmonary valve (Ref: Nelson 19th E/P1550)
- Patients of Eisenmenger syndrome become symptomatic usually after 3rd decade of life with initial mild presentations like cyanosis, fatigue and dyspnea which can progress to heart failure.
- The clinical findings can be a right ventricular heave, **loud single or narrow split S$_2$, loud P$_2$** and murmurs of tricuspid regurgitation and pulmonary insufficiency (early decrescendo diastolic murmur or **Ghram steel murmur**).

6. (c) ASO titre included in major criteria in Jones criteria (Ref: Nelson 19th E/P877, 1740)
- **ASO titre** is a **minor criteria** in Jones criteria.
- Only **80–85%** of patients with acute rheumatic fever have an **elevated ASLO titre,** hence it may not be elevated in 20 % cases of carditis.
- If the ASLO titres are raised but other Jones critera are not fulfilled then a diagnosis of rheumatic fever should never be made. This is because it may be a coincidental finding as in case of younger **school aged children** who had a group A streptococcal pyoderma in summer or unrelated group A streptococcal pharyngitis in winter.
- **Post streptococcal glomerulonephritis** is caused by streptococcal pharyngitis in winters or streptococcal skin infection (pyoderma) during winters. It is important to note here that **ASLO** title is raised after pharyngeal infection but it **rarely increases in case of skin infection.**

7. (a) Valvular stenosis (Ref: CPDT 19th E/P545)
- This gives rise to TOF, which primarily consists of four components i.e. **right ventricular outflow tract (infundibular stenosis>pulmonary valve stenosis) obstruction, right ventricular hypertrophy, ventricular septal defect** and **dextroposition of the aorta.**

8. (c) Intercostal arteries and superior epigastric arteries (Ref: nelson 19th E/P1519)
- In coarctation of aorta systolic or continuous murmurs may be heard over the left and right sides of the chest laterally and posteriorly due to formation of **collaterals** by periscapular, transverse cervical, **intercostal, superior** and **inferior epigastric artery** and internal mammary arteries.

9. **(a)** Erythromycin (Ref: CPDT 19th E/P556)

Antibacterial treatment and prophylaxis of rheumatic fever:

- The drug of choice for treatment is single **benzathine penicillin G**. However in case of penicillin allergy, **erythromycin** should be given.
- The drug of choice for prophylaxis is **benzathine penicillin G once in 21 days**. Other drugs like penicillin V, Sulfadiazine and erythromycin can be used.

10. **(d)** Prostaglandin inhibitors (Ref: Nelson 19th E/P1512)

- In premature infants if spontaneous closure doesn't occur then **prostaglandin inhibitor indomethacin (As prostaglandins cause vasodilation and interfere with its closure)**, 0.2 mg/kg at 12–24 hr intervals for three doses may induce pharmacologic closure by inhibiting prostaglandin synthesis.

11. **(c)** Can be associated with AR (Ref: Nelson 19th E/P876, Harrison 19thE/P)

Carey Coomb's murmur:

- It is heard in acute rheumatic fever due to flow through an edematous mitral valve.
- It is a short, low density, mid-diastolic murmur heard best at the apex.

Other named murmurs:

Murmur	Characteristics
Austin flint murmur in aortic regurgitation.	Apical low pitched mid diastolic murmur.
Graham Steel murmur in pulmonary regurgitation.	High pitched decrescendo early to mid-diastolic murmur.
Rytand's murmur in complete heart block.	Mid to late diastolic murmur.
Still's murmur in normal children and adolescents.	It is a benign grade 2, vibratory mid-systolic murmur at the lower left sternal border
Docks murmur in left anterior descending artery stenosis	Diastolic murmur similar to that of AR
Mill wheel or water wheel murmur due to air in the heart.	Splashing sounds are heard

12. **(b)** Tetralogy of Fallot (Ref: Nelson 19th E/P 1525)

- Pulmonary complications are seen with conditions associated with increased pulmonary blood flow.
- TOF is associated with decreased pulmonary blood flow due to right ventricular outflow obstruction.

13. **(c)** Predominantly left to right shunt (Ref: Nelson 19th E/P1524)

- TOF is a cyanotic heart disease characterized by right to left shunt.
- **Loud and harsh ejection systolic murmur is heard at 2nd intercostal space** in left sternal border due to turbulence through the right ventricular outflow tract. **Single loud second sound** corres-ponding to aortic valve closure is heard. A continuous murmur may be audible if prominent collaterals are present.
- **JVP** is usually normal.

14. **(c)** Holt Oram syndrome (Ref: Nelson 19E/P1503, Rudolph 22nd E/P1780)

Holt-Oram syndrome:

- It is an A.D disorder caused by TBX5 gene mutation, located in the 12th chromosome.
- It is associated with a wide range of congenital abnormalities
  - ❖ **Congenital heart diseases like ASD (more common), muscular VSD and 1st degree heart block**.
  - ❖ Phocomelia i.e. limb defects like hypoplastic or absent radii, triphalangeal thumb, fingerised thumb (unopposable).

Lesch-Nyhan syndrome:

- It is a X linked disorder of purine metabolism which causes deficiency of hypoxanthine guanine phospho-ribosyltransferase.
- Selective **neurotoxicity** seen in this syndrome can be attributed to the fact that HGPRT is abundantly found in CNS. The clinical findings are **mental retardation, cerebral palsy with early choreo-athetosis, spasticity and dystonia, dysarthria and compulsive self-biting.**

Rasmussen syndrome (Epilepsia partialis continua):

- This is an epileptic syndrome usually seen in children less than 10 years.
- It begins with GTCS followed by intractable focal seizures which poorly respond to antiepileptic drugs.
- In most of the patients the onset of disease is preceded by an infectious or inflammatory disease.
- The patient may develop **neurological deficits like hemiplegia, hemianopia and aphasia.**

Leopard syndrome (Multiple lentigenes syndrome):

- It is an autosomal dominant disorder in which **lentigines (brown macules of size less than 3mm)** are distributed all over the body symmetrically.
- It is also associated with *o*cular hypertelorism, pulmonary stenosis, abnormal genitals (cryptorchidism, hypogonadism, hypospadias), growth *r*etardation, sensorineural deafness and rarely with HOCM and pectus excavtum.

15. **(d)** Isoprenaline (Ref: Nelson 19th E/P1527)

Treatment of cyanotic spell: The main aim in treating a cyanotic spell is to increase oxygenation by providing oxygen and increasing pulmonary blood flow.

- Place infant on the abdomen in the knee-chest position.
- **Morphine** is useful in terminating a **prolonged and severe attack.**

- Beta blockers like **propranolol** are used for prophylaxis to reduce the frequency of attacks.
- Administration of oxygen relieves dyspnea.
- Drugs increasing systemic B.P like methoxamine or **phenylephrine**, improve right ventricular outflow, decrease the right-to-left shunt, and thus improve the symptoms. **Isoprenaline** by acting on beta 2 receptor will cause vasodilation and worsen the condition due to increase in right to left shunt.
- Development of metabolic acidosis warrants intravenous administration of **sodium bicarbonate**.

16. **(a)** Prostaglandin E1 (Ref: Nelson 19th E/P1512)
    - Remember: **P**rostaglandins maintain **p**atency of DA.
    - Prostaglandin E1 analogues like misoprostol and alprostadil can be used to maintain patency of ductus arteriosus.

17. **(a)** ASD (Ref: Nelson 19E/P1504)
ASD:

> "Pulmonary vascular resistance remains low throughout childhood, although it may begin to increase in **adulthood** and may eventually result in reversal of the shunt and **clinical cyanosis**."

- Children with ASD are usually asymptomatic, however large ASDs may present with CHF.
- The pulmonary blood flow is increased which can cause pulmonary hypertension and reversal of shunt but usually after 4th decade.

Cyanotic congenital heart diseases:
- **TOF — Cyanosis is seen in the later half of 1st year.**
- **Tricuspid atresia — Cyanosis is seen at birth.**
- **TGA.**
- Double outlet right ventricle.
- **TAPVC.**
- Truncus arteriosus.
- Double ventricle.
- **Hypoplastic left heart syndrome – Cyanosis is seen at birth.**
- **Eisenmenger complex.**

18. **(c)** Ventricular septal defect with pulmonary arterial hypertension (Ref: Nelson 19th E/P1504)
    - Clinical findings on examination secondary to **increased blood flow to the right side** of heart through ASD are a palpable **right ventricular systolic lift at the left sternal border, fixed and split 2nd heart sound and systolic pulmonic ejection click murmur.**

19. **(b)** Coarctation of aorta (Ref: Nelson 19th E/P1519)
    - The classical sign of coarctation is **radial-femoral pulse delay** i.e. femoral pulse is felt after radial (Normally femoral pulse can be felt earlier than radial). **Pulse in the upper limb is felt well than in the lower limb.**
    - The blood pressure in lower extremities is lower than the upper extremities (Normally B.P in lower limbs is 10–20 mmHg higher than in arms).
    - Inferior rib notching can also be seen with coarctation of aorta.

20. **(b)** Vascular changes in pulmonary circulation (Ref: Nelson 19th E/P1508)
    - Spontaneous closure is associated with muscular VSD and not membranous.
    - The cause of sudden improvement in CHF can be because of compensatory dilation of pulmonary blood vessels.

21. **(b)** Transposition of great vessels (Ref: Nelson 19th E/P1535)
    - Transposition of great vessels presents with cyanosis within first few hours or days after birth.
    - A loud second heart sound with **soft systolic ejection murmur** may be seen.
    - TOF does not present with cyanosis at birth, rather is seen towards end of 1 year.
    - ASD and VSD lead to right to left shunt which does not lead to cyanosis rather pulmonary plethora is seen.

22. **(d)** Ventricular septal defect (Ref: Nelson 19th E/P1550)
    - Large sized VSDs present with congestive heart failure commonly between 2–6 months.
    - ECG shows features of left ventricular hypertrophy and left axis deviation.
    - A loud holosystolic murmur can be heard at the lower left sternal border.

23. **(a)** Tricuspid atresia (Ref: Nelson 19th E/P1530)
    - All the mentioned options can cause central cyanosis but **left ventricular hypertrophy** is a feature that **distinguishes tricuspid atresia from other cyanotic heart diseases.**
    - Eisenmenger syndrome, TOF and TAPVC can be associated with **right ventricular hypertrophy.**

24. **(a)** Left to right shunt, pulmonary hypertension, right ventricular hypertrophy, right to left shunt. (Ref: Nelson 19th E/P1550)
Pathophysiology of acyanotic heart diseases: (See Flowchart 1)

25. **(c)** Communicable disease (Ref: Nelson19thE/P875, CPDT19thE/P554–55)
    - Rheumatic fever is more commonly encountered in developing countries because of presence of predisposing conditions like:
      ❖ **low socioeconomic status**
      ❖ overcrowding
      ❖ poor nutrition
      ❖ poor hygine

Flowchart 1

```
          Congenital defects with left to right shunt
                            │
                            ▼
   Movement of extra volume of blood to the right ventricle or/and atrium and
   subsequently to the lungs (no cyanosis, rather pulmonary plethora)
                            │
            ┌───────────────┴───────────────┐
            ▼                                ▼
   Delayed closure of pulmonary valve    Shunt murmurs due to passage of blood
   And early closure of aortic valve –   in conditions like VSD and PDA (because
   wide split S2                          of huge pressure difference between
                                          chambers) but not in ASD (pressure
                                          difference between chambers is minimal)
            │                                │
            ▼                                ▼
   Increased amount of blood in lungs causes medial   Increased blood return to
   hypertrophy and vasoconstriction which ultimately  left atrium and ventricle
   leads to pulmonary hypertension followed by right  can cause hypertrophy
   ventricular hypertrophy                            and left pericardial bulge
            │                                │
            ▼                                ▼
   Pulmonary pressure reaches systemic pressure and   Increased amount of blood flow
   blood starts flowing from right side of heart to left  through tricuspid valve causes
   side – Shunt reversal or Eisenmenger syndrome      mid-diastolic flow murmur
            │
            ▼
   This is when cyanosis can be seen in acyanotic CHDs
```

- It is usualy seen in the age group of **5–15 years**.
- The onset of rheumatic fever is preceded by infection of the upper respiratory tract by **group A β haemolytic streptococci**.

26. **(a)** Central cyanosis with clubbing (Ref: Nelson 19th E/P1524–25)

27. **(d)** Splitting of S_2 (Ref: Nelson 19th E/P1531)

   - Faulty embryogenesis leading to unequal division of the atrioventricular (A-V) canal causes A-V canal defect, which gives rise to a **small and atretic tricuspid valve**, a larger mitral valve, ASD, VSD and a **hypoplastic right ventricle.**

   - The deoxygenated blood is accumulated in the right atrium and flows to the right side of heart by an ASD and patent foramen ovale, where it is mixed with the oxygenated blood. Further from the left ventricle mixed blood is pumped in to aorta (systemic circulation) and right ventricle (pulmonary circulation) by a VSD.

   - Clearly volume overload of the left side of heart causes **left atrial and ventricular hypertrophy**, whereas **limited supply of blood for oxygenation in to pulmonary circulation** causes cyanosis at birth.

   - **Holosystolic murmur** is heard along the left sternal border. The **2nd heart sound is usually single.**

28. **(b)** ASD (Ref: Nelson 19th E/P1565)
   Congenital heart diseases causing endocarditis:
   - The CHDs like **VSD, aortic stenosis, TOF and PDA** are at increased risk of developing IE because of intracardiac high velocity ejection of blood causing endocardial damage.
   - ASD creates a low pressure shunt and hence endocardial damage and endocarditis is not seen.

29. **(c)** Pulmonary stenosis (Ref: Nelson 19th E/P1518)
   - **Males are more commonly affected**; however in **females** coarctation of aorta is commonly seen in association with **Turner syndrome**.
   - It can be associated with the other form of coarctation (**aortic arch hypoplasia and/or atresia**) and various congenital abnormalities like **bicuspid aortic valve (most common),** aberrant origin of subclavian artery, VSD and PDA.

30. **(a)** Split S_2 (Ref: Nelson 19th E/P1531)

31. **(d)** Pulmonary oligemia in chest X-ray (Ref: Nelson 19th E/P1509)
   - VSD results in left to right shunt which causes increased blood to the right side of heart and the lungs. This results in pulmonary plethora.

32. **(a)** Assessment of a child for presence of heart disease (Ref: Ghai 7th E/P399)
   - Nada's criteria are used for presence of heart disease in a child. Presence of a major criteria or two minor criteria is required for confirmation.

Major criteria	Minor criteria
• Grade 3 or > grade 3 Systolic murmur	• < Grade 3 systolic murmur
• Diastolic murmur	• Abnormal 2nd sound
• Cyanosis	• Abnormal ECG
• CHF	• Abnormal X-ray
	• Abnormal blood pressure

33. (a) Symptoms similar to pulmonary window (Ref: Nelson 19th E/P1511–12)

- Aortopulmonary window is a communication between ascending aorta and main pulmonary artery. When the communication is small the presentation is similar to PDA.
- Because of the anatomical defect, **PDA persisting beyond 1 week in mature infants rarely close spontaneously** or with pharmacological intervention (Prostaglandin inhibitors).
- **CHF** is the **most common cause of death in adolescents**, however they may present with other frequent complications like **infective endocarditis** and pulmonary or systemic embolism.

34. (a) Mitral regurgitation (MR) (Ref: CPDT 19th E/P554)

"Valvulitis is frequently seen, with the **mitral valve most commonly affected. Mitral insufficiency** is the most common valvular residua of acute rheumatic carditis. Mitral stenosis after acute rheumatic fever is rarely encountered until 5–10 years after the first episode. Thus, **mitral stenosis** is much more commonly seen in **adults** than in children."

35. (b) Acute glomerulonephritis (Ref: Nelson 19th E/P1593)

36. (d) Squatting (Ref: Nelson 19th E/P1525)

- **Blue spells or hypercyanotic episodes** are caused due to acute reduction in pulmonary blood flow by various reasons like prolonged crying and fever
- Dyspnoea occurs on exertion and the child acquires **a squatting position**, which increases the systemic B.P and increases blood flow to lungs through VSD.

37. (b) Right to left shunt (Ref: Nelson 19th E/P1504)

- ASD results in blood flow from the left side of the heart to right side i.e. left to right shunt.
- Osteum secundum is the most common type seen in 90% of cases.
- CHF is rarely seen with the ostium primum ASD.

38. (b) Bicuspid aortic valve (Ref: Nelson 19th E/P1518) Coarctation of aorta can be associated with:

- **Bicuspid aortic valve (most common)**
- Aberrant origin of subclavian artery
- VSD
- PDA.

39. (d) Coarctation of aorta (Ref: Nelson 19th E/P1518–19)

- Increased blood pressure in the upper limbs and decreased pulse in the lower limb makes the diagnosis of coarctation of aorta.

40. (d) Renal parenchymal disease (Ref: Nelson 19th E/P1593)

Hypertension in young children is usually secondary to systemic disorders like:

- Renal parenchymal disease — Most common cause is chronic glomerulonephritis.
- Coarctation of aorta.
- Endocrine disorders like pheochromocytoma.
- Renal artery stenosis.

41. (a) It is more common in males than females (Ref: Nelson 19th E/P1511)

- PDA is caused by **immaturity and hypoxia** (Causes vasodilation) in premature infants.
- **Rubella infection** in the first trimester of pregnancy is highly associated with PDA.
- PDA less than 5 mm may be treated by trans-catheter coil or an umbrella like device, whereas larger ones require surgical closure by **ligation and division of ductus** by thoracoscopic approach.
- PDA is two **times more common in females than males**.

42. (c) Fever (Ref: CPDT 19th E/P554)

Jones criteria for diagnosis of rheumatic fever:

Major criterias	Minor criterias
• Carditis	• Fever
• Polyarthritis	• Polyarthralgia
• Sydenhams chorea	• Previous rheumatic fever or rheumatic heart disease
• Subcutaneous nodules	• Elevated ESR, CRP
• Erythema marginatum	• Leucocytosis
	• Prolonged PR interval or 1st degree AV block.

- For diagnosis of rheumatic fever any 2 major criterias or 1 major and 2 minor criterias are required along with the concrete evidence of preceding streptococcal infection. The evidences of streptococcal infection are
  1. Increased titres of anti streptococcal antibodies like **antistreptolysin O**, antihyaluronidase or anti-DNAse B.
  2. Positive throat culture for group A strepto-coccus.

43. (b) TOF with ASD (Ref: Julia Fetal echocardiography/P221)

- TOF primarily consists of four components i.e. **right ventricular outflow tract (infundibulum) obstruction, right ventricular hypertrophy, ventricular septal defect** and **dextroposition of the aorta. Pentalogy of Fallot** consists of the features of tetralogy along with **ASD**.

44. (b) Atrial septal defect (Ref: Nelson 19th E/P1504)

Chest x-ray findings in ASD:

- **Enlarged right atrium and ventricle**
- Large pulmonary artery
- Increased pulmonary vascularity
- **Small aortic shadow.**

45. (c) ASD (Ref: Nelson 19th E/P1524)

- TOF primarily consists of four components i.e. **right ventricular outflow tract (infundibulum) obstruction, right ventricular hypertrophy, ventricular septal defect** and **dextroposition of the aorta.**
- **Pentalogy of Fallot** consists of the features of tetralogy along with **ASD.**

46. (a) Aorta to pulmonary artery (Ref: Nelson 19th E/P1527)

- **Corrective surgery for TOF** is done usually within 4–12 months of birth.
- **Blalock-Taussig shunt** (aortopulmonary shunt)— It joins **subclavian artery** to the homolateral branch of the **pulmonary artery.** Subclavian artery is a branch of **aorta.**

47. (b) Coarctation of aorta (Ref: Nelson 19th E/P1519)

- The classical sign of coarctation is **radial-femoral pulse delay** i.e. femoral pulse is felt after radial (Normally femoral pulse can be felt earlier than radial). **Pulse in the upper limb is felt well than in the lower limb.**

48. (a) Supracardiac type (Ref: Nelson 19th E/P1539)

- In **Supracardiac TAPVC** pulmonary vein connects to coronary sinus or superior vena cava by a vertical vein. It is the **most common type of TAPVC,** seen in 50% cases.
- In cardiac type pulmonary vein directly drains in to right atrium. It is seen in 25% cases.
- In infracardiac type Pulmonary vein connects to the inferior vena cava by ductus arteriosus. It is seen in 25% cases.
- In mixed type A combination of various connections can be seen. It is the **least common type** encountered.

49. (a) Return of left ventricle and right ventricle to normal size (Ref: Nelson 19th E/P1549–50)

- It is defined as an increase in the pulmonary vascular resistance by a ratio of pulmonary to systemic ratio of **more than 1.**
- X-ray shows a prominent pulmonary artery, **enlarged pulmonary vessels in the hilar areas which taper down at the periphery.**
- The best way of treatment is to prevent it in infancy by surgical approach because once the changes develop they never come back to normal.

50. (d) Tetralogy of Fallot (Ref: Nelson 19th E/P1525)

- Chest x-ray in patients of TOF shows **boot or wooden shoe shaped heart (Coeur en sabot) ,clear hilar areas and lung fields** because of diminished pulmonary blood flow, large aorta and a right sided aortic arch.

51. (b) Transposition of great vessels (Ref: Nelson 19th E/P1535–36)

Simple or isolated TGA:

- TGA is not associated with VSD or PAS. Baby presents with **cyanosis in first few hours or days** of life as the ductus arteriosus begins to close.
- Simple TGA is a **medical emergency** and treatment should be initiated as soon as the diagnosis is made. **Prostaglandin E1** is given to maintain the patency of ductus arteriosus. **Rashkind balloon atrial septostomy** *is* done if patient still remains hypoxemic on Pg E1 or delay in definite surgery is anticipated.

52. (b) Left atrial hypertrophy (Ref: Nelson 19th E/P1504)

- ASD is associated with right atrial and ventricular hypertrophy.
- Left atrial hypertrophy is not seen because blood is shunted through the defect to right atrium.

53. (d) VSD (Ref: Nelson 19th E/P15)

- Pulmonary complications and evidence of left ventricular hypertrophy and left axis deviation are consistent with the diagnosis of VSD.

54. (b) Descending aorta to left pulmonary artery (Ref: Ghai 7th E/P410)

Blalock-Taussig shunt	Between **subclavian artery** and **pulmonary artery.**
Pott's shunt	Between **descending aorta** and **pulmonary artery.**
Waterson's shunt	Between **ascending aorta** and **pulmonary artery.**

55. (b) Tricuspid atresia (Ref: Nelson 19th E/P1530–31)

- Tricuspid atresia causes left ventricular hypertrophy which differentiates it from other cyanotic heart diseases.

56. (d) Anomalous coronary artery (Ref: Nelson 19th E/P1546)

- In anomalous coronary artery arising from the pulmonary artery there is significant decrease in the blood flow to myocardium post birth. This can result in **myocardial ischemia, infarction and fibrosis.**
- The patient presents with CHF, cardiomegaly, cardiac aneurysms and mitral insufficiency due to left ventricular dysfunction.

57. (d) May cause a machinery murmur by its patency (Ref: Nelson 19th E/P1511)

- **Machinery like or thunder rolling murmur** is heard in PDA because of continuous passage of blood from aorta to pulmonary artery.
- In the full term infants, the physiological (functional) closure occurs within 10 to 15 **hours**, whereas the **anatomical closure** may take place only in the **3rd postnatal week.**
- Its closure is induced by decrease in prostaglandins and increase in oxygen concentration.
- It forms ligamentum arteriosum later after closure.

58. (b) VSD (Ref: Nelson 19th E/P1549)

- VSD is the most common type of congenital heart disease accounting for almost 25% cases.

59. (c) TAPVC (Ref: Nelson 19th E/P1539)

- In TAPVC X-ray shows an enlarged heart termed as **figure of eight or snowman**, which is caused by dilated left vertical vein, innominate vein, right superior vena cava along with dilated heart.

60. (d) Coarctation of aorta (Ref: Nelson 19th E/P1519, Ghai 7th E/P420)

- **Coarctation most commonly presents insidiously in the 60% of children** with no symptoms in infancy. The symptoms can be **exercise induced claudication and pain in lower limbs, headache** and **dyspnea.**

61. (a) Most common site is distal to the origin of the left subclavian artery (Nelson 19th E/P1518)

- Juxtaductal coarctation is the **most common type** which arises **distal to origin of left subclavian artery** near the origin of the ductus arteriosus.
- **Most commonly it presents insidiously in the 60% of children** with no symptoms in infancy.
- **Inferior rib notching** is seen due to dilated intercostal vessels.
- **Left ventricular hypertrophy** is seen due to increased afterload.

62. (c) Coarctation of aorta (Ref: Nelson 19th E/P1519)
X-ray findings in coarctation of aorta:

- A **"figure 3"** sign can be seen in chest X-ray because of prominence of aorta proximal to coarctation, indentation of aortic outline at coarctation and dilation of post-stenotic segment.
- **Notching of the inferior ribs** by large intercostal arteries can be seen.

63. (b) Left parasternal heave is due to increased pulmonary artery flow (Ref: Nelson 19th E/P1504)
Clinical findings of ASD: An **increase in blood flow to the right side** of heart through ASD produces findings like—

- A palpable **right ventricular systolic lift or heave at the left sternal border.**
- A **fixed and split 2nd heart sound.**
- A **systolic pulmonic ejection click murmur** is produced by the **increased flow across the right ventricular outflow tract into the pulmonary artery, not by low-pressure flow across the ASD.**

64. (a) Arthritis (Ref: Nelson 19th E/P876)

- The most common manifestation af rheumatic fever is **migratory polyarthritis** seen in almost **70% cases,** whereas **subcutaneous nodules** are the least common one seen only in **<1% cases.**

65. (a) Elevated pressure in left atrium (Ref: Nelson 19th E/P1504)

66. (b) Always associated with VSD (Ref: Nelson 19th E/P1539)

- Faulty connection of pulmonary vein directly with right atrium or indirectly by connection with various vessels draining in to right atriumleads to volume overload of right side of heart and lungs because of flow of both **oxygenated pulmonary venous blood** and **deoxygenated vena caval blood** in to right atrium.
- Further through foramen ovale or PDA this blood flows in to pulmonary artery via right ventricle and aorta via left ventricle. Hence the oxygen saturation is same in both the large vessels; however due to increased blood flow through the right heart, **total oxygen content is higher in pulmonary artery.**
- Infracardiac type is almost always obstructive.

67. (a) All pulmonary veins enter by a single trunk (Ref: Rudolph 22nd E/P1829)

- Though the pulmonary veins almost always join together to form a common vein before connecting with the right atrium or other vessels, it not an absolute phenomenon. Hence it is the best answer here.
- ASD is present but not always.
- Chest X-ray shows a figure of 8 or snowman heart configuration.
- Indeed TAPVS is a cyanotic CHD because of mixing of oxygenated and deoxygenated blood.

68. (b) Turner's (Ref: Nelson 19th E/P1518)

- **Males are more commonly affected;** however in **females** coarctation of aorta is commonly seen in association with **Turner syndrome.**

69. (c) Renal parenchymatous disease (Ref: Nelson 19th E/P1593)

70. (b) Aorta and pulmonary artery (Ref: Nelson 19th E/1511)

- Ductus arteriosus is an essential fetal structure that normally shunts blood from the **pulmonary artery to the aorta.**

71. (d) Liver enlargement (Ref: Nelson 19th E/P1583)
- On general examination edema (usually seen in eyelids and sacrum but lower **limbs are spared)**, **hepatomegaly** and splenomegaly is present most of the times.
- **JVP** is raised but **difficult to measure** in infants because of short neck.

72. (b), (c) and **(d)** Narrow splitting of 2nd heart sound, Lt axis deviation of ECG and Shunt murmur prominent

Ostium secundum ASD:
- **Most common type of ASD,** seen in 90% of cases. Located in the centre of septum and is caused by incomplete closure of hole of septum primum by septum secundum. May be associated with **partial anomalous pulmonary venous connection** or pulmonic stenosis.
- Clinical features and findings:
  - ❖ **Most commonly seen in females** and may be associated with **Holt oram syndrome**.
  - ❖ Usually defects under 6 mm in diameter close spontaneously, but larger defects may present as failure to thrive in younger and exercise intolerance in older children.
  - ❖ A palpable **right ventricular systolic lift or heave at the left sternal border** and a **fixed and widely split 2nd heart sound is seen.**
  - ❖ A **systolic pulmonic ejection click murmur** is produced by the **increased flow across the right ventricular outflow tract into the pulmonary artery, not by low-pressure flow across the ASD.**
- Diagnosis :
  - ❖ ECG shows changes corresponding to **right axis deviation** and right ventricular hypertrophy.
  - ❖ Chest X-ray shows
    - ❑ **Enlarged right atrium and ventricle**
    - ❑ Large pulmonary artery
    - ❑ Increased pulmonary vascularity
    - ❑ **Small aortic shadow**
- Treatment:
  Nonsurgical closure with an umbrella like device (e.g. amplatzer) is preferred over surgical closure. Elective closure is usually done **after the 1st year and before entry into school.**

73. (b) TGA (Ref: Nelson 19th E/P1535)
- Transposition of great vessels presents with cyanosis within first few hours or days after birth.
- TOF does not present with cyanosis at birth, rather is seen towards end of 1 year.
- TAPVC also does not present with cyanosis at birth though later minimal cyanosis can be seen.
- PDA leads to pulmonary plethora and no cyanosis is seen.

74. (a), (c) and **(e)** Rhabdomyoma, Atrial myxoma and Fibroma (Ref: Nelson 19th E/P1581)

"The most common benign cardiac tumors in children are **rhabdomyomas**, **fibromas** and **myxomas.**"

75. (c) TOF (Ref: Nelson 19E/P1485, Rudolph 21E/P1755)
Systolic ejection click murmur:
- It is usually seen because of opening snap of semilunar valve or suddern distention of pulmonary artery or aorta wall in systole.
- The various causes of systolic ejection click murmur are:
  - ❖ Valvular aortic stenosis
  - ❖ Bicuspid aortic valve
  - ❖ Truncus arteriosus
  - ❖ **TOF**
  - ❖ Valvular pulmonic stenosis
  - ❖ Idiopathic dilation of pulmonary artery
  - ❖ Pulmonary hypertension.
- Cyanosis in TOF is usually seen towards the end of 1st year of life. In this question acyanotic baby is of 4 weeks with ejection click murmur is present. Hence the answer is TOF.

76. (a) and **(c)** Non tender and Present on extensor surfaces (Ref: Nelson 19th E/P877, Rudolph 22nd E/P943)
Subcutaneous nodules in rheumatic fever:
- This is the **least common manifestation** of rheumatic fever **(<1%)**, which is exclusively seen with severe cases like **severe carditis**.
- **Nontender, nonpruritic, freely movable nodules** of size up to **2 cm** can be seen, which are located **predominantly on the extensor surfaces of joints**, scalp and spine.
- They tend to **occur in crops** and may be present for days to months after the onset of rheumatic fever.
- These are **not specific for rheumatic fever** as they can also be seen with RA and SLE.

77. (a), (b) and **(c)** Cyanosis at birth, CHF and VSD (Ref: Nelson 19th E/P1537)
Classification of TGA: (See Table 1)

78. (c) and **(d)** VSD and Blalock taussig shunt is between pulmonary artery and subclavian artery (Ref: Nelson 19th E/P1524)
- TOF is characterized by **right ventricular hypertrophy** and **right axis deviation** in ECG. Other features are **VSD**, right ventricular outflow obstruction and dextroposition of aorta.
- Blalock Taussig shunt is the surgical management of choice which connects pulmonary artery with subclavian artery.
- **Morphine** is useful in severe and prolonged attack.

Table 1

Simple or isolated TGA	TGA with VSD	TGA with VSD and Pulmonary artery stenosis
• TGA is not associated with VSD or PAS. • Baby presents with **cyanosis in first few hours or days** of life as the ductus arteriosus begins to close. • Severe hypoxemia is seen, however CHF is less frequent. • A **loud second heart soundwith soft systolic ejection murmur** may be seen.	• TGA is associated with VSD and at times along with PAS. • Cyanosis is usually delayed because of mixing of oxygenated and deoxygenated blood through VSD. • **CHF is a frequent** complication and it should be repaired within first months of life.	• This combination of anomalies may mimic TOF and present with similar features like cyanosis, exercise intolerance and growth retardation.

79. **(a), (c), (d)** and **(e)** Sodium nitroprusside strips, Pheochromocytoma mimics the condition, IV labetolol, hydralazine, and diaoxide are given, Nifedipine is used (Ref: Nelson 19th E/P1596)
   - Increased blood pressure along with altered sensorium and seizure are diagnostic of hypertensive crisis.
   - Drugs used for the management of hypertensive crisis are:
     ❖ Labetalol
     ❖ Nitroprusside
     ❖ Nifedipine
     ❖ Hydralazine
     ❖ Diazoxide
     ❖ Furosemide
   - Pheochromocytoma is also a cause of raised blood pressure in children and may present with same symptoms.
   - Most common cause of hypertension in infants and young children is secondary i.e. due to other systemic disorders. Primary or essential hypertension i.e. if cause is not known, is common in adolescents.

80. **(a), (b), (c)** and **(e) i.e. Renal artery stenosis, Coarctation of aorta, Glomerulonephritis and Pheochromocytoma (Ref: Nelson 19th E/P1593)**
   This patient has developed hypertensive encephalopathy. Hypertension in young children is usually secondary to systemic disorders like:
   - Renal parenchymal disease — Most common cause is chronic glomerulonephritis.
   - Coarctation of aorta.
   - Endocrine disorders like pheochromocytoma.
   - Renal artery stenosis

81. **(a), (d)** and **(e)** VSD, Taussig-Blalock shunt is between pulmonary and subclavian artery and Morphine is given for Cyanosis (Ref: Nelson 19th E/P1524–25)

82. **(d)** Erythema multiforme seen (Ref: Nelson 19th E/P877, Rudolph 22nd E/P943)
   - **Chorea** is **aggravated by pregnancy** and OCPs. It is commonly seen in prepubertal girls of 8–12 years of age. Unlike other presentations of chorea like carditis and arthritis which manifest within 3–4 weeks after infection, chorea takes months to develop. This is the reason it is usually **not associated with other features like arthritis.**
   - The subcutaneous nodules are **nontender**, non-pruritic and freely movable under the skin.
   - **Erythema marginatum** is seen in RF and not erythema multiforme.

83. **(a),** and **(d)** Polyarthritis and Most common valve involved is mitral (Ref: Nelson 19th E/P 876–77, Rudolph 22nd E/P942–43)
   - Rheumatic fever is a post infective autoimmune sequalea of β **haemolytic streptococcal infection** of the upper respiratory tract.
   - **Migratory polyarthritis** is the most common manifestation seen in 70% patients.
   - **Erythema marginatum** is seen only in <3% of patients. It is a characteristic rash of rheumatic fever involving trunk and extremities but the **face is spared**.
   - **Carditis** is the **second most common** manifestation seen in 50% patients. Endocardium is always involved and the most common valve affected is **mitral valve** (mitral insufficiency).

84. **(a)** α-Hemolytic Streptococci (Ref: CPDT 19th E/P560-61)
   - Infective endocarditis can be caused by a wide range of bacteria, viruses and fungi. However the most common causes are bacterias like **viridians streptococci (α hemolytic)** followed by *Staphylococcus aureus.*

CPDT 19th E/P560–61
"Common organisms causing IE are **viridians streptococci** (30–40 % of cases), *Staphylococcus aureus* (25–30%) and fungal agents (about 5%)."

85. **(a)** Turner syndrome (Ref: Nelson 19th E/P1483, Rudolph 22E/P1778)

Syndromes associated with ASD:
- **Ellis-van Creveld syndrome (Large ASD)**
- **Down's syndrome (Ostium primum defect)**
- **Halt-Oram syndrome (Ostium secundum defect)**

- **TAR syndrome**
- cri du chat syndrome
- Trisomy 18, 13
- Noonan syndrome
- VATER syndrome complex
- Hall-Hitner (CHARGE) syndrome
- Treacher Collins syndrome
- Cardiofaciocutaneous syndrome
- Carpenter syndrome
- Cornelia De Lange syndrome
- Costello syndrome
- Loey Dietz syndrome
- Mckusick- Kaufman syndrome
- Mowat-Wilson syndrome
- Peter's plus syndrome
- Rubenstein Taybi syndrome
- Simpson-Golabi-Behmel syndrome
- Smith-Lemeli-Opitz syndrome
- Sotos syndrome
- Townes-Brocs syndrome

Other causes of ASD:
- Phenytoin
- Maternal phenylketonuria

86. **(b), (d)** and **(e)** Tricuspid atresia, Eisenmenger complex and Tetralogy of Fallot (Ref: Nelson 19E)
   Cyanotic congenital heart diseases:
   - **TOF**
   - **Tricuspid atresia**
   - TGA
   - Double outlet right ventricle
   - TAPVC
   - Truncus arteriosus
   - Double ventricle
   - **Hypoplastic left heart syndrome – Cyanosis is seen at birth.**
   - **Eisenmenger complex.**

87. **(a)** Turner's syndrome (Ref: Nelson 19th E/P1500)
   Genetic causes of ASD:
   - Single gene mutation in genes can give rise to:
     - ❖ **Noonan syndrome** — Pulmonary stenosis and hypertrophic cardiomyopathy, **ASD.**
     - ❖ **Apert syndrome** — Coarctation of aorta and VSD.
     - ❖ **Holt-Oram syndrome** — ASD and VSD.
     - ❖ **Ellis-Van creveld syndrome** — Single atrium, ASD.
     - ❖ **TAR (Thrombocytopenia-Absent Radius) syndrome** — ASD and TOF.
     - ❖ **DiGeorge syndrome** — Cardiac outflow tract defects.
     - ❖ **Alagille syndrome** — Pulmonary artery stenosis, Tetralogy of Fallot.

- Chromosomal abnormalities can give rise to:
  - ❖ Cridu chat syndrome
  - ❖ **Down syndrome — ASD**
  - ❖ Trisomy 13
  - ❖ Trisomy 18

  VSD is the most common cardiac lesion seen in these conditions

  - ❖ **Turner syndrome** — Bicuspid aortic valve and coarctation of aorta are commonly seen.

88. **(a)** VSD (Ref: Nelson 19th E/P1549)
   - Eisenmenger complex is usually seen in patients with **VSD** but can be associated with ASD, PDA or any aortopulmonary connection.

89. **(a)** Streptococcal endocarditis (Ref: CPDT 19th E/ P560–61)
   - This is a case of RHD complicated with infective endocarditis.
   - Infective endocarditis is most commonly caused by viridians streptococci.

90. **(a)** CCF (Ref: Rudolph 22nd E/P1805)
   - Most common cause of death in PDA is congestive heart failure followed by infective endocarditis.

91. **(c)** Tricuspid atresia (Ref: Nelson 19th E/P1530)
   - Faulty embryogenesis leading to unequal division of the atrio-ventricular (A-V) canal causes A-V canal defect, which gives rise to a **small and atretic tricuspid valve**, a larger mitral valve, ASD, VSD and a **hypoplastic right ventricle**.
   - The deoxygenated blood is accumulated in the right atrium and flows to the right side of heart by an **ASD and patent foramen ovale**, where it is mixed with the oxygenated blood. Further from the left ventricle mixed blood is pumped in to aorta (systemic circulation) and right ventricle (pulmonary circulation) by a VSD.
   - Clearly volume overload of the left side of heart causes **left atrial and ventricular hypertrophy**, whereas **limited supply of blood for oxygenation in to pulmonary circulation** causes **cyanosis** at birth.

92. **(b)** and **(c)** Cyanotic heart disease and Aorta anterior to pulmonary artery (Ref: Nelson 19th E/P1535)
   - TGV causes ventriculo-arterial discordance, i.e. aorta arises from right ventricle (located on the **right anterior side of pulmonary artery**) and pulmonary artery from left ventricle.
   - Cyanosis can be seen within few hours or days of birth.

93. **(c)** Subacute bacterial endocarditis (Ref: 1509)
   - Patients of VSD are at an increased risk of infective endocarditis which can result in clubbing.

94. **(b)** Renal disease (Ref: Nelson 19th E/P1593)

95. **(a)** Small (Ref: Ghai 7th E/P402)
   Chest X-ray findings in ASD:
   - Enlarged right atrium and ventricle
   - Large pulmonary artery

- Increased pulmonary vascularity
- **Small aortic shadow.**

96. **(b), (c) and (d)** Osler nodes, Microscopic hematuria and Roth spots (Ref: CPDT 19th E/P391)

On general examination one can find various manifestations of vasculitis caused by **immune complexes** in patients of bacterial endocarditis.

- **Osler nodes** — Intradermal nodes in the pads of fingers and toes.
- **Janeway lesions** — Erythematous lesions on palms and soles.
- **Splinter haemorrhages** — Linear lesions beneath the nails.

- **Roth spot** — Retinal haemorrhages.
- **Glomerulonephritis** — It presents as **microscopic hematuria**.
- **Arthralgia, myalgia, clubbing and splenomegaly**

97. **(d)** Anterior MI (Ref: Nelson 19th E/P1519)

Complications of coarctation of aorta:

- Premature coronary artery disease
- **Heart failure**
- Hypertensive encephalopathy
- **Intracranial haemorrhage**
- Aortic aneurysm
- **Infective endocarditis or endarteritis.**

QUESTIONS OF OTHER EXAMINATIONS

1. **(d)** Tetralogy of Fallot (Ref: Nelson 19th E/P1524)
2. **(d)** Squatting (Ref: Nelson 19th E/P1525)
   - **Blue spells or hypercyanotic episodes** are caused due to acute reduction in pulmonary blood flow by various reasons like prolonged crying and fever.
   - Dyspnoea occurs on exertion and the child acquires **a squatting position**, which increases the systemic B.P and increases blood flow to lungs through VSD.
3. **(a)** Electrocardiogram (Ref: Ghai 7th E/P390)
   - This is a case of rheumatic heart disease complicated by infective endocarditis.
   - Infective endocarditis should be suspected in case of nonspecific symptoms like pallor, fever and weight loss.
   - **Urine examination** shows albuminuria and microscopic hematuria.
   - **Blood culture** should be done for diagnosis of the causative agent.
   - **Echocardiography** is done to detect the cardiac changes like vegetations.
4. **(c)** Paroxysmal supraventricular tachycardia (Ref: Ghai 7th E/P429)
   - Drug of choice for treatment of PSVT is adenosine and prophylaxis of PSVT is verapamil.
5. **(b)** Congenital heart disease (cyanotic) (Ref: Nelson 19th E/P1386)

"Infants with bilalateral choanal atresia who have difficulty with mouth breathing make vigorous attempts to inspire, often suck in their lips, and develop cyanosis. Distressed children then **cry (which relieves the cyanosis)** and become more calm with normal skin color, only to repeat the cycle after closing their mouths."

6. **(c)** Prostaglandin E1 (Ref: Nelson 19th E/P1528)
   - Prostaglandin E1 is administered to maintain the patency of ductus arteriosus in patients of cyanotic congenital heart diseases.

7. **(d)** Left ventricular hypertrophy (Ref: Nelson 19th E/P1524)
8. **(b)** Transposition of great arteries (Ref: Nelson 19th E/P1535)
   - Cyanosis within first few months of births can be seen with TGV.
   - The other findings which point towards TGV are cardiomegaly and ejection systolic murmur.
9. **(a)** 1 vein and 2 arteries (Ref: Ghai 6th E/P401)
   - Umbilical cord has 2 arteries and 1 vein i.e. the left vein.
10. **(d)** Absence of flow murmurs over scapular region (Ref: Ghai 7th E/P420)
11. **(b)** PDA with reversal of shunt (Ref: Satpathy Congenital heart diseases/P22)
    - Differential cyanosis is characterized by bluish discoloration of lower limbs with normal upper limbs.
    - It can be caused by PDA with pulmonary artery hypertension or reversal of shunt and severe coarctation of aorta.
    - Reversed differential cyanosis is characterized by bluish discoloration of upper limbs with normal lower limb. It can be seen with TGA associated with PDA and pulmonary hypertension with reversal of shunt at PDA level.
12. **(b)** Indomethacin therapy (Ref: Nelson 19th E/P1512)
    - Prostaglandin maintains patency of ductus arteriosus and prostaglandin synthesis inhibitor like indo-methacin induces closure.
13. **(b)** Pulmonary stenosis (Ref: Nelson 19th E/P1525)
    - **Loud and harsh ejection systolic murmur is heard at 2nd intercostal space** in left sternal border due to turbulence through the right ventricular outflow tract.
14. **(c)** Transposition of great vessels (Ref: Nelson 19th E/P1535)

15. **(c)** Transposition of great vessels (Ref: Nelson 19th E/P1535)

16. **(d)** Congenital heart disease (Ref: Nelson 19th E/P1582)

Heart failure can be caused by:
- CHDs (**most common cause in infants**).
- RHD (**most common cause in children beyond 5 years of age**).
- Infective endocarditis.
- Myocarditis.
- Arrhythmia.

17. **(c)** Endocarditis (Ref: Ghai 7th E/P380–82)
- Carditis is the most common cause of morbidity and mortality in patients of rheumatic fever.
- Endocarditis is almost always present whereas pericarditis and myocarditis are less commonly seen.

18. **(b)** Osteum secundum (Ref: Nelson 19th E/P1504)

19. **(d)** Tetralogy of Fallot (Ref: Nelson 19th E/P1524)
- VSD, ASD and PDA cause left to right shunt which results in pulmonary plethora.
- TOF results in right to left shunting and cyanosis.

20. **(a)** Left ventricular hypertrophy (Ref: Nelson 19th E/P1504)

21. **(a)** 3 weeks (Ref: CPDT19th E/P555)
In a case of carditis in rheumaticfever:
- **Steroid** is given for **3 weeks**.
- **Aspirin** is started at 3rd week and given for **8 weeks**.

22. **(d)** Heart block (Ref: Avery disease of newborn/P875)
- Maternal SLE can lead to transfer of antibodies to the fetus and inflammatory reaction in the A-V node can lead to heart block in the newborn.

23. **(b)** Fallot's tetralogy (Ref: Nelson 19th E/P 1524)

24. **(d)** Pedal edema (Ref: Ghai 7th E/P375)

25. **(d)** Rheumatic carditis (Ref: Ghai 7th E/P380)

26. **(a)** Spontaneous closure occurs in some term infants (Ref: Nelson 19th E/P1511)
- Spontaneous closure is seen in preterm infants but not in term infants who have an anatomical defect.
- Increased flow of blood to lungs may develop pulmonary hypertension.
- CHF and recurrent pulmonary infections are frequently associated with PDA.
- Anatomic existence of PDA seen in term infants is an indication for surgery that should be done before child attains 1 year of age.

27. **(a)** Balloon septostomy (Ref: Nelson 19th E/P1535–36)
- Simple **TGA** is a **medical emergency** and treatment should be initiated as soon as the diagnosis is made.

- **Prostaglandin E1** is given to maintain the patency of ductus arteriosus.
- **Rashkind balloon atrial septostomy** *is* done if patient still remains hypoxemic on Pg E1 or delay in definite surgery is anticipated.

28. **(b)** Coxscakie B (Ref: Nelson 19th E/P1577)
- Myocarditis and pericarditis in infant can be caused by Coxscakie B and adeno virus.

29. **(d)** Hypoplastic left heart syndrome (Ref: CPDT 19th E/P549)
Hypoplastic left heart syndrome:
- Hypoplastic left syndrome is caused by different lesions of the left heart. Stenosis or atresia of the mitral and aortic valve is commonly seen. There is hypertrophy and enlargement of the right side of heart.
- The patient's condition worsens towards the end of first week due to closure of ductus arteriosus. If treatment is not started death occurs in the first week.
- Chest X-ray reveals cardiomegaly. ECG shows right axis deviation.
- Pg E1 is administered to maintain the patency of ductus arteriosus. Then Norwood procedure can be done followed by Blalock-Taussig shunt.

30. **(d)** None (Ref: Ghai 7th E/P391)

31. **(b)** Calcified mitral stenosis (Ref: Park Pediatric cardiology/P113–14)
Indications of Balloon valvuloplasty:
- **Pulmonary valve stenosis.**
- **Aortic valve stenosis.**
- **Mitral stenosis without calcification.**

32. **(a)** Cardiac deformities (Ref: Nelson 19th E/P1500)
- Lithium intake by mother can cause cardiac defects like Ebstein anomaly.

33. **(d)** Ebstein's anomaly of tricuspid valve (Ref: Ghai 7th E/P412)
- Intracardiac ECG with simultaneous pressure recording is done for diagnosis of Ebstein's anomaly.

34. **(a)** Carditis (Ref: CPDT 19th E/P555)
- *Steroids are given in rheumatic fever when there is severe carditis or heart failure.*
- *Steroid of choice is prednisolone at a dose of 2mg/kg/d for 2 weeks followed by 1 mg/kg/d in the third week, and aspirin is started at a dose of 50 mg/kg/d.*
- ***Prednisolone is stopped at the end of 3rd week*** *and aspirin is continued for 8weeks or until CRP is negative and ESR is going downhill.*

35. **(b)** Acute glomerulonephritis (Ref: Nelson 19th E/P1593)

36. (b), (c) and **(d)** Osler nodes, Microscopic hematuria and Roth spots (Ref: CPDT 19th E/P391)

On general examination one can find various manifesta-tions of vasculitis caused by **immune complexes** in patients of bacterial endocarditis.

- **Osler nodes** — Intradermal nodes in the pads of fingers and toes.

- **Janeway lesions** — Erythematous lesions on palms and soles.

- **Splinter haemorrhages** — Linear lesions beneath the nails.

- **Roth spot** — Retinal haemorrhages.

- **Glomerulonephritis** — It presents as **microscopic hematuria**.

- **Arthralgia, myalgia, clubbing and splenomegaly**

37. (a) Pulmonary edema (Ref: Nelson 19th E/P1582)

- Pulmonary edema is seen in left sided heart failure and not right sided.

5

Central Nervous System

CONGENITAL DEFECTS OF CNS

The formation of the CNS can be divided in to two periods of 0–28 days and post 28 days:

- **0–28 days** of gestation is the period of **neural tube formation and closure**. Any abnormality in this phase can lead to neural tube defects like spina bifida occulta, meningocele, **myelomeningocele, encephalocele, anencephaly,** dermal sinus, tethered cord, syringomyelia, diastometamyelia and lipoma involving the conus medullaris and filum terminale.
- **Post 28 days** there is **proliferation and migration of neuronal cells** to their proper site. Any abnormality in this phase can cause disorders in neuronal migration like lissencephaly, schizencephaly, porencephaly and holoprosencephaly.

NEURAL TUBE DEFECTS (NTD)

The primary cause for NTD is not known, however many predisposing factors like hyperthermia, drugs (anticonvulsants, antifolate), malnutrition **(folic acid deficiency),** radiation exposure and genetic factors (mutation in folate dependent pathways) have been attributed to its cause. NTDs allow fetal substances like α **fetoprotein** and **acetylcholinesterase** in to amniotic fluid, which are used as prenatal biochemical markers for diagnosis.

Spina Bifida Occulta

- This is usually a self-limiting defect of the vertebral bodies caused by inability of the neural tube to separate from the overlying ectoderm.
- Most common presentation is benign dermal lesions like **patches of hair**, lipoma, pigmented macules, hemangioma or a dermal sinus in the **middle of lower back.**

Meningocele

- This is caused by herniation of meninges through a defect in the posterior vertebral arches.
- In females there may be associated genital tract abnormalities like rectovaginal fistula and vaginal septa.

Myelomeningocele

- This is the **most severe form of NTD** characterised by herniation of the meninges along with the spinal cord. The most common site of location is **lumbosacral region**. The clinical presentation depends on the site of location.
- Lower sacral lesions cause **bladder** and **bowel incontinence** with perineal anaesthesia.
- Midlumbar lesions cause **flaccid paralysis of lower limbs,** constant urinary dribbling, **laxed anal sphincter** and a higher incidence of lower limb deformities like club feet and subluxation of hip joint.
- **Hydrocephalus** can be seen in 80% cases and is commonly associated with **type II Chiari defect**.
- Treatment comprises of early surgical repair (within 3 days) of the defect to prevent infection. This is followed by shunt placement for hydrocephalus. Broad spectrum antibiotic from birth till closure is indicated.

- The most common post-operative complication is **wound dehiscence** which can be followed by CSF leak if a shunt is not placed. The baby is at a high risk of fecal contamination of the wound and in case of CSF leak, meningitis is unavoidable. In this case a **CSF study should be done with biochemical parameters and culture.**

Encephalocele

- This is protrusion of the cerebral cortex, cerebellum or brain stem through a cranial defect cranium bifidum.
- The most common location is the **occipital region.**
- Hydrocephalus can be seen due to **aqueductal stenosis, Chiari malformation** or the **Dandy-Walker syndrome.**

Anencephaly

- This is due to failure of development of cerebral hemispheres and cerebellum.
- It may be associated with **cleft palate** and **congenital heart defects.**

Neuronal Migration Defects

Neuronal migration defects are caused by a defect in the **radial glial fibres** which attach to the neurons and help in migration to proper site. Most of these defects are associated with severe **intractable seizures, developmental delay and neonatal hypotonia.**

Lissencephaly or Agyria

- It is characterised by absence of cerebral convolutions, a four layered cortex (normally there are 6 layers), enlarged lateral ventricles, microcephaly and microopthalmia.
- When associated with **Miller-Dieker syndrome** the baby has a characteristic facies with prominent forehead, bitemporal hallowing, anteverted nostrils, micrognathia and a prominent upper lip.

Schizencephaly

- It is characterised by unilateral or bilateral clefts in the cerebral hemispheres.
- The baby presents with cognitive deficits and congenital spastic quadriparesis (bilateral clefts) or hemiparesis (unilateral cleft).

Porencephaly

- It is characterised by presence of **cysts in the brain** because of **developmental defect or acquired lesions caused by infarction or injury.**
- Most common site of location is **sylvian fissure**.
- True porencephalic cysts connect with the subarachnoid space but pseudoporencephalic cysts which are caused by abnormalities of vascular system(infarction, haemorrhage) duringperinatal or postnatal period do not connect.

Holoprosencephaly

- This is caused by defect in the cleavage of prosencephalon.
- The baby might have facial abnormalities like cyclopia, cebocephaly, single central incisor tooth and premaxillary agenesis.

CRANIOSYNOSTOSIS

Craniosynostosis is a developmental defect of the skull caused by early fusion of the cranial sutures. The different types of craniosynostosis that can be seen based on the suture involved are scaphocephaly, plagiocephaly, brachycephaly, trigonocephaly and turricephaly.

Scapocephaly

This is the **most common** type of craniosynostosis which is caused by early fusion of **sagittal sutures.** It is commonly seen in **males.**

Plagiocephaly

It can be associated with Chotzen syndrome.

- **Frontal plagiocephaly:** This is **2nd most common type** of craniosynostosis which is caused by early fusion of **coronal** and **sphenofrontal sutures**. It is more commonly seen in **females.**
- **Occipital plagiocephaly:** It is most commonly caused by positioning during infancy or by early fusion of lambdoid sutures.

Brachycephaly

This is seen because of early fusion of **both coronal sutures**. It can be associated with Crouzon syndrome and Apert syndrome.

Trigonocephaly

This is caused by early fusion of **metopic suture** which gives a keel shaped forehead and hypertelorism.

Turricephaly

This is a cone shaped skull because of early closure of coronal, sphenofrontal and frontoethmoidal sutures. It is associated with Pfeiffer syndrome.

Kleeblatschadel Deformity

This is a cloverleaf shaped skull that can be seen in Carpenter syndrome.

HYDROCEPHALUS

Hydrocephalus is a condition characterised by increased CSF volume (Normal volume=50 ml in infants) due to increased production (choroid plexus papilloma), obstruction to flow (non- communicating hydrocephalus) or decreased absorption of CSF (communicating hydrocephalus). CSF is predominantly produced by choroid plexus in the lateral ventricles, which then passes subsequently through foramen of **Monroe** to third ventricle and **cerebral aqueduct** to fourth ventricle. Then via foramen of **Luschka** and **Magendi,** CSF reaches the basal cisterns which connect the spinal and cranial subarachnoid space. Finally absorption of CSF takes place in the subarachnoid space by the arachnoid villi.

Non-communicating Hydrocephalus

Non-communicating hydrocephalus is caused by obstruction to the flow of CSF at various levels (aqueduct, posterior fossa). This is the **most common type of hydrocephalus** seen in children which is caused by aqueductal stenosis, Chiari malformation, Dandy-Walker malformation and space occupying lesions.

- **Aqueductal stenosis:** This is the **most common cause** of non-communicating hydrocephalus. Being a long and narrow tract of CSF flow, aqueduct is more prone to develop stenosis. The different causes of stenosis can be
  - ❖ Genetic (X linked recessive) — This is a **rare cause of hydrocephalus** which may be associated with congenital anomalies like neural tube defects.
  - ❖ Gliosis of the aqueduct caused by **meningitis (mumps)** and subarachnoid haemorrhage are relatively **more common cause of aqueductal stenosis**.
- **Chiari malformation:** The cause is displacement of cerebellar tonsils in to the cervical canal resulting in compression of the medulla. Type I usually presents in adulthood without hydrocephalus, but **type II, the most common type** presents with hydrocephalus and a myelomeningocele in the infancy.
- **Dandy-Walker malformation:** A cystic malformation of the cerebellum and fourth ventricle is seen because of atresia of foramen of Luscha and Magendie.
- Mass lesions like vein of Galen malformation, tumors, abscess and hematoma also can cause obstructive hydrocephalus.

Communicating Hydrocephalus

Communicating hydrocephalus is usually caused by various factors like blood, inflammatory exudates and cells that decrease the absorption of CSF by arachnoid villi.

- **Subarachnoid haemorrhage:** This is the **most common cause** of communicating hydrocephalus.
- **Infections:** Pneumococcal and tubercular meningitis produce thick exudates that block CSF absorption.
- Leukemic infiltrates also can block the CSF absorption.

Clinical Findings of Hydrocephalus

- The most common appreciable sign of hydrocephalus is **rapid increase in the size of head along with a bulging anterior fontanel**, dilated scalp veins and frontal bossing.
- **Papilledema** is seen in older children but **usually absent in infants** because of open sutures which can absorb the increase in ICT.
- **Setting sun eye sign:** This is because of downward eye deviation.
- **Crack pot sound** on percussion of skull (**Macewen sign**) can be heard, which is because of suture separation.

Clinical Features of Hydrocephalus

- Infants usually present with irritability, vomiting, drowsiness and refusal to feed.
- In older children early morning **headache**, visual abnormalities (**diplopia** and blurred vision), **gradual personality change** and **deterioration of academic performance** can be seen.

Diagnosis

- X-ray shows a **"beaten silver"** appearance of the skull due to increased convolutional markings.
- USG is more preferred in infants; however CT scan or MRI should be done to establish the cause of hydrocephalus.

Treatment

- Medical management (diuretics) is preferred for temporary relief but are not effective for long term management.
- For long term benefit interventional procedures are done:
  - ❖ Different shunts like ventriculo-atrial, ventriculo-peritoneal and externalised shunt can be established.
  - ❖ Endoscopic third ventriculostomy also can be done.

SEIZURE AND EPILEPSY IN CHILDHOOD

Seizure is characterised by a paroxysmal motor, sensory or behavioural activity caused by synchronous discharge of cortical neurons. Epilepsy is a tendency to develop recurrent unprovoked seizures i.e. which are not provoked by other factors like fever, metabolic derangements (hypoglycemia or hyponatremia), CNS insult (stroke, trauma or meningitis). Seizures can be classified as partial seizures and generalised seizures based on their etiopathogenesis and presentation.

Generalised Seizures

Generalised seizures are caused by abnormal firing of thalamic neurons mediated by calcium channels, which depolarises whole of the cortex. Thus antiepileptic that block calcium channels are most preferred for treatment. The different types of generalised seizures are absence seizures, myoclonic seizures, clonic seizures, tonic seizures, generalised tonic clonic seizures (GTCS) and atonic seizures.

Absence Seizures

Absence seizure can be classified as simple absence seizure and complex absence seizure.

- **Simple/Typical absence seizure (Petit mal seizures):**
  - ❖ SAS is characterised by a **brief state of staring** lasting less than 30 seconds, which may be associated with other features like blinking of eyes, upward deviation of eyes and slackening of facial muscles. Most of the times it can be **precipitated by hyperventilation.**
  - ❖ It is seen in **children after 5 years of age** and is more common in female child. Most of the times these children have **poor school performance** due to intermittent episodes during classes.
  - ❖ It is not associated with falls, aura or **post ictal confusion.**
  - ❖ EEG shows a characteristic **3 Hz spike wave discharge.**

- **Complex/Atypical absence seizure:**
  - ❖ Apart from the general features of SAS, CAS also has myoclonic movements of face, fingers or extremities and loss of body tone.
  - ❖ **Rolandic spikes** (centrotemporal spikes) are characteristic.
- **Treatment:** The most preferred drug for treatment of absence seizures is **sodium valproate**. However because of its increased risk of hepatotoxicity in **children less than 2 year, ethosuximide** is more preferred in this age group.

Myoclonic Epilepsies

In myoclonic epilepsy repetitive seizures are seen which are characterised by brief muscular contraction with loss of body tone. Depending on the presentation they can be classified as benign myoclonus of infancy, typical myoclonic epilepsy, complex myoclonic epilepsy, **juvenile myoclonic epilepsy** and progressive myoclonic epilepsy.

- **Juvenile myoclonic epilepsy (Janz syndrome):**
  - ❖ JME begins in the age group of 12–16 years with bilateral **myoclonic jerks (myoclonus)** in **early morning period** which later progress to **GTCS and absence seizures in only 25% of patients**. It can be precipitated by sleep deprivation.
  - ❖ Family history of epilepsy is common and the gene locus for JME is chromosome 6p21.
  - ❖ EEG shows a **4–6 Hz irregular spike and wave discharges (fast spikes)** enhanced by photo stimulation. **Neurological examination is normal.**
  - ❖ Out of all drugs that block the thalamic calcium channels JME responds best to **valproate** but recurrence rate is very high on discontinuation. This makes the therapy mandatory for **lifelong**. Other drugs which are effective in treating JME are **topiramate, zonisamide and lamotrigine.**

Infantile Spasms

Infantile spasms are characterised by a symmetric contraction of the body muscles. They can be classified based on clinical presentation and etiology.

- **Clinical classification:**
  - ❖ **Flexor spasm** — This is characterised by flexion of hips and neck tensing of shoulders, which is referred to as **"jack knife seizures"** or **"salaam seizures"**.
  - ❖ **Extensor spasm** — This is the least common type of infantile spasm.
  - ❖ **Mixed spasm** — This is the most common type of infantile spasm.
- **Etiological classification:** Based on etiology it can be classified as cryptogenic and symptomatic infantile spasm

Cryptogenic infantile spasm	Symptomatic infantile spasm
• The cause of spasm can't be identified.	• The cause is related to various factors like neurodegeneration, infection, trauma and congenital defects.
• Prognosis is good.	• **Mental retardation** is seen in 90% cases.
• 20% cases are cryptogenic.	• **Most common type** and accounts for 80% cases

- **Diagnosis:** EEG shows a high voltage, slow wave activity called as **hypsarrhythmia**.
- **Treatment:** The **drug of choice** for infantile spasms is **ACTH**. Vigabatrin though equipotent, is not preferred because it can cause irreversible visual field defects.

Partial Seizures

Partial seizures are caused by a focal abnormality in the cortex like infarct, tumor, or infective lesions like NCC. These lesions irritate the cortical neurons which lead to epileptogenic activity mediated by sodium channels. Thus the best drug to treat this condition is a sodium channel blocker i.e. **carbamazepine**. Partial seizures can be of two type **simple partial seizure** and **complex partialseizure (temporal lobe epilepsy).**

- Features of simple and complex partial seizures:

Simple partial seizure (SPS)	Complex partial seizure (CPS)
In SPS **motor activity** characterised by tonic or clonic movement of face, neck or extremities **without loss of consciousness**. *Aura can be present. ***Automatism is not seen.** Lasts 10-20 seconds. **Postictal confusion absent.**	In CPS **motor activity** characterised by tonic or clonic movement of face, neck or extremities with **loss of consciousness.** Aura can be present. **Automatism is characteristic.** Lasts 1-2 minutes. **Postictal confusion present.**

*Aura is presence of some unusual feeling, chest discomfort, headache or hallucinations (auditory, visual or **gustatory**).

*Automatism is presence of some movements like smacking of lips, chewing, swallowing after loss of consciousness in CPS.

- Partial seizures respond best to anticonvulsants blocking sodium channels like carbamazepine, oxcarbazepine, phenytoin, levetiracetam, and Zonisamide. The drug of choice for partial seizures is **carbamazepine**.

Febrile Seizures

Febrile seizure is the most common seizure disorder in children characterised by rapid increase in body temperature to **more than 39°C.** The most common cause is acute respiratory illness, which makes the winter time as most common period for febrile seizures. The most common age group affected is **9 months to 5 years;** however the peak age is 18 months.

- **Clinical presentation:**
  - ❖ The seizure is usually generalised tonic- clonic in nature which lasts for a period of **less than 5 minutes** in most cases. Based on the different associated features febrile seizures can be classified as simple and complex febrile seizures.
  - ❖ A **simple febrile seizure** is a single and brief seizure episode which has a benign outcome.
  - ❖ A **complex febrile seizure** is characterised by presence of different atypical features like **seizure duration more than 15 minutes, more than one seizure a day and focal seizures in post-ictal period.**
  - ❖ **Recurrent seizure** is a feature of febrile seizures which can be seen in **30-50%** of patients. The risk factors for the same are **early age of onset (<12 months), family history of febrile seizures,** short duration of fever, seizure following lower temperature (<40°C), **developmental delay,** abnormal neurological conditions (cerebral palsy or mental retardation) and **presence of atypical features (complex febrile seizure).**
- **Prognosis:** Simple febrile seizure is associated with a favourable outcome, whereas complex febrile seizure is associated with an increased risk of status epilepticus associated mesial temporal lobe sclerosis, mental retardation and developmental delay.
- **Diagnosis:** The aim is to find out the cause of fever and rule out other CNS infections.
  - ❖ Neurological imaging is done in cases of complex febrile seizures.
  - ❖ Lumbar puncture is more important in patients younger than 18 months as physical findings of CNS infections are less reliable.
  - ❖ Serum electrolytes and blood glucose should be done to rule out hyponatremia and hypoglycaemia.
  - ❖ **EEG is normal** in patients of simple febrile seizure; however 3 Hz spikes can be seen in complex febrile seizure patients.
- **Treatment:** The drug of choice for an acute episode is diazepam by rectal route or intra venous route.
- **Prophylaxis:**
  - ❖ **Intermittent prophylaxis — Diazepam** by oral route at the onset of fever is the preferred method for both simple and complex febrile seizures.
  - ❖ Continuous prophylaxis — Anticonvulsants effective in febrile seizure like **phenobarbitone** and **valproate** are indicated if febrile seizures are complex or prolonged and medical reassurance (prophylactic diazepam at onset of fever) fails to relieve family anxiety. This is continuous prophylaxis and the duration of treatment is seizure free period of 1 year or till 5 years of age.
  - ❖ Measures to lower the temperature like sponging and **antipyretics don't have any role** in prophylaxis.

Neonatal Seizures

Neonatal seizures can be classified based on their presentation as focal, multifocal, myoclonic, tonic and **subtle seizures (most common type)**. **Subtle seizures** are characterised by movements of upper limb ("swimming", "boxing" or "hooking") and lower limb ("bicycling"); sucking, lip smacking and apnoea. These are caused by a wide range of pathological abnormalities and hence require a multidimensional approach for management.

- **Causes of neonatal seizures:**
    - ❖ **Hypoxic ischemic encephalopathy** is the **most common cause of neonatal seizures** and is associated with **worst prognosis**. Seizures develop within first 24 hours because of cerebral edema.
    - ❖ In neonatal period various metabolic abnormalities can cause seizure:
        - ❑ **Hypoglycemia** — It develops within 24 hours after birth and **Seizure with mental retardation** can be seen.
        - ❑ **Hypocalcemia** — It can be early onset hypocalcemia (within 72 hours) and late onset hypocalcemia. Seizures are usually caused by early onset hypocalcemia and are associated with a **better neurological outcome.**
        - ❑ Hypo and Hypernatremia
    - ❖ Metabolic diseases like galactosemia, hyperglycinemia and urea cycle disorders can cause seizures.
    - ❖ Benign familial neonatal seizures start at 2nd–3rd day of life, but most commonly present on 5th day (**Fifth day fits**). It is associated with a favourable outcome.
    - ❖ **Pyridoxine** dependent seizures are seen shortly after birth, which are resistant to anticonvulsants. Pyridoxine deficiency leads to depletion of inhibitory neurotransmitter GABA, which is the primary cause for seizure. The best treatment is pyridoxine replacement.
    - ❖ Withdrawal of certain drugs like barbiturates, benzodiazepines and opioids can cause seizure.
    - ❖ Congenital brain abnormalities like neuronal migration defects and neurodegenerative disorders can also cause seizures. The prognosis is poor.
- The drug of choice for neonatal seizures is **phenobarbitone.**

Status Epilepticus

Status epilepticus is defined as a condition in which the duration of one seizure is 30 minutes or multiple seizures occur in 30 minutes without regaining of consciousness.

- **Cause:** It can be precipitated by many causes but in children 50% of cases are because of either infection (sepsis, meningitis, encephalitis) or metabolic abnormalities (hypoglycaemia, hypocalcemia, **hyponatremia**). Most common age group affected is children **less than 2 years of age** and most common cause is febrile seizure. It is a medical emergency and requires prompt management.
- **Treatment:**

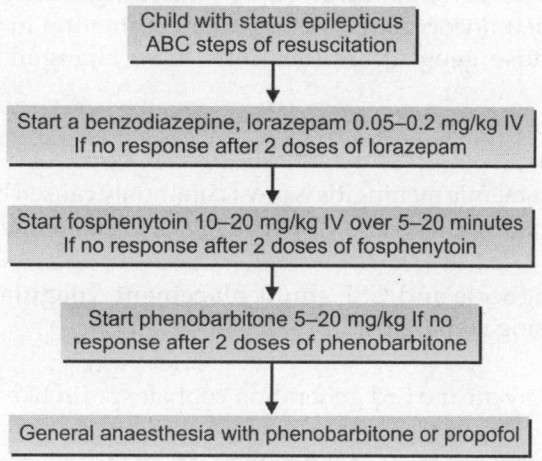

Fig. 5.1

Valproate is preferred in place of phenytoin if it is a case of absence status epilepticus.

CNS INFECTIONS

CNS infections are **most commonly caused by viruses** followed by bacteria and then fungi and parasites. Depending on the extent of involvement infections of CNS can be classified as **meningitis, encephalitis, meningoencephalitis and brain abscess**. These are one of the major treatable causes of morbidity and mortality in children. Hence prompt diagnosis and treatment is always desired.

Meningitis

- **Clinical features:**
  - ❖ The most common presentation of meningitis is nonspecific signs and symptoms like lethargy, irritability, refusal to feed, skin lesions (petechiae, purpura or rash) and headache.
  - ❖ Meningeal irritation presents as nuchal rigidity (rare in neonate), meningismus and some clinical signs of Kernig and Brudginski. **Kernig sign** is positive if flexion of hip at 90° and extension of leg causes pain whereas **Brudginski** sign is positive if flexion of the neck leads to flexion of hips and knees. **Meningismus** refers to a reflex tension of back and neck muscle to avoid the pain caused by extension of inflamed meninges.
  - ❖ **Seizures** are the **most common complication**, seen in almost 1/3rd cases of meningitis and should be differentiated from a febrile seizure (seizure occurs with onset of fever). The other complications that can be seen are **subdural effusions**, **abscess**, subarachnoid haemorrhage, cortical infarction and necrosis, cranial nerve palsies (II,IV,VII,VIII), raised ICT and hydrocephalus. Hydrocephalus can be seen because of aqueductal stenosis or arachnoid villi blockade due to inflammatory exudates.
- **Diagnosis:** Diagnosis of meningitis is confirmed by the study of CSF. The different findings seen in CSF are —

Cause of meningitis	Cells	Protein	Glucose	ICT
Bacterial	Neutrophils	Increased	Decreased	Increased
Tubercular	Lymphocytes	Increased	Decreased	Increased
Viral	Lymphocytes	Normal to slightly increased	Normal	Normal to slightly increased

Bacterial Meningitis

- The cause of bacterial (septic) meningitis in children is diverse and varies according to different age groups and presence of risk factors. Overall 80% of infections are caused by *N. meningitidis, S. pneumonae and H. infuenzae*.
  - ❖ **Etiology based on age group:**
    - ❑ Neonates (0–28 days) — The most common cause of neonatal meningitis is the group B Streptococcus i.e. **streptococcus agalctiae followed by E. coli.** Other causative organisms are enterococci, **Klebsiella** and **Listeria monocytogenes**.
    - ❑ 2 months-12 years — In the **developing countries like India**, the most common cause of meningitis in this particular age group is *S. pneumonae* **followed by N.meningitidis and** *H. influenzae*. However due to widespread successful pneumococcal and H.infuenza vaccination in the **developed countries**, the most common pathogen in those geographic locations have changed to *N. meningitidis* **followed by** *S. pneumoniae*.
    - ❑ In adults i.e. age >20 years *S. pneumoniae* is the most common agent.
  - ❖ **Etiology based on risk factors:**
    - ❑ In children with occult bacteraemia meningitis is most commonly caused by *N. meningitidis*.
    - ❑ In children with **splenic abnormalities** and **CSF leakage**, *S. pneumoniae* is the commonest pathogen causing bacterial meningitis.
    - ❑ Babies with myelomeningocele and CSF shunt placement, coagulase negative staphylococci are the commonest organism causing meningitis.
- **Treatment:**
  - ❖ For empirical therapy Vancomycin and 3rd generation cephalosporin like ceftriaxone or cefotaxime should be used.
  - ❖ When diagnosis is confirmed the treatment of choice is based on the sensitivity of the organism to any particular antibiotic.
  - ❖ **S.pneumoniae** sensitive to beta lactam antibiotics are treated by **penicillin** or a **3rd generation cephalosporin** for 10–14 days. In case of resistance **vancomycin** should be used.

❖ *H. influenzae* is treated by **amoxicillin** for a period of 10 days. In case of resistance extended spectrum cephalosporins are given. **Dexamethasone** decreases the incidence of hearing loss and should be given 1-24 hours before administration of antibiotics.

❖ **Penicillin** is the drug of choice for *N. meningitidis* and *L. monocytogens*.

❖ Gram negative organisms like **Pseudomonas**, *E.coli* and *Klebsiella* should be treated with a **combination of ceftazidime and an aminoglycoside** for 3 weeks.

Tubercular Meningitis

- The most common age group affected is children from **6 months to 4 years** of age.
- The cause of tubercular meningitis is usually a **"Rich focus"** located in the cortex or meninges, which is a caseous lesion formed by dissemination of the primary infection. This lesion discharge tubercle bacilli in to subarachnoid space which forms inflammatory exudate which causes cerebral pathologies like vasculitis, **infarction**, edema and hydrocephalus. Brain stem is commonly involved and can present as **3rd, 6th and 7th cranial nerve palsies**.
- **SIADH** may be associated with tubercular meningitis which can further affect the outcome.
- **Clinically it can be divided in to three stages:**
  ❖ **First stage** — It is characterised by nonspecific symptoms like drowsiness, fatigue, fever and irritability. Treatment at this stage has the best outcome.
  ❖ **Second stage** — It is characterised by specific signs and symptoms of meningitis like nuchal rigidity, positive Kernig and Brudginski signs, seizures, hypotonia and cranial nerve palsies.
  ❖ **Third stage** — It is characterised by hemiplegia, paraplegia, coma and death. Treatment at this phase has the worst outcome.
- **Diagnosis:**
  ❖ Examination and culture of CSF is the best diagnostic method as tuberculin test and chest radiograph is normal in majority of patients. The CSF shows **lymphocytes, decreased glucose or hypoglycorrachia i.e. glucose less than 40mg/dl and increased protein levels**. Culture and staining of CSF should be done for definite diagnosis.
  ❖ CT or MRI shows **basilar enhancement** and **communicating hydrocephalus**.

Viral Meningoencephalitis

Viruses are the most common cause of CNS infection and most of them have an acute or subacute course. Most of the viruses that infect meninges have some degree of brain parenchymal infection and hence the term viral (aseptic) meningoencephalitis is apt here. The common viruses capable causing meningoencephalitis are **enteroviruses**, herpes simplex virus type 1 and 2, human herpes virus-6 and mumps virus. Rarely respiratory viruses (adenovirus, influenza and parainfluenza virus), rubella, rubeola and rabies virus or by live vaccinations against **polio, measles**, mumps or rubella can also cause meningoencephalitis.

- **Enteroviruses:** These are the **most common cause** of viral meningoencephalitis.
- **HSV:** HSV usually affects the **temporal lobe** and thus focal seizures or focal findings in CT, MRI or EEG involving the temporal lobe are diagnostic for HSV infection. Unlike other viral infections with a normal or slightly elevated CSF protein levels, in **HSV protein levels can be very high.**
  ❖ **HSV-1** is a predominant cause of sporadic encephalitis in **children and adults**. Unlike other viruses it causes **focal involvement.**
  ❖ **HSV-2** is a primary cause in **neonates**, who acquire the virus from the genital tract of mother. In this case there is **diffuse involvement** of the brain.
- **VZV:** The most common manifestation of VZV CNS infection is **cerebellar ataxia.**
- **HHV-6:** It is a cause of meningoencephalitis in **immunocompromised patients.**
- **Mumps:** It is associated with a **milder meningoencephalitis** but **hearing loss** can be seen due to 8th cranial nerve damage. Unlike other viral infections the **CSF glucose level is low.**

Brain Abscess

- Brain abscess can be caused secondarily to embolization because of **right to left shunt CHD (TOF)**, meningitis and infections of other origins like ear, teeth and eye. Though a wide range of organisms are responsible, **citrobacter** is the most common cause of brain abscess. These lesions are usually single.
- The clinical presentation starts with generalised symptoms like **fever** and lethargy which can progress to specific CNS symptoms like seizures and hemiparesis.

- **Diagnosis:**
  - ❖ MRI is the investigation of choice; however CT can also be used for diagnosis.
  - ❖ EEG shows focal slowing.
  - ❖ Lumbar puncture is contraindicated as it can cause cerebellar herniation. The CSF is usually normal and CSF study does not add to diagnosis.
- **Treatment:**
  - ❖ Antibiotics are the initial management of choice.
  - ❖ Surgical excision is required if:
    - ❑ Size of abscess is more than 2.5 cm
    - ❑ Gas is present inside abscess
    - ❑ Multiple lesions are present
    - ❑ Lesion is in posterior fossa
    - ❑ Fungal cause of lesion is established.

NEUROCUTANEOUS DISORDERS OR PHAKOMATOSES

The neurocutaneous disorders are a group of autosomal dominant inherited disorders characterised by abnormal growth of various tissues. The disorders included are neurofibromatosis, tuberous sclerosis, Sturge-Weber disease, von Hippel-Lindau disease, PHACE syndrome, ataxia telangiectasia, linear nevus syndrome, hypomelanosis of Ito and incontinentia pigmenti.

Neurofibromatosis

Neurofibromatosis or von Recklinghausen disease is caused by faulty neural crest differentiation and migration. Based on the gene involved and clinical presentation they can be of 2 types NF1 and NF2. Gene for NF1 is located in **17th** chromosome and NF2 is located in **22nd** chromosome.

Neurofibromatosis 1

This is the most common neurocutaneous disorder characterised by a wide range of clinical presentations.
- **Clinical findings:**
  - ❖ **Café au lait spots** are lesions seen in all patients during early childhood (first 2 years of life) are hallmark of NF1. They are usually located on the trunk and extremities (**face is spared**). For diagnosis 6 lesions with a diameter of more than 5 mm should be present.
  - ❖ Benign cutaneous neurofibromas are purple colour lesions that are collection of Schwann cells, fibroblasts and mast cells seen at the time of puberty or pregnancy. Itching can be present but they are not painful.
  - ❖ Plexiform neurofibromas are premalignant neurofibromas which are associated with peripheral nerve sheaths and are commonly located in orbital or temporal region of face. They can transform in to **nerofibrosarcomas**.
  - ❖ Intertriginous freckling usually involves the axillary and the inguinal areas.
  - ❖ Lisch nodules are iris hamartomas.
  - ❖ **Optic gliomas** — Patients with these benign pilocytic astrocytomas are usually **asymptomatic**.
  - ❖ Skeletal features — Sphenoid wing dysplasia (**mostly unilateral**), long bone bowing and dystrophic scoliosis (**most common**) can be seen.
- **Complications:**
  - ❖ Speech and language delays can be seen in half of the cases.
  - ❖ CNS complications like seizures (CPS and GTCS), hydrocephalus, macrocephaly, moyamoya disease and cerebral infarction can be seen.
  - ❖ Tumors like neurofibrosarcoma, astrocytoma, rhabdomysarcoma, meningioma, pheochromocytoma and **juvenile myelomonocytic leukaemia (juvenile chronic myelogenous leukaemia; JCML)** can be seen.
- **Diagnosis:** For diagnosis of NF1 any one of the clinical findings of neurofibromatosis along with family history should be present.

Neurofibromatosis 2

- For diagnosis of NF2 **bilateral acoustic neuromas** (VIIIth nerve tumor) should be present along with a positive family history. Other classical features of NF1 are less commonly seen.
- Posterior subcapsular lenticular opacities are seen in half of the patients.

Tuberous sclerosis

Tuberous sclerosis (Bourneville's disease) is caused by mutation of TSC genes. TSC1 gene is located in **9th** chromosome and TSC2 gene in **16th** chromosome. The clinical findings in tuberous sclerosis can be classified as major and minor findings.

- **Major clinical findings:**
  - ❖ **Skin lesions** — The different skin lesions that can be seen are **hypopigmented macules (ashleaf macules), sebaceous adenomas**, shagreen patches and subungual or periungual fibromas.
  - ❖ Retinal lesions like mulberry tumors and hamartomas can be seen.
  - ❖ **CNS manifestations** — **Seizures**(infantile spasms, myoclonic epilepsies), **cognitive and behavioural impairment** can be seen (autism).
  - ❖ **Tumors** — **Malignant astrocytoma**, rhabdomyosarcoma of heart, renal angiomyolipoma and pulmonary lymphangiomyomatosis can be seen.
- Minor clinical findings like bone and renal cysts, rectal polyps, confetti skin lesions and neuronal migrational defects can be seen.
- **Diagnosis** — For diagnosis either 2 major findings or 1 major plus 1 minor is required.
- **Treatment** — Recently Everolimus has been approved for treatment of T.S associated tumors.

Sturge-Weber Syndrome

Sturge-Weber syndrome is caused by a faulty vasculogenesis which leads to poor vascularisation of the cerebral cortex and hypervascularisation of surrounding membranes (pia and arachnoid mater). This leads to atrophy and calcification of the cortex.

- **Clinical findings and management:**
  - ❖ **Port-wine stain (facial nevus)** — This is a capillary malformation characterised by unilateral pink-purple macular lesion seen on **ophthalmic and maxillary distribution of the trigeminal nerve** in the head and neck region (**upper face and eyelid is always involved**) and at times in mucous membranes. This is a **permanent lesion**, which in adulthood can give cobblestone appearance. These lesions should be distinguished from salmon patch which is a **transient vascular lesion**. The best treatment is **flashlamp-pumped-pulse dye laser**.
  - ❖ **Seizures** — Focal tonic-clonic seizures are seen opposite to the side of nevus. If seizures are refractory to medication, hemispherectomy is done.
  - ❖ Transient stroke like episodes can be seen due to cortical vein thrombosis.
- **Complications:**
  - ❖ Mental retardation can be seen in half of the patients.
  - ❖ Ipsilateral bupthalmos and glaucoma can be seen.
- **Diagnosis:**
  - ❖ X-ray skull shows a characteristic **rail-track or serpentine** calcified lesions.

Von Hippel-Lindau disease

VHL is an autosomal dominant disorder caused by germline mutation in the VHL gene in 3rd chromosome.

- **Clinical findings:**
  - ❖ **Cerebellar hemangioblastomas** — These capillary malformations in the cerebellum present with symptoms of raised ICT.
  - ❖ **Retinal angiomas** —These angiomas are usually located in the peripheral retina and do not affect vision, however they can cause retinal detachment.
  - ❖ **Renal cell carcinoma** — This is the most common cause of death.
  - ❖ Pheochomocytoma and various cystic lesions in kidney, liver and pancreas can be seen.

Incontinentia Pigmenti

Incontinentia pigmenti or Bloch – Sulzberger disease is caused by a random X inactivation of an X linked dominant gene. It is lethal in males and hence more frequently can be seen in females.

- **Clinical presentation:**
  - ❖ Cutaneous manifestation that can be seen are linear erythematous streaks and vesicular plaques on the limbs and trunk, **verrucous plaques** due to keratinization of dry blisters and hypopigmented and hairless patches primarily on the flexor aspects of legs.

❖ CNS abnormalities like seizures, microcephaly and MR can be seen.

❖ Ocular abnormalities like microopthalmia, strabismus, optic nerve atrophy and cataracts can be seen.

❖ Other abnormalities like dental, nail and skeletal defects can be seen.

ENCEPHALOPATHY

Encephalopathy is a disorder of CNS which can be static (**cerebral palsy**) or progressive (**mitochondrial encephalopathies**). It can be caused by infections, toxins, metabolic syndromes and perinatal hypoxia. **Microcephaly** is commonly associated with encephalopathies.

Cerebral Palsy

A cerebral palsy is a motor dysfunction caused by CNS injury which is often associated with seizures, mental retardation, hearing, speech, visual abnormalities and posture abnormality (**extensor posture**). CP can be classified as spastic CP, extrapyramidal CP (athetoid CP), atonic CP and ataxic CP.

Spastic Cerebral Palsy

This is the **most common** form of CP which can present in three different clinical forms i.e. hemiparetic CP (spastic hemiplegia), double hemiparetic CP (spastic quadriplegia), diplegic CP (spastic diplegia).

Spastic hemiplegia	Spastic diplegia	Spastic quadriplegia
• Usually caused by **large vessel (MCA) strokes**. • Spastic weakness of one side of body is seen in following order of severity i.e. **arms>legs>face**. • Seizures (partial complex) can be seen in **1/3rd patients**. • MR is seen in 25% patients. • MRI shows cerebral hemisphere atrophy with contralateral ventricular dilation.	• Most common cause is **premature birth**. • Bilateral spastic weakness of **legs>arms** is seen. This causes lagging of legs while crawling (**commando crawling**). • Seizures are rarely seen. • MR is rarely seen. • **Periventricular leukomalacia is the characteristic finding in MRI.**	• Most common cause is **birth asphyxia.** Severe spastic weakness of all 4 limbs is seen in following order of severity i.e. **arms>legs**. • Seizure is seen in **half of the patients.** • Most commonly associated with **MR**. • Associated supranuclear bulbar palsies can cause drooling of saliva and **aspiration pneumonia**. • Periventricular leukomalacia and multicystic cortical encephalomalacia can be seen in MRI.

Athetoid Cerebral Palsy

• Athetoid CP is caused by birth asphyxia and kernicterus.

• Most common presentation is **dystonia** or **athetosis**; however it may also present with sudden myoclonic jerks, postural instability, gait and speech impairment.

• Seizures and MR can be seen.

• On general examination the tone is variable and can range from the **'lead pipe' rigidity** to **hypotonia**.

• MRI shows lesions in the basal ganglia called as **status marmoratus**.

Ataxic Cerebral Palsy

• It is the second most common type of CP after spastic CP.

• Ataxic CP is commonly associated with other forms of CP like spastic diplegia (mixed CP).

• Ataxia, nystagmus and hypotonia are commonly seen.

• Lesions in the **forebrain** are more commonly seen than in the cerebellum in MRI.

Hypotonic Cerebral Palsy

• Hypotonic CP can be caused by parasagittal brain infarction and maternofetal hyperthermia.

• The baby presents with marked **hypotonia (floppy child)**, weakness and head lag.

• On examination a characteristic sign called as **Forster sign** is seen. When the examiner holds the baby in vertical position by placing hand on armpits, hip and leg flexion can be seen.

Mitochondrial Encephalopathies

Mitochondrial encephalopathies are a group of disorders caused by mutation of mitochondrial DNAs. The various disorders included in it are MELAS (mitochondrial encephalopathy, lactic acidosis and stroke like episodes), MERRF (myoclonus epilepsy with ragged red fibres), Leigh subacute necrotising encephalopathy, LHON (Leber hereditary optic neuropathy), KSS (Kearns-Sayre Syndrome), NARP (ATPase 6 mutation) and **Reye syndrome.**

Reye Syndrome

Reye syndrome is characterised by acute encephalopathy and hepatic dysfunction. It is preceded by **viral infections** like **varicella, influenza (type b>a), adenovirus**, EBV and is strongly related to use of **aspirin.** Mortality is seen in a major group of patients (30–40%) because of **cerebral edema.**

- Clinical findings correlate to mitochondrial toxicity resulting in abnormality in the metabolic role played mitochondria like urea genesis and ketogenesis.
- **Diagnosis:**
  - ❖ The various laboratory findings in Reye syndrome are —
    - ❑ **Increased ALT and AST more than 3 times normal.**
    - ❑ Increased blood ammonia — Blood ammonia level correlates with the prognosis of disease.
    - ❑ **Hypoglycemia.**
    - ❑ Prolonged INR.
    - ❑ **Normal bilirubin.**
    - ❑ **PT is normal or increased.**
  - ❖ Liver biopsy shows **microvesicular hepatic steatosis.**
  - ❖ CSF pressure is elevated along with decreased glucose (**hypoglycorrachia**) but proteins and cell count are normal.
- Treatment is usually symptomatic and consists of **glucose administration** for hypoglycaemia and **mannitol** infusion for increased CSF pressure.

MENTAL RETARDATION

Mental retardation is characterised by an **IQ less than 70** and **adaptive skills 2 SD below the mean**. MR is more common in **males.** The overall prevalence of MR is 2.5 % and **prevalence of mild MR** is **2.1%** and sever MR is 0.3–0.5%.

Mental retardation	Intelligence quotient ( )IQ
Mild MR	50–69
Moderate MR	35–49
Severe MR	20–34
Profound MR	<20

- **Classification:** Based on the intelligence quotient (IQ) mental retardation can be classified in to four categories.
- **Etiology:**
  - ❖ Mild mental retardation is commonly caused by environmental factors; however some biological causes cannot be ruled out.

Environmental factors	Biological factors
• **Inadequate maternal education** • **Poverty** • **Malnutrition**	• **Genetic syndromes** • Prematurity • Perinatal insult • Maternal drug abuse • Sex chromosomal abnormalities

  - ❖ Severe mental retardation is commonly caused by various biological abnormalities like **tuberous sclerosis,** preventable condition like iodine deficiency (**hypothyroidism and cretinism**), metabolic diseases caused by enzyme deficiencies (**PKU**, Tay-Sachs disease, **homocystinemia**, histidinemia), congenital CNS defects (microcephaly, porencephaly, lissencephaly), **hypoxia**, radiation, intrauterine infections (rubella, toxoplasma, HIV, syphilis, CMV and herpes) trisomy 13, 15 and 21 (Edward, Patau and **Down syndrome**); and other chromosomal disorders like Klinefelter and **fragile X syndrome.**

Mnemonic: THICK CORTEX

- T — **Tuberous sclerosis**
- H — **Hypothyroidism**
- I — **Intrauterine infections**
- C — **Cerebral palsy**
- K — **Klinefelter syndrome**
- C — **Congenital CNS defects**
- O — **Oxygen decreased (Hypoxia)**
- R — **Radiation**
- T — **Trisomy 13, 15, 21**
- E — **Enzyme deficiencies** causing metabolic syndromes
- X — **Fragile X syndrome**

- **Diagnosis :** Various scales can be used for different age groups.
  - ❖ **Children 0 – 3.5 years** — For this age group **Barley Scales of Infant Development II (BSID II)** are used.
  - ❖ **Children older than 3 years** — For this age group **Wechsler scale** are used.
  - ❖ **Nonverbal patient** — For this group **Leiter-R scale** is used.

MULTIPLE CHOICE QUESTIONS

1. **2-month-old girl present with verrucous plague on the trunk: What is your most probable diagnosis?**
   [AIIMS Nov. 08]
   a. Incontinentia pigmentosa
   b. Darier disease
   c. Cogenital nevus
   d. Ichthyosis

2. **The drug of choice for absence seizures:**
   [AIIMS Nov. 06]
   a. Valproate   b. Gabapentin
   c. Carbamazepine   d. Phenytoin

3. **A newborn presents with congestive heart failure, on examination has bulging anterior fontanelle with a bruit on auscultation. Transfontanelle USG shows a hypoechoic midline mass with dilated lateral ventricles. Most likely diagnosis is:**
   [AIIMS Nov. 06, AI 07]
   a. Medulloblastoma
   b. Encephalocele
   c. Vein of Galen malformation
   d. Arachnoid cyst

4. **Which one of the following is the characteristic feature of juvenile myoclortic epilepsy?**
   [AIIMS May 06]
   a. Myoclonic seizures frequently occur in morning
   b. Complete remission is common
   c. Response to anticonvulsants is poor
   d. Associated absence seizures are present in majority of patients

5. **All are features of absence seizures except:**
   [AIIMS May 05]
   a. Usually seen in childhood
   b. 3-Hz spike wave in EEG
   c. Postictal confusion
   d. Precipitation by hyperventilation

6. **A neonate develops signs of meningitis at seven days of birth. The presence of which of the following infectious agent in the maternal genital tract can be the causative agent of this disease:**
   [AIIMS May 04]
   a. *Neisseria gonorrhoea*   b. *Chlamydia trachomatis*
   c. *Streptococcus agalactiae* d. *Haemophilous ducreyi*

7. **Which one of the following is the most common tumor associated with type 1 neurofibromatosis:**
   [AIIMS 03]
   a. Optic nerve glioma
   b. Meningioma
   c. Acoustic schwannoma
   d. Lowgrade astrocytoma

8. **An infant presents with hypotonia and hypo-reflexia. During his intrauterine period there was polyhydramnios and decreased fetal movements. Most probable diagnosis is:**   [AIIMS May 02]
   a. Spinal muscular atrophy
   b. Congenital myasthenia
   c. Congenital myotonia
   d. Muscular dystrophy

9. A 6-year-child with acute onset of fever of 104°F developed febrile seizures and was treated. To avoid future recurrences of seizure attacks what should be given: [AIIMS May 01]
   a. Paracetamol 400 mg+ phenobarbitone daily
   b. Oral diazepam 6 hourly
   c. Paracetamol 400 mg 6 hourly
   d. I.V diazepam infusion over 12 hours

10. CSF examination of a patient shows high protein, markedly low sugar, low chloride and increased neutrophils. The diagnosis is: [AIIMS Nov. 99]
    a. Viral meningitis
    b. Meningococcal meningitis
    c. Tuberculous meningitis
    d. Fungal meningitis

11. Aseptic meningitis is caused by all except :
                                   [AIIMS June 98]
    a. Mumps   b. Polio
    c. Measles   d. Coxsackie virus

12. A triad of seizure, mental retardation and sebaceous adenoma is seen in: [AIIMS June 97]
    a. Congenital syphilis
    b. Tuberous sclerosis
    c. Toxoplasmosis
    d. Linear sebaceous nevus syndrome

13. Which type of cerebral palsy is commonly associated with scoliosis and orthopaedic problems?
                                   [AIIMS June 97]
    a. Spastic quadriplegia
    b. Anterior cerebral palsy
    c. Spastic diplegia
    d. Atonic cerebral palsy

14. Brachycephaly is due to fusion of:
                              [AIIMS Feb. 97, AI96]
    a. Parietal suture
    b. Saggital suture
    c. Lambdoid suture
    d. Coronal suture

15. Which among the following is the most common tumour associated with neurofibromatosis in a child?   [AI 11]
    a. Juvenile myelomonocytic leukemia
    b. Acute lymphoblastic leukemia
    c. Acute monocytic leukemia
    d. Acute myeloid leukemia

16. Which of the following is the most common cause of meningoencephalitis in children?   [AI 10, 11]
    a. Mumps   b. Arbovirus
    c. HSV   d. Enterovirus

17. A 2-year-old child is brought by parents with history of seizures and developmental delay. He has multiple hypopigmented macules over the back. What is the most probable diagnosis? [AI 10]

    a. Neurofibromatosis type 1
    b. Tuberous sclerosis
    c. Sturge Weber's syndrome
    d. Linear sebaceous nevus syndrome

18. Following can be used in the treatment of myoclonic seizures except: [AI 10]
    a. Valproate   b. Carbamazepine
    c. Topiramate   d. Zonisamide

19. A school going boy was noted with vacant stare several times a day. There was no history of fever, seizures and neurological deterioration. What is the diagnosis?   [AI 2010]
    a. Atonic seizures   b. Absence seizures
    c. Myoclonic seizures d. School phobia

20. Which of the following is NOT associated with increase in the risk of seizures in future in a child with febrile seizures?   [AI 2010]
    a. Developmental delay
    b. Late age of onset
    c. Complex partial seizures
    d. Family history positive

21. Most common sequalae due to periventricular leukomalacia: [AI 09]
    a. Spastic diplegia   b. Spastic quadriplegia
    c. Mental retardation d. Seizures

22. CSF picture in tubercular meningitis is: [AI 07]
    a. Increased protein, increased sugar, increased lymphocyte
    b. Increased protein, decreased sugar, increased lymphocyte
    c. Decreased protein, increased sugar, increased lymphocyte
    d. Decreased protein, decreased sugar, increased lymphocyte

23. Jitteriness can be distinguished from seizures by all of the following except: [AI 07]
    a. Sensitivity to stimuli
    b. Frequency of movement
    c. Abnormality of gaze
    d. Autonomic disturbances

24. Most common organism causing meningitis in a 1 year old child is: [AI 07, PGI June 2007]
    a. Listeria
    b. E. coli
    c. H. influenza
    d. Streptococcus pneumonae

25. A newborn presents with congestive heart failure, on examination has bulging anterior fontanelle with a bruit on auscultation. Transfontanelle USG shows a hypoechoic midline mass with dilated lateral ventricles. Most likely diagnosis is:
                                 [AIIMS Nov. 06, AI 07]

a. Medulloblastoma
b. Encephalocele
c. Vein of Galen malformation
d. Arachnoid cyst

26. **The following bacteria are most often associated with acute neonatal meningitis except:** [AI 05]
    a. *Escherichia coli*
    b. *Streptococcus agalactiae*
    c. *Neisseria meningitidis*
    d. *Listeria monocytogenes*

27. **Which one of the following is the common cause of congenital hydrocephalus?** [AI 05]
    a. Craniosynostosis
    b. Intrauterine meningitis
    c. Aqueductal stenosis
    d. Malformations of great vein of Galen

28. **All of the following are neural tube defects except:** [AI 04]
    a. Myelomeningocoele   b. Anencephaly
    c. Encephalocele   d. Holoprosencephaly

29. **Bacterial meningitis in children (2 months-12 years of age) is usually due to the following organisms except:** [AI 04]
    a. *Streptococcus pneumoniae*
    b. *Neisseria meningitidis*
    c. *Haemophilus influenzae type B*
    d. *Listeria monocytogenes*

30. ***Haemophilus influenzae* has been isolated from the CSF of a two year old boy suffering from meningitis. The strain is beta-lactamase producing and resistant to chloramphenicol. The most appropriate anti-microbial in such a situation is:** [AI 04]
    a. Trimethoprim-sulfamethoxazole combination
    b. Ciprofloxacin
    c. Third-generation cephalosporin
    d. Vancomycin

31. **A 10 month old child presents with two weeks history of fever, vomiting and alteration of sensorium Cranial CTscan reveals basal exudates and hydrocephalus, the most likely etiological agent is:** [AI 04, 95]
    a. *Mycobacterium tuberculosis*
    b. *Cryptococcus neoformans*
    c. *Listeria monocytogenes*
    d. *Streptococcus pneumonia*

32. **A 25 years old woman had premature rupture of membranes and delivered a male child who became lethargic and apneic on the 1st day of birth and went into shock. The mother had a previous history of abortion 1 year back. On vaginal swab culture growth of b-hemolytic colonies on blood agar was found. On staining these were found to be gram-positive cocci. Which of the following is the most likely etiological agent?** [AI 04]

a. *Streptococcus pyogenes*
b. *Streptococcus agalactiae*
c. Peptostreptococci
d. *Enterococcus faecium*

33. **Absence seizures are characterised on EEG by:** [AI 03]
    a. 3 Hz spike and wave
    b. 1–2 Hz spike and wave
    c. Generalised polyspikes
    d. Hypsarrythmia

34. **Most common cause of pyogenic meningitis in 6 month to 2 years of age is:** [AI 01, 98]
    a. *Staphylococcus aureus*
    b. Pneumococcus
    c. *Streptococcus pneumonia*
    d. *H. influeuenzae*

35. **Neural tube defects are prevented by:** [AI 99]
    a. Pyridoxin   b. Folic acid
    c. Thiamine   d. Iron

36. **Increase acetylcholinestrase in amniotic fluid indicates:** [AI 99]
    a. Open neural tube defects
    b. Esophageal atresia
    c. Down's syndrome
    d. Edward's syndrome

37. **Porencephaly refers to:** [AI 99]
    a. Fetal alcohol syndrome
    b. Dandy-walker-syndrome
    c. Vascular lesion due to degenerative vessel disease and head injury
    d. Neural tube defects

38. **Most common cause of hydrocephalus in children is:** [AI 98, SGPGI 04]
    a. Post inflammatory obstruction
    b. Buddchiary syndrome
    c. Brain tumor
    d. Perinatal injury

39. **Commonest cause of non-communicating hydro-cephalus in children is:** [AI 96]
    a. Congenital anomaly
    b. Perinatal injury
    c. Post inflammatory obstruction
    d. Brain tumors

40. **Brachycephaly is due to fusion of:** [AIIMS Feb. 97, AI96]
    a. Parietal suture   b. Saggital suture
    c. Lambdoid suture   d. Coronal suture

41. **Which of the following statements is false about sacral myelomeningocele?** [AI 95]
    a. Spasticity of the lower limb is seen
    b. Hydrocephalus is seen
    c. Bladder incontinence may be seen
    d. Lax anal sphincter is present

42. **IQ between 50–70 indicates:**   [AI 95]
    a. Mild metal retardation
    b. Moderate retardation
    c. Severe retardation
    d. Profound retardation

43. **Which of the following is a preventable cause of mental retardation:**   [AI 95]
    a. Hypothyroidism   b. Down syndrome
    c. Cerebral palsy   d. ALL of the above

44. **The CSF findings in TB meningitis include:**   [AI 94, 07]
    a. High sugar + low protein
    b. Low sugar + high protein and Lymphocytosis
    c. High sugar + high chloride
    d. Low sugar + high protein and Lymphopenia

45. **True about infantile tremor syndrome:**   [PGI June 09]
    a. Hyperpigmentation of extremities
    b. Fine tremor
    c. Cortical atrophy
    d. Self-limiting disorder
    e. More common in girls

46. **A newborn of 7 days old presented with meningitis. Most common cause:**   [PGI Nov. 08]
    a. *E. coli*
    b. Streptococcal pneumonia
    c. *N. meningitides*
    d. *Streptococcus agalactiae*
    e. *H. influenzae*

47. **Neurological complications of meningitis include all of the following except :**   [PGI June 08]
    a. Seizures
    b. Increased intracranial pressure
    c. Cerebral hamartoma
    d. Subdural effusions
    e. Brain abscess

48. **Condition associated with MR:**   [PGI June 08]
    a. Trisomy 21   b. Fragile - X
    c. Homocystinemia   d. Phenylketonuria
    e. Tuberous sclerosis

49. **Bulging anterior fontanelle is/are seen in:**   [PGI 08]
    a. Rickets   b. CMV infection
    c. Scurvy   d. Hypothyroidism
    e. Tetracycline therapy

50. **True about juvenile myoclonic epilepsy:**   [PGI Dec. 07]
    a. DOC is Sodium Valproate
    b. Mental retardation
    c. Seizure can develop
    d. Neurological examination abnormal
    e. Life long treatment needed

51. **Neonatal meningitis is caused by:**   [PGI Nov. 07]
    a. Group 'A' Streptococcus
    b. Group 'B' Streptococcus
    c. *E. coli*
    d. *H. influenza*
    e. *Klebsiella*

52. **Most common organism causing meningitis in a 1 year old child is:**   [AI 07, PGI June 2007]
    a. Listeria
    b. *E.coli*
    c. *H. influenza*
    d. *Streptococcus pneumoniae*

53. **Mild MR – Feature are:**   [PGI June 06]
    a. Present in 5-10% population
    b. Incidence in low socioeconomic group
    c. Present in 2 years
    d. Genetic background present

54. **True about juvenile myoclonic epilepsy:**   [PGI June 05]
    a. Focal seizure
    b. Generalised seizure
    c. Myoclonus
    d. Response to sodium valproate
    e. Spike and waves in EEG

55. **Features of cerebral palsy:**   [PGI June 05]
    a. Athetosis   b. Spasticity
    c. Saturday night palsy   d. Mixed palsy
    e. Rigidity

56. **True about Reye's syndrome:**   [PGI June 05]
    a. Microvesicular fatty infiltration
    b. Hepatic encephalopathy
    c. Brain edema
    d. Hypoglycemia

57. **Reye's syndrome is characterised by:**   [PGI Dec. 03]
    a. Viral infection is seen
    b. Present as deep jaundice
    c. Cerebral edema
    d. Microvesicular fatty infiltration

58. **True regarding febrile convulsion:**   [PGI Dec. 00]
    a. Carbamazepine is good drug to treat it
    b. Patients with family h/o FC have increased incidence of recurrence
    c. Long-term neurological deficits are common
    d. Usually last for short while

59. **4 years old male child had febrile seizures, best prophylaxis:**   [PGI June 00]
    a. Paracetamol 6 hourly
    b. Paracetamol and diazepam
    c. Diazepam
    d. Phenobarbitone

60. **Most common cause of neonatal meningitis:**
    [PGI Dec. 99]
    a. Staphylococcus
    b. *E. coli*
    c. *H. influenza*
    d. Pneumococcus

61. **CNS tumors seen in von Hippel-Landau syndrome is:**
    [PGI Dec. 99]
    a. Meningioma
    b. Cerebellar hemangioblastoma
    c. CNS lymphoma
    d. Glioma

62. **Brain tumor is associated with all except:**
    [PGI Dec. 99]
    a. Tuberous sclerosis
    b. von Hippel Landau disease
    c. Neurofibromatosis
    d. Sturge Weber disease

63. **Closure of anterior fontanelle is delayed in all except:**
    [PGI 98]
    a. Down syndrome
    b. Osteogenesis imperfect
    c. Hypogonadism
    d. Hypothyroidism

64. **Not found in cerebral palsy:**
    [PGI June 98]
    a. Hypotonicity
    b. Microcephaly
    c. Ataxia
    d. Flaccid paralysis

65. **Preventable conditions of mental retardation are:**
    [PGI 87]
    a. Down syndrome
    b. Phenylketonuria
    c. Cretinism
    d. Cerebral palsy

66. **Reye's syndrome is characterised by encephalitis, fatty liver and following biochemical changes except:**
    [PGI 79, 83]
    a. Moderate elevation of SGOT and SGPT
    b. Hypoglycemia
    c. Hypoglycorrachia
    d. Hyperuricemia

67. **Most common cause of hydrocephalus in children is:**
    [AI 98, SGPGI 04]
    a. Post inflammatory obstruction
    b. Buddchiary syndrome
    c. Brain tumor
    d. Perinatal injury

68. **Sturge Weber syndrome is associated with:**
    [Delhi 96]
    a. Portwine stain
    b. Cavernous hemangioma
    c. Lymphangioma
    d. Hemangiosarcoma

69. **All of the following are features of juvenile myoclonic epilepsy, except:**
    a. Myoclonus on awakening
    b. Generalised tonic-clonic seizure
    c. Automatism
    d. Absence seizure

70. **True about febrile convulsions is:**
    a. Recurrent in nature
    b. Follows high temperature
    c. No spontaneous remission
    d. Occurs at 6 years onwards

71. **Myoclonic seizures typically seen in:**
    a. SSPE
    b. Cerebellar lesions
    c. Pontine lesions
    d. Thalamic lesions

72. **Absence seizures are seen in:**
    a. Grand mal epilepsy
    b. Myoclonic epilepsy
    c. Petitmal epilepsy
    d. Hyperkinetic child

73. **Which is true regarding febrile seizures?**
    a. 50% recurrence
    b. Long term phenytoin required
    c. Interictal EEG normal
    d. Status epilecticus is common

74. **All are the signs of hydrocephalus in a neonate except:**
    a. Enlarged head
    b. Sunset sign
    c. Crack pot sign
    d. Depressed fontanel

75. **A neonate develops encephalitis without any skin lesions. Most probable causative organism is:**
    a. HSV 1
    b. HSV 2
    c. Meningococci
    d. Streptococci

QUESTIONS OF OTHER EXAMINATIONS

1. **Neural tube defects have which of the following inheritance patterns?**
   [UPSC 09]
   a. Autosomal dominant
   b. Autosomal recessive
   c. X-linked recessive
   d. Multifactorial

2. **Commonest cause of convulsions in a child with fever is:**
   [UPSC 08]
   a. Febrile convulsions
   b. Meningitis
   c. Epilepsy
   d. Hypothyroidism

3. **Not cause of neonatal seizures:**
   [APPG 08]
   a. Pyridoxine deficiency
   b. Hypokalemia
   c. Hypoxia
   d. None

4. **Commonest cause of obstructive hydrocephalus in children is:**
   [UP 07, 05]
   a. Aqueductal stenosis
   b. Aqueductal gliosis
   c. Subarachnoid haemorrhage
   d. Tubercular meningitis

5. **Which type of shift in intracranial content is common in children with progressive hydrocephalus?**
   [Karnataka 06]
   a. Transforaminal herniation
   b. Upward cerebellar herniation

   c. Unilateral transtentorial herniation

   d. Central transtenorial herniation

6. **Mesial temporal lobe epilepsy is associated with:**
   [NIMHANS 06]
   a. Simple partial
   b. Generalised tonic clonic
   c. Complex partial
   d. Atonic seizures

7. **The following are recognised signs of raised cranial tension in 9 month old infant except:** [SGPGI 05]
   a. Bulging fontanel   b. Diplopia
   c. Papilledema   d. Increase in head size

8. **Banana sign seen in foetal brain suggests:**
   [COMEDK 05]
   a. Renal agenesis   b. Encephalocele
   c. Spina Bifida   d. Porencephaly

9. **Management of typical febrile seizures include except:** [DPG 10, Karnataka 05]
   a. Sponging
   b. Paracetamol ibuprofen
   c. Intermittent diazepam
   d. Prophylactic phenobarbitone

10. **Carbamazepine is drug of choice in:** [MAHE 05]
    a. Absence attacks   b. Partial complex seizures
    c. Myoclonus   d. Infantile spasms

11. **Wide open anterior fontanel is found in following diseases except:** [COMEDK 05]
    a. Rickets
    b. Cretinism
    c. Osteogenesis imperfect
    d. Craniosyntosis

12. **Porencephaly is seen in:** [APPGE 04]
    a. Trisomy 13
    b. Fetal alcohol syndrome
    c. Down syndrome
    d. Dandy-Walker syndrome

13. **Acquired extracanial infection that causes aqueductal stenosis is:** [UPSC 04]
    a. Bacterial endocarditis
    b. Mumps
    c. Measles
    d. Staphylococcal septicaemia

14. **A child in status epilepticus should not be given:**
    [JIPMER 04]
    a. Clonazepam   b. Phosphenytoin
    c. Lamotrigine   d. Diazepam

15. **A 25-year-old man with congenital cyanotic heart disease reports to emergency with history of headache. On examination there is systolic murmur best heard on the left side of the sternum in the fourth intercostal space; the second sound is not split. Temperature is 37.5°C. What is the most likely diagnosis:** [ICS 2000]

a. Cortical vein thrombosis
b. Pyogenic septicaemia
c. Cerebral abscess
d. Encephalitis

16. **Scapocephaly is due to premature closure of:**
    [Orissa 99]
    a. Coronal suture   b. Metopic suture
    c. Saggital suture   d. Lambdoid suture

17. **8 days old neonate with extensor posture:** [TN 99]
    a. Cerebral palsy
    b. Hypoxic ischemic encephalopathy
    c. Malnutrition
    d. Infection

18. **Drug of choice for neonatal convulsions:**
    [Jipmer 98]
    a. Valproate   b. Phenytoin
    c. Phenobarbitone   d. Carbamazepine

19. **All of the following are true about Reye's syndrome except:** [UP 97]
    a. It frequently complicates viral infections
    b. Prothrombin time is prolonged
    c. Disease may be precipitated by salicylates
    d. Deep jaundice is present

20. **All of the following are true of febrile seizures except:** [AP 97]
    a. Most commonly seen between 9 months and 5 years
    b. Do not last more than 10 minutes
    c. Almost invariably develop in to epilepsy
    d. Prognosis is good

21. **Neonatal seizures in the following disorders is associated with poor prognosis except:** [UP 97]
    a. Hypoglycemia
    b. Intraventricular haemorrhage
    c. Hypocalcemia
    d. Meningitis

22. **In children with cerebral edema which one of the following corticosteroids will be effective:**
    [UPSC 96]
    a. Hydrocortisone   b. Prednisolone
    c. Dexamethasone   d. Betamethasone

23. **IQ (Intelligent quotient) of child means:** [Delhi 96]
    a. The creative efficiency of a child
    b. The capability of a child to perform intellectual tasks in relation to other children of same age
    c. The efficiency of memory of child
    d. Quantification of memory of child

24. **Untrue about acute febrile convulsions:** [AMU 95]
    a. Focal in nature
    b. EEG normal after 2 weeks
    c. Usually occur below 6 years of age

25. **The common type of cerebral palsy seen in hospitals is:** [CUPGEE 95]
    a. Spastic
    b. Monoplegic
    c. Quadriplegic
    d. Diplegia

26. **Reye's syndrome is caused by all except:** [Kerala 95]
    a. Adenovirus
    b. RSV
    c. Herpes
    d. Influenza

27. **Mental retardation is not seen in:** [Kerala 94]
    a. Down syndrome
    b. Cretinism
    c. Hypopitutarism
    d. Birth asphyxia

28. **Which is incorrect about Reye's syndrome?** [Jipmer 91]
    a. Bilirubin more than 3 mg
    b. Normal prothrombin time

c. Cerebral edema
d. Microfatty changes in liver without inflammatory changes

29. **Rapid antigen tests for meningitis organisms in a child can be done on the following specimens except:**
    a. Blood
    b. CSF
    c. Urine
    d. Throat swab

30. **All are seen in Reye's syndrome except:**
    a. Aminoaciduria
    b. Metabolic acidosis
    c. Increased serum transaminases
    d. Respiratory alkalosis

31. **Which of the following has the worst prognosis?**
    a. Rolandic epilepsy
    b. Versive epilepsy
    c. Abscence epilepsy
    d. Infantile spasms

ANSWERS

1. (a) Incontinentia pigmenti (Ref: Nelson 19th E/P 2178)
- Incontinentia pigmenti is seen in females as it is lethal in males:
  - ❖ Cutaneous manifestation can be divided in to 4 phases
  - ❖ First phase is characterised by linear erythematous streaks and vesicular plaques on the limbs and trunk, which usually lasts from birth till 4 months.
  - ❖ Second phase is characterised by **verrucous plaques** due to keratinization of dry blisters.
  - ❖ Third stage is characterised by pigmentation of skin that can involve any part of body and it disappears by 16 years of age.
  - ❖ Fourth stage is characterised by hypopigmented and hairless patches primarily on the flexor aspects of legs.

2. (a) Valproate (Ref: CPDT 19th E/P686)

3. (c) Vein of Galen malformation (Ronald Clinical Paediatric Neurology/P375)
  Vein of Galen malformation (VGAM):
- VGAM is a misnomer as it is malformation of the precursor of vein of Galen i.e. median prosencephalic vein of Markowsky. So the vein of Galen never forms in a VGAM.
- This is a large midline arterio-venous malformation that shunts a significant amount of blood in to the venous circulation. It is more common in males.
- **Clinical presentation:**
  - ❖ **CHF** — It is the most common presentation in neonates because of increased venous return to the right side of heart. It begins as right sided heart failure but later biventricular failure develops.
  - ❖ **Hydrocephalus** — It develops because of the venous hypertension which decreases the CSF absorption (non-communicating hydrocephalus). In neonates it presents with fullness of fontanels. Communicating hydrocephalus can be rarely seen because of aqueductal stenosis.
  - ❖ Cerebral calcification and haemorrhage can be seen in some cases.
- **Diagnosis:**
  - ❖ CECT or MRI shows enlargement of lateral and 3rd ventricles if there is aqueductal stenosis.
  - ❖ X-ray chest shows an enlarged heart with a normal shape.
  - ❖ A cranial bruit can be heard on auscultation.
- **Treatment:** Embolization of VGAM is the current treatment of choice.

4. (a) Myoclonic seizures frequently occur in the morning (Ref: Nelson 19th E/P1998)
- JME begins with bilateral myoclonic jerks in **early morning period** which later progress to **GTCS and absence seizures in 25% patients.**
- **JME responds well** to anticonvulsant **valproate**, however on discontinuation the relapse rate is very high. Hence **lifelong therapy with valproate is required.**

5. (c) Postictal confusion (Ref: Nelson 19th E/P1997)
Absence seizure:

"Immediately after the seizure, patients resume preseizure activity with **no indication of postictal impairment.**"

6. (c) *Streptococcus agalctiae* (Ref:Nelson 19th E/P2038)
- Neonatal meningitis are most commonly caused by the pathogens of maternal genital tract like strepto-coccus agalactiae and E.coli.

7. (a) Optic nerve glioma (Ref: Nelson 19th E/P2016)
Tumors seen in Neurifibromatosis 1:
- **Optic nerve glioma** — This can be seen in 15% of patients.
- Neurofibrosarcoma
- Astrocytoma
- Rhabdomysarcoma
- Meningioma
- Pheochromocytoma
- **Myelogenous leukemia** can be seen.

9. (b) Oral diazepam 6 hourly (Ref: Rudolph 22nd E/P2205, CPDT 19th E/P298, Nelson 19th E/P1994)
- **Diazepam** given at the onset of fever by **oral route** at a dose of **0.5 mg/kg 2–3 times a day** is the preferred prophylactic management.
- The factors limiting use of diazepam are its side-effect like sedation and the fact that fever is often preceded by seizure.

10. (b) Meningococcal meningitis (Ref: CPDT 19th E/P728)
CSF findings in different types of meningitis:

Cause of meningitis	Cells	Protein	Glucose	ICT
Bacterial	Neutrophils	Increased	Decreased	Increased
Tubercular	Lymphocytes	Increased	Decreased	Increased
Viral	Lymphocytes	Normal to slightly increased	Normal	Normal to slightly increased

11. (d) Coxscakie virus (Ref: Nelson 19th E/P2045)

Causes of viral or aseptic meningoencephalitis:

- Enteroviruses
- Herpes simplex virus type 1 and 2
- Human herpes virus-6
- **Mumps virus**
- Influenza and parainfluenza virus
- Adeno virus
- Rubella virus
- Rubeola virus
- Rabies virus
- Live vaccinations against **polio, measles,** mumps or rubella.

12. (b) Tuberous sclerosis (Ref: Nelson 19th E/P2017)

Major clinical findings in Tuberous sclerosis:

- Skin lesions like **ash leaf macules (hypopigmented), sebaceous adenomas,** shagreen patches and sub-ungual or periungual fibromas.
- CNS manifestations like **Seizures, cognitive and behavioural impairement**(autism).

13. (a) Spastic quadriplegia (Lovell and Winter's paediatric orthopaedics vol. 1/p559)

"In patients with mild hemiplegia scoliosis occurs in fewer than 5%; in patients with severe **spastic quadriplegia** its occurrence is much greater in the range of, **50–75%.**"

14. (d) Coronal suture (Ref: Nelson 19th E/P1992)

Synostosis	Sutures involved
Scapocephaly	Saggital
Frontal Plagiocephaly	Coronal and sphenofrontal Lambdoid
Occipital Plagiocephaly	suture
Brachycephaly	**Both coronal**
Turricephaly	Coronal, sphenofrontal and fronto-ethmoidal
Trigonocephaly	Metopic

15. (a) Juvenile myelomonocytic leukemia (Ref: Nelson 19th E/P733)

- Juvenile chronic myelogenous leukemia (JCML) also called as juvenile myelomonocytic leukemia is associated with NF1 and monosomy 7.
- It is associated with a poor prognosis.
- Treatment of choice is stem cell therapy.

16. (d) Enterovirus (Ref: Nelson 19th E/p2044)

Causes of viral or aseptic meningoencephalitis:

- **Enteroviruses** — These are the most common cause of meningoencephalitis.
- Herpes simplex virus type 1 and 2
- Human herpes virus-6

- **Mumps virus**
- Influenza and parainfluenza virus
- Adeno virus
- Rubella virus
- Rubeola virus
- Rabies virus

17. (b) Tuberous sclerosis (Ref: Nelson 19th E/P2017)

18. (c) Carbamazepine (Ref: CPDT 19th E/P686)

Drugs used for treatment of various seizure types:

Seizure type	Drugs
Juvenile Myoclonic epilepsy	• **Valproate** • **Lamotrigine** • **Topiramate** • **Zonisamide**
GTCS	Infants • Phenobarbitone Children >1 year • Valproic acid - DOC • Carbamazepine· Phenytoin • Topiramate • Lamotrigine
Partial seizure	• **Carbamazepine - DOC** • Oxcarbazepine • Phenytion • Lamotrigine • Gabapentine • Topiramate • Levetiracetam • Zonisamide
Absence seizure	• **Valproic acid - DOC** • Ethosuximide • Lamotrigine • Zonisamide • Topiramate • Levetiracetam • Acetazolamide • Ketogenic diet
Infantile spasms	• **ACTH - DOC** • Vigabatrin • Valproic acid • Topiramate • Lamotrigine • Ketogenic diet
Neonatal seizures	• **Phenobarbitone- DOC** • Phenytoin • Diazepam

19. (b) Absence seizure (Ref: Nelson 19th E/P1997)

- Absence seizure is characterised by a brief state of staring lasting less than 30 seconds, which may be associated with other features like blinking of eyes, upward deviation of eyes and slackening of facial mucles.

20. (b) Late age of onset (Ref: CPDT 19th E/P697)
- Increased risk of recurrence is seen in following cases:
  1. **Early age of onset (<12 months)**
  2. **Family history of febrile seizures**
  3. Short duration of fever
  4. Seizure following lower temperature (<40°C)
  5. **Developmental delay**
  6. Abnormal neurological conditions (cerebral palsy or mental retardation)
  7. **Presence of complex features** (seizure duration more than 15 minutes, more than one seizure a day and focal seizures in post ictal period).

21. (a) Spastic diplegia(Ref: Rudolph 22nd E/P2178–81)
- Periventricular leukomalacia is characteristically seen in spastic diplegia; however it can also be seen with spastic quadriplegia.

22. (b) Increased protein, decreased sugar, increased lymphocyte (Ref: CPDT 19th E/P728)
CSF findings in different types of meningitis:

Cause of meningitis	Cells	Protein	Glucose	ICT
Bacterial	Neutrophils	Increased	Decreased	Increased
Tubercular	**Lymphocytes**	**Increased**	**Decreased**	Increased
Viral	Lymphocytes	Normal to slightly increased	Normal	Normal to slightly increased

23. (b) Frequency of movement (Ref: Nelson 19th E/P560)
Jitteriness:
- It is the most common involuntary movement of healthy full term infant, which is characterised by rhythmic movements of flexors and extensors.
- It is exaggerated by crying and stimuli like examination.
- It is abnormal if it persists beyond 2nd week of life.
- Causes of jitteriness can be sepsis, intracranial hemorrhage, hypoxic encephalopathy, hypoglycemia, hypocalcemia, hypomagnesemia, prenatal exposure to maternal marijuana, and the narcotic abstinence syndrome.
- Differential diagnosis — It should be differentiated from a seizure activity as the later requires prompt management.

Jitteriness	Seizures
Precipitated by crying and stimuli like examination.	Not sensitive to stimuli.
Abnormal eye movements and apnea not seen.	Abnormal eye movements and apnea are frequently seen.
Autonomic disturbance never seen.	Autonomic disturbance like urinary and bowel incontinence can be seen.

24. (d) *Streptococcus pneumoniae* (Ref:Nelson 19th E/P2038)
Common causes of meningitis in different age groups:
- **Neonates (0–28 days)** — Most common cause is *Streptococcus agalactiae* followed by *E.coli*. Other causative organisms are enterococci, Klebsiella and *Listeria monocytogenes.*
- **2 months-12 years** — Most common cause in **India is** *S. pneumoniae* followed by *N. meningitidis* and *H. influenzae* but in developed countries is *N. meningitidis* followed by *S. pneumoniae.*
- In adults i.e. age >20 years *S.pneumoniae* is the most common agent.

25. (c) Vein of Galen malformation (Ronald Clinical Paediatric Neurology/P375)
Vein of Galen malformation (VGAM):
- VGAM is a misnomer as it is malformation of the precursor of vein of Galen i.e. median prosencephalic vein of Markowsky. So the vein of Galen never forms in a VGAM.
- This is a large midline arterio-venous malformation that shunts a significant amount of blood in to the venous circulation. It is more common in males.
- **Clinical presentation:**
  ❖ **CHF** — It is the most common presentation in neonates because of increased venous return to the right side of heart. It begins as right sided heart failure but later biventricular failure develops.
  ❖ **Hydrocephalus** — It develops because of the venous hypertension which decreases the CSF absorption (non-communicating hydrocephalus). In neonates it presents with fullness of fontanels. Communicating hydrocephalus can be rarely seen because of aqueductal stenosis.
  ❖ Cerebral calcification and haemorrhage can be seen in some cases.
- **Diagnosis:**
  ❖ CECT or MRI shows enlargement of lateral and 3rd ventricles if there is aqueductal stenosis.
  ❖ X-ray chest shows an enlarged heart with a normal shape.
  ❖ A cranial bruit can be heard on auscultation.
- **Treatment:** Embolization of VGAM is the current treatment of choice.

26. (c) Neisseria meningitides (Ref:Nelson 19th E/P2038)
Causes of neonatal meningitis:
- *Streptococcus agalactiae*
- *E.coli*
- *Enterococci*
- *Klebsiella*
- *Listeria monocytogenes.*

27. (c) Aqueductal stenosis (Ref: Rudolph 22nd E/P2174)
- Aqueductal stenosis is the most common cause of congenital hydrocephalus, which is responsible for 20% cases with an incidence of 0.5–1% per 1000 births.

28. (d) Holoprosencephaly (Ref: Nelson 19th E/P1987)

Neural tube defects	*Neuronal migration defects*
• Spina bifida occulta	• Lissencephaly
• Meningocele	• Schizencephaly
• **Myelomeningocele**	• Porencephaly
• **Encephalocele**	• **Holoprosencephaly**
• **Anencephaly**	
• Dermal sinus	
• Tethered cord	
• Syringomyelia	
• Diastometamyelia	
• Lipoma involving the conus medullaris and filum terminale	

29. (d) Listeria monocytogens (Ref:Nelson 19th E/P2038) Common causes of meningitis in different age groups:
- **Neonates (0–28 days)** — Most common cause is *Streptococcus agalctiae* followed by *E.coli*. Other causative organisms are enterococci, *Klebsiella* and *Listeria monocytogens*.
- **2 months-12 years** — Most common cause in **India** is *S. pneumoniae* followed by *N. meningitidis* and *H. influenzae* but in developed countries is *N. meningitidis* followed by *S. pneumonae*.
- In adults i.e. age >20 years *S. pneumonae* is the most common agent.

30. (c) Third generation cephalosporin (Ref: Nelson 19th E/P2042)

Treatment of bacterial meningitis:
- *S.pneumonae* sensitive to beta lactam antibiotics are treated by **penicillin** or a **3rd generation cephalosporin** for 10–14 days. In case of resistance **vancomycin** should be used.
- *H. influenzae* is treated by **Amoxycillin** for a period of 10 days. In case of resistance **extended spectrum cephalosporins** are given. **Dexamethasone** decreases the incidence of hearing loss and should be given 1–24 hours before administration of antibiotics.
- **Penicillin** is the drug of choice for *N. menigitidis* and *L. monocytogenes*.
- Gram negative organisms like **pseudomonas**, *E.coli* and *Klebsiella* should be treated with a **combination of ceftazidime and an amino-glycoside** for 3 weeks.

31. (a) *Mycobacterium tuberculosis* (Ref: Nelson 19th E/P966)

Diagnosis of tubercular meningitis:
- Examination and culture of CSF is the best diagnostic method as tuberculin test and chest radiograph is normal in majority of patients. The CSF shows lymphocytes, decreased glucose or hypoglycorachia i.e. glucose less than 40 mg/dl and increased protein levels. Culture and staining of CSF should be done for definite diagnosis.
- CT or MRI shows basilar enhancement and communicating hydrocephalus.

32. (a) *Streptococcus agalactiae* (Ref:Nelson 19th E/P2038)
- Beta haemolytic colonies and gram positive cocci on staining leaves no dobut that it is a case of neonatal meningitis caused by *Streptococcus agalactiae*.
- Neonatal meningitis is most commonly caused by streptococcus agalctiae followed by *E.coli*.

33. (a) 3 Hz spike and wave (Ref: Nelson 19th E/P1997)
- In typical absence seizure EEG shows a characteristic **3 Hz spike wave discharge.**
- In atypical absence seizure EEG shows a slow spike wave discharge at 2–2.5 Hz.
- Hypsarrythmia are characteristic for infantile spasms.

34. (a) Pneumococcus (Ref: Nelson 19th E/P2038)

35. (a) Folic acid (Ref: Nelson 18th E/P2445)

Prophylaxis of NTD:
- 0.4 mg of folic acid is given prophylactically during pregnancy.
- If it's a high risk pregnancy i.e. with previous history of NTD, then 4 mg of folic acid is started 1 month before conception.

36. (a) Open neural tube defects (Ref: Nelson 19th E/P1983)
- Neural tube is open at both ends, and the neural canal communicates freely with the amniotic cavity for some time .
- Failure of closure of the neural tube allows excretion of fetal substances like **α-fetoprotein and acetylcholinesterase** into the amniotic fluid, serving as biochemical markers for a neural tube defect.

37. (c) Vascular lesion due to degenerative vessel disease and head injury (Ref: Nelson 19th E/P1987)
- Porencephaly refers to formation of cystic lesions in the brain due to congenital defects of neuronal migration or acquired lesions like brain infarction.

38. (a) Post inflammatory obstruction (Ref: Rudolph 22nd E/P2174)
- Most common type of hydrocephalus in children is **obstructive or non-communicating** one. Out of various causes **aqueductal stenosis** is the most common cause of non communicating hydrocephalus and the causes can be
  - ❖ Genetic (X linked recessive)
  - ❖ Gliosis of the aqueduct caused subarachnoid haemorrhage and **meningoencephalitis.**

39. (c) Post inflammatory obstruction (Ref: Nelson 19th E/P1990)

"In a small percentage of cases, aqueductal stenosis is inherited as a sex-linked recessive trait. These patients occasionally have minor neural tube closure defects, including spina bifida occulta. Rarely, aqueductal stenosis is associated with neurofibromatosis. *Aqueductal gliosis* may also give rise to hydrocephalus. As a result of **neonatal meningitis** or a subarachnoid hemorrhage in a premature infant, the ependymal lining of the aqueduct is interrupted and a brisk glial response results in complete obstruction."

- Most common cause of non-communicating hydro-cephalus is aqueductal stenosis.
- Aqueductal stenosis is most commonly caused by meningitis and subarachnoid haemorrhage.

40. (d) Coronal suture (Ref: Nelson 19th E/P1992)

Synostosis	Sutures involved
Scapocephaly	Saggital
Frontal Plagiocephaly	Coronal and sphenofrontal Lambdoid
Occipital Plagiocephaly	suture
Brachycephaly	**Both coronal**
Turricephaly	Coronal, sphenofrontal and fronto-ethmoidal
Trigonocephaly	Metopic

41. (a) Spasticity of the lower limbs is seen (Ref: Nelson 19th E/P1985)

The clinical presentation of myelomeningocele depends on the site of location.

- Lower sacral lesions cause **bladder** and **bowel incontinence** with perineal anesthesia.
- Midlumbar lesions cause **flaccid paralysis of lower limbs**, constant urinary dribbling, **laxed anal sphincter** and a higher incidence of lower limb deformities like club feet and subluxation of hip joint.

42. (a) Mild mental retardation (Ref: CPDT 19th E/P95)

Mental retardation	Intelligence quotient (IQ)
Mild MR	50–69
Moderate MR	35–49
Severe MR	20–34
Profound MR	<20

43. (a) Hypothyroidism (Ref: Nelson 19th E/P 139)
- Out of all the given causes only **hypothyroidism** can be prevented by iodine supplementation of the mother in endemic areas of iodine deficiency.

44. (b) Low sugar + high protein and Lymphocytosis (Ref: CPDT 19th E/P728)

CSF findings in different types of meningitis:

Cause of meningitis	Cells	Protein	Glucose	ICT
Bacterial	Neutrophils	Increased	Decreased	Increased
Tubercular	**Lymphocytes**	**Increased**	**Decreased**	Increased
Viral	Lymphocytes	Normal to slightly increased	Normal	Normal to slightly increased

45. (a), (c) and **(d)** Hyperpigmentation of extremities, Cortical atrophy and Self limiting disorder (Ref: Ghai 7th E/P558–59)

Infantile tremor syndrome:
- It is a **self-limiting disorder** characterised by behavioural abnormalities, coarse tremors and pigmentation changes. It is **more common in boys** in the age group of 5 months to 3 years.
- The cause is still not established but the various predisposing conditions thought to be linked are infections of CNS (meningoencephalitis), malnutrition, low socioeconomic group, vitamin B12 deficiency and magnesium deficiency.
- **Clinical featutes:**
  - ❖ **Behavioural abnormalities** — Apathy, vacant looks, inability to recognise mother and decreased interest in the surrounding can be seen.
  - ❖ **Tremor** — **Fine generalised tremors** can be seen which disappear on sleep.
  - ❖ **Pigmentation abnormalities** — **Hyperpigmentation of skin** and brown discolouration of hair can be seen.
- **Diagnosis:**
  - ❖ Blood analysis may show anemia and hypomagnesemia.
  - ❖ CSF is usually normal.
  - ❖ **Cortical atrophy** can be seen on imaging.
  - ❖ Epiliptiform discharges can be seen in EEG.

46. (a) and **(d)** *E.coli* and *Streptococcus agalactiae* (Ref: Nelson 19th E/P2038)

Common causes of meningitis in different age groups:
- **Neonates (0–28 days)** — Most common cause is *Streptococcus agalctiae* **followed by E.coli.** Other causative organisms are enterococci, Klebsiella and *Listeria monocytogenes.*
- **2 months-12 years** — Most common cause in **India** is *S.pneumoniae* followed by *N.meningitidis* and *H.influenzae* but in developed countries is N.meningitidis followed by S.pneumoniae.
- In adults i.e. age >20 years *S.pneumonae* is the most common agent.

47. (c) Cerebral hamartoma (Ref: Nelson 19th E/P2041, CPDT 19th E/P730)

Complications of meningitis:

- **Seizures** — Most common complication and seen predominantly in neonates.
- **Subdural effusions** — Most commonly seen with *S.pneumonae*.
- **Abscess**
- Subarachnoid haemorrhage
- Cortical infarction and necrosis
- Cranial nerve palsies (II, IV, VII, VIII)
- **Raised ICT and pappiledema**
- Hydrocephalus.

48. All (Ref: Ghai 7th E/P562)

Kindly refer text.

49. (a), (b) and **(e)** Rickets, CMV infection and Tetracycline therapy (Ref: Rudolph 22nd E)

Causes of bulging anterior fontanel can be remembered as

HEAD:

H — **Hyperparathyroidism, Hydrocephalus**
E — **Elevated ICT** seen in meningoenecephalitis (HSV, **CMV**, rubella), tumor, subdural hematoma, pseudotumorcerebri
A — **Adrenal insufficiency**
D — vitamin **D** deficiency (Rickets) and **Drugs** (**tetracycline**, vitamin A, quinolones, amiodarone, glucocorticoids)

50. (a), (c) and **(d)** DOC is sodium valproate, Seizure can develop and Lifelong treatment needed (Ref: Nelson 19th E/P1998)

- The cause of JME is calcium channel mediated overfiring of thalamic neurons. Hence the best way to treat (DOC) is to block the thalamic calcium channels by **sodium valproate.**
- JME responds well to valproate but on discontinuation relapse rate is very high, which makes **anticonvulsant treatment mandatory for lifelong.**
- GTCS and absence seizure can be seen in 25% of patients.

51. All (Ref:Nelson 19th E/P2038)

Common causes of meningitis in different age groups:

- **Neonates (0–28 days)** — Most common cause is *Streptococcus agalactiae* followed by *E.coli.* Other causative organisms are enterococci, *Klebsiella* and *Listeria monocytogenes.*
- **2 months-12 years** — Most common cause in **India** is *S. pneumoniae* followed by *N.meningitidis* and *H.influenzae* but in developed countries is *N. meningitidis* followed by *S. pneumoniae.*
- In adults i.e. age >20 years *S. pneumoniae* is the most common agent.

52. (d) *Streptococcus pneumoniae* (Ref:Nelson 19th E/P2038)

Common causes of meningitis in different age groups:

- **Neonates (0–28 days)** — Most common cause is *Streptococcus agalctiae* followed by *E.coli.* Other causative organisms are enterococci, *Klebsiella* and *Listeria monocytogens.*
- **2 months-12 years** — Most common cause in **India** is *S.pneumonae* followed by *N.meningitidis* and *H.influenzae* but in developed countries is *N. meningitidis* followed by *S. pneumoniae.*
- In adults i.e. age >20 years *S.pneumoniae* is the most common agent.

53. (b) and **(d)** Incidence in low socioeconomic group and Genetic background present (Ref: Nelson 19th E/P139)

- Mild MR is seen in 2.1% of population.
- Most common predisposing cause of mild MR is environmental factors like poverty, malnutrition, inadequate maternal education seen in low socio-economic group.
- Biological causes like genetic disorders can also cause mild MR.

54. (b), (c), (d) and **(e)** Generalised seizure, Myoclonus, Response to sodium valproate, Spike and waves in EEG (Ref: Nelson 19th E/P1998)

- Three types of seizures that can be seen in JME are **myoclonic seizures, GTCS** and **absence seizures.**
- **JME responds best to valproate.**
- **Nelson 19th E/P1998**

"The EEG shows a 4–6/sec irregular spike and wave pattern which is enhanced by photic stimulation."

55. (a), (b), (d) and **(e)** Athetosis, Spasticity, Mixed palsy and Rigidity (Ref: Nelson 19th E/P2024–25, Rudolph 22nd E/P2178-81)

- Athetosis is the most common presentation of extrapyramidal CP. It can also be seen at times with spastic quadriplegia and then it is called as mixed cerebral palsy.
- Spasticity is seen in the spastic palsies.
- Rigidity is a feature of extrapyramidal CP.

56. (a), (b), (c) and **(d)** Microvesicular fatty infiltration, Hepatic encephalopathy, Brain edema, Hypoglycemia (Ref: Rudolph 22nd E/P1506)

- Reye syndrome is characterised by **acute encephalopathy and hepatic dysfunction.**
- Most common cause of death is **cerebral edema.**
- Laboratory changes that can be seen are **hypoglycaemia**, hyperammonemia, increased liver transaminases and PT.
- **Microvesicular hepatic steatosis** can be seen in liver biopsy.

57. (a), (c) and **(d)** Viral infection is seen, cerebral edema and Microvesicular fatty infiltration (Ref: Rudolph 22nd E/P1506)
- Reye's syndrome is preceded by **viral infections** like **varicella, influenza (type b>a)**, **adenovirus**, EBV and is strongly related to use of **aspirin**.
- Most common cause of death is **cerebral edema**.
- **Microvesicular fatty steatosis** can be seen in liver biopsy.

58. (b) and **(d)** Patients with family h/o FC have increased incidence of recurrence and usually last for short while (Ref: CPDT 19th E/P697)
- 90% of the febrile seizures last less than 5 minutes.
- Increased risk of recurrence is seen in following cases:
  1. **Early age of onset (<12 months).**
  2. **Family history of febrile seizures.**
  3. Short duration of fever.
  4. Seizure following lower temperature (<40°C).
  5. **Developmental delay.**
  6. Abnormal neurological conditions (cerebral palsy or mental retardation).
  7. **Presence of complex features** (seizure duration more than 15 minutes, more than one seizure a day and focal seizures in post ictal period).

59. (c) Diazepam (Ref: Rudolph 22nd E/P2205, CPDT 19th E/P298, Nelson 19th E/P1994)
- Diazepam given at the onset of fever by oral route at a dose of 0.5 mg/kg 2–3 times a day is the preferred prophylactic management.
- The factors limiting use of diazepam are its side-effect like sedation and the fact that fever is often preceded by seizure.

60. (b) *E.coli* (Ref:Nelson 19th E/P2038)
- Neonatal meningitis is most commonly caused by streptococcus agalctiae followed by *E.coli.*

61. (b) Cerebellar hemangioblastoma (Ref: Nelson 19th E/P2019)
Tumors seen in Von hippel landau disease:
- **Cerebellar hemangioblastomas** — These capillary malformations in the cerebellum present with symptoms of raised ICT.
- **Retinal angiomas** — These angiomas are usually located in the peripheral retina and do not affect vision, however they can cause retinal detachment.
- **Renal cell carcinoma** — This is the most common cause of death.

62. (d) Sturge Weber disease (Ref: Nelson 19th E/P2017-19) Kindly refer text for details.

62. (c) Hypogonadism (Ref: Nelson 19th E/P 525) Causes of large anterior fontanelle can be remembered as **CHOPRAS:**

- **C** — Cleidocranial dystosis, Chromosomal trisomy of 13, 15, 21 (**Down syndrome**)
- **H** — **Hypothyroidism**, Hdrocephalus, Hypophosphatasia
- **O** — **Osteogenesis Imperfecta**
- **P** — Pyknodystosis, Prematurity
- **R** — Rickets, Rubella (congenital)
- **A** — Achondroplasia
- **S** — Syndromes like Apert syndrome, Hallerman-Heriff syndrome, Russel Silver syndrome, Kenny syndrome

Also remember:
- **Third fontanelle** can be seen in **Down syndrome.**
- **Small fontanelles** can be seen in **hyperthyroidism, craniosyntosis, microcephaly** and **wormian bones.**

64. (d) Flaccid paralysis (Ref: Nelson 19th E/P2024-25, Rudolph 22nd E/P2178-81)

CPDT 19th E/P748
"Microcephaly is frequently present in CP."

- Hypo tonicity is a feature of hypotonic CP.
- Ataxia is seen in ataxic CP.
- Flaccid paralysis is seen in damage to the motor neurons of the spinal cord and not in CP.

65. (c) Cretinism (Ref: Ghai 7th E/P 562)
- Iodine deficiency can cause hypothyroidism and cretinism, both of which can be prevented by iodine supplementation.

66. (d) Hyperuricemia (Ref: Rudolph 22nd E/P1506–07)
- Damage to mitochondria leads to defect in urea genesis and hence **hypouricemia** will be seen.

67. (a) Post inflammatory obstruction (Ref: Rudolph 22nd E/P2174)
- Most common type of hydrocephalus in children is **obstructive or non-communicating** one. Out of various causes **aqueductal stenosis** is the most common cause of non communicating hydrocephalus and the causes can be
  ❖ Genetic (X linked recessive)
  ❖ Gliosis of the aqueduct caused subarachnoid haemorrhage and **meningoencephalitis**.

68. (a) Portwine stain (Ref:Nelson 19th E/P2017)
Clinical findings in Sturge Weber syndrome:
- **Port-wine stain (facial nevus)**
- Seizures
- Transient stroke like episodes
- Mental retardation
- Ipsilateral bupthalmos and glaucoma

69. (c) Automatism (Ref: Nelson 19th E/P1997-98)
- Automatism is a feature of complex partial seizure characterised by movements like smacking of lips, chewing, swallowing after loss of consciousness.
- Juvenile muclonic epilepsy is associated with GTCS and absence seizure in 25% cases.

70. (a) Recurrent in nature (Ref: Nelson 19th E/P1994)
Febrile seizures:

"Approximately 30–50% of children have recurrent seizures with later episodes of fever and a small minority have numerous recurrent seizures."

- It is seen in the initial rising phase of temperature i.e. when it is low.
- It is benign in nature and usually self limiting.
- Most common age group affected is 9 months to 5 years.

71. (a) SSPE

- Myoclonic seizures are characteristically seen in SSPE in the second stage of disease.
- In the myoclonic stage "**suppression-burst episodes**" can be seen in EEG in which high-amplitude slow and sharp waves recur at intervals of 3–5 sec on a slow background.

72. (a) Petitmal epilepsy (Ref: Nelson 19th E/P1997)

73. (a) 50% recurrence (Ref: Nelson 19th E/P 1994)

- Recurrence is seen in 30–50% patients.
- Carbamazepine and phenytoin are ineffective in prophylaxis.
- EEG is normal but certain changes like 3/s spike wave discharges may be seen in complicated febrile seizure.
- Status epilepticus is rarely seen in febrile seizure.

74. (d) Depressed fontanel (Ref: Nelson 19th E/P1990)

- **Clinical findings of hydrocephalus.**
- The most common appreciable sign of hydrocephalus is rapid **increase in the size of head along with a bulging anterior fontanel**, dilated scalp veins and frontal bossing.
- **Setting sun eye sign** — This is because of downward eye deviation.
- **Crack pot sound** on percussion of skull (**Macewen sign**) can be heard, which is because of suture separation.

75. (b) HSV 2 (Ref: Nelson 19th E/P2045)

HSV meningoencephalitis:

- HSV usually affects the **temporal lobe** and thus focal seizures or focal findings in CT, MRI or EEG involving the temporal lobe are diagnostic for HSV infection. Unlike other viral infections with a normal or slightly elevated CSF protein levels, in **HSV protein levels can be very high**.
- ❖ **HSV-1** is a predominant cause of sporadic encephalitis in **children and adults**. Unlike other viruses it causes **focal involvement**.
- ❖ **HSV-2** is a primary cause in **neonates**, who acquire the virus from the genital tract of mother. In this case there is **diffuse involvement** of the brain.

QUESTIONS OF OTHER EXAMINATIONS

1. (d) Multifactorial (Ref: Nelson 19th E/P1983)

"Although the precise cause of neural tube defects remains unknown, evidence suggests that many factors, including radiation, drugs, malnutrition, chemicals, and genetic determinants (mutations in folate-responsive or folate-dependent pathways), may adversely affect normal development of the CNS from the time of conception."

2. (a) Febrile convulsions (Ref: Nelson 19th E/P1994)

"**Febrile convulsions, the most common seizure disorder during childhood**, generally have an excellent prognosis but may also signify a serious underlying acute infectious disease such as sepsis or bacterial meningitis."

3. (b) Hypokalemia (Ref: Nelson 19th E/P2472–23)

4. (a) Aqueductal stenosis (Ref: Rudolph 22nd E/P2174)

- Aqueductal stenosis is the most common cause of congenital hydrocephalus, which is responsible for 20% cases with an incidence of 0.5–1% per 1000 births.

5. (d) Central transentorial herniation (Ref: Black Neurosurgery P71)

"Although this mass (Central transtentorial herniation) can be caused by any bilateral central mass, the major cause is **acute hydrocephalus** supratentorially."

6. (c) Complex partial (Ref: Nelson 19th E/P1998)
Complex partial seizure:

"Radiographic studies including CT scanning and especially MRI are most likely to identify an **abnormality in the temporal lobe** of a child with **CPS**. These lesions include **mesial temporal sclerosis**, hamartoma, postencephalitic gliosis, subarachnoid cysts, infarction, arteriovenous malformations, and slow-growing glioma."

7. (c) Papilledema (Ref: Nelson 19th E/P1991)

"Papilledema is observed in older children but is **rarely present in infants** because the cranial sutures separate as a result of the increased pressure."

8. (c) Spina bifida (Ref: Principles and practice of pediatric neurosurgery P349)

Ultrasonographic findings myelomeningocele (NTD):

- **Lemon sign** — Two frontal bone appear convex inwards.
- **Banana sign** — Elongated curved posterior fossa due to Chiari malformation.

9. (d) Prophylactic phenobarbitone (Ref: CPDT 19th E/P698)

"Anticonvulsants are not recommended after an uncomplicated febrile seizure."

- **Prophylaxis of febrile seizure:**
  ❖ Diazepam by oral route at the onset of fever is the preferred method for both simple/typical and complex/atypical febrile seizures.
  ❖ Anticonvulsants effective in febrile seizure like phenobarbitone and valproate are only indicated if febrile seizures are complex or prolonged and medical reassurance (prophylactic diazepam at onset of fever) fails to relieve family anxiety.

10. (b) Partial complex seizures (Ref: Nelson 19th E/P1997)

- DOC for partial seizures is carbamazepine.
- DOC for generalised seizures like absence seizures, Myoclonic seizures and GTCS is valproate.
- DOC for infantile spasms is ACTH.

11. (d) Craniosyntosis (Ref: Nelson 19th E/P 525)

12. (d) Dandy-Walker syndrome (Ref: Nelson 19th E/P1987)

13. (b) Mumps (Ref: Nelson 19th E/P1990)

"Intrauterine viral infections may also produce aqueductal stenosis followed by hydrocephalus, and **mumps meningoencephalitis** has been reported as a cause in a child."

14. (c) Lamotrigine (Ref: CPDT 19th E/P697)

15. (c) Cerebral abscess (Ref: Nelson 19th E/P2047–48) Kindly refer text for details on brain abscess.

16. (c) Saggital suture (Ref: Nelson 19th E/P1992)

Synostosis	Sutures involved
Scapocephaly	**Saggital**
Frontal plagiocephaly	Coronal and sphenofrontal
Occipital plagiocephaly	Lambdoid suture
Brachycephaly	Both coronal
Turricephaly	Coronal, sphenofrontal and frontoethmoidal
Trigonocephaly	Metopic

17. (a) and **(b)** Cerebral palsy and Hypoxic ischemic encephalopathy (Ref: Rudolph 22nd E/P2178)

- Posture abnormalities like extensor posture is seen in cerebral palsy.
- Hypoxic ischemic encephalopathy is a common cause of cerebral palsy.

18. (c) Phenobarbitone (Ref: CPDT 19th E/P684)

- Start with IV/IM **phenobarbitone**; if patient doesn't respond then add phenytoin IV at a dose of 20 mg/kg.

19. (d) Deep jaundice is present (Ref: Rudolph 22nd E/P1506–07)

20. (c) Almost invariably develop in to epilepsy (Ref: Rudolph 22nd E/P2205)

"Outcome of febrile seizures is usually **favourable**, but **2% to 10%** of children with febrile seizures experience subsequent **epilepsy**."

21. (c) Hypocalcemia (Ref: Ghai 7th E/P531)

22. (c) Dexamethasone (Ref: Ghai 7th E/P541)

23. (b) The capability of a child to perform intellectual tasks in relation to other children of same age (Ref: Ghai 7th E/P 562)

24. (a) Focal in nature (Ref: Nelson 19th E/P 1994)

"The seizure is usually **generalized, is tonic-clonic** and lasts a few seconds to 10-min, and is followed by a brief postictal period of drowsiness."

25. (a) Spastic (Ref: CPDT 19th E/P748)

"The most common form of cerebral palsy (75% of cases) involves **spasticity** of the limbs."

26. (b) RSV (Ref: Rudolph 22nd E/P1506–07)

Reye's syndrome is usually preceded by viral infections like:

- **Varicella**
- **Influenza**
- **Adenovirus**
- EBV

27. (c) Hypopitutarism (Ref: Ghai 7th E/P562)

28. (a) Bilirubin more than 3 mg (Ref: Rudolph 22nd E/P1506–07)

- **Bilirubin is normal**.
- PT is either **normal** or increased.

29. (a) Blood (Ref: Nelson 19th E/P835)

Rapid antigen test for bacterial infections:

- **Latex agglutination test** is used for diagnosis of various organisms.
  - ❖ Group A Streptococcus in **pharynx by throat swab.**
  - ❖ *H. influenza, Streptococcus agalactiae* and pneumoniae and *Nisseria meningitides* in **CSF**.
- **Binax NOW urinary antigen test** is used for diagnosis of *Streptococcus pneumoniae* in **urine**.

30. (a) Aminoaciduria (Ref: Rudolph 22nd E/P1506–07)

- Lactic acidosis and compensatory metabolic alkalosis can be seen.

31. (d) Infantile spasms (Ref: CPDT 19th E/P685–87)

- Rolandic epilepsy is also called as **bening epilepsy** with cntrotemporal spikes (BECTS), in which GTCS can be seen. Treatment is not required if seizures are infrequent.
- Versive seizures are seen in simple partial seizure, which consists of head turning and conjugate eye movement.
- Absence seizure is associated with a favourable outcome.
- **Infantile spasms** are frequently associated with **mental retardation.**

6

Neuromuscular Diseases

Neuromuscular diseases are caused by any abnormality in the motor unit, which consists of the motor neuron in spinal cord, nerve fibres of the motor neuron innervating the muscles, the neuromuscular junction and the muscle fibres.

DISEASES OF MOTOR NEURONS

The motor neuron disorders or anterior horn cell diseases that are common in children are spinal muscular atrophy and poliomyelitis.

Spinal Muscular Atrophy

SMA is caused by mutation of SMN1 gene, which results in failure of cessation of apoptosis of motor neurons in the fetus. This results in progressive motor neuron apoptosis from fetal period till death. Based on severity of disease they are classified in to 4 types i.e. SMA1 or Werdnig-Hoffman disease, SMA2, SMA3 or Kugelberg-Welander disease and SMA4 (adult type).

- **Clinical presentation and findings:**
  - ❖ **Muscle weakness** — Hypotonia and weakness of **proximal muscle** of legs>arms can be seen. The intercostal respiratory muscles are also involved. Muscular hypertrophy can be seen in place of atrophy.
  - ❖ **Fasciculations** — This is a sign of denervation that can be seen in skeletal muscles but is more marked in the **tongue muscles.**
  - ❖ Cardiac involvement and **MR are not seen.**
  - ❖ Hypotonia can be detected in infants by various signs like **frog leg posture,** head lag and slip-through on vertical suspension.
  - ❖ **Deep tendon reflexes are decreased** or absent.
- **Diagnosis:**
  - ❖ SMN gene mutation detection in blood is the definitive diagnostic procedure.
  - ❖ EMG shows fibrillation potentials.

DISEASES OF THE NERVE FIBRES

The nerve fibre disorders or neuropathies can be hereditary (HSMN) and acquired (toxic neuropathy, GBS, Bell palsy).

Hereditary Motor Sensory Neuropathies

These neuropathies are characterised by predominant motor fibres involvement along with sensory and autonomic fibres. They can be classified in to 3 types i.e. **HMSN I (Peroneal muscular atrophy or Charcot-Marie-Tooth disease),** HSMN II and HSMN III (Dejerine-Sottas disease).

Peroneal Muscular Atrophy

It is an AD disease characterised by abnormality in the peripheral myelin protein gene located in 17th chromosome.

- **Clinical presentation:**
  - ❖ The peroneal and tibial nerves are most severely affected which results in muscle wasting of the anterior compartment of legs. This gives an **inverted champagne bottle or stork (a bird) like appearance** to the leg because of preserved proximal muscles and severe distal muscle wasting.
  - ❖ Pes cavus and foot drop can cause gait disturbance.
- **Diagnosis:** Sural nerve biopsy is diagnostic which gives a characteristic **onion bulb formation**.

Guillain-Barre Syndrome

GBS is a postinfectious, autoimmune, demyelinating neuropathy with predominant involvement of the **motor nerve fibres**, which presents as an **acute ascending flaccid paralysis**. The preceding events of GBS are infections caused by Campylobacter, *H. pylori, Mycoplasma pneumoniae*, West Nile virus, hepatitis B virus, CMV, EBV and immunization with vaccines against rubies, influenza, polio and meningococcus. The contributing pathologic process is production of **antiganglioside antibodies (anti GM1 and GD1).**

- **Clinical presentation and finding:**
  - ❖ Weakness usually begins in the lower limbs and gradually moves upwards to involve the other muscles of body (trunk, upper limb, **face** and bulbar). This pattern is characteristically called as **Landry ascending paralysis**. There is symmetric involvement of **proximal** and **distal muscles**. Extraocular muscles are usually spared but can be involved in another variant called as **Miller-Fisher syndrome**, which involves external opthalmoplegia, ataxia and areflexia.
  - ❖ The other features can be urinary incontinence, paraesthesia and dysphagia.
  - ❖ **Deep tendon reflexes are usually lost.**
  - ❖ Congenital GBS presents with severe hypotonia, weakness and areflexia. Treatment is usually not required.
  - ❖ GBS has a very benign course and **spontaneous recovery** is seen in most cases. Deep tendon reflexes are the last to recover.
- **Diagnosis:** The CSF finding of increased proteins with a **normal cell count (albumino cytological dissociation)** is characteristic for GBS.
- **Treatment:** Treatment of choice for GBS is **intravenous immunoglobulin (IVIG)**. If patient fails to respond then plasmapheresis and immunomodulators (**steroids are ineffective**) can be used.

DISEASES OF NEUROMUSCULAR JUNCTION

The neuromuscular junction is critical for mediation of action potential from the nerve to the muscle. When action potential depolarises the presynaptic membrane, intraneuronal calcium increases due to opening of calcium channels. This leads to release of Ach in to synaptic cleft which acts on Ach receptor and causes muscle contraction. The different abnormalities in neuromuscular junction can be caused by block of calcium channels by botulinum toxin (infant botulism) and Ach receptor by antibodies (myasthenia gravis).

Myasthenia Gravis

Myasthenia gravis is an autoimmune disease characterised by autoantibodies against the Ach receptors. Thymus is thought to play a role in the antibody production and **thymoma** can be seen in some cases (thymoma is common in adults). Girls are more commonly affected than boys.

- **Clinical presentation:** Clinically in children MG can be classified in to Neonatal MG, congenital MG and juvenile MG.
  - ❖ **Neonatal and Congenital MG:**
    - ❑ Neonatal MG is caused by maternal anti Ach receptor antibodies which are transferred to the fetus but congenital MG is caused by a genetic abnormality causing alteration in the Ach receptor (**no anti Ach receptor antibodies**).
    - ❑ Baby may have constant **hypotonia** and is referred to as "floppy infant". Floppy infant is a nonspecific term as it can also be seen in spinal muscular atrophy and infant botulism.
    - ❑ **Reflexes are usually preserved.**
  - ❖ **Juvenile MG:**
    - ❑ Juvenile MG is caused by production of anti Ach receptor antibody production in children. Other autoimmune conditions like JRA, Hashimoto thyroiditis and SLE can be associated.

❑ It may present with fatigue of muscles of mastication, swallowing and respiration; however in children **ocular features like ptosis and diplopia are more typical** but **pupillary response is normal**. Usually distal muscle weakness is seen but in rare cases **proximal muscle involvement can be seen**.

❑ Many other disorders like Guillain-Barre syndrome and myopathies may present like MG, but what differentiates the latter is its **diurnal variation in weakness** (more towards the end of the day) and **fluctuating pattern of weakness (patient suddenly may become asymptomatic)**. The **weakness increases with activity**.

- **Diagnosis:**
  - ❖ **Ocular ice pack test** — MG worsens with heat and improves with cold. Hence application of ice cold pack to the ptotic eye relieves the ptosis. It is a highly sensitive test.
  - ❖ **Tests with cholinergic drugs:**
    - ❑ **Edrophonium or Tensilon test**
    - ❑ Neostigmine test.
  - ❖ **Antibody detection** — Anti Ach receptor antibodies and anti- MUSK (muscle specific kinase) antibodies can add to the diagnosis.

- **Treatment:**
  - ❖ Cholinergic drugs like **pyridostigmine (drug of choice)** and neostigmine are used to alleviate the symptoms; however anticholinergic drug like atropine can be added to minimise the cholinergic side-effects. Neonatal MG requires a short term treatment. Congenital MG responds poorly as the Ach receptors are modified.
  - ❖ Immunomodulators like steroids, mycophenolate mofetil, and azathioprine are also used.
  - ❖ Plasmapheresis and IVIG can be used to remove the circulating antibodies and neutralise them respectively.
  - ❖ **Thymectomy** can be done in juvenile MG but not in neonatal or congenital MG. It is useful if Anti Ach receptor antibody level is very high or symptoms are there for <2years.

Infantile Botulism

- Botulism is caused by **clostridium botulinum**, which is an anaerobic, spore forming, gram positive bacteria. Infantile botulism is usually seen from **3 to 6 months** of life when introduction of formula feed and solid foods alter the microflora of intestine.
- The baby presents with constipation, **severe hypotonia (floppy infant)**, poor suck, mewing cry and apnea.
- Demonstration of botulinum toxin in stool by neutralisation bioassay is diagnostic.
- Electromyography (EMG) shows **BSAP** (Brief, small, abundant potential) abnormalities.
- Treatment is started only with human **intravenous botulism immunoglobulin**. (Antitoxin is used for food borne botulism).

DISEASES OF MUSCLE FIBRES

The diseases of muscle fibres, also called as myopathy consists of congenital abnormalities in development of muscles and dystrophy of muscles. Most of the muscular diseases are associated with proximal muscle weakness, elevated CPK, cardiac abnormalities and mild MR.

Muscular Dystrophies

These are primary, progressive and degenerative disease of the muscle fibres. The different subtypes are Duchenne, Becker, Emery-Dreifuss, myotonic, limb-girdle and fascioscapulohumeral muscular dystrophies.

Duchenne Muscular Dystrophy

DMD is an X linked recessive disorder characterised by mutation of the dystrophin gene responsible for production of a **sarcolemmal protein dystrophin**. It is most common inherited neuromuscular disease.

- **Clinical presentation:**
  - ❖ **Muscle weakness** — The **proximal muscles** of limbs are more affected, which gives a characteristic **Trendelenburg** or **waddling gait**. Because of proximal muscle weakness of leg (thigh muscles), the compensatory overuse of **calf muscle** leads to **hypertrophy**. Weakness of the respiratory (pulmonary infections, decreased respiratory reserve) and pharyngeal muscles (aspiration) can also be seen. Extraocular muscles are spared.
  - ❖ **Cardiomyopathy** is seen in majority of patients and is an important cause of mortality after respiratory failure.
  - ❖ Other features that can be seen are skeletal abnormalities (scoliosis), epilepsy and mild mental retardation (almost in all patients).

- **Clinical signs:**
  - ❖ **Gower sign** — The child uses hand support to push themselves in to upright position from sitting because of proximal muscle weakness of legs.
- **Diagnosis:**
  - ❖ **CPK levels are elevated many fold** than the normal level (<160 IU/L) but **gradually decreases as the age progresses** due to decrease in muscle mass.
  - ❖ Blood PCR for the dystrophin gene mutation is the definite diagnosis.
  - ❖ Muscle biopsy show characteristic changes of myopathy; however it is less preferred as it is an invasive method.
- **Treatment:** Apart from supportive treatment, prednisolone has been seen to improve the muscular strength.

Becker Muscular Dystrophy

BMD is similar to DMD in etiology, but the only difference is presence of partial expression of dystrophin protein which gives this disease a lesser severity.

Scapulohumeral Muscular Dystrophy

SHMD or Emery-Dreifuss muscular dystrophy is an X linked recessive disorder characterised by mutation of emerin gene, which leads to decreased production of **nuclear membrane protein emerin**.
- **Clinical presentation and findings:**
  - ❖ **Muscle weakness** — It is confined to scapulohumeroperoneal distribution. Contractures can be seen but muscle hypertrophy is not seen.
  - ❖ **Cardiomyopathy** — It is severe and mortality is usually caused by heart block or ventricular fibrillation.
  - ❖ MR is not seen and CPK levels are also normal.

Myotonic Muscular Dystrophy

MMD is an autosomal dominant disease caused by abnormal **CTG trinucleotide repetition** in the DM gene located in the **19th chromosome**. The characteristic finding with this type of dystrophy is association of multiple organ disorders.
- **Clinical presentation:**
  - ❖ **Muscle weakness** — Unlike other dystrophies it starts with **involvement of distal muscles** (thenar and hypothenar weakness). Facial muscle weakness gives the baby a **V shaped upper lip** and tongue is atrophic (speech abnormality).
  - ❖ **Myotonia** — This is the characteristic feature which can be seen in the patient as contraction of muscle followed by a slow relaxation.
  - ❖ Cardiac abnormalities like heart block and arrhythmias can be seen.
  - ❖ Endocrine abnormalities like hypothyroidism>hyperthyroidism, adrenal insufficiency, DM and frontal baldness can be seen.
  - ❖ Other abnormalities like immunologic impairment, cataracts and mild MR can be seen.
- **Diagnosis:**
  - ❖ Blood DNA analysis for CTG repeat is diagnosis.
  - ❖ EMG shows features of myotonia.
  - ❖ CPK levels are usually normal.

Limb-Girdle Muscular Dystrophy

- This is a group of muscular dystrophies which have predominantly AR inheritance and are caused by mutation of several sarcolemmal protein that decreases production of several proteins like adhalen, **dysferlin, caveolin-3 or calpain-3, sarcoglycans (α, β, γ and δ),** fukutin, titin and telethronin.
- It usually presents in the late childhood i.e. towards the end of first decade.
- **Clinical presentation:**
  - ❖ **Muscle weakness** — Apart from hip and shoulder girdle muscles, the neck muscles are also universally involved.
  - ❖ Other features like **cardiac involvement** and **MR are usually not seen.**

Fascioscapulohumeral Muscular Dystrophy

FSMD or Landouzy-Dejerine disease is an AD disorder which can be associated with **Mobius syndrome.**

- **Clinical presentation:**
  ❖ **Muscle weakness** — Asymmetric weakness in the fascioscapulohumeral distribution is characteristic. Facial weakness can be seen as a round mouth with protruded lips and inability to close eyes during sleep. Scapular muscle dystrophy and weakness presents as scapular winging.
  ❖ Other features that can be seen are hearing loss, retinal vasculopathy, spine deformities (lordosis and kyphoscoliosis).

Congenital Muscular Dystrophies

CMD involves a group of disorder which present at birth but usually are benign in nature. It is usually caused by absence of a **sarcolemmal protein merosin** which is also found in CNS.
- **Clinical presentation:**
  ❖ **Muscle weakness** — The baby is hypotonic at birth and multiple contractures (arthrogryposis) can also be seen.
  ❖ **CNS defects** — As merlin is present in CNS, certain CNS defects can be seen like holoprosencephaly, lissencephaly, agenesis of corpus callosum and cerebellar hypoplasia.

MULTIPLE CHOICE QUESTIONS

1. **Duchenne's dystrophy; investigation of choice:**
   [AIIMS Nov. 08]
   a. Serum creatinine
   b. Nerve conduction study
   c. ESR
   d. CPK

2. **Which of the following is not a limb girdle dystrophy?** [AIIMS Nov. 06]
   a. Sarcoglycan dystrophy b. Dystrophin dystrophy
   c. Dysferlin dystrophy   d. Calpain dystrophy

3. **An infant presents with hypotonia and hyporeflexia. During his intrauterine period there was polyhydramnios and decreased fetal movements. Most probable diagnosis is:** [AIIMS May 02]
   a. Spinal muscular atrophy
   b. Congenital myasthenia
   c. Congenital myotonia
   d. Muscular dystrophy

4. **All of the following are associated with proximal muscle weakness except:** [AIIMS May 02]
   a. Spinomuscular atrophy
   b. Duchenne muscular dystrophy
   c. Polymyositis
   d. Myotonic dystrophy

5. **10 years old Ramu has increasing muscle weakness and raised CPK levels. The most likely defect is in plasma membrane of:** [AIIMS Nov. 01]
   a. Nerves   b. Muscle fibres
   c. Basement membrane d. All body cells

6. **Give the most probable diagnosis of a 1-year-old child of normal intelligence with features of hypotonia. On examination there are tongue fasciculations and he keeps his body in a frog like position:** [AIIMS Nov. 00]
   a. Guillian Barre Syndrome
   b. Limb girdle atrophy
   c. Down's syndrome
   d. Spinal muscular atrophy

7. **All are clinical features of myasthenia gravis except:**
   [AIIMS Feb. 97]
   a. Spontaneous remission
   b. Absent deep tendon reflexes
   c. Proximal muscle involvement
   d. Worsen by exertion

8. **Thymoma is associated with:** [AI 08 2k, 94]
   a. Myasthenia gravis
   b. Scleroderma
   c. Oesophageal atresia
   d. Hypergammaglobulinemia

9. **Duchenne Muscular Dystrophy is a disease of:**
   [AI 04, Manipal 09]
   a. Neuromuscular junction
   b. Sarcolemmal proteins
   c. Muscle contractile proteins
   d. Disuse atrophy due to muscle weakness

10. **Gene for myotonic dystrophy is coded on chromosome number:** [AI 99]
    a. 19
    b. 20
    c. 21
    d. 24

11. **Drug of choice for myasthenia gravis:** [PGI Dec. 99]
    a. Gallamine
    b. Succinylcholine
    c. D. tubocurare
    d. Pyridostigmine

QUESTIONS OF OTHER EXAMINATIONS

1. Gower sign is classical of one of the following condition:
   a. Congenital myopathy
   b. Werdig-Hoffman disease
   c. Duchenne muscular dystrophy
   d. Guillain-Barre syndrome

2. A child was brought to the paediatrician with complaints of closing of eyelids towards the evening. He also has recently developed difficulty in swallowing food. What would be the diagnostic approach for the condition?
   a. Electromyography
   b. Nerve conduction study
   c. Ocular ice pack test
   d. Serum CPK levels

3. Most common clinical finding in juvenile myasthenia gravis is:
   a. Ptosis
   b. Dysphagia
   c. Dysarthria
   d. Proximal muscle weakness

4. Which of the following can be used for diagnosis of Guillain Barre syndrome?
   a. Antimyelin antibody
   b. Anti ganglioside antibody
   c. Anti MUSK antibody
   d. CPK level

5. Treatment of choice for Guillain Barre syndrome is:
   a. Steroids
   b. Plamapheresis
   c. IVIG
   d. Azathioprine

6. Onion bulb appearance on nerve biopsy can be seen in:
   a. Spinal muscular atrophy
   b. Peroneal muscular atrophy
   c. Guillain Barre syndrome
   d. Axonal neuropathy

7. Mobius syndrome can be associated with:
   a. Spinal muscular atrophy
   b. Facioscapulohumeral muscular dystrophy
   c. Limb Girdle muscular dystrophy
   d. Myotonic muscular dystrophy

8. Most common muscle to undergo hypertrophy in Duchenne muscular dystrophy:
   a. Tongue
   b. Thenar
   c. Thigh
   d. Tarsal

9. An infant of 5 months brought to you with a history of constipation and difficulty in sucking and swallowing. After taking history it was learnt that the baby was recently started on solid food. What is the most probable cause?
   a. Infantile spinal muscular atrophy
   b. Myasthenia gravis
   c. Congenital myotonic dystrophy
   d. Botulism

ANSWERS

1. (d) CPK (Ref: Rudolph 22nd E/P2243)
Diagnosis of DMD:
- **CPK levels are elevated many fold** than the normal level (<160 IU/L). However it is not specific for DMD.
- Blood PCR for the dystrophin gene mutation is the definite diagnosis.
- Muscle biopsy show characteristic changes of myopathy; however it is less preferred as it is an invasive method.

2. (b) Dystrophin dystrophy (Ref: Rudolph 22nd E/P2245)
LGMD classification:

Type	Gene location	Protein
LGMD1A	5	Myotilin
LGMD1B	1	Lamin A/C
LGMD1C	3	Caveolin-3
LGMD1D	6	—
LGMD1E	7	—
LGMD2A	15	**Calpain-3**
LGMD2B	2	**Dysferlin**
LGMD2C	13	γ sarcoglycan
LGMD2D	17	α sarcoglycan
LGMD2E	4	β sarcoglycan
LGMD2F	5	δ sarcoglycan
LGMD2G	17	Telethronin
LGMD2H	9	TMCP 32
LGMD2I	19	Fukutin related protein
LGMD2J	2	Titin

Note: All LGMD1 subtypes are AD inherited, whereas LGMD2 are AR inherited.

3. (a) Spinal muscular atrophy (Ref: Rudolph 22nd E/P2228–29)
All these disorders can present in intrauterine period with polyhydramnios due to poor swallowing and decreased fetal movements. Hypotonia can be seen with all but reflexes are lost only in spinal muscular atrophy.
- **SMA** — It presents typically with hypotonia and decreased or absent reflexes.
- **Muscular dystrophy** — The muscular dystrophies usually present after the infancy.
- **Congenital myotonia** — It may present at birth with sever hypotonia but reflexes are preserved.
- **Congenital myasthenia gravis** — Baby presents with severe hypotonia but reflexes are preserved.

4. (d) Myotonic dystrophy (Ref: Nelson 19th E/P2065)
- Proximal muscle weakness is a rule in muscle dystrophies but the exception is myotonic muscular dystrophy which is associated with distal muscle weakness.

5. (b) Muscle fibre (Ref: Rudolph 22nd E/P2241)
- Increasing muscle weakness and Raised CPK levels point towards muscular dystrophy.
- Muscular dystrophy is caused by defects in the muscle fibres e.g. dystrophin, a sarcolemmal protein deficiency in Duchenne and Becker muscular dystrophy.

6. (d) Spinal muscular atrophy (Ref: Rudolph 22nd E/P2228)
Spinal muscular atrophy:
- Hypotonia can be detected in infants by various signs like **frog leg posture**, head lag and slip-through on vertical suspension.
- **Deep tendon reflexes are decreased** or absent.
- **Muscle weakness** — Hypotonia and weakness of **proximal muscle** of legs>arms can be seen. The intercostal respiratory muscles are also involved. Muscular hypertrophy can be seen in place of atrophy.
- **Fasciculations** — This is a sign of denervation that can be seen in skeletal muscles but is more marked in the **tongue muscles.**

7. (b) Absent deep tendon reflexes (Ref: Rudolph 22nd E/P2236)
- The weakness in MG is fluctuating in nature and spontaneous improvement can be typically seen.
- Deep tendon reflexes can be diminished but are never lost.
- Usually distal muscles of limbs are involved but rarely it can mimic myopathy by involving the proximal muscles.
- Weakness in MG typically increases on activity.

8. (a) Myasthenia gravis (Ref: Nelson 19th E/P2073)
- Thymoma is usually seen in adult MG but can be rarely seen in children with MG.

9. (b) Sarcolemmal protein (Ref: Function and Genetics of Dystrophin and Dystrophin-Related Proteins in Muscle, Derek J. Blake)
- Dystrophin is located at the muscle sarcolemma in a membrane-spanning protein complex that connects the cytoskeleton to the basal lamina.
- Although the precise function of dystrophin is unknown, the lack of protein causes membrane destabilization and the activation of multiple pathophysiological processes, many of which converge on alterations in intracellular calcium handling.

10. (a) 19 (Ref: Rudolph 22nd E/P2244)
Muscular dystrophies and genetic cause:

Muscular dystrophy	Genetic cause
Duchenne and Becker	X linked recessive disorder causes mutation of dystrophin gene.
Scapulohumeral or Emery-Driefuss	X linked recessive inheritance causes mutation of emerin geneAD and AR inheritance by mutation of lamin A/C genes in chromosome 1.
Myotonic	AD inheritance causes repetation of CTG trinucleotide in 19th chromosome.
LGMD	AD and AR inheritance can cause mutation of multiple genes.
Facioscapulohumeral	AD inheritance causes deletion of D4Z4 in 4th chromosome.
Congenital	Mutation of merosin gene on 6th chromosome.

QUESTIONS OF OTHER EXAMINATIONS

1. (c) Duchenne muscular dystrophy (Ref: Rudolph 22nd E/P2241)

- **Gower sign** — The child uses hand support to push themselves in to upright position from sitting because of proximal muscle weakness of legs.

2. (c) Ocular ice pack test (Ref: Rudolph 22nd E/P2237)

- Closing of eyelids towards the evening and dysphagia hint towards myasthenia gravis.
- **Ocular ice pack** test is now a days more preferred than edrophonium test because of its high sensitivity and lack of cholinergic side effects.

3. (a) Ptosis (Ref: Rudolph 22nd E/P2237)

"Ptosis is the most common JMG finding."

4. (b) Anti ganglioside antibody (Ref: Nelson 19th E/P2081)

- Anti ganglioside antibodies against GM1 and GD1 can be seen in Guillain Barre syndrome.

5. (c) IVIG (Ref: Nelson 19th E/P2081)

11. (d) Pyridostigmine (Ref: CPDT 19th E/P742)

- Cholinergic drugs are the preferred drugs to alleviate the symptoms. Pyridostigmine is the drug of choice.
- Certain drugs which can block the neuromuscular transmission are contraindicated in myasthenia gravis.
  - ❖ **Succinylcholine**
  - ❖ **Tubocurare**
  - ❖ Vecuronium
  - ❖ D-Penicillamine
  - ❖ Antibiotics like aminoglycosides.

- Treatment of choice for GBS is IVIG. Plasmapheresis and immunomodulators are used if patient does not respond to IVIG. Steroids are ineffective in treating GBS.

6. (b) Peroneal muscular atrophy (Ref: Nelson 19th E/P2077)

- Onion bulb formation is the name given to schwann cell proliferation around the axon seen in peroneal muscular atrophy. This is an interstitial hypertrophic neuropathy.

7. (b) Facioscapulohumeral muscular dystrophy (Ref: Nelson 19th E/P2067)

- Facioscapulohumeral muscular dystrophy can be associated with Mobius syndrome.

8. (a) Tongue (Ref: Nelson 19th E/P2061)
- Order of muscle hypertrophy in DMD is **calves> tongue> forearm**.

9. (d) Botulism (Ref: Nelson 19th E/P948)
- An infant presenting with bulbar symptoms and constipation with recent history of starting solid food indicates towards botulism.
Kindly refer text for details on infant botulism.

7

Gastrointestinal System

ESOPHAGEAL DISORDERS

Tracheoesophageal Fistula

Tracheoesophageal fistula (TEF) can be classified in to five types based on the presence of esophageal atresia and location of the fistula.

Type A-Esophageal atresia without TEF	Type B-Proximal TEF fistula	Type C-Proximal esophageal atresia with distal TEF	Type D-Both proximal and distal fistula	Type E-Isolated TEF (H or N type fistula)
• 2nd most common type • No gas in abdomen	• No gas in abdomen	• **Most common type** • Gas in abdomen present	• Least common type • Gas in abdomen present	• Distal gas present

The most common type of TEF is type C which is characterised by presence of **esophageal atresia in the proximal part and fistula in the distal part**. TEF is most commonly associated with CVS abnormalities, however other conditions like VACTERL, hypospadias, undescended testis, duodenal atresia, aqueductal stenosis, Goldenhar syndrome and CHARGE syndrome can be associated.

Clinical Presentation

- TEF is associated with polyhydramnios because of inability of the foetus to swallow the amniotic fluid.
- After birth neonates present with **frothing, excessive drooling** and coughing **with feeds**. This is followed by cyanosis and **respiratory distress.**
- H or N type fistulas usually present later than other types with recurrent pneumonia due to aspiration.

Diagnosis

- A **nasogastric tube** is inserted and inability to pass it confirms the diagnosis of TEF.
- **X-ray** shows a coiled tube in the atretic end and gas in the abdomen in type C,D and E TEF.
- **Prenatal USG** shows polyhydramnios, microgastria and **absent stomach bubble**.

Treatment

- Surgical repair of the fistula and end to end anastomosis of esophagus is the mainstay of treatment if the distance between both ends is less than 3 cm. If the gape is more, then a gastrostomy is done and the esophageal repair by conduits (stomach, jejunum or colon) is delayed by 2–3 months.
- The earliest complication of surgery is **anastomotic leak** and the most common one is **stricture formation** at the site of anastomosis. Other complications that can be seen are GERD, Barret esophagus and esophageal cancer.

DISORDERS OF STOMACH

Hypertrophic Pyloric Stenosis

The cause of hypertrophic pyloric stenosis has been attributed to decrease NO synthase production, enteric denervation and loss of interstitial cells of Cajal. It is the **most common surgical cause of nonbilious vomiting in infants**. **Males (first born)** are more commonly affected than females.

Clinical Presentation

- The infant typically presents with **forceful, projectile**, postprandial **nonbilious vomiting** between **2–4 weeks of age.** After vomiting child is **hungry** and has a **voracious appetite.**
- Long term vomiting may lead to dehydration, weight loss and constipation. Initial loss of HCl leads to **hypochloremic hypokalemic metabolic alkalosis.** Initially protons are saved to compensate for alkalosis. But continuous loss of **sodium**, **potassium** and **chloride** leads to compensatory loss of protons in urine to save the other ions, which leads to **paradoxical aciduria.**
- Unconjugated hyperbilirubinemia may be seen due to decreased glucose absorption, which results in decreased activity of glucuronyl transferase.

Diagnosis

- **Ultrasonography** is the most specific and sensitive diagnostic method for pyloric stenosis. A pyloric thickness of >4mm and a length of >14mm is diagnostic.
- Upper gastrointestinal contrast is the definitive method which shows **string sign, double tract sign** and **shoulder sign**.
- On examination a visible **peristalsis mass from left to right** can be seen and a mobile **olive shaped pyloric mass** can be palpated in 80-90% of cases. **Feeding** is useful for diagnosis as it increases the peristalsis and **palpation of mass is easier.**

Treatment

- **Ramstedt pyloromyotomy** is the surgical treatment of choice.
- Electrolyte abnormality should be corrected before surgery.

DISORDERS OF INTESTINE

Intestinal Obstruction

Intestinal obstruction can be caused by intrinsic defects like atresia, stenosis, meconium ileus and aganglionosis; and extrinsic defects like malrotation, bands, hernias and intestinal duplications. **Intestinal atresia** is the most common cause of neonatal intestinal obstruction, the most common site being **jejunoileal segment (50%)** followed by **duodenum (45%).** Malrotation is the second most common cause followed by meconium ileus.

Clinical Presentation

The presenting symptoms of intestinal obstruction are feeding intolerance, abdominal distention, bilious emesis and failure to pass meconium stool.

- Distension of bowel due to accumulation of food, swallowed air and secretions can be seen which is followed by decrease in intestinal motility. The most important component of distention is **swallowed air.**
- These factors lead to **bilious vomiting** which is the most characteristic symptom of intestinal obstruction.
- Pain in proximal obstruction is typically located in the epigastrium and periumbilical area, whereas it is diffuse in distal obstruction.
- Meconium stools can be initially passed in proximal obstruction but not in distal obstruction.

Diagnosis

The mainstay of diagnosis of intestinal obstruction is plain abdominal X-ray.

- Fluid gas levels are seen in complete intestinal obstruction.

- Meconium ileus shows a **ground glass appearance** and meconium peritonitis shows **calcification.**
- Duodenal obstruction caused by **duodenal atresia**, duodenal duplication, **peritoneal bands, pancreatic pseudocyst**or **annular pancreas** presents with a **double bubble sign** that shows gas filled stomach and duodenum, whereas rest of intestine is gasless.
- Intestinal atresia gives a **Christmas tree appearance** on contrast radiography which shows coiling of ileum around right colic or ileocolic artery.
- **Volvulus** is diagnosed by barium contrast study; however if perforation is suspected a water soluble contrast should be used and a **plain abdominal X-ray** should be done to demonstrate gas under the diaphragm.

Treatment

- The Initial management is aimed at stabilizing the patient by giving IV fluids.
- This is followed by nasogastric decompression.
- After establishing the diagnosis selective management is done based on the cause of obstruction.

Intussusception

Intussusception is a disorder characterised by invasion of one part of intestine **(intussuceptum)** in to another part of intestine **(intussuscipiens) i.e. the outer part**. The most common type is **ileocolic** whereas **multiple intuccusception** is least common type . It is the most common cause of **intestinal obstruction** in **children above 3 months and under 6 years**. Males are more commonly affected than females. Disorders causing intussusception are **Meckel's diverticulum, intestinal polyps**, lymphomas, **duplication cysts**, parasites and viral infections causing **hypertrophy of Peyer patches.** Since viral infections of intestine is common in children, **hypertrophy of Peyer patch** is most common cause of intussusception.

Clinical Presentation

- The baby presents with **acute onset intermittent abdominal pain** caused by **recurrent obstruction** followed by vomiting.
- Mucosal ischemia and damage leads to passage of blood in stool and called as **currant jelly stools**.
- Complications like perforation and peritonitis may be seen.

Diagnosis

- On palpation a **sausage shaped mass** and emptiness in the right iliac fossa **(dance sign)** can be felt.
- Barium enema and air enema is both useful for diagnosis and treatment. It shows **claw sign** and **coiled spring sign.**
- USG and CT with contrast shows **target sign.**
- X-ray of abdomen shows air, proximal bowel dilation and distal air outlining the intussuceptum.

Treatment

- Correction of intussusception by **barium enema** is the initial **management of choice.**
- If correction does not occur by enema then surgical correction is required.

Hirschsprung Disease

Hirschsprung disease or **congenital aganglionic megacolon** is caused by **defective migration of the neural crest cells in to the mesodermal layers of gut**. This leads to **absence of ganglions** in the **submucosal** and **myenteric plexus** of intestine, which results in decreased peristalsis and contraction of the involved segment. **Infants** and **children** are commonly involved; however rarely can be seen in **adults**. The inheritance patterns can be both **AD** and **AR**. The most common part involved is **rectosigmoid**; however rest of colon and **small intestine** can also be involved. Males are more commonly affected. It is associated with Down syndrome, MEN 2A, Santos syndrome and Waardenburg syndrome.

Clinical Presentation

- The newborns characteristically present with **delayed passage of meconium** followed by bilious vomiting and **abdominal distension.**
- Enterocolitis is usually seen in between 2 and 4 weeks, which is characterised by fever, **bloody stools** and protein loss.
- The complications that can be seen are intestinal perforation, constipation and **rectal bleeding.**

Diagnosis

- The definitive diagnostic procedure is **intestinal biopsy** which shows **absence of ganglions**, nerve trunk hypertrophy and staining shows increased acetylcholinesterase activity in the involved segment.
- **Barium enema** shows a **contracted involved segment** with **dilation of the normal proximal segment**.
- Rectal manometry shows failure of the internal anal sphincter to relax after dilation of the rectum. An abnormal test is not absolutely diagnostic but a **normal test excludes the disorder**.

Treatment

- **Diversion colostomy** is done initially to gain time if patient is not fit for surgery.
- Surgical resection of the aganglionic segment and anastomosis of the normal segments is the treatment of choice. The different surgical options used for the same are **Swenson**, **Duhamel**, **Soave** and **Boley** procedures.

Disorders of Malabsorption

Celiac Disease

Celiac disease is a malabsorption syndrome characterised by intestinal hypersensitivity to **gliadin** part of gluten in **wheat**, **rye**, **barley** and **oats**. Gliadin activates T helper cells which damages the proximal small intestine mucosa and causes crypt hyperplasia and villous atrophy. Immunologic mechanism is supported by the fact that increased incidence is seen with disorders like **NIDDM**, Addison's disease, **pernicious anemia**, autoimmune thyroiditis, sjogren syndrome, Ig A nephropathy, and collagen vascular disease. Other disorders associated are **dermatitis herpetiformis**, Turner syndrome, Williams syndrome and Down syndrome. The **strongest association** of celiac disease is seen with **HLA DQ2** followed by HLA DQ8; however other HLA subtypes like **B8**, DR3 and DR7 can also be associated.

- **Clinical presentation:**
  - ❖ The child presents with diarrhoea after 6 months of age when grains containing gladin is introduced in to feed. Anorexia, weight loss and failure to thrive can be seen.
  - ❖ CNS manifestation like ataxia and seizures can be seen.
  - ❖ Symptoms of deficiency of **iron, folic acid** and **fat soluble vitamins** (A, D, E, K) can be seen.
- **Diagnosis:**
  - ❖ The mainstay of diagnosis is based on the **histopathological findings** and **symptom resolution on gluten restriction**. Small intestinal biopsy shows **villi atrophy** and **crypt hyperplasia (decreased villi to crypt ratio), decreased brush border epithelium and mucosa, intraepithelial lymphocytes** and **plasma cells in lamina propria.**
  - ❖ The most specific and sensitive test for screening is **anti-tissue transglutaminase antibodies**. The other antibodies that can be seen are antiendomysial, anti gliadin and anti reticulin antibodies.
  - ❖ **D-xylose test** — After 60 minutes of oral D-xylose intake a blood level of less than 20 mg/dl can be seen in celiac disease.
  - ❖ **Fecal fat content** — A 3 day fecal fat excretion of more than 15% of total intake is useful for diagnosis.
- **Treatment:**
  - ❖ The mainstay of treatment is administration of **gluten free diet** lifelong.

Lactase Deficiency

Lactase deficiency is the most common enzyme deficiency in humans. Congenital lactase deficiency can be caused by mutation of lactase gene in chromosome 2. Acquired lactase deficiency is a normal physiological conditions characterised by downregulation of lactase enzyme after weaning from breast milk. **Secondary lactase deficiency** can also be seen due to **viral intestinal infection**, inflammatory disease, radiation and drugs. Patient presents with diarrhoea, bloating and abdominal pain and vomiting after ingestion of milk and milk products. **Reducing substances** and **organic acids** are seen in stool. Diagnosis can be confirmed by improvement of symptoms on exclusion of milk products, lactase breath test and demonstration of decreased lactose activity in small intestine.

Diarrhoea

Acute diarrhoea is defined as passage of **watery stools three or more times in one day**. It is the most common cause of **under-five mortality** in India. The most common cause of diarrhoea is viruses, among which **rota virus** is the most common cause. The other viruses responsible are **adenovirus, calcivirus** (norovirus or Norwalk agent), astrovirus and enteroviruses. The most common bacterial cause of diarrhoea is *E.coli;* however other bacterias like Shigella and Salmonella can also cause diarrhoea.

- **Persistent diarrhoea** is the one which continues for **14 days or more**.
- **Dysentery** is the form of diarrhoea in which **bloody stools** are passed. Dysentery is most commonly caused by **shigella**; however other bacterias like *E. coli* (EHEC, EIEC), *Campylobacter jejuni*, *Yersinia enterocolitis*, *A. hydrophilia* and *E. histolytica* are also responsible.
- **Intractable diarrhoea** is a form of chronic diarrhoea for more than 14 days along with failure to gain weight and in which **no bacterial pathogen can be identified**. The cause of diarrhoea is not known, known but with ineffective treatment (microvillus atrophy, tufting enteropathy, congenital enterocyte heparin sulphate deficiency) and known but has partially effective treatment (autoimmune enteropathy, lactose intolerance, **cystic fibrosis**, **cow milk protein intolerance**, **secretory tumors**).

DISORDERS OF LIVER

Cholestatic Jaundice

Cholestasis can be caused by various intrahepatic and extrahepatic disorders.

Intrahepatic Cholestasis

Intrahepatic cholestasis is caused by disorders of liver like hepatitis caused by infections (**hepatitis B and C**; HSV, HIV, CMV, HHV6, toxoplasma, treponema), toxins, metabolic diseases (fructosemia and galactosemia), congenital disorders (Alagille syndrome); and the rest of the cases for which cause cannot be identified belongs to the category of idiopathic neonatal hepatitis or giant cell hepatitis. The patient has increased aminotransferases (ALT and AST), LDH, prolonged clotting time and mixed hyperbilirubinemia.

- **Idiopathic neonatal hepatitis:** This is the **most common cause of neonatal intrahepatic cholestasis**. It is associated with various disorders like progressive familial intrahepatic cholestasis (PFIC), Niemann-Pick disease, α_1 **antitrypsin deficiency** and Alagille syndrome. When associated with PFIC, neonatal hepatitis is characterised by a **low level of gamma glutamyl transpeptidase (GGT)**. Liver biopsy shows multinucleated giant cells; however it is not specific as can also be seen in other types of hepatitis.
- Alagille syndrome is caused by mutation of Jagged1 gene located on chromosome 20. It is characterised by absence or decreased bile ducts in liver.

Extrahepatic Cholestasis

Extrahepatic cholestasis can be caused by biliary atresia, choledochal cyst and mechanical obstruction to the common duct. **Serum GGT, alkaline phosphatase** and **5′ nucleotidase** levels are raised. Aminotransferases are moderately raised as compared to intrahepatic cholestasis. **Conjugated bilirubin** level is raised.

- **Extrahepatic biliary atresia:** The patient usually presents within 3 months of life with symptoms of cholestasis like **jaundice**, **acholic stools** and hepatosplenomegaly. Later the child can develop clubbing, xanthomas and rachitic rosary. **HIDA** scan shows absence or **decreased intestinal secretion of nucleotide**; however it is not diagnostic as the same can also be seen in intrahepatic cholestasis. USG shows a small gall bladder and triangular cod sign (cone shaped fibrotic mass). **Percutaneous liver biopsy** is the **most specific and definitive diagnostic procedure** to differentiate between intrahepatic and extrahepatic biliary disorders. The treatment of choice is **Kasai's procedure** (hepatoportoenterostomy).
- **Choledochal cyst:** In neonates the choledochal cyst which are symptomatic are usually associated with atresia of distal common duct and present like biliary atresia. Females are more commonly affected. Treatment of choice is excision of cyst and choledocho-Roux-en-Y jejunal anastomosis.

Portal Hypertension

Portal hypertension is characterised by an increase in portal venous pressure of more than 10–12 mmHg or 5 mmHg more than inferior vena caval pressure. It is the **most common cause of gastrointestinal bleeding in children**. Based on the location of cause it can be classified as prehepatic, intrahepatic and suprahepatic portal hypertension.

Prehepatic Portal Hypertension

Prehepatic portal hypertension is caused by **extrahepatic portal vein obstruction (EHPVO)** commonly caused by intraluminal obstruction like thrombosis (trauma or hypercoagulable states) or extraluminal obstruction by tumor or pancreatic mass. **EHPVO is the most common cause of portal vein hypertension in India.** The child presents with symptoms of gastrointestinal variceal bleeding **(hematemesis, malena)** and splenomegaly. **Hepatomegaly** and **ascites** is usually not seen.

Noncirrhotic portal fibrosis (NCPF) can have both intrahepatic and prehepatic involvement and hence can cause both type of portal hypertension. Portal vein involvement **presents as prehepatic portal hypertension and has similar presentation**.

Intrahepatic Portal Hypertension

Intrahepatic portal hypertension can be caused by **cirrhosis**, **veno-occlusive disease**, congenital hepatic fibrosis and noncirrhotic portal fibrosis. It is the most common cause of portal hypertension in developed countries. The child presents with **hepatosplenomegaly**, **ascites**, gastrointestinal variceal bleeding symptoms **(hematemesis and malena)** and symptoms of liver involvement.

Suprahepatic Portal Hypertension

Suprahepatic portal hypertension is caused by intraluminal obstruction (thrombosis) or extraluminal compression of hepatic veins **(Budd-Chiari syndrome)**. The **presentation is similar to that of intrahepatic portal hypertension.**

Wilson Disease

Wilson disease or hepatolenticular degeneration is an **autosomal recessive** disorder caused by mutation of **ATP7B gene** present on **long arm of chromosome 13**, which codes for a p type ATP responsible for copper excretion and incorporation in to ceruloplasmin in the liver. This mutation leads to accumulation of copper in the liver followed by other organs like CNS and eye.

Clinical Presentation

- Hepatic involvement can present initially as **acute hepatitis or chronic liver disease** and progress to cirrhosis. Hepatomegaly, splenomegaly, jaundice and symptoms of portal hypertension can be seen.
- The earliest manifestation of CNS involvement is decrease in school performance associated with **emotional liability.** This can be followed by other manifestations of basal ganglia involvement like tremors, dysarthria and drooling of saliva.
- **Psychiatric features** like depression, anxiety and psychosis can be seen.
- Ocular involvement is usually seen in **older children** as **Kayser-Fleischer (K-F) ring** and **sunflower cataract.** K-F ring is seen as **brown colour bands in the descement membrane** of cornea.
- The other presentations are **coombs negative haemolytic anemia, Fanconi syndrome** and cardiomyopathy.

Diagnosis

- **Serum ceruloplasmin (<20 mg/dl)** and **copper levels** are **decreased**.
- **Urinary copper** excretion is **increased** i.e. more than 150 mcg/dl.
- **Liver biopsy** shows **increased tissue copper** of more than 250 mcg/dl and mallory bodies.
- Hypouricemia, increased bilirubin levels and decreased alkaline phosphatase can be seen.

Treatment

- **D-penicillamine** or trientene hydrochloride is the treatment of choice for Wilson disease.
- **Zinc acetate** can be given for **maintenance therapy** to reduce copper absorption.

MULTIPLE CHOICE QUESTIONS

1. Hirschsprung disease is due to: [AIIMS Nov. 09]
   a. Loss of ganglionic cells in sympathetic chains
   b. Atrophy of longitudinal muscles
   c. Failure of migration of neural crest cells form cranial to caudal direction
   d. Malformed taenia coli

2. A robust male baby with vigorous feeding and immediate vomiting at 2 months of age. Most probable diagnosis is: [AIIMS Nov. 09]
   a. Paralytic ileus
   b. Hirschprung's disease

c. Brain tumor

d. Congenital hypertrophic pyloric stenosis

3. **Most common biochemical abnormality in congenital hypertrophic pyloric stenosis:**

[AIIMS Nov. 09, 06, 02]

a. Hypochloremic metabolic alkalosis

b. Hyperchloremic metabolic acidosis

c. Hypochloremic metabolic acidosis

d. Hyperchloremicmetabolic alkalosis

4. **A male infant presented with distension of abdomen shortly after birth with passing of less meconium. Subsequently a full-thickness biopsy of the rectum was performed. The rectal biopsy is likely to show:** [AIIMS Nov. 04, Nov. 09]

a. Fibrosis of submucosa

b. Lack of ganglion cells

c. Thickened muscularis propria

d. Hyalinization of the muscular coat

5. **In a child with active liver failure, the most important prognosis factor for death is:** [AIIMS May 06]

a. Increasing transaminases

b. Increasing bilirubin

c. Increasing prothrombin time

d. Gram-negative sepsis

6. **In a child presenting with obstructive jaundice all are seen except:** [AIIMS Nov. 06]

a. Gamma glutamyl transpeptidase

b. Alkaline phosphatase.

c. Glutamate dehydrogenase

d. 5'Nucleotidase

7. **The diagnosis of congenital megacolon is confirmed by:** [AIIMS Nov. 05]

a. Clinical features   b. Barium enema

c. Rectal biopsy   d. Recto-sigmoidoscopy

8. **Which of the following circulating antibodies has the best sensitivity and specificity for the diagnosis of celiac disease?** [AIIMS May 05]

a. Anti-endomysial antibody

b. Anti-tissue transglutaminase antibody

c. Anti gladin antibody

d. Anti-reticulin antibody

9. **A 12-year-old girl has history of recurrent bulky stools and abdominal pain since 3 years of age. She has moderate pallor and her weight and height are below 3rd percentile. Which one of the following is the most appropriate investigation to make a specific diagnosis?** [AIIMS Nov. 04]

a. Small intestinal biopsy

b. Barium studies

c. 24 hours fecal fat estimation

d. Urinary D-xylose test

10. **A neonate is being investigated for jaundice. A liver biopsy shows features of a "Giant Cell/ Neonatal hepatitis". Which one of the following conditions usually results in this case?** [AIIMS Nov. 04]

a. Congenital hepatic fibrosis

b. Hemochromatosis

c. Alpha-1-antitrypsin deficiency

d. Glycogen storage disease Type 1

11. **All of the following statements about Wilson's disease are true except:** [AIIMS May 04]

a. It is an autosomal recessive disorder

b. Serum ceruloplasmin level is <20 mg/dl

c. Urinary copper excretion is <100 mg/dl

d. Zinc acetate is effective as maintenance therapy

12. **Congenital hypertrophic pyloric stenosis usually presents:** [AIIMS May 04]

a. Within 2 days after birth

b. Around 1 week after birth

c. Around 2 weeks after birth

d. Around 2 months after birth

13. **A 6-month-old infant presents to the 'diarrhea clinic' unit with some dehydration. The most likely organism causing diarrhea is:** [AIIMS Nov. 03]

a. Entamoeba histolytica

b. Rotavirus

c. Giardia lamblia

d. Shigella

14. **The following cereals should be avoided in patients with celiac diseases, except:** [AIIMS Nov. 03]

a. Wheat   b.Barely

c. Maize   d.Rye

15. **Portal hypertension in children in India is commonly due to:** [AIMS Nov. 03]

a. Indian childhood cirrhosis

b. Extrahepatic portal venous obstruction

c. Idiopathic portal hypertension

d. Hepatic out flow tract obstruction

16. **A newborn baby had normal APGAR score at birth and developed excessive frothing and choking on attempted feeds. The investigation of choice is:**

[AIIMS May 03]

a. Esophagoscopy

b. Bronchoscopy

c. MRI chest

d. X-ray chest and abdomen with the red rubber catheter passed per orally into esophagus

17. **In neonatal cholestasis, if the serum gamma-glutamyl transpeptidase is more than 600IU/L the most likely diagnosis is:** [AIIMS Nov. 02]

a. Neonatal hepatitis   b. Choledochal cyst

c. Hypothyroidism   d. Biliary atresia

18. **Failure to pass meconium within 48 hours of birth in a newborn with no obvious external abnormality should lead to the suspicion of:** [AIIMS Nov. 02]
    a. Anal atresia
    b. Congenital pouch colon
    c. Congenital aganglionosis
    d. Meconium ileus

19. **A 40-year-old male presents with recurrent bouts of vomiting since 9 months because of pyloric obstruction. The compensatory biochemical change is :** [AIIMS May 01]
    a. Respiratory alkalosis
    b. Respiratory acidosis
    c. Paradoxical aciduria with hyponatremia and hypochloremia
    d. Metabolic acidosis

20. **A neonate presents with jaundice and clay white stools. On liver biopsy giant cells are seen. Most likely diagnosis is:** [AI 01, AIIMS Nov. 01]
    a. Physiological jaundice
    b. Neonatal hepatitis with extrabiliary atresia
    c. Neonatal hepatitis with physiological jaundice
    d. Extrabiliary atresia

21. **All are false except one in case of hypertrophic pyloric stenosis:** [AIIMS June 2000]
    a. Symptomatic within one week
    b. Lump is always clinically palpable
    c. T/t of choice is Finney's pyloroplasty
    d. Ultrasonography is the diagnostic test

22. **A boy comes with complaints of vomiting, bloated abdomen and abdominal pain. He has history of attending ice-cream eating competition last night. He also has past history of similar episodes following ingestion of milk and milk products. The likely cause:** [AIIMS Nov. 99]
    a. Pancreatic amylase deficiency
    b. Lactase deficiency
    c. Salivary amylase deficiency
    d. Food poisoning

23. **A 2-months-old exclusively breast fed child develops jaundice since birth, acholic stool high conjugated bilirubin in blood and absent urobilinogen in urine. The likely cause is :** [AIIMS Nov. 99]
    a. Hypothyroidism
    b. Congenital biliary atresia
    c. Neonatal hepatitis
    d. Breast milk jaundice

24. **Aganglionic segment is encountered in which part of colon in case of Hirschsprung's disease:** [AIIMS Nov. 99]
    a. Distal to dilated segment
    b. In whole colon
    c. Proximal to dilated segment
    d. In the dilated segment

25. **True statement regarding Hirschsprung's disease:** [AIIMS June 99]
    a. Giant ganglia are present
    b. Mucosa is involved and show foldings
    c. Manometry excludes the disease
    d. Rectal biopsy is contraindicated in infants

26. **A 6-year-old boy presenting with palpable abdominal mass in the epigastrium. The clinical diagnosis is (There is no bile in vomitus):** [AIIMS Dec. 98]
    a. Duodenal atresia   b. Choledochal cyst
    c. Pyloric stenosis   d. Esophageal atresia

27. **All can cause diarrhea except:** [AIIMS June 98]
    a. Rotavirus   b. Calci virus
    c. Reo virus   d. Adenovirus

28. **Neonatal cholestasis is seen in :** [AIIMS June 98]
    a. Chronic hepatitis
    b. Hepatitis B and C
    c. Glycogen storage disorders
    d. Mucopolysaccharidosis

29. **Not true regarding Hirschsprung disease is:** [AIIMS Nov. 97]
    a. Autosomal dominant
    b. Absent ganglionic cells in myenteric plexus
    c. Absent ganglionic cells in submucous plexus
    d. Rectal biopsy is diagnostic

30. **Most important cause of abdominal distension in intestinal obstruction:** [AIIMS Dec. 95]
    a. Cases produced by bacterial activity
    b. Cases diffused from blood
    c. Swallowed air
    d. Products of digestion

31. **Most common cause of acute intestinal obstruction in neonate is:** [AIIMS 92]
    a. Jejunal atresia   b. Malrotation
    c. Duodenal atresia   d. Acute intussusception

32. **In celiac sprue there is a deficiency of all except:** [AIIMS 91]
    a. Vitamin A   b. Vitamin B12
    c. Folic acid   d. Iron

33. **Which is not a feature of Wilson's disease in child?** [AIIMS 91]
    a. Fanconi syndrome   b. Sensory changes
    c. Hemolytic anemia   d. Chronic active hepatitis

34. **Following procedures are done for correction of Hirschsprung disease:** [AIIMS 87, Jipmer 81]
    a. Duharnel's   b. Soave's
    c. Swenson's   d. Bayar's

35. **Infective diarrhoea in infancy is commonly due to:** [AIIMS 83]
    a. Pseudomonas   b. E.coli
    c. Klebsiella   d. Shigella

36. **Recurrent abdominal pain in children is most often due to:** [AIIMS 83]
    a. Round worms
    b. Emotional/Behavioural problems
    c. Amebiasis
    d. Giardiasis

37. **A neonate presents with fever, lethargy, abdominal distension, vomiting and constipation. Clinically he was diagnosed as volvulus neonatarum with suspected perforation. Best investigation would be:** [AI 10]

    a. Plain X-ray
    b. Barium enema
    c. Upper GI endoscopy
    d. Barium meal follow through

38. **True about Wilson's disease:** [AI 10]
    a. Increase in urinary copper and increased serum ceruloplasmin and copper
    b. Increased serum ceruloplasmin levels with increased urinary copper
    c. Elevated hepatic copper level and increased serum ceruloplasmin levels
    d. Increased in urinary copper and decreased serum ceruloplasmin

39. **A patient presents with chronic small bowel diarrhoea, duodenal biopsy shows villous atrophy. Anti endomysial antibodies and Ig A TTG antibodies are positive. What is the treatment of choice?** [AI 07]

    a. Gluten free diet   b. Antibiotics
    c. Loperamide   d. 5-ASA

40. **One of the intestinal enzymes that is generally deficient in children following an attack of severe infectious enteritis is:** [AI 05]
    a. Lactase   b. Trypsin
    c. Lipase   d. Amylase

41. **A 12-year-old girl with mood and emotional liability has a golden brown discolouration of descement membrane. Most likely diagnosis is:** [AI 04]
    a. Fabry's disease
    b. Wilson's disease
    c. Glycogen storage disease
    d. Acute rheumatic fever

42. **Which one of the following is most suggestive of neonatal small bowel obstruction?** [AI 03]
    a. Generalized abdominal distension
    b. Failure to pass meconium in the first 24 hours
    c. Bilious vomiting
    d. Refusal of feeds

43. **Gluten sensitive enteropathy is most strongly associated with:** [AI 03]
    a. HLA-DQ2   b. HLA-DR4
    c. HLA-DQ3   d. Blood group 'B'

44. **A 7-year-old girl from Bihar presented with three episodes of massive hematemesis and melena. There is no history of jaundice. On examination, she had a large spleen, non-palpable liver and mild ascites. Portal vein was not visualized on ultrasonography. Liver function tests were normal and endoscopy revealed esophageal varices. The most likely diagnosis is:** [AI 03]
    a. Kala azar with portal hypertension
    b. Portal hypertension of unknown etiology
    c. Chronic liver disease with portal hypertension
    d. Portal hypertension due to extrahepatic obstruction

45. **A 2-month-baby presents with history of jaundice, turmeric colored urine and pale stools since birth. Examination reveals liver span of 10 cm, firm in consistency and spleen of 3 cm. The most specific investigation for establishing the diagnosis would be:** [AI 03]
    a. Liver function tests
    b. Ultrasound abdomen
    c. Preoperative cholangiogram
    d. Liver biopsy

46. **Which is the most characteristic of congenital hypertrophic pyloric stenosis?** [AI 03]
    a. Affects the first born female child
    b. The pyloric tumor is best felt during feeding
    c. The patient is commonly marasmic
    d. Loss of appetite occurs early

47. **The most common genetic cause of liver disease in children is:** [AI 02]
    a. Hemochromatosis
    b. α1 antitrypsin deficiency
    c. Cystic fibrosis
    d. Glycogen storage disease

48. **The histological features of celiac disease include all of the followings except:** [AI 02]
    a. Crypt hyperplasia
    b. Increase in thickness of the mucosa
    c. Increase in intraepithelial lymphocytes
    d. Increase in inflammatory cells in lamina propyria

49. **A 10 month old infant presents with acute intestinal obstruction. Contrast enema X-ray shows the intussusceptions, likely cause is:** [AI 02]
    a. Peyer's patch hypertrophy
    b. Meckel's diverticulum
    c. Mucosal polyp
    d. Duplication cyst

50. **A newborn has dribbling after feeds. He has respiratory distress and froths at the mouth. Diagnosis is:** [AI 01]
    a. Tracheoesophageal fistula
    b. Tetralogy of fallot
    c. Respiratory distress syndrome
    d. None of the above

51. **Ramu, a 8 years old boy presents with upper GI bleeding. On examination, he is found to have splenomegaly; there are no signs of ascites, or hepatomegaly; esophageal varices are found on UGId. Most likely diagnosis is :** [AI 01]
    a. Budd chiari syndrome
    b. Non cirrhotic portal fibrosis
    c. Cirrhosis
    d. Veno-occlusive disease

52. **Which is true regarding congenital hypertrophic pyloric stenosis?** [AI 01]
    a. More common in girls
    b. Hypochloremic alkalosis
    c. Heller's myotomy is the procedure of choice
    d. Most often manifests at birth

53. **A neonate presents with jaundice and clay white stools. On liver biopsy giant cells are seen. Most likely diagnosis is:** [AI 01, AIIMS Nov. 01]
    a. Physiological jaundice
    b. Neonatal hepatitis with extrabiliary atresia
    c. Neonatal hepatitis with physiological jaundice
    d. Extrabiliary atresia

54. **Pseudopancreatic cyst in a child is commonly due to:** [AI 99]
    a. Annular pancreatitis
    b. Drug induced pancreatic
    c. Traumatic pancreatic
    d. Choledochal cyst

55. **In children presence of increased fecal fat excretion and increased fecal nitrogen levels is a feature of all except:** [AI 99]
    a. Pancreatic insufficiency
    b. Bacterial overgrowth syndrome
    c. Coeliac sprue
    d. Ulcerative colitis

56. **Most common type of intussusception is:** [AI 99]
    a. Ileo-colic
    b. Ileo-ieal
    c. Colo-colic
    d. Caecocolic

57. **Most common cause of portal hypertension in children is:** [AI 98]
    a. Extrahepatic compression
    b. Budd chiari syndrome
    c. Veno-occlusive disease
    d. Post necrotic

58. **Most common cause of cholestatic jaundice in newborn is:** [AI 97]
    a. Hypoplasia of biliary tract
    b. Neonatal hepatitis
    c. Choledochal cyst
    d. Physiological

59. **The most common cause of diarrhoea in children is:** [AI 95]
    a. *Vibrio cholera*
    b. *E.coli*
    c. Rota virus
    d. Pneumococcus

60. **Which is not true about intussusception:** [AI 91]
    a. Common in neonates
    b. Fever always presents
    c. Not associated with tumors of intestine
    d. Usually relieved by barium enema

61. **Blood and mucous are seen in stool with all except:** [AI 89]
    a. *E. histolytica*
    b. *Shigella*
    c. *E.coli*
    d. *V. cholera*

62. **Diarrhea in children is caused by:** [PGI June 09]
    a. AIDS
    b. Nanvalle
    c. Rotavirus
    d. *E . coli*

63. **True about Hirschsprung disease:** [PGI June 08]
    a. Aganglionic segment is contracted not dilated
    b. Descending colon is most common site
    c. Barium enema is diagnostic
    d. Barium enema shows calcification

64. **What a patient of gluten hypersensitivity can consume?** [PGI Dec. 06]
    a. Rice
    b. Barley
    c. Oat
    d. Corn
    e. Rye

65. **A child is brought by mother with H/O massive hematemesis with H/O drug intake previously with NSAIDs and on Rx. Associated with moderate splenomegaly diagnosis is:** [PGI Dec. 06]
    a. Esophageal varices
    b. Duodenal ulcer
    c. Drug induced gastritis
    d. Peptic ulcer

66. **Celiac disease associated with:** [PGI Dec. 06]
    a. Dermatitis herpetiformis
    b. Type 1 DM
    c. Lymphoma
    d. Atrophic gastritis
    e. IBD

67. **Features of pyloric stenosis:** [PGI June 2006]
    a. Hypokalemic alkalosis
    b. Peristalsis right to left
    c. Commonly caused by carcinoma stomach
    d. Retention vomiting present
    e. Commonly females involved

68. **Hirschsprung disease true are:** [PGI June 2006]
    a. Sometimes found in adult
    b. Dilated segment involved
    c. Auerbach's plexus absent
    d. Sometimes involve small intestine
    e. Bleeding PR is usual presentation

69. **Double bubble sign in children is seen in A/E:** [PGI Dec. 04]
    a. Ladds band
    b. Annular pancreas
    c. Pancreatic pseudocyst
    d. Diaphragmatic hernia

70. **True about diarrhea:** [PGI Dec. 03]
    a. Defined as passage of 2–3 formed stool/day
    b. Blood mixed with mucous stool is defined as dysentery
    c. Rotavirus is the most common organism in children
    d. Persistent diarrhea is defined if duration is more than 21 days

71. **True about extrahepatic biliary atresia:**
    [PGI June 03]
    a. Acholic stool
    b. Unconjugated hyperbilirubinemia
    c. Conjugated hyperbilirubinemia
    d. Absence of nucleoid in duodenum in HIDA scan
    e. Jaundice is presenting feature

72. **A 6-month-old baby with H/O bloody diarrhoea of 2 days duration with abdominal distention and on examination the baby screams, diagnosis is:**
    [PGI Dec. 03]
    a. Intussusception   b. HUS
    c. Appendicitis   d. *Ac. enterocolitis*

73. **Hirschsprung disease:** [PGI June 02]
    a. Is seen in infants and children only
    b. Absence of ganglia in the involved segment
    c. The involved segment is dilated colon
    d. Bleeding PR is presenting feature
    e. Surgery is used in therapy

74. **Congenital pyloric stenosis causes:** [PGI Dec. 02]
    a. Bilious vomiting   b. Non-bilious vomiting
    c. Projectile vomiting   d. Non projectile vomiting
    e. Forceful

75. **Celiac sprue diagnosed by:** [PGI Dec. 02]
    a. Intestinal biopsy
    b. Unequivocal response to gluten restriction
    c. Finding of organism
    d. Improvement of dapsone treatment
    e. H/O fat malabsorption

76. **The grain which can be safely used in celiac sprue is:** [PGI Dec. 01]
    a. Corn   b. Rye
    c. Soyabean   d. Rice
    e. Barley

77. **True about Hirschsprung's disease:** [PGI June 01]
    a. Pathology of myenteric plexus of Auerbach
    b. Blood in stools
    c. May involve small intestine rarely
    d. Involved segment of the intestine is dilated
    e. Present only in infant in children

78. **Infant with blood in stool and mass in abdomen, diagnosis is:** [PGI June 01]
    a. Intussusception
    b. Volvulus

c. Idiopathic abdominal epilepsy
d. Hirschprung's disease

79. **True about pyloric stenosis:** [PGI June 01]
    a. Hypokalemia   b. Hyponatremia
    c. Metabolic acidosis   d. Hypochloremia
    e. Hypocalcemia

80. **Features of intussusception are:** [PGI June 01]
    a. Pincer sign   b. Target sign
    c. Dove sign   d. Coiled spring sign
    e. Dance sign

81. **Proved association of celiac sprue is with:**
    [PGI Dec. 2000]
    a. Dermatitis herpetiformis
    b. Scleroderma
    c. Pemphigus
    d. Pemphigoid

82. **Recurrent obstruction, mass per rectum and diarrhoea in child:** [PGI June 2000]
    a. Intussusception   b. Rectal prolapse
    c. Internal hernia   d. Haemorrhoids

83. **Intractable diarrhea in children is caused by all except:** [PGI June 00]
    a. Cystic fibrosis   b. Giardiasis
    c. Secreting tumors   d. Milk allergy

84. **In celiac disease A/E:** [PGI June 00]
    a. Gliadin is cause
    b. Associated with HLA-B$_8$
    c. Decreased villi to crypt ratio
    d. Increased brush border

85. **The commonest type of tracheoesophageal fistula is:** [PGI 99]
    a. Proximal end blind; distal end communicating with trachea
    b. Distal end blind; proximal end communicating with trachea
    c. Both ends blind
    d. Both ends open

86. **Investigation of choice in Hirschsprung disease is:**
    [PGI Dec. 98]
    a. Rectal manometry
    b. Rectal examination
    c. Rectal biopsy
    d. Barium enema

87. **What is intussuscipiens:** [PGI Dec. 97]
    a. The entire complex of intussusception
    b. The entering layer
    c. The outer layer
    d. The process of reducing the intussusception

88. **Commonest cause of intestinal obstruction in children is:** [PGI 88]
    a. Intussusception   b. Volvulus
    c. Hernia   d. Adhesions

89. **Regarding congenital hypertrophic pyloric stenosis all are correct except:** [PGI 87]
    a. Weight loss
    b. Diarrhoea
    c. Visible peristalsis
    d. Remsted's operation is done

90. **Cause of liver cirrhosis in childhood include:** [PGI 81, 84]
    a. Alpha-1 antitrypsin deficiency
    b. Celiac disease
    c. Phenylketonuria
    d. Cow's milk intolerance

91. **The least common type of intussusception is:** [PGI 81, AP 89]
    a. Multiple   b. Colocolic
    c. Ileoileal   d. Ileocolic

92. **All of the following are features of Wilson's disease, except:**
    a. Hemolytic anemia   b. Testicular atrophy
    c. Chorea   d. Chronic active hepatitis

93. **Commonest cause of intussusception is:** [TN 90]
    a. Submucous lipoma
    b. Meckel's diverticulum
    c. Hypertrophy of submucous patches
    d. Polyp

QUESTIONS OF OTHER EXAMINATIONS

1. **Oesophageal atresia may occur as a part of VACTER group of anomalies. What does 'TE' stand for?** [UPSC 10]
   a. Tetralogy of Fallot
   b. Thoracic empyema
   c. Tracheo-esophageal fistula
   d. Talipesequinovarus

2. **The gene for Wilson's disease is on:** [Maharashtra 10]
   a. Long arm of chromosome 13
   b. Long arm of chromosome 6
   c. Short arm of chromosome 13
   d. Short arm of chromosome 6

3. **In a child with acute liver failure, the important abnormal serum biochemical test that indicates poor prognosis is:** [COMED 09]
   a. Increasing transaminases
   b. Increasing bilirubin
   c. Increasing prothrombin time
   d. Reversal of albumin globulin ratio

4. **Claw sign is seen in:** [APPG 08]
   a. Intussusception   b. Volvulus
   c. Both   d. None

5. **Most common cause of persistent diarrhoea in children?** [APPG 08]
   a. Rota virus   b. E coli
   c. Cholera bantii   d. Salmonella

6. **Wilson's disease is characterised by:** [COMED 08]
   a. Low serum ceruloplasmin and low urinary copper
   b. Low serum ceruloplasmin and high urinary copper
   c. High serum ceruloplasmin and low urinary copper
   d. High ceruloplasmin and high urinary copper

7. **Antigladin antibodies are detectable in:** [COMED 08]
   a. Tropical sprue   b. Whipple's disease
   c. Celiac disease   d. Intestinal lymphoma

8. **A young boy presents with failure to thrive. Biochemical analysis of duodenal aspirate after a meal reveals a deficiency of enteropeptidase (enterokinase). The level of which one of the following enzymes will be affected?** [UPSC 07]
   a. Amylase   b. Pepsin
   c. Lactose   d. Trypsin

9. **The most common type of tracheoesophageal fistula is:** [MAHE 07]
   a. Esophageal atresia without tracheoesophageal fistula
   b. Esophageal atresia with proximal tracheoesophageal fistula
   c. Esophageal atresia with distal tracheoesophageal fistula
   d. Esophageal atresia with proximal and distal fistula

10. **With reference to Hirschsprung's disease which one of the following statements is correct?** [UPSC 07]
    a. It is initially treated by colostomy
    b. In neonatal period it is best confirmed by barium enema
    c. It is associated with high incidence of genito-urinary tract anomalies
    d. It is characterised by absence of ganglion cells in the transverse colon

11. **Celiac sprue causes malabsorption syndrome due to:** [UPSC 07]
    a. Coliform infection of small bowel
    b. Lactase deficiency
    c. Hypersensitivity to dietary gluten
    d. Ischemia of celiac artery

12. **A two-year-old child presents with persistent diarrhoea acidic stools and presence of reducing substances in the fresh stools. What is the most probable diagnosi?** [UPSC 07]

a. Cystic fibrosis
b. Lactose intolerance
c. Rotavirus induced diarrhoea
d. Intestinal tuberculosis

13. **The commonest cause of vomiting in a one month old infant is:**   [KCET 06]
   a. Pyloric stenosis   b. Cardiac achalasia
   c. Aerophagy   d. Gastroesophagial reflux

14. **A newborn with recurrent vomiting, cyanosis after each feed is likely to be suffering from:** [APPGE 05]
   a. Tracheoesophageal fistula
   b. Tetralogy of fallot
   c. Congenital hypertrophic pyloric stenosis
   d. ARDS

15. **Congenital Wilson's disease is characterised by:**
                    [SGPGI 05]
   a. KF ring is present at birth
   b. May present as acute hepatitis
   c. Decreased urinary copper excretion
   d. Decreased hepatic copper concentration

16. **Absent stomach bubble on antenatal ultrasonography is an important finding for antenatal diagnosis of:**
   a. Congenital heart disease in foetus
   b. Oesophageal atresia in foetus
   c. Omphalocele in foetus
   d. Spina bifida in foetus

17. **Following procedures are done for correction of Hirschsprung disease:**   [AIIMS 87, Jipmer 81]
   a. Duharnel's   b. Soave's
   c. Swenson's   d. Bayar's

18. **Hirschsprung's disease is treated by:**   [AP 98]
   a. Colostomy
   b. Excision of aganglionic segment
   c. Colectomy
   d. Sodium chloride wash

19. **Intrahepatic cholestasis is seen in:**   [MP 98]
   a. Galactosemia   b. Hypercalcemia
   c. Haemochromatosis   d. Cystic fibrosis

20. **Most common cause of dysentery is:**   [Jipmer 98]
   a. Shigella dysenterie   b. E.histolytica
   c. Salmonella   d. Campylobacter

21. **All of the following are recognised features of Wilson's disease except:**   [UP 97]
   a. Psychological disturbances
   b. Increased ceruloplasmin levels
   c. Increased copper content of liver
   d. Histopathological features of chronic active hepatitis

22. **Most common cause of severe hematemesis in child is:**   [UPSC 85, Jipmer 87]
   a. Portal hypertension
   b. Peptic ulcer
   c. Mallory Weiss syndrome
   d. None of the above

23. **All of the following are features of Wilson's disease, except:**
   a. Hemolytic anemia   b. Testicular atrophy
   c. Chorea   d. Chronic active hepatitis

24. **Colic generally disappear by the age of:** [UPSC 83]
   a. 1 year   b. 2 years
   c. 4 months   d. 8 months

ANSWERS

1. **(c)** Failure of migration of neural crest cells form cranial to caudal direction (Ref: Rudolph 22nd E/P1436)
   - Hirschsprung disease or **congenital aganglionic megacolon** is caused by **defective migration of the neural crest cells in to the mesodermal layers of gut**.

2. **(d)** Congenital hypertrophic pyloric stenosis (Ref: Rudolph 22nd E/P1420)
   - In congenital hypertrophic pyloric stenosis infant typically presents with projectile nonbillious vomiting between **2 and 4 weeks of age.**
   - After vomiting child is **hungry** and has a **voracious appetite**.

3. **(a)** Hypochloremic metabolic alkalosis (Ref: Rudolph 22nd E/P1420)
   - Long term vomiting pyloric stenosis may lead **hypochloremic metabolic alkalosis.**

4. **(b)** Lack of ganglion cells (Ref: Rudolph 22nd E/P1436)
   - Less passage of meconium after birth along with abdominal distention indicates towards Hirschsprung disease.
   - Diagnosis is confirmed by biopsy which shows absence of ganglionic cells.

5. **(d)** Gram negative sepsis (Ref: Nelson 19th E/P1343)
   Factors associated with increased mortality in liver failure are:
   - **Sepsis**
   - Severe haemorrhage
   - Renal failure
   - Age <1 year
   - Stage 4 encephalopathy
   - Need for dialysis before transplantation

6. **(c)** Glutamate dehydrogenase (Ref: CPDT 19th E/P618)
   - In obstructive jaundice patient presents with acholic or pale stools.
   - **Serum GGT, alkaline phosphatase** and **5′ nucleotidase** levels are raised.
   - Aminotransferases are moderately raised as compared to intrahepatic cholestasis.

7. **(c)** Rectal biopsy (Ref: Rudolph 22nd E/P1436)

8. **(b)** Anti-tissue transglutaminase antibody (Ref: CPDT 19th E/P602)

"The most sensitive and specific screening test for celiac disease in Ig A sufficient patients is a **tissue transglutaminase antibody test**."

9. **(a)** Small intestinal biopsy (Ref: CPDT 19th E/P600-01)
   - This is a case of malabsorption syndrome.
   - Malabsorption syndromes are characterised by diarrhoea, vomiting, anorexia, abdominal distension, bulky stool with fats.
   - Tests for specific diagnosis are:
     1. Sweat chloride test for cystic fibrosis.
     2. **Intestinal mucosal biopsy** for celiac disease, intestinal lymphangectasia, giardiasis and inflammatory bowel disease.
     3. Liver and gall bladder function test.
     4. Pancreatic stimulation test.

10. **(c)** Alpha-1-antitrypsin deficiency (Ref: CPDT 19th E/P615)
    - **Idiopathic neonatal hepatitis** is the most common cause of neonatal intrahepatic cholestasis.
    - It is associated with various disorders like progressive familial intrahepatic cholestasis (PFIC), Niemann-Pick disease, α_1 antitrypsin deficiency and Alagille syndrome.
    - Liver biopsy shows **multinucleated giant cells**; however it is not specific as can also be seen in other types of hepatitis.

11. **(c)** Urinary copper excretion is <100 mg/dl (Ref: CPDT 19th E/P632)
    - Wilson disease or hepatolenticular degeneration is an **autosomal resessive** disorder caused by mutation of **ATP7B gene** present on **long arm of chromosome 13.**
    - **Serum ceruloplasmin (<20 mg/dl)** and copper levels are decreased.
    - Urinary copper excretion is increased i.e. **more than 150 mcg/dl.**
    - **Liver biopsy** shows **increased tissue copper** of more than 250 mcg/dl.
    - **Zinc acetate** can be given for **maintenance therapy** to reduce copper absorption.

12. **(c)** Around 2 weeks after birth (Ref: CPDT 19th E/P580)
    - Hypertrophic pyloric stenosis presents with nonbilious vomiting between 2 and 4 weeks of age.

13. **(b)** Rotavirus (Ref: CPDT 19th E/P593)
    - The most common cause of diarrhoea is viruses, among which **rota virus** is the most common cause. The other viruses responsible are adenovirus, calcivirus (norovirus or Norwalk agent), astrovirus and enteroviruses.
    - The most common bacterial cause of diarrhoea is *E. coli*; however other bacterias like Shigella, Salmonella, Campylobacter and Yersinia.

14. (c) Maize (Ref: Nelson 19th E/P1264)
- Celiac disease is a malabsorption syndrome chara-cterised by intestinal hypersensitivity to gliadin part of gluten in **wheat, rye, barley** and **oats.**

15. (b) Extrahepatic portal venous obstruction (Ref: Ghai 7th E/P289)
- Extrahepatic portal vein obstruction is the most common cause of portal hypertension in India.

16. (d) X-ray chest and abdomen with the red rubber catheter passed per orally into esophagus (Ref: Rudolph 22nd E/P1401)
- A **nasogastric tube is inserted** and inability to pass it confirms the diagnosis of TEF.
- **X-ray** shows a **coiled tube in the atretic end** and gas in the abdomen in type C, D and E TEF.

17. (d) Biliary atresia (Ref: CPDT 19th E/P618)
- In extrahepatic biliary atresia patient presents with acholic or pale stools.
- **Serum GGT**, alkaline phosphatase and 5' nucleo-tidase levels are raised.
- Aminotransferases are moderately raised as compared to intrahepatic cholestasis.

18. (c) Congenital aganglionosis (Ref: Rudolph 22nd E/P1436)
- Delayed passage of meconium after birth is chara-cteristically seen with Hirschsprung disease or congenital aganglionic megacolon.

19. (c) Paradoxical aciduria with hyponatremia and hypochloremia (Ref: Rudolph 22nd E/P1420)
- Initial loss of HCl leads to **hypochloremic metabolic alkalosis**.
- To maintain the concentration of other vital ions in body there is compensatory loss of protons in urine, which leads to **paradoxical aciduria**.

20. (b) Neonatal hepatitis with extrabiliary atresia (Ref: CPDT 19th E/P617)
- Clay coloured stools is more characteristic for **extrabiliary atresia.**
- Giant cells are not specific for any liver disease as it can be seen in many conditions.

21. (d) Ultrasonography is the diagnostic test (Ref: Rudolph 22nd E/P1420, CPDT 19th E/P580)
- It presents with nonbilious vomiting between 2 to 4 weeks.
- A mobile olive shaped mass is palpable but not in all cases.
- Treatment of choice is Ramstedt's pyloro-myotomy.
- Ultrasonography is the most specific and sensitive diagnostic method for pyloric stenosis. A pyloric thickness of >4 mm and a length of >14 mm is diagnostic.

22. (b) Lactase deficiency (Ref: CPDT 19th E/P603)
- Complaints of vomiting, bloated abdomen and abdominal pain following intake of milk product i.e. ice cream confirms the diagnosis of lactase deficiency.

23. (b) Congenital biliary atresia (Ref: CPDT 19th E/P617)

24. (a) Distal to the dilated segment (Ref: Rudolph 22nd E/P1437)

25. (c) Manometry excludes the disease (Ref: Rudolph 22nd E/P1436)

26. (c) Pyloric stenosis (Ref: Rudolph 22nd E/P1420)

27. (c) Reo virus (Ref: CPDT 19th E/P594)
- The most common cause of diarrhoea is viruses, among which **rota virus** is the most common cause. The other viruses responsible are **adeno-virus, calcivirus** (norovirus or Norwalk agent), astrovirus and enteroviruses.

28. (b) Hepatitis B and C (Ref: CPDT 19th E/P609) Intrahepatic cholestasis is caused by disorders of liver like :
- Infections (**hepatitis B and C**; HSV, HIV, CMV, HHV6, toxoplasma, treponema).
- Toxins.
- Metabolic diseases (fructosemia and galactosemia).
- Congenital disorders (Alagille syndrome).
- Idiopathic neonatal hepatitis or giant cell hepatitis.

29. None (Ref: Rudolph 22nd E/P1436)
- This is an old question and at that time inheritance pattern was not clear. But now it is clear that Hirschsprung disease can be sporadic or inherited as AD or AR pattern.
- Ganglionic cells are absent in both submucosal and myenteric plexus.
- Rectal biopsy is indeed diagnostic of Hirschsprung disease.

30. (c) Swallowed air (Ref: Rudolph 22nd E/P1394)
- The most important component causing abdo-minal distention is swallowed air.

31. (c) Duodenal atresia (Ref: CPDT 19th E/P583, Puri Pediatric surgery P416)

Puri Pediatric surgery P416
"**Meconium ileus** accounts for 9–33% of all neonatal intestinal obstructions with an incidence of 1:2500 newborns, representing the **third most common cause of neonatal small bowel obstruction** after **ileal and duodenojejunal atresia** and **malrotation**."

32. (b) Vitamin B12 (Ref: CPDT 19th E/P602)
- Iron and fat soluble vitamin (A, D, E, K) deficiency is seen in celiac sprue.
- Vitamin B12 deficiency will not be seen as it is absorbed from terminal ileum and celic disease involves duodenum.

33. (b) Sensory changes (Ref: Nelson 19th E/P1322)

34. (d) Bayar's (Ref: Rudolph 22nd E/P1437)

35. (b) *E.coli* (Ref: Ghai 7th E/P261)

36. (b) Emotional/Behavioural problems (Ref: Ghai 7th E/P258)

"The perception of recurrent abdominal pain is the summation of sensory, **emotional** and **cognitive** input."

37. (a) Plain X-ray (Ref: Jonathan common surgical diseases P171)
- A water soluble contrast study should be used in place of barium for the diagnosis of volvulus because if perforation is present then barium can cause peritonitis.
- This is a case of volvulus with perforation, hence barium cannot be used.
- Plain abdominal X-ray is an ideal choice as it can easily detect the gas under diaphragm and confirm perforation.

38. (d) Increased in urinary copper and decreased serum ceruloplasmin (CPDT 19th E/P632)

Diagnosis of Wilson's disease:
- **Serum ceruloplasmin (<20 mg/dl)** and **copper levels** are **decreased.**
- **Urinary copper** excretion is **increased** i.e. more than 150 mcg/dl.
- **Liver biopsy** shows **increased tissue copper** of more than 250 mcg/dl and mallory bodies.

39. (a) Gluten free diet (Ref: CPDT 19th E/P603)
- Small bowel diarrhoea and villous atrophy along with positive anti endomysial and anti-tissue trans-glutaminase antibody test confirms the diagnosis of celiac disease.
- The mainstay of treatment for celiac disease is gluten free diet lifelong.

40. (a) Lactase (Ref: CPDT 19th E/P603)
- Secondary lactase deficiency can be seen due to viral gastroenteritis; however it is a self-limiting disease.

41. (b) Wilson's disease (Ref: CPDT 19th E/P632)
- Feature of CNS involvement i.e. mood and emotional liability and ocular involvement as brown dis-colouration of descement membrane is seen in Wilson disease.

42. (c) Bilious vomiting (Ref: Walker Pediatric GIT diseases Volime1/P563)

"Vomiting — **Bile-stained vomiting is characteristic of intestinal obstruction** distal to ampulla of vater, and if present, obstruction must be excluded."

43. (a) HLA-DQ2 (Ref: Rudolph 22nd E/P1440)

"Celiac disease is strongly associated with **HLA-DQ2** molecule, which is present in 90% of all individuals with confirmed diagnosis. Most individuals with celiac disease who do not posses the DQ2 molecule carry the **HLA-DQ8** molecule"

44. (d) Portal hypertension due to extrahepatic obstruction (Ref: Ghai 7th E/P289)

Prehepatic portal hypertension:
- Prehepatic portal hypertension is caused by **extrahepatic portal vein obstruction (EHPVO)** commonly caused by intraluminal obstruction like thrombosis (trauma or hypercoagulable states) or extraluminal obstruction by tumor or pancreatic mass.
- The child presents with symptoms of **gastrointestinal variceal bleeding** (**hematemesis, malena**) and **splenomegaly.**
- Hepatomegaly and ascites is usually not seen.

45. (d) Liver biopsy (Ref: Nelson 19th E/P1317)
- **Percutaneous liver biopsy** is the most specific and definitive diagnostic procedure to differentiate between intrahepatic and extrahepatic biliary disorders.
- USG, HIDA and laboratory values though useful in diagnosis are not specific as the findings can be seen in both types of cholestasis.

46. (b) The pyloric tumor is best felt during feeding (Ref: Rudolph 22nd E/P1420, Nelson 19th E/P1229)
- First born male child is more commonly involved.
- Feeding is useful for diagnosis as peristalsis can be seen and mass can be palpated.
- Because of early diagnosis and treatment chronic complications of malnutrition are not seen.
- After vomiting child's appetite is voracious.

47. (b) α1 antitrypsin deficiency (Ref: CPDT 19th E/P615)
- The most common cause liver disease is idiopathic neonatal hepatitis which is associated with genetic disorders like Niemann-Pick disease, Alagille syndrome and **α1 antitrypsin deficiency.**

48. (b) Increase thickness of mucosa (Ref: CPDT 19th E/P603)

Small intestinal biopsy — Biopsy is the definitive diagnostic procedure for celiac disease that shows
- Villi atrophy and crypt hyperplasia (decreased villi to crypt ratio).
- Decreased brush border epithelium.
- Intraepithelial lymphocytes.
- Plasma cells in lamina propria.
- Loss of mucosa and brush border epithelium.

49. (a) Peyer's patch hypertrophy (Ref: CPDT 19th E/P584)
- All of the mentioned options can cause intestinal obstruction, however Peyer's patch hypertrophy is relatively more common caused by viral infections and introduction of new food proteins.

50. (a) Tracheoesophageal fistula (Ref: Rudolph 22nd E/P1401)
- Neonates with TEF characteristically present with frothing and excess drooling after feeds. This is followed by coughing, cyanosis and respiratory distress.

51. (b) Non cirrhotic portal fibrosis (Ref: CPDT 19th E/P635, Ghai 7th E/P289)
- Budd chiari syndrome, cirrhosis and veno-occlusive disease will present with hepatomegaly and ascites.
- Non cirrhotic portal fibrosis with prehepatic portal hypertension presents with splenomegaly but hepatomegaly and ascites is not seen.

52. (b) Hypochloremic alkalosis (Ref: Rudolph 22nd E/P1420)
- Congenital hypertrophic pyloric stenosis is more common in males.
- Repeated vomiting leads to hypochloremic metabolic alkalosis.
- Ramstedt's pyloromyotomy is the procedure of choice. Heller's myotomy is done for achalasia cardia.
- Most commonly presents between 2 and 4 weeks of age.

53. (b) Neonatal hepatitis with extrabiliary atresia (Ref: CPDT 19th E/P617)
- Clay coloured stools is more characteristic for **extrabiliary atresia.**
- Giant cells are not specific for any liver disease as it can be seen in many conditions.

54. (c) Traumatic pancreatic cyst (Ref: Ghai 7th E/P260)
- Most common cause of pancreatitis in children is trauma.

55. (c) Ulcerative colitis (Ref: Rudolph 22nd E/P1440)
  Causes of fat in stool:
- **Pancreatic insufficiency.**
- Decreased bile production or secretion – Cirrhosis, bile duct obstruction or biliary atresia, **celiac disease**
- Congenital absence of bile synthesis.
- **Bacterial overgrowth syndrome** — It causes dehydroxylation of bile salts.
- Disruption of enterohpatic cycle of bile salts in disorders affecting distal ileum — **Crohn disease**, Intestinal lymphoma or tuberculosis.

56. (a) Ileocolic (Ref: Rudolph 22nd E/P1428)

57. (a) Extrahepatic compression (Ref: Ghai 7th E/P289)
- Extrahepatic portal vein obstruction is the most common cause of portal hypertension in India.

58. (b) Neonatal hepatitis (Ref: CPDT 19th E/P615)

59. (c) Rota virus (Ref: CPDT 19th E/P594)

60. (d) Usually relieved by barium enema (Ref: Rudolph 22nd E/P1428)

- Common age of presentation is from 3 months to 6 years and is rarely seen in neonates.
- Fever is present if perforation and peritonitis occurs.
- Lymphoma of intestine is the most common cause of intussusception in children older than 6 years.
- Barium enema is the initial management of choice as most of the cases respond.

61. (d) *V. cholera* (Ghai 7th E/P261)
- Campylobacter, *Yersinia enterocolitica, A. hydrophilia, E. histolytica* and *E.coli* (EIEC and EHEC) are associated with dysentery.

62. (c) and (d) Rotavirus and *E.coli* (Ref: CPDT 19th E/P594)
- The most common cause of diarrhoea is viruses, among which **rota virus** is the most common cause. The other viruses responsible are adenovirus, calcivirus (norovirus or Norwalk agent), astrovirus and enteroviruses.
- The most common bacterial cause of diarrhoea is *E.coli;* however other bacterias like Shigella, Salmonella, Campylobacter and Yersinia.

63. (a) Aganglionic segment is contracted not dilated (Ref: Rudolph 22nd E/P1436)
- Barium enema shows contraction of aganglionic segment and dilation of segment proximal to it.
- Rectal biopsy is diagnostic for Hirschsprung disease.
- Most commonly rectosigmoid part is involved.

64. (a) and **(d)** Rice and Corn (Ref: CPDT 19th E/P602)
The grains containing gladin which cannot be used in celiac sprue are:
- Wheat
- Barley
- Rye
- Oat

65. (a) Esophageal varices (Ref: Ghai 7th E/P289)
- Among the given options esophageal varices will be associated with splenomegaly in case of portal hypertension.

66. (a), (b) and **(d)** Dermatitis herpetiformis, Type 1 DM, Atrophic gastritis (Ref: Nelson 19th E/P1265, Rudolph 22nd E/P1441)
  Disorders associated with celiac disease:
- **NIDDM**
- Addison's disease
- **Pernicious anemia**
- Autoimmune thyroiditis
- Sjogren syndrome
- Ig A nephropathy
- Collagen vascular disease
- **Dermatitis herpetiformis**
- Turner syndrome
- Williams syndrome
- Down syndrome.

67. **(a)** Hypokalemic alkalosis (Ref: Rudolph 22nd E/P1420)
   - Hypochloremic hypokalemic alkalosis can be seen.
   - Peristalsis is seen from left to right.
   - Males are commonly involved.
   - Vomiting is seen just after feeding and is not retention vomiting which is seen hours after feeding.
   - The cause of hypertrophic pyloric stenosis has been attributed to decreased NO synthase production, enteric denervation and loss of interstitial cells of Cajal.

68. **(a), (c)** and **(d)** Sometimes found in adult, Auerbach's plexus absent, Sometimes involve small intestine (Ref: Rudolph 22nd E/P1436)
   - Hirschsprung disease thought commonly seen in infants and children; adults can also be involved.
   - Contracted segment is involved and the dilated segment which is proximal to involved on is normal.
   - Submucosal and myenteric plexus are absent.
   - Thought rectosigmoid part is most commonly involved, small intestine can be rarely involved.
   - Bleeding PR is an unusual symptom seen only in 5% patients.

69. **(d)** Diaphragmatic hernia (Ref: CPDT 19th E/P582)
   - Duodenal obstruction caused by **duodenal atresia**, duodenal duplication, **peritoneal bands**, **pancreatic pseudocyst** or **annular pancreas** presents with a **double bubble sign** that shows gas filled stomach and duodenum whereas rest of intestine is gasless.

70. **(b)** and **(c)** Blood mixed with mucous stool is defined as dysentery, Rotavirus is the most common organism in children (Ref: Ghai 7th E/P260)
   - Diarrhoea is passage of **loose stools** 3 times or more in a day.
   - Dysentery is diarrhoea characterised by passage of bloody stools.
   - Rotavirus is the most common cause of diarrhoea in children.
   - Persistent diarrhoea is passage of loose stools for **14 days** or more.

71. **(a), (c), (d)** and **(e)** Acholic stool, Conjugated hyperbilirubinemia, Absence of nucleoid in duodenum in HIDA scanand Jaundice is presenting feature (Ref: CPDT 19th E/P617)
   - In extrahepatic biliary atresia jaundice may be seen in the neonatal period.
   - Conjugated hyperbilirubinemia is seen.
   - Since bile doesn't reach intestine, stool is acholic.
   - HIDA scan shows decreased secretion of nucleotide in to intestine.

72. **(a)** Intussusception (Ref: Rudolph 22nd E/P1428)
   - In intussusception baby presents with **acute onset intermittent abdominal pain** followed by vomiting.
   - Mucosal ischemia and damage leads to passage of blood in stool and called as **currant jelly stools.**

73. **(b), (d)** and **(e)** Absence of ganglia in the involved segment, Bleeding PR is presenting feature, Surgery is used in therapy (Rudolph 22nd E/P1436)
   - Hirschsprung disease is commonly seen in infants and children; however can also be seen in adults.
   - It is characterised by absence of ganglionic cells in submucosal and myenteric plexus.
   - The involved segment is contracted and segment proximal to it is dilated.
   - Rectal bleeding is present in some cases. (Ref: Rudolph 22nd E/P1436)

"About 5% children present with chronic constipation, 3% with intestinal perforation during the neonatal period, **5% with rectal bleeding from an anal fissure**, and 5% with hydroureter from urethral compression."

   - Surgical removal of the aganglionic segment and anastomosis of normal segments is the mainstay of treatment.

74. **(b), (c)** and **(e)** Non-bilious vomiting, Projectile vomiting, Forceful (Ref: Rudolph 22nd E/P1420)
   - The infant typically presents with **forceful, projectile**, postprandial **nonbilious vomiting** between **2–4 weeks of age.**

75. **(a)** and **(b)** Intestinal biopsy and unequivocal response to gluten restriction (Ref: Rudolph 22nd E/P1442)

"Revised criteria for the diagnosis of celiac disease published by the European society of pediatric gastroenterology and Nutrition in 1990 and endorsed by North American Society of Pediatric Gastroenterology and Nutrition in 2005 lists 2 mandatory requirements for the diagnosis of celiac disease: (1) **Identification of characteristic histologic findings on small intestinal mucosal histology in a symptomatic patient** and (2) **Complete symptom resolution on a strict gluten free diet.**"

76. **(a), (c)** and **(d)** Corn, Soybean and Rice (Ref: CPDT 19th E/P602)

The grains containing gladin which cannot be used in celiac sprue are:
   - Wheat
   - Barley
   - Rye
   - Oat

77. (a), (b) and (c) Pathology of myenteric plexus of Auerbach, Blood in stools, May involve small intestine rarely (Ref: Rudolph 22nd E/P1436)
- Hirschsprung disease is characterised by absence of ganglionic cells in submucosal and myenteric plexus.
- Bloody stools can be seen.

Rudolph 22nd E/P1436↓ "Enterocolitis most commonly occurs in second to fourth week of life and is characterised by fever; abdominal distension; and explosive foul smelling and sometimes **bloody stool**."

- Most commonly rectosigmoid part is involved however rest of the colon and small intestine can also be involved.
- Involved segment is contracted and segment proximal to it is dilated.
- Commonly seen in infants and children but adults can also be involved.

78. (a) Intussusception (Ref: Rudolph 22nd E/P1428)
- On palpation a **sausage shaped mass** can be felt in intussusception.
- Mucosal ischemia and damage leads to passage of blood in stool and called as **currant jelly stools.**

79. (a), (b) and (d) Hypokalemia, Hyponatremia and Hypochloremia (Ref: Rudolph 22nd E/P1420, CPDT 19th E/P580–81)
- In pyloric stenosis long term vomiting may lead to dehydration, weight loss and constipation. Initial loss of HCl leads to **hypochloremic hypokalemic metabolic alkalosis.**
- Initially protons are saved to compensate for alkalosis. But continuous loss of **sodium**, **potassium** and **chloride** leads to compensatory loss of protons in urine to save the other ions, which leads to para-doxical aciduria.

80. (b), (d) and (e) Target sign, Coiled spring sign and Dance sign (Ref: Rudolph 22nd E/P1428–29, Nelson 19th E/P1242)
- On palpation a **sausage shaped mass** and emptiness in the right iliac fossa **(dance sign)** can be felt.
- USG and CT with contrast shows **target sign.**
- Barium enema and air enema is both useful for diagnosis and treatment. It shows claw sign or **coiled spring sign.**

81. (a) Dermatitis herpetiformis (Ref: Nelson 19th E/P1264)
- **Dermatitis herpetiformis** can be associated with celiac disease which presents with **maculopapular rash.**

82. (a) Intussusception (Ref: Rudolph 22nd E/P1428)
- Here the key word is recurrent obstruction.
- Intussusception presents with recurrent abdominal pain due to recurrent obstruction.

83. (b) Giardiasis (Ref: Elzouki Clinical paediatrics volume1/P1862)
- **Intractable diarrhoea** is a form of chronic diarrhoea for more than 14 days along with failure to gain weight and in which **no bacterial pathogen can be identified**.
- The cause of diarrhoea is not known, known but with ineffective treatment (microvillus atrophy, tufting enteropathy, congenital enterocyte heparin sulphate deficiency) and known but has partially effective treatment (autoimmune enteropathy, lactose intolerance, **cystic fibrosis**, **cow milk protein intolerance**, **secretory tumors**).

84. (d) Increased brush border (Ref: Nelson 19th E/P1264)
- Gladin present in food is responsible for the cytotoxic damage of intestine in celiac disease.
- Most strong association of celiac disease is seen with HLA DQ2followed by HLA DQ8; however other HLA subtypes like B8, DR3 and DR7 can also be seen.
- Normally villi are longer than crypts but in celic disease villous atrophy leads to reversal of villi to crypt ratio.
- **Brush border epithelium is decreased** in celiac disease which leads to malabsorption.

85. (a) Proximal end blind; distal end communicating with trachea (Ref: Rudolph 22nd E/P1401)
- The most common type of TEF is type C which is characterised by presence of **esophageal atresia in the proximal part and fistula in the distal part.**

86. (c) Rectal biopsy (Ref: Rudolph 22nd E/P1436)
Diagnosis of Hirschsprung disease:
- The definitive diagnostic procedure is **intestinal biopsy** which shows **absence of ganglions**, nerve trunk hypertrophy and staining shows increased acetylcholinesterase activity in the involved segment.
- **Barium enema** shows a **contracted involved segment** with **dilation of the normal proximal segment**.
- Rectal manometry shows failure of the internal anal sphincter to relax after dilation of the rectum. An abnormal test is not absolutely diagnostic but a **normal test excludes the disorder**.

87. (b) The entering layer (Ref: Rudolph 22nd E/P1428)
- Intussusception is a disorder characterised by invasion of one part of intestine (intussuceptum) in to **another part of intestine (intussuscipiens) i.e. the outer part.**

88. (a) Intussusception (Ref: Rudolph 22nd E/P1428)

89. (b) Diarrhoea (Ref: Rudolph 22nd E/P1420)

90. (a) Alpha 1 antitrypsin deficiency (Ref: CPDT 19th E/P633)

Causes of liver cirrhosis in children:
- Hepatitis
- Inborn errors of metabolism (galactosemia and fructosemia)
- Wilson disease
- Hemochromatosis
- **Alpha 1 antitrypsin deficiency**
- Biliary atresia
- Choledochal cyst
- Drugs
- Parasites (Liver flukes).

91. **(a)** Multiple (Ref: Bailey and love 24th E/P1195)

92. **(b)** Testicular atrophy (Ref: Nelson 19th E/P1322)

93. **(c)** Hypertrophy of submucous patches (Ref: Rudolph 22nd E/P1428)

QUESTIONS OF OTHER EXAMINATIONS

1. **(c)** Tracheo-esophageal fistula (Ref: Rudolph 22nd E/P1401)
   VACTERL group of anomalies:
   - Vertebral anomalies
   - Atresia of intestine
   - Cardiac malformations (ASD, VSD, PDA)
   - **Tracheo-Esophageal fistula**
   - Renal anomalies
   - Limb defects

2. **(a)** Long arm of chromosome 13 (Ref: Nelson 19th E/P1321)
   - Wilson disease or hepatolenticular degeneration is an **autosomal recessive** disorder caused by mutation of **ATP7B gene** present on **long arm of chromosome 13**, which codes for a p type ATP responsible for copper excretion and incorporation in to ceruloplasmin in the liver.

3. **(b)** Increasing bilirubin (Ref: CPDT 19th E/P634)

"Patients with **a rising bilirubin**, a vitamin K resistant coagulopathy or diuretic resistant ascites usually survive less than 1–2 years."

4. **(a)** Intussusception (Ref: Rudolph 22nd E/P1428)
   - Barium enema and air enema is both useful for diagnosis and treatment of intussusception. It shows **claw sign** and **coiled spring sign.**

5. **(a)** Rota virus (Ref: CPDT 19th E/P594)

6. **(b)** Low serum ceruloplasmin and high urinary copper (Ref: Nelson 19th E/P1322)

7. **(c)** Celiac disease (Ref: CPDT 19th E/P602)

8. **(d)** Trypsin (Ref: Harper 28th E/P462)

"In the small intestine, trypsinogen, the precursor of **trypsin**, is activated by **enteropeptidase**, which is secreted by duodenal epithelial cells."

9. **(c)** Esophageal atresia with distal tracheoesophageal fistula (Ref: Rudolph 22nd E/P1401)
   - The most common type of TEF is type C which is characterised by presence of **esophageal atresia in the proximal part and fistula in the distal part**.

10. **(a)** It is initially treated by colostomy (Ref: CPDT 19th E/P588)

11. **(c)** Hypersensitivity to dietary gluten (Ref: CPDT 19th E/P602)

12. **(b)** Lactose intolerance (Ref: CPDT 19th E/P603)
Lactase deficiency:

"Stools are liquid or frothy, with a pH below 4.5 owing to presence of **organic acids. Reducing substances** are present in fresh stools."

13. **(a)** Pyloric stenosis (Ref: Rudolph 22nd E/P1420)

14. **(a)** Tracheoesophageal fistula (Ref: Rudolph 22nd E/P1401)

15. **(b)** May present as acute hepatitis (Ref: Nelson 19th E/P1322)
   - KF ring is usually seen in older children.
   - Hepatic involvement can present initially as **acute hepatitis** or chronic liver disease and progress to cirrhosis.
   - Urinary copper excretion is increased.
   - Hepatic copper concentration is increased.

16. **(b)** Oesophageal atresia in foetus (Ref: Rudolph 22nd E/P1401)

17. **(d)** Bayar's (Ref: Rudolph 22nd E/P1437)

18. **(b)** Excision of aganglionic segment (Ref: Rudolph 22nd E/P1437)

19. **(a)** Galctosemia (Ref: CPDT 19th E/P613)

20. **(a)** Shigella dysenterie (Ref: Ghai 7th E/P261)

21. **(b)** Increased ceruloplasmin levels (Ref: Nelson 19th E/P1322)

22. **(a)** Portal hypertension (Ref: Ghai 7th E/P289)

23. **(b)** Testicular atrophy (Ref: Nelson 19th E/P1322)

24. **(c)** 4 months (Ref: Newton's Baby colic P5)
   - Colic in children generally disappears by the age of 3 months.

Kidney and Urinary Tract

8

CONGENITAL MALFORMATIONS

Embryological development of kidney starts with the formation of urogenital ridge from the intermediate mesoderm. The urogenital ridge gives rise to the three embryological steps of kidney development i.e. pronephros, mesonephros and metanephros. The non-functional pronephros containing rudimentary epithelial cords (nephrotomes) develops at 3rd week of gestation at the cranial end. The pronephros regresses to functional mesonephros and mesonephric (Wolffian) duct at 4th week. At 5th week metanephros develops and it stimulates formation of ureteric bud from mesonephric duct. The **ureteric bud** forms the **collecting system of kidney** whereas **metanephros** forms **nephrons.** Abnormalities in the renal embryogenesis lead to agenesis and dysgenesis of kidney. These disorders are more common in males than females.

Renal Agenesis

- Unilateral renal agenesis is associated with compensatory hypertrophy and overfunctioning of other kidney. These patients have increased incidence of contralateral vesicoureteral reflux and ureteropelvic junction obstruction, ipsilateral absent vas deferens, ureter and trigone of bladder and a **single umbilical artery.** It may be associated with Mayer-Rokitansky-Kuster-Hauser syndrome in females.
- Bilateral renal agenesis or **Potter syndrome** is characterised by a characteristic facies (**flat nose**, widely separated eyes with epicanthal folds and low set ears), **oligohydramnios** and pulmonary hypoplasia.

Renal Dysgenesis

Renal dysgenesis is characterised by presence of abnormal and undifferentiated tissues and can present as dysplasia, hypoplasia and cysts. In cystic dysplasia if cysts are present in entire kidney then it is called as multicystic dysplastic kidney. **Multicystic dysplastic kidney** is the **most common form of renal cystic disease in infants** and is also the **most common cause of an abdominal mass in neonate.** Mostly it is **unilateral** and associated with hypertension and Wilms tumor. Vesicoureteric reflux can be seen in normal kidney.

Autosomal Recessive Polycystic Kidney Disease

Autosomal recessive polycystic kidney disease (ARPKD) is caused by mutation of **PKHD1 gene** which results in transformation of collecting ducts in to **fusiform cysts.**

Clinical Presentation

- The patient has **bilaterally enlarged kidneys** and associated extrarenal involvement.
- **Liver** is the most common extrarenal site of involvement characterised by **fibrosis and cysts**; however cysts of **pancreas, spleen** and biliary tree (Caroli disease) can also be seen.
- Lung underdevelopment leads to oligohydramnios and potter facies.
- Complications like portal hypertension, urinary tract infection, hypertension, growth retardation and ascending cholangitis can be seen.

Diagnosis

- Prenatal USG shows a **salt and pepper appearance** of the kidney.
- MRI of kidney shows **radially arranged fusiform dilated collecting ducts**.

Treatment

- The treatment of complications, dialysis and transplantation of cystic organs (liver and kidney) is the most that can be done.

Nephronopthisis

Nephronopthisis is an autosomal recessive disorder caused by mutation of NPHP gene. In this disorder cysts are characteristically located in the corticomedullary junction. The patient usually presents with **polyuria**, **polydipsia**, **anemia** and **growth retardation**. The other associated features are retinitis pigmentosa, cerebellar vermis aplasia, coloboma of eye, hepatic fibrosis and cone-shaped epiphysis. The patient does not develop hypertension due to **salt loss in the urine**. USG shows **small kidneys** and lack of corticomedullary differentiation.

DISORDERS OF GENITOURINARY TRACT

Ectopic Ureter

Ectopic ureter is more common in **females** than in males. The most common site of ectopic ureter opening is **urethra** i.e. **posterior urethra in males** and urethra near the bladder neck in females. In males the other sites of opening are vas deferens, **seminal vesicles** and **distal trigone of bladder**; and the patient presents with **urinary tract infection** without incontinence. In females the other sites of opening are bladder neck, vagina, uterus and fallopian tube; and the presenting symptom is **urinary incontinence**.

Vesicoureteral Reflux

Vesicoureteral reflux is defined as retrograde flow of urine from bladder in to ureter and renal pelvis. The primary reflux is due to anatomic defect of the ureterovesical junction and is associated with other congenital anomalies like multicystic dysplastic kidney and renal agenesis. Secondarily reflux can be seen due to neuropathic bladder, ureteral duplication and posterior urethral valves. **Prenatal Vesicoureteral reflux** seen as hydropnephrois in USG is **more common in newborn males**; however in **older children** i.e. 2–3 years of age the incidence is higher in **females.**

Clinical Presentation

- Vesicoureteral reflux is the most common cause of **recurrent urinary tract infection.**
- Infection is followed by **renal scarring**, hypertension and growth retardation.

Diagnosis

- **Voiding cystourethrogram (VCUG)** – A contrast radionucleotide VCUG is done to confirm the diagnosis.

Treatment

- The initial management of choice is **daily antibiotic prophylaxis** till the spontaneous resolution of reflux or 5 years of age or child attains bladder control.
- Surgical intravesical and extravesical ureteral reimplantation is reserved for patients who do not respond to medical management.

Posterior Urethral Valves

Posterior urethral valves are congenital obstructive lesions of leaflets in the verumontanum of prostatic urethra. These are the **most common cause of urinary obstruction in a male infant** and most common type of obstructive lesion causing renal failure.

Clinical Presentation

- Obstruction to urine flow creates a backpressure which leads to prostatic urethra dilation, bladder hypertrophy and trabeculation, vesicoureteric reflux and renal changes like hydronephrosis and dysplasia.
- The neonates have a **weak urinary stream, a palpable distended bladder, dribbling of urine** and **increased risk for UTI.**
- The good prognostic factors are a normal prenatal USG with visualisation of corticomedullary junction and serum creatinine <0.8–1.0 mg/dl after bladder decompression. The poor prognostic factors are oligohydramnios, prenatal hydronephrosis, serum creatinine >1.0 mg/dl, renal cysts and diurnal incontinence beyond 5 years of age.

Diagnosis

- The investigation of choice is **voiding cystourethrogram (VCUG)** which shows a **dilated prostatic urethra** and filling defects of the valves.
- Prenatal diagnosis can be done by USG which shows bilateral hydroureteronephrosis and a **keyhole** appearance.

Treatment

- The initial management of choice is insertion of a feeding tube and decompression of the bladder.
- After the serum creatinine level decreases a transurethral ablation of the leaflets is done. If serum creatinine level does not decrease, initially vesicotomy is done and ablation follows once serum creatinine is normalised.

Ureterocele

Ureterocele is an obstructive lesion characterised by narrowing of ureteral orifice and cystic dilation of the terminal ureter. It is more common in girls and associated with duplication of ureter. In case of males a single ureter can be associated. Vesicoureteric reflux, **unilateral hydronephrosis** and UTI can also be seen in these patients. VCUG is the investigation of choice which shows a **filling defect in bladder, cobra head appearance of ureterocele** and **drooping lilly** appearance of kidney. USG kidney shows **hydroureter** and **hydronephrosis**. The initial management of choice is endoscopic transurethral incision of ureteroceles.

Urinary Tract Infection

Males are more commonly affected during **infancy** and females after infancy. UTI is most commonly caused by *E.coli.* Urinary stasis is the most important cause in children and conditions like Vesicoureteral reflux and posterior urethral valves are commonly associated. Uncircumcised boys are at increased risk of UTI.

Clinical Presentation

- The newborns and infants have nonspecific symptoms like fever, jaundice, vomiting, failure to thrive and jaundice.
- Older children have more specific symptoms. Cystitis can present as dysuria, frequency and urgency and pyelonephritis presents with fever, vomiting and flank pain.
- Inflammation of kidney i.e. pyelonephritis results in scars and complications like hypertension and renal failure.
- **Xanthogranulomatous pyelonephritis** is most commonly caused by **proteus**; and is associated with staghorn renal calculus or other obstructive lesions. Children from **infancy till16 years** of age are commonly affected. In **children focal renal involvement is seen** as compared to diffuse involvement in adults. It is characterised by granulomatous inflammation and presence of histiocytes and foamy cells around yellow colour nodules. In children **partial nephrectomy** is usually sufficient for the focal disease.

Diagnosis

- Urine sample is collected for both microscopic analysis and culture. In older children midstream clean catch is sufficient but in **infants suprapubic aspiration should be done** as it is the most uncontaminated urine specimen.
- Microscopic analysis showing pyuria i.e. **>5 W.B.Cs/hpf** is suggestive of infection; however it is **not confirmatory** as **pyuria can be seen without infection** and **infection can be present without pyuria**.
- **Deep stick test for nitrite** and **leucocyte esterase** can add to diagnosis but are **not specific** for UTI. **WBC casts are specific for pyelonephritis,** as casts are seen only if renal parenchyma is involved.

- Microscopic examination of urine showing **1 bacterium per oil-immersion field on gram stain** is also a **specific test** as it equals to 100,000 bacteria/ml of urine.
- Urine culture is the mainstay of diagnosis. For diagnosis **>100,000 colonies** or >10,000 colonies with symptomatic child is required.
- **VCUG** should be done to rule out the obstructive lesions. It is indicated in a **male child with more than one UTI** and a **female child with more than two UTIs within 6 months.**
- DMSA scan can be done to confirm the diagnosis of pyelonephritis.

Treatment

- Empirical treatment should be started with trimethoprim-sulfamethoxazole in uncomplicated UTI and **IV 3rd generation cephalosporin or aminoglycoside in complicated UTI.** After urine culture antimicrobial therapy is directed against the specific pathogen.

GLOMERULAR DISEASES

Glomerular diseases can be broadly classified as **glomerulonephritis, nephrotic syndrome** and **hemolytic uremic syndrome.**

Glomerulonephritis

Most common cause of glomerulonephritis is immune mediated injury caused by immune complexes and glomerular antigen mediated damage. It is characterised by the triad of **hematuria**, azotemia and hypertension.

Ig A nephropathy

Ig A nephropathy or **Berger's disease** is the **most common cause of glomerulonephritis worldwide**. Most common age group affected are in their **2nd and 3rd decade** and **males** are more commonly affected. The patient usually presents with **recurrent gross macroscopic hematuria preceded 24–48 hours by upper respiratory tract infection**. This is followed by microscopic hematuria and some proteinuria. Most of the cases resolve spontaneously; however some cases may progress to renal dysfunction. Renal biopsy is shows **mesangial proliferation** and Ig A deposition; however it is not specific as same changes can also be seen in HSP. Ig A levels is not used for diagnosis as they are elevated only in minority of cases. The treatment is aimed at treating hypertension (ACE inhibitors, angiotensin receptors blockers), immune mediated injury (**corticosteroids** and immunomodulators) and inflammation (fish oil).

Acute Poststreptococcal Glomerulonephritis

Acute poststreptococcal glomerulonephritis is caused by autoimmune injury **only due to selective nephritogenic strains of streptococcus**. The patient develops glomerulonephritis with **streptococcal pharyngitis** usually in winter after 1–2 weeks of infection and with **streptococcal pyoderma** in summer after 3–6 weeks of infection. The most common age of presentation is 5–12 years and is rarely seen before 3 years of age. The patient presents with **gross hematuria with a smoky, cola or tea colour urine**; edema and hypertension. Complications that can be seen are **hypertensive encephalopathy**, pulmonary haemorrhage, cerebral vasculitis, **hyperkalemia**, hypophosphatemia and **acidosis**. The diagnosis is based on the clinical findings along with evidence of recent poststreptococcal infection and a **low C3 level**. **RBC casts** on urine analysis is a characteristic finding. The treatment is usually supportive because most of the cases resolve spontaneously and **rarely may progress to renal failure**. **Penicillin** is usually given for infection however it **does not alter the course or risk of glomerulonephritis.**

Henoch-Schönlein Purpura

HSP is a self-limiting systemic vasculitis syndrome characterised by **purpuric rash, arthritis, abdominal pain** and glomerulonephritis. Renal involvement manifests as **hematuria** (microscopic>gross) after 1–3 weeks of upper respiratory tract infection. Ureteritis can also be seen followed by stricture and hydronephrosis. Diagnosis is confirmed by presence of **palpable purpura with a normal platelet count** along with at least one of the following: **abdominal pain, arthritis or arthralgia, mesangial Ig A deposition on renal biopsy**. Renal biopsy changes are similar to Ig A nephropathy. The nephritis resolves spontaneously and only requires supportive treatment. Glucocorticoids may reduce the severity of nephritis.

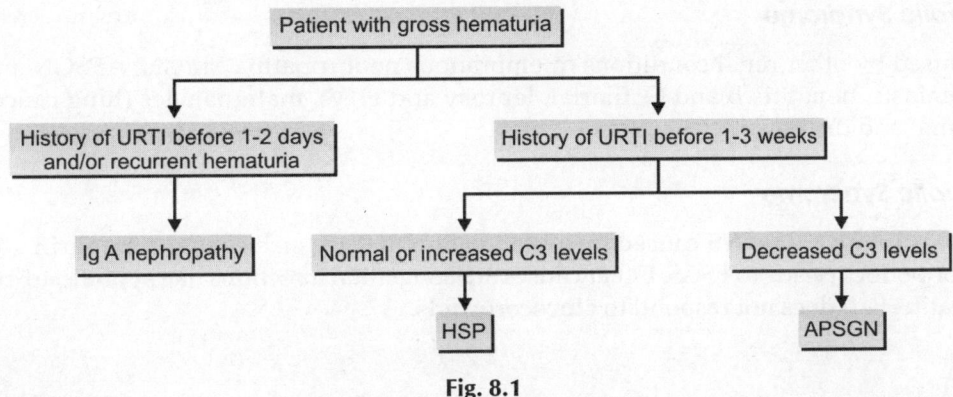

Fig. 8.1

Hemolytic Uremic Syndrome

Hemolytic uremic syndrome (HUS) is the **most common cause of acute renal failure and most common type of leucocytoclastic vasculitis** in young children. In most of the cases it is preceded by 1 week with gastroenteritis caused by **shigella** in developing countries and shiga like toxin producing **E.coli** strain in developed countries. Gastroenteritis manifests as vomiting, diarrhoea, fever and abdominal pain. This infection leads to **microthrombi formation** and manifests as classical triad of HUS i.e. **microangiopathic hemolytic anemia**, **thrombocytopenia** and **uremia**. Severity of renal involvement is variable but about half of the patients develop **oliguria** and need **dialysis**. **Neurologic involvement** is common and presents as hypersomnolence, seizures and coma. **Hepatomegaly**, pancreatitis and cardiac involvement can also be seen. Peripheral smear shows **fragmented RBCs**, helmet cells and **burr cells**. Mild reticulocytosis, significant **leucocytosis**, hypoalbuminemia and low serum haptoglobin can be seen. Treatment is mainly supportive.

Nephrotic Syndrome

Nephrotic syndrome (NS) is combination of clinical findings like **massive proteinuria**, **hypoalbuminemia**, **edema**, **hyperlipidemia** and **lipiduria**. It can be broadly classified as primary or idiopathic NS, secondary NS and congenital NS.

Primary Nephrotic Syndrome

Primary nephrotic syndrome consists of 3 clinical entities named **minimal change disease (MCD) or lipoid nephrosis**, mesangial proliferation and **focal segmental glomerulosclerosis (FSGS)**. It is more common in males. **Minimal change disease** is the **most common cause of nephrotic syndrome in children** and is the **most responsive of all to steroids**. It is characterised by **fusion of foot processes or podocytes** in electron microscopy. **Mesangial proliferation** is associated with Ig A and Ig M deposition and effacement of podocytes. **Focal segmental glomerulosclerosis** is the **most common cause of steroid resistant NS**. It is an AR disorder characterised by mutation of **NPHS2 gene** which codes for slit diaphragm protein podocin. It shows Ig M and C3 deposition and scarring of the glomerular tuft.

- **Clinical presentation:** The patient presents with dependent edema prominent in the eyelids, scrotum and labia. The most important cause of edema is primary sodium and water retention due to renal insensitivity to ANP; however decreased oncotic pressure and secondary sodium and water retention do play a role. Most of the cases are preceded by upper respiratory tract infection. Microscopic hematuria and hypertension can be rarely seen. The **most common complication of NS is bacterial peritonitis** and most common causative agent is **pneumococcus**. Thromboembolic events can be associated due to **increase in fibrinogen and thrombin**; and **decrease in AT III and protein C and S**. **Hypocalcemia** can be seen due to loss of calcium binding protein as well as vitamin D3.
- **Diagnosis:** Urine analysis shows massive proteinuria with a protein excretion of more than **40 mg/m^2/hr** in children and a protein creatinine ratio of more than 2. Serum albumin level is decreased, cholesterol and triglyceride levels are increased and complement levels are normal. **Renal biopsy is not indicated** for treatment of **MCD** however it should be done for FSGS.
- **Treatment:** The **mainstay of treatment is glucocorticoids**. Prednisolone is given daily for 4–6 weeks followed by alternate day tapering dose till 8 weeks. Patient who relapse on alternate day period or within 28 days of stopping prednisolone are called as **steroid dependent**. Patients who fail to respond within 8 week are called as **steroid resistant**. Steroid resistant or dependent patients should be treated with **cyclophosphamide**; however if toxicity is a limiting factor then **cyclosporine** is preferred. High dose pulse methylprednisolone, ACE inhibitors and angiotensin receptor blockers may also be beneficial.

Secondary Nephrotic Syndrome

Secondary NS is caused by other renal conditions (membranous nephropathy, MPGN, APSGN and HSP), infections (malaria, schistosomiasis, hepatitis B and C, filarial, leprosy and HIV), malignancies (lung cancer, GIT cancer and Hodgkin's lymphoma) and drugs.

Congenital Nephrotic Syndrome

Most common cause is **Finnish type NS** caused by mutation of **NPHS1** which codes for **nephrin**. Mutation of NPHS 2 gene which codes for podocin leads to FSGS. Other causes are congenital infections like syphilis, toxoplasmosis, rubella, CMV, HIV and hepatitis B. It does not respond to glucocorticoids.

RENAL FAILURE

Acute Renal Failure

ARF is characterised by an acute decline in the GFR which leads to accumulation of BUN and creatinine. It is not a disease rather is a consequence of various diseases and based on that it can be classified as prerenal, renal and postrenal. Prerenal ARF is caused by any disease that leads to contraction of the blood volume and subsequently decreases the glomerular filtration pressure. Renal ARF can be caused by diseases of kidney like APSGN, HSP, **HUS**, MPGN, lupus nephritis, anti GBM disease and acute tubular necrosis. Postrenal ARF is caused by obstructive lesions of the urinary tract like posterior urethral valve, ureteropelvic junction obstruction, tumors and stones.

Clinical Presentation

- The patient presents with progressive accumulation of BUN and creatinine. This differentiates it from CRF in which there is a steady rise of nitrogen products.

Diagnosis

- The important part of diagnosis is to find out the exact type of renal failure as the management depends on it. The signs and symptoms of the diseases associated with each type of renal failure add to the diagnosis.
- Prerenal ARF can be distinguished from renal ARF by certain urinary values.

Values	Prerenal ARF	Renal ARF
Urinary specific gravity	>1020	<1012
Urine/plasma creatinine	>40	<20
Urine sodium	<20	>40
FENa	<1%	>2%
Urine osmolarity	>500 mOsm/kg	<350 mOsm/kg

Complications

- The complications that can be seen are hyperkalemia, hypocalcemia, dilutional hyponatremia, metabolic acidosis, hypertension, anemia due to hemodilution and neurological symptoms.

Treatment

- Treatment is usually aimed at the etiology of ARF and the complications associated with it.

RENAL TUBULAR DISORDERS

Bartter Syndrome

Bartter syndrome is an autosomal recessive disorder caused by mutation of gene coding for basolateral chloride channel (ClC-Kb). The patient losses ions like sodium, chloride, potassium and calcium in the urine. Calcium loss in urine may lead to **nephrocalcinosis**. Loss of protons in the urine leads to **metabolic alkalosis**. A history of polyhydramnios can be present and the baby has a typical facies with a triangular face, protruding ears, strabismus and drooping mouth. The patient presents with recurrent episodes of dehydration and failure to thrive. Clinical features along with **decreased**

serum sodium, potassium (usually <2.5 mmol/L) and chloride is sufficient for diagnosis. Treatment is aimed at adequate hydration and potassium supplementation. Indomethacin might be of some importance due to inhibition of prostaglandin synthesis.

Gitleman Syndrome

Gitleman syndrome is an autosomal recessive disorder caused by mutation of genes encoding sodium chloride cotransporter (NCCT). The patient presents with hypocalciuria, hypomagnesemia, hypokalemia and metabolic alkalosis. The patient presents with recurrent muscle cramps and growth retardation. Treatment is aimed at correcting hypomagnesemia and hypokalemia.

MULTIPLE CHOICE QUESTIONS

1. A 3-month-old infant presents with bilateral medullary nephrocalcinosis. All of the following can cause medullary nephrocalcinosis except:

    [AIIMS May 09]
    a. Hyperoxaluria
    b. Bartter syndrome
    c. Prolonged use of furosemide
    d. ARPKD

2. A child develops non-blanching macules and papules on lower extremities, mild abdominal pain and skin biopsy showed IgA deposition. Most appropriate diagnosis is: [AIIMS May 09]
    a. Drug induced vasculitis
    b. HSP
    c. Wegener's granulomatosis
    d. Kawasaki disease

3. A 3-year-old male had non blanching rashes over the shin and swelling of knee joint with hematuria +++ and protein +. Microscopic analysis of his renal biopsy specimen is most likely to show:

    [AIIMS Nov. 08]
    a. Tubular necrosis
    b. Visceral podocyte fusion
    c. Mesangial deposits of IgA
    d. Basement membrane thickening

4. Baby born at 30 weeks for 18 years old primigravida of weight 2 kg which died after 48 hours. APGAR scores were 5 and 8 at 1 and 5 minutes. On autopsy bilateral enlarged kidney with multiple radially arranged cysts. Which of the following finding is expected to be associated with?   [AIIMS June 08]
    a. Imperforate anus   b. Hepatic cyst and fibrosis
    c. Absence of ureter   d. Holoprosencephaly

5. Most common cause of renal artery stenosis in children in India is: [AIIMS May 07]
    a. Takayasu aortoarteritis
    b. Fibromedial hypertrophy
    c. Fibrointimal hyperplasia
    d. Polyarteritisnodosa

6. The most common gene defect in idiopathic steroid resistant nephrotic syndrome:

    [AIIMS May 07, Nov. 06]
    a. ACE   b. NPHS 2
    c. HOX 11   d. PAX

7. In Schwartz formula for calculation of creatinine clearance in a child, the constant depends on the following except: [AIIMS Nov. 06]
    a. Age
    b. Method of estimation of creatinine
    c. Mass
    d. Severity of renal failure

8. The most common gene defect in idiopathic steroid resistant nephrotic syndrome:

    [AIIMS Nov. 06; May 07]
    a. ACE   b. NPHS 2
    c. HOX 11   d. PAX

9. A boy suffering from acute pyelonephritis, most specific urinary finding will be: [AIIMS Nov. 06]
    a. Leukocyte esterase test
    b. WBC casts
    c. Nitrite test
    d. Bacteria in Gram stain

10. A 3-year-old boy presents with fever, dysuria and gross hematuria. Physical examination shows a prominent suprapubic area which is dull on percussion. Urine analysis reveals red blood cells but no proteinuria. Which of the following is the most likely diagnosis?   [AIIMS May 06]
    a. Acute glomerulonephritis
    b. Urinary tract infections
    c. Posterior urethral valves
    d. Teratoma

11. Which of the following statements is true of primary grade IV-V vesicoureteric reflux in young children?   [AIIMS May 06]
    a. Renal scarring usually begins in the midpolar region
    b. Postnatal scarring may occur even in the absence of urinary tract infections

c. Long term outcome is comparable in patients treated with antibiotic prophylaxis or surgery

d. Oral amoxicillin is the choice antibiotic for prophylaxis

12. **Henoch-Schönlein purpura is characterized by the deposition of the following immunoglobulin around the vessels:** [AIIMS Nov. 05]
    a. IgM   b. IgG
    c. IgA   d. IgE

13. **A 2-month-old girl has failure to thrive, polyuria and medullary nephrocalcinosis affecting both kidneys. Investigations shows blood pH 7.48, bicarbonate 25 mEq/l, potassium 2 mEq/l, sodium 126 mEq/l and chloride 88 mEq/l. The most likely diagnosis is:** [AIIMS Nov. 04]
    a. Distal renal tubular acidosis
    b. Primary hyperaldosteronism
    c. Bartter syndrome
    d. Pseudohypoaldosteronism

14. **An 8 day old breast fed baby presents with vomiting, poor feeding and loose stools. On examination the heart rate is 190/minute, blood pressure 50/30 mm Hg, respiratory rate 72 breaths/minute and capillary refill time of 4 seconds. Investigations show hemoglobin level of 15g/dl, Na 120 mEq/L, K$^+$ 6.8 mEq/L, bicarbonate 15 mEq/L, urea 30 mg/dL and creatinine 0.6 mg/dL. The most likely diagnosis is:** [AIIMS Nov. 04]
    a. Congenital adrenal hyperplasia
    b. Acute tubular necrosis
    c. Congenital hypertrophic pyloric stenosis
    d. Renal tubular acidosis

15. **A 9 years old boy has steroid dependent nephrotic syndrome for the last 5 years. The patient is markedly cushingoid with blood pressure of 120/86 mmHg and small subcapsular cataracts. The most appropriate therapy of choice is:** [AIIMS Nov. 04]
    a. Long-term furosemide with enalapril
    b. Cyclophosphamide
    c. Intravenous immunoglobulin
    d. Intravenous pulse corticosteroids

16. **Which of the following is the most appropriate method for obtaining a urine specimen for culture in an 8 month old girl:** [AIIMS May 04]
    a. Suprapubic aspiration
    b. Indwelling catheter sample
    c. Clean catch void
    d. Urinary bag sample

17. **An 8-year-old boy during a routine check-up is found to have E. coli 1,00,000 cc/ml on a urine culture. The urine specimen was obtained by midstream clean-catch void. The child is asymptomatic. Which is the most appropriate next step in the management?** [AIIMS May 04]

a. Treat as an acute episode of urinary tract infection
b. No therapy
c. Prophylactic antibiotics for 6 months
d. Administer long-term urine alkalinizer

18. **Vesicoureteric reflux is more common in:**
    [AIIMS May 04]
    a. Newborn females   b. Older girls
    c. Older boys   d. Only during pregnancy

19. **The treatment of choice for primary grade V vesicoureteric reflux involving both kidneys in a 6-month-old boy is:**
    [AIIMS Nov. 04, AIIMS May 03]
    a. Antibiotic prophylaxis
    b. Ureteric reimplantation
    c. Cystoscopy followed by subureteric injection of Teflon
    d. Bilateral ureterostomies

20. **A 9 years old child has steroid dependant nephrotic syndrome for the last 5 years. He has received corticosteroids almost continuously during this period and has cushingoid features. The blood pressure is 120/86 mmHg and there are bilateral subcapsular cataracts. The treatment of choice is:** [AIIMS May 03]
    a. Levamisole
    b. Cyclophosphamide
    c. Cyclosporine A
    d. Intravenous pulse corticosteroids

21. **A child with recurrent urinary tract infections is most likely to show:** [AI 05, AIIMS Nov. 03]
    a. Posterior urethral valves
    b. Vesicoureteric reflux
    c. Neurogenic bladder
    d. Renal and ureteric calculi

22. **A 12 years old boy is referred for evaluation of nocturnal enuresis and short stature. The blood pressure is normal. The blood urea is 112 mg/dl, creatinine 6 mg/dl, sodium 119 mEq/L, potassium 4 mEq/L, calcium 7 mg/dl, phosphate 6 mg/dl and alkaline phosphatase 400 U/l. Urinalysis shows trace proteinuria with hyaline casts; no red and white cells are seen. Ultrasound shows bilateral small kidneys and the micturating cysto-urethrogram is normal. The most likely diagnosis is:**
    [AIIMS May 03, Nov. 03]
    a. Alport's syndrome
    b. Medullary sponge kidney
    c. Chronic glomerulonephritis
    d. Nephronopthisis

23. **One year old male child presented with poor urinary stream since birth. The investigation of choice for evaluation is:** [AIIMS May 03]
    a. Voiding cystourethrography (VCUG)
    b. USG bladder

c. Intravenous urography

d. Uroflowmetry

24. A 10-year-old boy is having polyuria, polydipsia, laboratory data shows (in mEq/L)

Na–154

K–4.5

HCO_3–22

Serum osmolarity–295

Blood urea–50

Urine specific gravity–1.005

The diagnosis is: [AIIMS May 02]

a. Diabetes insipidus   b. Renal tubular acidosis

c. Bartter syndrome   d. Recurrent UTI

25. 12 years of old Shyam presented with gross hematuria with 80% dysmorphic RBC's days after aattack of upper respiratory tract infection diagnosis is: [AIIMS Nov. 01]

a. Microangiopathic thrombotic anemia

b. IgA Nephropathy

c. PSGN

d. HS purpura

26. An 8-years-old child suffering from recurrent attacks of polyuria since childhood presents to the pediatrics OPD. On examination the child is short statured vitals and BP are normal. Serum Creatinine – 6 mg%, HCO_3–16 mEq, Na–134. On USG bilateral small kidneys are seen. Diagnosis is:

[AIIMS May 01]

a. Reflux nephropathy

b. Nephronopthisis

c. Polycystic kidney disease

d. Medullary cystic kidney disease

27. A five-year-old male child presents with complaints of fever and abdominal distension. He is having vomiting for the last five days. On examination there are 6–8 Pus Cell/hpf in urine. WBC count shows 78% neutrophils. What is the best line of management? [AIIMS Nov. 00]

a. Send urine for culture and sensitivity and wait for results.

b. Send urine for culture and sensitivity and start IV antibiotics immediately

c. Send urine for culture, do an USG and start chloroquine

d. Radio nucleotide studies

28. A child presents with abdominal colic and hematuria. On ultrasonography a stone 2.5 cm in diameter is seen in the renal pelvis. The next step in management of this case is: [AIIMS Nov. 00]

a. Pyelolithotomy   b. Nephroureterostomy

c. Conservative   d. ESWL

29. Ig A nephropathy is seen in: [AIIMS June 2000]

a. Membranous glomerulonephritis

b. Mesangioproliferative glomerulonephritis

c. Focal glomerulonephritis

d. Crescentic glomerulonephritis

30. T/t of choice for grade IV vesicoureteric reflux with recurrent UTI: [AIIMS June 2000]

a. Cotrimaxozole

b. Bilateral reimplantation of ureter

c. Injection of collagen in the ureter

d. Endoscopic resection of ureter

31. A 2-year-old child comes with 1 year H/O generalised edema. His B.P is 107/70 mm, urine examination shows hyaline cast, proteinuria +++, WBC and RBC are nil, the likely diagnosis is:

[AIIMS Nov. 99]

a. Selective proteinuria

b. Uremia

c. Focal segmental glomerulosclerosis

d. Low serum complement level

32. Ectopic ureter opening is not located in:

[AIIMS Nov. 98]

a. Bulbar urethra   b. Prostatic urethra

c. Seminal vesicle   d. Bladder neck

33. In case of vesicoureteric reflux which of the following will be investigation of choice: [AIIMS Nov. 98]

a. Micturating cystourethrogram

b. IVP

c. Cystography

d. Radionucleotide study

34. All of the following are decreased in nephrotic syndrome, except:

[AIIMS June 98, Dec. 95, AI 97]

a. Serum transferrin

b. Serum fibrinogen

c. Serum ceruloplasmin

d. Serum albumin

35. A child with 22-25 stools/day, 3 day old pneumonitis, no passage of urine from 36 hours, low B.P, blood ph 7.21, urine Na 18 mEq/L, S. Urea 120, serum creatinine 1.2 indicate: [AIIMS May 95]

a. Acute cortical necrosis

b. Acute tubular necrosis

c. Prerenal azotemia

d. Acute medullary necrosis

36. Unilateral renal agenesis is associated with:

[AIIMS May 95, 93]

a. Polycystic disease of pancreas

b. Hepatic cysts and fibrosis

c. Single umbilical artery

d. Hypogonadism

37. In nephrotic syndrome the essential feature is:

[AIIMS 83]

a. Proteinuria   b. Hypoalbuminemia

c. Hyperlipidemia   d. Edema

38. A 7-year-old girl is brought with complaints of generalised swelling of the body. Urinary examination reveals grade 3 proteinuria and the presence of hyaline and fatty casts. She has no history of hematuria. Which of the following statements about her condition is true? **[AI 09]**
    a. No Ig G deposits or C3 deposition on renal biopsy
    b. C3 levels will be low
    c. Ig A nephropathy is likely diagnosis
    d. Alport's syndrome is the likely diagnosis

39. True about infantile polycystic kidney disease include the following except: **[AI 08]**
    a. Autosomal dominant
    b. Hepatic cysts
    c. Renal cysts present at birth
    d. Periportal fibrosis

40. A-6-yr child presents with recurrent episodes of gross hematuria for 2 yrs. He is likely to have: **[AI 08]**
    a. IgA nephropathy
    b. Wilms tumor
    c. Henoch-Schönlein Purpura (HSP)
    d. Neuroblastoma

41. A six-year-old male baby presents to a hospital with recurrent gross hematuria for 2 years. There is no h/o burning micturition or pyuria. Urine routine examination demonstrated no pus cells and urine culture was sterile. Serum C3 levels were normal. What is the most probable diagnosis? **[AI 08]**
    a. Wilm's tumor
    b. IgA nephropathy
    c. Post-streptococcal glomerulonephritis
    d. Urinary tract infection

42. The Finnish type of congenital nephrotic syndrome occurs due to gene mutation affecting the following protein: **[AI 06]**
    a. Podocin   b. Alpha-actinin
    c. Nephrin   d. CD2 activated protein

43. The most common cause of renal scarring in a 3 year old child is: **[AI 05]**
    a. Trauma
    b. Tuberculosis
    c. Vesicoureteral reflux induced pyelonephritis
    d. Interstitial nephritis

44. A child with recurrent urinary tract infections is most likely to show: **[AI 05, AIIMS Nov. 03]**
    a. Posterior urethral valves
    b. Vesicoureteric reflux
    c. Neurogenic bladder
    d. Renal and ureteric calculi

45. Which of the following is the most common renal cystic disease in infant? **[AI 05]**
    a. Polycystic kidney
    b. Simple renal cyst

    c. Unilateral renal dysplasia
    d. Calyceal cyst

46. Polycystic disease of the kidney may have cysts in all of the following organs except: **[AI 04]**
    a. Lung   b. Liver
    c. Pancreas   d. Spleen

47. Which one of the following statements is false with regard to pyuria in children? **[AI 03]**
    a. Presence of more than 5 WBC/hpf (high power field) for girls and more than 3 WBC/hpf for boys
    b. Infection can occur without pyuria
    c. Pyuria may be present without urinary tract infection
    d. Isolated pyuria is neither confirmatory nor diagnostic for urinary tract infection

48. Which of the following statement is false with regard to Xanthogranulomatous pyelonephritis in children: **[AI 03]**
    a. Often affects those younger than 8 year of age
    b. It affects the kidney focally more frequently than diffusely
    c. Boys are affected more frequently
    d. Clinical presentation is children is same as in adults

49. UTI in infant, true about: **[PGI Dec. 03]**
    a. Common in female infants
    b. If two episodes of UTI in females of 7 years occur, then cystometric evaluation needed
    c. If two episodes of UTI in male of 5 year occur then cystometric evaluation needed

50. Which one of the following is the most common cause of abdominal mass in neonates? **[AI 03]**
    a. Neuroblastoma
    b. Wilm's tumor
    c. Distended bladder
    d. Multicystic dysplastic kidneys

51. A six months old girl is having recurrent UTI. Ultrasound abdomen shows bilateral hydro-nephrosis. MCU (Micturating cystourethrogram) shows bilateral Grad IV vesicoureteral reflux. The treatment of choice is: **[AI 02]**
    a. Endoscopic injection of polyteflon at the ureteric orifices
    b. Ureteric reimplantation
    c. Bilateral ureterostomy
    d. Prophylactic antibiotics

52. Most common cause of urinary obstruction in a male infant is: **[AI 01]**
    a. Anterior urethral valves
    b. Posterior urethral valves
    c. Stone
    d. Stricture

53. A 5 years old child presents with a calculus of size 2 cm in the upper ureter. He also complains of hematuria. USG shows no further obstruction in the urinary tract. TT of choice for this patient would be: [AI 01]
    a. Ureterolithotomy   b. Endoscopic removal
    c. ESWL   d. Observation

54. A 5 years old child suffering from nephrotic syndrome is responding well to steroid therapy. What would be the most likely finding on light microscopy? [AI 01]
    a. No finding
    b. Basement membrane thickening
    c. Hypercellular glomeruli
    d. Fusion of foot processes

55. True about poststreptococcal glomerulonephritis is: [AI 2000]
    a. 50% of cases occur after pharyngitis
    b. Early treatment of pharyngitis eliminates the risk of pharyngitis
    c. Glomerulonephritis secondary to skin infection is more common in summer
    d. Recurrence is seen

56. A 4-month-old female presents with grade IV Vesicoureteral reflux without dilation of urinary bladder. The treatment of choice is: [AI 2000]
    a. Septran + Follow up
    b. Reimplantation of ureter
    c. Injection of collagen at ureteric orifices
    d. Bilateral ureterostomy

57. A 6-years-old girl presents with recurrent echo infection in urine. Ultrasound of abdomen shows Hydroureter and Hydronephrosis. Micturating cystourethrogram shows filling defect in urinary bladder. The likely diagnosis is: [AI 00]
    a. Sacrococcygeal Teratoma
    b. Vesicoureteric Reflux-grade II
    c. Duplication of Ureter
    d. Ureterocele

58. A 3-year-old male child diagnosed to have acute UTI developed left flank pain, on ultrasonogram the left ureter was found to be duplicated. The most probable site of opening of ectopic ureter will be: [AI 99]
    a. Prostatic urethra   b. Vas deferens
    c. Seminal vesicle   d. Trigone of bladder

59. Marker for the renal vasculitis in children is: [AI 98]
    a. Increased IgA level
    b. Low complement level
    c. Antineutrophilic cytoplasmic antibody titre
    d. Increase antinuclear antibody

60. Best response to steroids is observed with: [AI 96]
    a. Focal glomerulonephritis
    b. Lipoid nephrosis
    c. Membranous GN
    d. Membranoproliferative GN

61. Most common cause of hemolytic uremic syndrome is: [AI 96]
    a. E.coli   b. Shigella
    c. Salmonella   d. Pseudomonas

62. In shigella dysentery associated with hemolytic uremic syndrome, the false statement is: [AI 95]
    a. Leucocytosis
    b. Neurological abnormalities
    c. Hepatic failure
    d. Thrombotic angiopathy

63. All are seen in in Henoch schonlein purpura except: [AI 94]
    a. Thrombocytopenia   b. Glomerulonephritis
    c. Arthralgia   d. Abdominal pain

64. Nephrotic syndrome in children is caused by: [PGI Dec. 08]
    a. Minimal change disease
    b. RPGN
    c. MPGN
    d. FSGS
    e. Membranous nephritis

65. Which of the following is/are not the features of Henoch-Schönlein purpura (HSP): [PGI Dec. 08]
    a. Abdominal pain   b. Splinter haemorrhage
    c. Thrombocytopenia   d. Epistaxis
    e. Arthritis

66. Which of the following is included in definition of Nephrotic syndrome: [PGI June 04]
    a. Microalbuminuria
    b. Massive proteinuria
    c. Microscopic hematuria
    d. Edema
    e. Hyperlipidemia

67. True about Nephrotic syndrome in a child: [PGI June 03]
    a. Minimal Change disease is commonest cause
    b. Proteinuria of 4 gm/m²/hr is characteristic
    c. Cyclosporine and Azathioprine is mainstay of therapy
    d. Pretreatment biopsy is done in all cases
    e. Spontaneous bacterial peritonitis is associated with it

68. Nephrotic syndrome is characterised by: [PGI Dec. 02]
    a. Proteinuria   b. Hyperlipidemia
    c. Oedema   d. Hematuria
    e. Lipiduria

69. **Renal causes of acute renal failure include:**
    [PGI Dec. 01]
    a. Minimal change disease
    b. Renal amyloidosis
    c. Preeclampsia
    d. Malignant hypertension
    e. Hemolytic uremic syndrome

70. **Post-streptococcal glomerulonephritis is associated with:** [PGI Dec. 01]
    a. Follows skin and throat infection
    b. Antibiotic treatment induces remission
    c. Is a cause of chronic renal failure in majority of children
    d. Low complement level occurs
    e. Caused by all serotypes

71. **Recurrent gross hematuria is seen in:**
    [PGI Dec. 2000]
    a. Alport's syndrome   b. Ig A nephropathy
    c. Focal segmental GN   d. DM

72. **Characteristic of acute G.N:**   [PGI June 2000]
    a. RBC cast   b. Hemoglobinuria
    c. Proteinuria   d. Broad cast

73. **Child with BP 190/110, pedal edema ++; facial edema ascites - absent. Gross hematuria diagnosis is:** [PGI June 00]

    a. Acute GN   b. Nephrotic syndrome
    c. Renal thrombosis   d. Renal amyloidosis

74. **All are true about minimal change GN except:**
    [PGI Dec. 99]
    a. Selective proteinuria
    b. Ig G deposition in mesangium
    c. Common in age group of 2–9 years
    d. Responds to steroids

75. **Which is seen in nephrotic syndrome:** [PGI June 99]
    a. Low serum calcium   b. Raised AT-III
    c. Low lipid   d. Platelet activation

76. **Which is seen in nephrotic syndrome:** [PGI June 99]
    a. Low serum phosphate
    b. Normal level of 1, 25 dihydroxy vitamin D3
    c. Low serum calcium
    d. Increased hydroxyproline in urine

77. **A child has diarrhea since 8 days. He is dehydrated and urine output is reduced. Which of the following is not correct regarding the renal failure in this patient?**
    a. Urinary sodium > 40 mEq/L
    b. Urinary osmolality > 500 mOsmol/kg
    c. FeNa<l%g
    d. BUN/Creatinine >20

QUESTIONS OF OTHER EXAMINATIONS

1. **An infant with severe dehydration secondary to diarrhoea suddenly presents with proteins and blood in urine. The most probable diagnosis is:**
   [DPG 09]
   a. Renal vein thrombosis
   b. Pyelonephritis
   c. Acute glomerulonephritis
   d. Lower nephrosis

2. **Which of the following is not seen in Henoch-Schönlein purpura:** [DPG 08]
   a. Purpura   b. Abdominal pain
   c. Seizure   d. Arthralgia

3. **Most common infection in a child nephrotic syndrome:** [MAHE 07, 08]
   a. Spontaneous bacterial pneumonitis
   b. Pneumonia
   c. UTI
   d. Cellulitis

4. **Straining ad dribbling of urine in a male infant with recurrent urinary tract infection should lead to suspicion of:** [UPSC 07]
   a. Vesico-ureteric reflux
   b. Posterior urethral valve

   c. Pelvic ureteric junction obstruction
   d. Phimosis

5. **A four-year-old presents with mild fever, malaise, purpura, arthritis, abdominal and microscopic hematuria. What would be the most likely diagnosis?** [UPSC 07]
   a. Thrombasthenia
   b. Idiopathic thrombocytopenia
   c. Systemic lupus erythematous
   d. Henoch-Schönlein purpura

6. **A 3-year-old child presents with four days history of puffiness of face, fever and tea coloured urine. During the course of his disease, he can have any of the complications except:** [UPSC 06]
   a. Hypokalemia
   b. Hypertensive encephalopathy
   c. Acute renal failure
   d. Acidosis

7. **Potter syndrome is associated with:** [MAHE 05]
   a. Renal anomalies
   b. Severe oligohydramnios
   c. Flattened nose
   d. All of the above

8. **Malformations of the following organ system of the fetus are found to be most commonly associated with single umbilical artery:** [SGPGI 05]
   a. Central nervous system
   b. Cardiovascular
   c. Genitourinary
   d. Skeletal

9. **A 3-year-old girl presents with recurrent UTI. On USG shows hydronephrosis with filling defect and negative shadow of bladder with no ectopic orifice:** [UP 04]
   a. Vesicoureteric reflux
   b. Hydronephrosis
   c. Ureterocele
   d. Sacrococcygeal teratoma

10. **RBC cast in urine is seen in:** [UPSC 2000, JIPMER 93]
    a. Nephrotic syndrome
    b. Renal amyloidosis
    c. CRF
    d. Glomerulonephritis

11. **Unilateral hydronephrosis is due to:** [AMC 99]
    a. Bladder neck contracture
    b. Stricture urethra
    c. Carcinoma of prostate
    d. Ureterocele

12. **Cylindrical dilation of renal tubules is seen in:** [Jipmer 95]
    a. Polycystic disease of kidney
    b. Medullary cystic disease
    c. Wilms tumor
    d. Lipoid nephrosis

13. **Posterior urethral valve is diagnosed on micturating cytometrogram by:** [KCET 95]
    a. Dilation of posterior urethra
    b. Bladder neck contracture
    c. Vesico-ureteric reflux
    d. Bladder wall hypertrophy

14. **Choose among the following the most important lab finding in nephrotic syndrome:** [TN 95]
    a. B-J protein
    b. Hyperkalemia
    c. Hypoalbuminemia
    d. Hypercholesterolemia

15. **The commonest type of renal lesion in children is:** [TN 95]
    a. Lipoid nephrosis
    b. MPGN
    c. FSGS
    d. Diffuse glomerulosclerosis

16. **Which is incorrect about hemolytic uremic syndrome:** [JIPMER 91]
    a. Always fatal
    b. Burr cells are present
    c. Acute renal failure
    d. Viral Prodrome

17. **Ectopic ureter may be frequently associated with:** [Jipmer 81, AMU 89]
    a. Oliguria
    b. Dysuria
    c. Bilateral hydroureter
    d. Paradoxical incontinence

ANSWERS

MULTIPLE CHOICE QUESTIONS

1. **(d)** ARPKD (Ref: Rudolph 22nd E/P1740)
   Causes of medullary nephrocalcinosis in children:
   - Hypercalciuria.
   - **Hyperoxaluria.**
   - Drugs like **furosemide**, methylxanthines, vitamin D, glucocorticoids, gentamicin and thiazides.
   - **Bartter syndrome.**
   - Distal RTA.

2. **(b)** HSP (Ref: Rudolph 22nd E/P1721)
   - Diagnosis of HSP is confirmed by presence of **palpable purpura with a normal platelet count** along with at least one of the following: **abdominal pain, arthritis or arthralgia, mesangial Ig A deposition on renal biopsy**.

3. **(c)** Mesangial deposits of Ig A (Ref: Rudolph 22nd E/P1720–21)
   - Purpura, joint swelling and hematuria confirm the diagnosis of HSP.
   - In HSP Ig A deposits can be seen on renal biopsy.

4. **(b)** Hepatic cyst and fibrosis (Ref: Rudolph 22nd E/P1702)
   - **Liver** is the most common extrarenal site of involvement characterised by **fibrosis and cysts**; however cysts of pancreas, spleen and biliary tree (Caroli disease) can also be seen.

5. **(a)** Takayasu aortoarteritis (Ref: Sternberg's surgical pathology/P1929)
   - Most common cause of renal artery stenosis in adults is atherosclerosis.
   - Most common cause of renal artery stenosis in children in India is Takayasu's aortoarteritis and in western countries is fibromuscular dysplasia.

6. **(b)** NPHS2 (Ref: Rudolph 22nd E/P1725)
   - Most common cause of steroid resistant NS is FSGS which is caused by mutation of NPHS2 gene which codes for podocin.

7. **(d)** Severity of renal failure (Ref: Gary Pediatric emergency/P1115)
   - Schwartz formula for creatinine clearance i.e.
     $$C_{cr} = K \times L/S_{cr}$$
   - K is a constant that depends on age, muscle mass and method of creatinine evaluation.
   - L is the length of baby.

8. **(b)** NPHS 2 (Ref: Rudolph 22nd E/P1724)
   - Steroid resistant nephrotic syndrome (SRNS) is most commonly seen in focal segmental glomerulosclerosis (FSGS).
   - FSGS is an AR disorder caused by mutation of NPHS2 gene which codes for slit diaphragm protein podocin.

9. **(d)** Bacteria in gram stain (Ref: Rudolph 22nd E/P952)
   - Microscopic examination of urine showing **1 bacterium per oil-immersion field on gram stain** is also a **specific test** as it equals to 100,000 bacteria/ml of urine.
   - The sensitivity is 82% and specificity is 92% for UTI.

10. **(c)** Posterior urethral valves (Ref: Rudolph 22nd E/P1743)
    - This is a case of posterior urethral valves which has been complicated with UTI.
    - Urine retention leads to bladder distention which causes prominent suprapubic area.

11. **(b)** Postnatal scarring may occur even in the absence of urinary tract infections (Ref: Nelson 18th E/P2229)
    - **Renal scarring** is not only caused by **infection** but also by **compression force on kidney** due to elevated bladder pressure.

12. **(c)** Ig A (Ref: Rudolph 22nd E/P1720–21)
    - HSP is characterised by mesangial deposition of Ig A.

13. **(c)** Bartter syndrome (Ref: Nelson 19th E/P1763)
    - This is a case of alkalosis and nephrocalcinosis with decrease in serum potassium, sodium and chloride which is sufficient to make a diagnosis of Bartter syndrome.
    - In primary hyperaldosteronism serum sodium is always elevated
    - In distal renal tubular acidosis there is metabolic acidosis.
    - In pseudohypoaldosteronism serum potassium is increased.

14. **(b)** Acute tubular necrosis (Ref: IAP 4th E/P738)
    - The most common causes of acute tubular necrosis is renal hypoperfusion followed by ECF volume contraction in acute gastroenteritis, severe renal vasoconstriction, nephrotoxic agents, shock and sepsis.
    - In this case the patient has gastroenteritis followed by sever hypotension which has lead to tubular necrosis. Hence this is a case of acute tubular necrosis.

15. **(b)** Cyclophosphamide (Ref: Nelson 19th E/P1756)
    - Patient who relapse on alternate day period or within 28 days of stopping prednisolone are called as **steroid dependent**. Patients who fail to respond within 8 week are called as **steroid resistant**.

- Steroid resistant or dependent patients should be treated with **cyclophosphamide;** however high dose pulse methylprednisolone, immunomodulators (Cyclosporine, tacrolimus or mycophenolate mofetil), ACE inhibitors and angiotensin receptor blockers may also be beneficial.
- Pulse methyl prednisolone should not be given as he has developed long term side effects of steroids.

16. (a) Suprapubic aspiration (Ref: CPDT 19th E/P671)

"In infants and young children, bladder catheterisation or **suprapubic collection** is necessary in most cases to avoid contaminated samples."

17. (a) Treat as an acute episode of urinary tract infection (Ref: Nelson 19th E/P1787)
- Urine culture is the mainstay of diagnosis. For diagnosis **>100,000 colonies** or >10,000 colonies with symptomatic child is required.
- Hence this is a case of UTI and should be treated with antibiotics.

18. (b) Older girls (Ref: Nelson 19th E/P1791)
- Vesicoureteral reflux in **newborns** is more common in **males** i.e. about 90% of cases.
- In **older children females** are more commonly affected with the average age of 2–3 years.

19. (a) Antibiotic prophylaxis (Ref: Nelson 19th E/P1791/ P1793)

Treatment of Vesicoureteral reflux:
- The initial management of choice is **daily antibiotic prophylaxis** till the spontaneous resolution of reflux or 5 years of age or child attains bladder control.
- Surgical intravesical and extravesical ureteral reimplantation is reserved for patients who do not respond to medical management.

20. (b) Cyclophosphamide (Ref: Nelson 19th E/P1756)
- Patient who relapse on alternate day period or within 28 days of stopping prednisolone are called as **steroid dependent.** Patients who fail to respond within 8 week are called as **steroid resistant.**
- Steroid resistant or dependent patients should be treated with **cyclophosphamide;** however high dose pulse methylprednisolone, immunomodulators (Cyclosporine, tacrolimus or mycophenolate mofetil), ACE inhibitors and angiotensin receptor blockers may also be beneficial.
- Pulse methyl prednisolone should not be given as he has developed long term side effects of steroids.

21. (b) Vesicoureteric reflux (Ref: Nelson 19th E/P1791)
- In children primary vesicoureteric reflux is most common cause of recurrent urinary tract infection.
- Secondary causes of vesicoureteric reflux like neurogenic bladder and posterior urethral valves are less common cause of reflux.

22. (d) Nephronopthisis (Ref: Rudolph 22nd E/P1704-05)
- The patient of Nephronopthisis have polyuria, polydipsia and night time fluid intake.
- Growth retardation and **anaemia** is also seen.
- There is salt loss and hence hypertension usually does not develop.
- USG shows a normal to small size kidneys and loss of corticomedullary differentiation.

23. (a) Voiding cystourethrography (Ref: Rudolph 22nd E/P1743)

Diagnosis of posterior urethral valves:
- The investigation of choice is **voiding cysto-urethrogram (VCUG).**
- Prenatal diagnosis can be done by USG which shows bilateral hydroureteronephrosis and a keyhole appearance.

24. (a) Diabetes insipidus (Ref: Nelson 19th E/P1763)
- A serum osmolarity of >290 mOsm/kg is seen in diabetes insipidus.
- The other supporting findings are polydipsia, polyuria and a decreased urinary specific gravity.

25. (b) Ig A nephropathy (Ref: CPDT 19th E/P658)
- Gross hematuria can be seen in Ig A nephropathy, PSGN and HSP, but what goes in favour of IgA nephropathy here is the onset of hematuria after 1 day of upper respiratory tract infection.
- After upper respiratory tract infection symptoms of Ig A nephropathy appear 1–2 days whereas that of HSP and PSGN appears after 1–3 weeks.

26. (b) Nephronopthisis (Ref: Rudolph 22nd E/P1704-05)
- The patient of Nephronopthisis have polyuria, polydipsia and night time fluid intake.
- Growth retardation and **anaemia** is also seen.
- There is salt loss and hence hypertension usually does not develop.
- USG shows a normal to small size kidneys and loss of corticomedullary differentiation.

27. (b) Send urine for culture and sensitivity and start IV antibiotics immediately (Ref: Nelson 19th E/ P1787)
- Emperical treatment should be started with trimethopsin-sulfamethoxazole in uncomplicated UTI and 3rd generation cephalosporin or aminoglycoside in complicated UTI.
- After urine culture antimicrobial therapy is directed against the specific pathogen.
- This is a case of complicated UTI and hence 1V antibiotics should be started after sending urine sample for culture.

28. (a) ESWL (Ref: Rudolph 22nd E/P1740)
Treatment of renal and ureteral stones:

Renal stones<1 cm	ESWL
Renal stones>2cm	Percutaeous nephrolithotomy
Lower pole stones	**ESWL**
Proximal Ureteral stone	**ESWL**
Distal ureteral stone	Ureteroscopy

29. (b) Mesangioproliferative glomerulonephritis (Ref: Nelson 19th E/P1738)
- Ig A nephropathy is a type of mesangio-proliferative glomerulonephritis.

30. (a) Cotrimaxozole (Ref: Nelson 19th E/P1793)

31. (a) Selective proteinuria (Ref: Nelson 19th E/P1755)
- This is a case of nephrotic syndrome which is characterised by selective proteinuria.

32. (a) Bulbar urethra (Ref: Rudolph 22nd E/P1741)
- The most common site of ectopic ureter opening is **urethra** i.e. **posterior urethra in males** and urethra near the bladder neck in females.
- In males the other sites of opening are vas deferens, **seminal vesicles** and **distal trigoneof bladder**; and the patient presents with **urinary tract infection** without incontinence.
- In females the other sites of opening are bladder neck, vagina, uterus and fallopian tube; and the presenting symptom is **urinary incontinence**.

33. (a) Micturating cystourethrogram (Ref: Nelson 19th E/P1791)

34. (b) Serum fibrinogen (Ref: Nelson 19th E/P1756)
- Thromboembolic events can be associated due to **increase in fibrinogen** and thrombin; and decrease in AT III and protein C and S.

35. (c) Prerenal azotemia **(Ref: Nelson 19th E/P1768)**
- The patient develops anuria secondary to depletion of blood volume and hence is a case of prerenal ARF or azotemia.

36. (c) Single umbilical artery (Ref: Nelson 19th E/P1784)
Unilateral renal agenesis is associated with:
- Contralateral vesicoureteral reflux and uretero-pelvic junction obstruction.
- Ipsilateral absent vas deferens, ureter and trigone of bladder.
- **Single umbilical artery.**
- Mayer-Rokitansky-Kuster-Hauser syndrome in female.

37. (a) Proteinuria (Ref: Nelson 19th E/P1755)
- Most important feature of nephrotic syndrome is proteinuria.

38. (a) No Ig G deposits or C3 deposition on renal biopsy (Ref: Nelson 19th E/P1755–57)

- This is clearly as case of nephrotic syndrome in which complements level is normal and neither complement nor Ig G deposition is seen.

39. (a) Autosomal dominant (Ref: Rudolph 22nd E/P1701)
- Infantile polycystic kidney disease is an autosomal recessive disorder characterised by mutation of PKHD1 gene.

40. (a) IgA nephropathy (Ref: Rudolph 22nd/P1716)
- Recurrent gross hematuria can be seen in both IgA nephropathy and HSP, but what goes in favour of IgA nephropathy in this question is absence of other features of HSP like rash, arthralgia and abdominal pain.
- After upper respiratory tract infection symptoms of Ig A nephropathy appear 1–2 days whereas that of HSP appears after 1–3 weeks.

41. (b) Ig A nephropathy (Ref: CPDT 19th E/P658)
- Gross hematuria can be seen with both Ig A nephro-pathy and PSGN, but what goes in favour of Ig A nephropathy is a normal serum C3 levels. Usually serum C3 levels are decreased in PSGN.

42. (c) Nephrin (Ref: Nelson 19th E/P1757)
Congenital nephrotic syndrome can be caused by mutation of NPHS1 and NPHS2 genes.
- NPHS1 gene codes for nephrin and its mutation leads to Finnish type nephrotic syndrome.
- NPHS2 gene codes for podocin and its mutation leads to FSGS.

43. (c) Vesicoureteral reflux induced pyelonephritis (Ref: Nelson 19th E/P1791)
- Vesicoureteral reflux is the most common cause of **recurrent urinary tract infection.**
- Infection is followed by **renal scarring**, hyper-tension and growth retardation.

44. (b) Vesicoureteric reflux (Ref: Nelson 19th E/P1791)
- In children primary vesicoureteric reflux is most common cause of recurrent urinary tract infection.
- Secondary causes of vesicoureteric reflux like neurogenic bladder and posterior urethral valves are less common cause of reflux.

45. (c) Unilateral renal dysplasia (Ref: Nelson 19th E/P1794)
- **Multicystic dysplastic kidney** is the **most common form of renal cystic disease in infants** and is also the **most common cause of an abdominal mass in neonate**.

46. (a) Lung (Ref: Rudolph 22nd E/P1702)
- **Liver** is the most common extrarenal site of involve-ment characterised by **fibrosis and cysts**; however cysts of **pancreas**, **spleen** and biliary tree (Caroli disease) can also be seen.

47. (a) Presence of more than 5 WBC/hpf (high power field) for girls and more than 3 WBC/hpf for boys (Ref: CPDT 19th E/P671)

- Microscopic analysis showing pyuria i.e. **>5 W.B.Cs/hpf** is suggestive of infection; however it is **not confirmatory** as **pyuria can be seen without infection** and **infection can be present without pyuria.**

48. (a) Often affects those younger than 8 year of age (Ref: Jeffrey's Pediatric urology/P 60–61)

- **Xanthogranulomatous pyelonephritis** is most commonly caused by **proteus**; and is associated with staghorn renal calculus or other obstructive lesions.
- Children from **infancy till 16 years** of age are commonly affected.
- In **children focal renal involvement is seen** as compared to diffuse involvement in adults.
- It is characterised by granulomatous inflammation and presence of histiocytes and foamy cells around yellow colour nodules.
- In children **partial nephrectomy** is usually sufficient for the focal disease.

49. (b) and (c) If two episodes of UTI in females of 7 years occur, then cystometric evaluation needed and If two episodes of UTI in male of 5 year occur then cystometric evaluation needed (Ref: Nelson 19th E/P1787)

- **Males** are more commonly affected during **infancy** and females after infancy.
- **VCUG** should be done to rule out the obstructive lesions. It is indicate in a **male child with more than one UTI** and a **female child with more than two UTIs within 6 months.**

50. (d) Multicystic dysplastic kidneys (Ref: Nelson 19th E/P1784)

- Multicystic dysplastic kidney is the most common cause of an abdominal mass in a newborn.

51. (d) Prophylactic antibiotics (Ref: Nelson 19th E/P1793)
Treatment of Vesicoureteral reflux:
- The initial management of choice is **daily antibiotic prophylaxis** till the spontaneous resolution of reflux or 5 years of age or child attains bladder control.
- Surgical intravesical and extravesical ureteral re-implantation is reserved for patients who do not respond to medical management.

52. (b) Posterior urethral valves (Rudolph 22nd E/P1743)

"Posterior urethral valves are the most common cause of lower urinary obstruction in male infants and the most common cause of obstructive uropathy leading to childhood renal failure."

53. (b) ESWL (Ref: Rudolph 22nd E/P1740)

54. (d) Fusion of foot processes (Ref: Nelson 19th E/P1755)

- Most responsive cause of nephrotic syndrome is minimal change disease which is characterised by effacement or fusion of the foot processes or podocytes.

55. (c) Glomerulonephritis secondary to skin infection is more common in summer (Ref: Nelson 19th E/P1740)

- The patient develops glomerulonephritis with **streptococcal pharyngitis** usually in **winter** after 1–2 weeks of infection and with **streptococcal pyoderma** in **summer** after 3–6 weeks of infection.
- **Penicillin** is usually given for infection however it **does not alter the course or risk of glomerulonephritis.**
- **Recurrence** is very rarely seen.

56. (a) Septran + Follow up (Ref: Nelson 19th E/P1793)

57. (d) Ureterocele (Ref: Nelson 19th E/P1799)

- VCUG is the investigation of choice for ureterocele which shows a **filling defect in bladder** and **drooping lilly** appearance of kidney. USG kidney shows **hydroureter** and **hydronephrosis.**

58. (a) Prostatic urethra (Ref: Nelson 19th E/P1799)

- The most common site of ectopic ureter opening is **urethra** i.e. posterior urethra in males and urethra near the bladder neck.

59. (a) Increased Ig A levels (Ref: Rudolph 22nd E/P1720-21)

- Renal vasculitis is seen in HSP which is characterised by raised Ig A levels.

60. (b) Lipoid nephrosis (Ref: Nelson 19th E/P1755)

- Best response to steroid is seen with MCD, also called as lipoid nephrosis.

61. (a) Shigella (Ref: Nelson 18th E/P2207)

- In most of the cases HUS is preceded by 1 week with gastroenteritis with **shigella** in developing countries and a shiga like toxin producing **E.coli** strain in developed countries.

62. (c) Hepatic failure (Ref: Rudolph 22d E/P1728)

- Hepatomegaly is seen in 40% cases of HUS; however hepatic failure is usually not seen.
- Significant leucocytosis and mild reticulocytosis can be seen.
- Neurological abnormalities like hypersomnolence, seizures and coma can be associated.

63. (a) Thrombocytopenia (Ref: Rudolph 22nd E/P1721)

- HSP is characterised by purpura in the presence of normal platelet count.

64. (a), (c) and (d) Minimal change disease, MPGN and FSGS (Ref: Nelson 19th E/P1755–57)

- Primary nephrotic syndrome consists of 3 clinical entities named **minimal change disease (MCD)**, mesangial proliferation and **focal segmental glomerulosclerosis (FSGS)**.

- Secondary NS is caused by other renal conditions like membranous nephropathy, **MPGN**, APSGN and HSP.

65. **(b), (c)** and **(d)** Splinter haemorrhage, Thrombocytopenia, Epistaxis (Ref: Rudolph 22nd E/P1720-21)
    - Diagnosis of HSP is confirmed by presence of **palpable purpura with a normal platelet count** along with at least one of the following: **abdominal pain, arthritis or arthralgia, mesangial Ig A deposition on renal biopsy.**

66. **(b), (d)** and **(e)** Massive proteinuria, Edema and Hyperlipidemia (Ref: Rudolph 22nd E/P1722)
    - Nephrotic syndrome (NS) is combination of clinical findings like **massive proteinuria, hypoalbuminemia, edema** and **hyperlipidemia.**

67. **(a)** and **(e)** Minimal Change disease is commonest cause, Spontaneous bacterial peritonitis is associated with it (Ref: Nelson 19th E/P1755–57, Rudolph 22nd E/P1725)
    - MCD is the most common cause of NS in children.
    - Proteinuria of more than 40 mg or .4 gm /m² /hr is characteristic.
    - Glucocorticoids are the mainstay of therapy.
    - Pretreatment biopsy should be done in resistant cases like FSGS and is not required in MCD.
    - Spontaneous bacterial peritonitis is the most common complication associated.

68. **(a), (b), (c)** and **(e)** Proteinuria, Hyperlipidemia, Oedema and Lipiduria (Ref: Nelson 19th E/P1755–57)
    - Nephrotic syndrome (NS) is combination of clinical findings like **massive proteinuria, hypoalbuminemia, edema, hyperlipidemia** and **lipiduria.**

69. **(e)** Hemolytic uremic syndrome (Ref: Nelson 19th E/P1768)
    Renal ARF can be caused by diseases of kidney like:
    - APSGN
    - HSP
    - **HUS**
    - MPGN
    - Lupus nephritis
    - Anti GBM disease
    - Acute tubular necrosis.

70. **(a)** and **(d)** Follows skin and throat infection and Low complement level occurs (Ref: Rudolph 22nd E/P1712)
    - Acute poststreptococcal glomerulonephritis is caused by autoimmune injury only due to **selective nephritogenic strains of streptococcus.**
    - The patient develops glomerulonephritis with **streptococcal pharyngitis** usually in winter after 1–2 weeks of infection and with **streptococcal pyoderma** in summer after 3–6 weeks of infection.

- The diagnosis is based on the clinical findings along with evidence of recent poststreptococcal infection and a **low C3 level.**
- The treatment is usually supportive because most of the cases resolve spontaneously and **rarely may progress to renal failure.**
- **Penicillin** is usually given for infection however it **does not alter the course of glomerulonephritis.**

71. **(b)** Ig A nephropathy (Ref: CPDT 19th E/P658)
    - Recurrent gross hematuria is seen in Ig A nephropathy.

72. **(a)** RBC cast (Ref: Rudolph 22nd E/P1714)
    - RBC casts are characteristic of acute glomerulonephritis.

73. **(a)** Acute GN (Ref: Rudolph 22nd E/P1714)
    - Gross hematuria, edema and hypertension are sufficient to make a diagnosis of acute glomerulonephritis.

74. **(b)** Ig G deposition in mesangium (Ref: Nelson 19th E/P1755–57)
    - Ig G deposition is not seen in MCD.
    - It is most commonly seen in age group of 2–6 years.

75. **(a)** Hypocalcemia (Ref: IAP Textbook of pediatrics 4th E/P749)

"**Hypocalcemia** is seen due to reduction in protein bound calcium secondary to hypoalbuminemia. Occasionally, low ionized calcium levels are seen, which results from urinary loss of vitamin D binding globulin and 25-hydroxyvitamin D3 and may cause tetany."

76. **(a)** and **(c)** Low serum phosphate and low serum calcium (Ref: IAP Textbook of pediatrics 4th E/P749)

"**Hypocalcemia** is seen due to reduction in protein bound calcium secondary to hypoalbuminemia. Occasionally, low ionized calcium levels are seen, which results from **urinary loss of vitamin D binding globulin and 25-hydroxyvitamin D3** and may cause tetany."

- Vitamin D is essential for absorption of **calcium** and **phosphorous** and loss of vitamin may cause deficiency of both.

77. **(d)** Urinary sodium > 40 mEq/L (Ref: Rudolph 22nd E/P1709)
    - This is clearly a case of prerenal ARF caused by diarrhoea and dehydration. The features of prerenal ARF are:

Values	Prerenal ARF
Urinary specific gravity	>1020
Urine/plasma creatinine	>40
Urine sodium	**<20**
FENa	**<1%**
Urine osmolarity	**>500 mOsm/kg**

1. (a) Renal vein thrombosis (Ref: CPDT 19th E/P660)
- Renal vein thrombosis may result from sepsis or dehydration in infants.
- The infant presents with sudden development of abdominal mass accompanied by hematuria and proteinuria.
  Anticoagulation with heparin is the treatment of choice.

2. (c) Seizure (Ref: Rudolph 22nd E/P1721)

3. (a) Spontaneous bacterial pneumonitis (Ref: Nelson 19th E/P1756)

4. (b) Posterior urethral valve (Ref: Rudolph 22nd E/P1743)
- Dribbling of urine and recurrent urinary tract infection is seen in posterior urethral valve.

5. (d) Henoch-Schönlein purpura (Ref: Rudolph 22nd E/P1721)

6. (a) Hypokalemia (Ref: Rudolph 22nd E/P1714)

"In patients with more severe renal insufficiency, **hyperkalemia**, hypophosphatemia and acidosis are likely to occur and will require medical management."

7. (d) All of the above (Ref: Nelson 19th E/P1783)
Bilateral renal agenesis or Potter syndrome is associated with:
- Characteristic facies — **Flat nose**, widely separated eyes with epicanthal folds and low set ears
- **Oligohydramnios**
- Pulmonary hypoplasia

8. (c) Genitourinary (Ref: Nelson 19th E/P1784, Keeling Neonatal and fetal pathology/P72)
Single umbilical artery is associated with:
- Maternal diabetes mellitus
- Maternal smoking
- Preterm and LBW infants
- Congenital anomalies — VACTERAL anomalies, **genitourinary anomalies** (most commonly associated), esophageal and anorectal atresia
- Trisomy 21, 13 and 18; and Zell-Weger syndrome

9. (c) Ureterocele (Ref: Rudolph 22d E/P1742)

10. (d) Glomerulonephritis (Ref: Nelson 19th E/P1740)

11. (d) Ureterocele (Ref: Rudolph 22nd E/P1742)

12. (a) Polycystic kidney disease (Ref: Rudolph 22nd E/P1701)

13. (a) Dilation of prostatic urethra (Ref: Nelson 19th E/P1802)

14. (c) Hypoalbuminemia (Ref: Ref: Nelson 19th E/P1755)

15. (a) Lipoid nephrosis (Ref: Nelson 19th E/P1755)

16. (a) Always fatal (Ref: Rudolph 22nd E/P1727)
- Mortality of 3–5 % is associated with HUS.
- It is the most common cause of renal failure in young children.
- Though E.coli is the most common cause some viruses like Coxscakie, Echo, influenza, varicella, HIV and EBV can also be the causative agent.

17. (d) Paradoxical incontinence (Ref: Nelson 19th E/P1799)

Respiratory System

9

The pediatric airway is **short** and **narrow**; and larynx is more anterior than adults and extends from C_2–C_4. The narrowest part of pediatric airway is **subglottis** and the epiglottis is of **omega shaped**.

DISORDERS OF AIRWAY OBSTRUCTION

The disorders causing airway obstruction can be broadly classified based on obstruction during inspiration and expiration. Airway obstruction in children presents with stridor (high pitch inhalational sound), hoarseness and retractions of intercostal and suprasternal muscles.

Inspiratory Obstructive Disorders

Inspiratory obstruction can be caused by congenital disorders like laryngomalacia, laryngeal web, atresia, cleft and cyst; layryngocele, and subglottic hemangioma. Acquired disorders causing obstruction are infectious diseases like laryngotracheobronchiolitis (croup), acute epiglottitis and bacterial tracheitis (pseudomembranous croup); and **vocal cord paralysis**.

Laryngomalacia

Laryngomalacia is a congenital disorder characterised by underdevelopment of supraglottic structures. It is the **most common cause of stridor in infants**. The stridor characteristically **worsens in supine position**. Direct laryngoscopy shows an inspiratory collapse of an **omega shaped epiglottis**. It resolves spontaneously and do not require any treatment.

Laryngotracheobronchiolitis (Croup)

This is the most common infectious cause of stridor in children. The most common cause is **parainfluenza type I virus**; however RSV, adenovirus, influenza virus, rubeola virus and mycoplasma pneumonae can also cause croup. The characteristic presentation is a harsh cough called as "**barking seal or dog**". X ray of neck shows **steeple sign** caused by tapering of subglottic airway. **Mild cases i.e. no stridor at rest** and seen on **crying**, agitation and activity can be treated with **hydration** and **corticosteroids (I/M dexamethasone or inhaled budesonide)**. Treatment of moderate and severe cases i.e. stridor at rest consists of **oxygenation, nebulization with epinephrine** and **corticosteroids (I/M dexamethasone or inhaled budesonide)**. Nebulization with epinephrine is used to relieve the acute symptoms of upper airway obstruction. The mainstay of treatment is **corticosteroids** which not only decrease the symptoms but also improve the outcome.

Epiglottitis

Acute epiglottitis or supraglottitis is most commonly caused by *H. influenzae;* however in patients with vaccination the common cause are pneumococcus, staphylococcus aureus and group A beta haemolytic streptococci. It presents suddenly with high fever, throat pain and muffled voice or "**hot potato**". The child prefers to sit and lean forward with neck extension for better airway and such a position is called as "**sniffing dog position**" or "**tripod position**". X ray of the neck shows a characteristic **"thumb print"** sign because of round and thick epiglottis. The mainstay of treatment is securing airway by **endotracheal intubation** followed by **antibiotic therapy**.

Bacterial tracheitis

Bacterial tracheitis is most commonly caused by **Staphylococcus aureus**. The patient presents like croup and epiglottitis. Subglottic stenosis and steeple sign can also be seen as in case of epiglottitis. The mainstay of treatment is antibiotic therapy along with proper airway management.

Expiratory Obstructive Disorders

Expiratory obstruction to airway can be caused by foreign body aspiration, GERD, tracheomalacia, bronchomalacia, bronchopulmonary dysplasia, bronchiectasis and bronchiolitis obliterans.

Foreign Body Aspiration

Most of the children are below 3 years of age and the most common object causing obstruction are nuts. The most common site of foreign body lodgement is **right bronchus**. Most commonly children present **acutely with coughing followed by respiratory distress, aphonia, drooling and stridor. Unilateral wheeze** or **decreased breath sounds** on examination confirms the diagnosis. If the foreign body is located in lower respiratory tract it is removed by **rigid bronchoscopy** and if in upper respiratory tract it can be removed by **Heimlich maneuverer** or **Magill forceps**. The complications that can be seen on delayed removal are pneumonia, bronchiectasis, hemoptysis and atelectasis.

Bronchiolitis Obliterans

The predisposing condition for bronchiolitis obliterans are infections (most common is adenovirus), inflammatory diseases (JRA, SLE, SJS), inhalation of toxic gases, chronic rejection in lung transplant patients and graft versus host disease in bone marrow transplantation. The basic pathology is obstruction of the airway due to inflammation and fibrosis. The classical presentation in case of respiratory infection is **initial improvement followed by deterioration manifesting as fever, cough, respiratory distress, cyanosis and dyspnea**. Chest X ray and CT scan shows **hyperlucency** with patchy infiltrates. Pulmonary function test shows **obstructive pattern**.

INFECTION OF THE AIRWAY

Bronchiolitis

Acute bronchiolitis is most commonly caused by **respiratory syncytial virus (RSV)**; however other microorganisms like parainfluenza virus, human metapneumovirus, **influenza virus**, adenovirus, **mycoplasma**, chlamydia and pneumocystis jiroveci can also cause bronchiolitis. It is most commonly seen in **children less than 3 years of age**. The child usually presents with fever, sneezing and rhinorrhea followed by more severe symptoms like cough, dyspnea, tachypnea, apnea and **wheezing**. These children are at higher risk for development of **bronchial asthma**. Chest X ray usually shows **hyperinflation** and patchy atelectasis. **WBC count is within normal limits**. Bronchodilators (β_2 agonists, anticholinergics), epinephrine nebulization and corticosteroids are used for **symptomatic management**. Antiviral drug **ribavirin** is given by aerosol is the drug of choice for bronchiolitis caused by **RSV**.

Pneumonia

Pneumonia is inflammation of parenchyma of the lungs caused by bacteria, viruses and other factors causing insult like aspiration (**right upper lobe involvement**), drugs and chemicals. The most common cause of bacterial pneumonia is **pneumococcus**. The most common virus causing pneumonia is **respiratory syncytial virus**; however other viruses like **influenza, parainfluenza**, adenovirus, rhinovirus and metapneumovirus account for some cases. Atypical pneumonia commonly seen in children > 5 years of age can be caused by organisms like chlamydia, mycoplasma and pneumocystis.

Clinical Presentation

- Pneumonia is often preceded by symptoms of upper respiratory tract infection like cough and rhinorrhoea. This is followed by fever which is higher in bacterial pneumonia as compared to viral. The other findings are tachypnea, cyanosis, retraction of respiratory muscles.

- **Staphylococcal pneumonia** is associated with severe parenchymal destruction characterised by **pneumatoceles, pneumothorax, empyema**, microabscess and cavitation.
- **Slow resolving pneumonia** is characterised by the presence of symptoms and x ray features of pneumonia beyond the expected time after treatment. The initial investigation of choice is a **repeat X-ray**. This should be followed by **bronchoscopy** to rule out endobronchial obstruction which is a common cause of slow resolving pneumonia.
- **Recurrent pneumonia** is characterised by >2 episodes of pneumonia in a year or >3 episodes of pneumonia overall with normalisation of X-ray finding in between.

Diagnosis and Classification

- Chest X-ray — **Lobar consolidation** is seen in **pneumococcal pneumonia**. Staphylococcal pneumonia shows extensive parenchymal destruction. **Viral pneumonia** usually shows **hyperinflation of lungs** and **peribronchial cuffing**.
- Definitive diagnosis of bacterial and viral infection is established by isolation of the organism from blood, pleural fluid or lungs.
- **Culture of sputum is not useful** for diagnosis.
- **Classification:**

Classification	Presentation
No pneumonia	• Cough and cold
	• No chest indrawing and fast breathing
Pneumonia	Tachypnea i.e. RR
	• ≥60 in <2 months
	• ≥50 in 2–12 months
	• **≥40 in 12–60 months**
Severe pneumonia	• Chest indrawing
Very severe pneumonia	• Severe chest indrawing
	• Cyanosis
	• **Inability to feed**
	• **Nasal flaring**
	• **Temperature >38.5°C**
	• Grunting
	• Intermittent apnea
	• **Difficulty breathing**

Treatment

- No pneumonia and pneumonia are treated at home with home remedies and antibiotics respectively. **Severe pneumonia** and **very severe pneumonia** require **hospitalization** and antibiotic therapy.
- The mainstay of bacterial pneumonia is antibiotic therapy. The first treatment of choice for children less than 5 years of age is **amoxicillin**. If resistance is suspected then other agents active against MRSA like vancomycin and against beta lactamase producing pneumococci like amoxicillin + clavulinic acid should be considered. Since in children older than 5 years **atypical organisms** are common a **macrolide** like **erythromycin** or **azithromycin** should be added to the regimen.
- Antibiotic therapy is stopped if viral pneumonia is suspected.

BRONCHIAL ASTHMA

Bronchial asthma is an allergic disorder of the airway characterised by bronchoconstriction, edema of bronchi and increased mucous production. All these three factors are responsible for obstruction of the airway. The strongest association of asthma is seen with **atopic dermatitis**; however other conditions can be associated like allergic rhinitis and conjunctivitis. The other precipitating factors are allergens (dust mite, animal dander, cockroach, soil mold and pollen grain), tobacco smoke, cold air, exercise and some foods. Childhood asthma usually **improves with age.**

Clinical Presentation

The most characteristic presentation of asthma is **wheeze**; however other symptoms like cough, **cyanosis**, shortness of breath or **dyspnea** and chest tightness can also be seen.

Diagnosis

- **Pulmonary function test** — A decrease in FEV_1 of less than 20% and vital capacity and increase in residual volume, fractional residual capacity and total lung capacity is consistent with asthma. An increase of FEV_1 of more than 12% or 200ml after beta agonist administration is diagnostic of asthma.
- **Peak expiratory flow rate (PEFR)** — A diurnal variation of PEFR of more than 20% is seen in asthma.
- **Bronchoprovocation challenge** — Worsening of symptoms on exposure to methacholine, histamine and cold or dry hair is seen with asthma.
- **Exercise challenge** — Worsening of symptoms on exercising can be seen.
- **Exhaled NO (FE_{NO})** — Increased NO can be used for diagnosis.
- Chest X-ray shows flattening of diaphragm and peribronchial thickening.

Treatment

Treatment of bronchial asthma is divided in to two categories, i.e. for persistent asthma and for an acute attack.

Persistent Asthma

- **Inhaled corticosteroids** are the drug of choice for persistent asthma. Systemic corticosteroids are used for treatment of exacerbations.
- **Long acting β_2 agonists** are drug of choice for prophylaxis of **exercise induced asthma**.
- Other drugs used for persistent asthma are theophylline, **omalizumab (anti Ig E Ab)**, leukotriene synthesis inhibitor **(zileuton)** and leukotriene receptor antagonists **(monteleukast, zafirleukast)**.

Acute Attack

- **Oxygen therapy** is preferred for initial management in an acute attack.
- **Short acting β_2 agonists** are drug of choice for an acute attack.
- Other drugs used for treatment of acute attack are anticholinergics, **oral corticosteroids**, **intravenous theophylline** and epinephrine.

CONGENITAL LUNG DEFECTS

The different congenital defects of lung are pulmonary hypoplasia and aplasia, cystic adenomatoid malformation, pulmonary sequestration, bronchogenic cysts, congenital pulmonary lymphangiectasia and lung hernia (**"Sibson hernia"**).

Congenital Cystic Adenomatoid Malformation of Lung (CCAM)

CCAM is caused by embryological defect of terminal bronchial structures. There are 5 types of CCAM i.e. CCAM 0–5.

CCAM 0	CCAM1	CCAM 2	CCAM 3	CCAM 4
• Also called acinar dysplasia • Incompatible with life	• Most common type • Best prognosis • Cyst spaces are lined by pseudostratified ciliated columnar epithelium	• 2nd most common type • Generally cause **respiratory distress** in first month of life • Are associated with ❖ Renal agenesis ❖ Cardiovascular defects ❖ **Diaphragmatic hernia** ❖ Syringomyelia	• Occur exclusively in males • Expand a whole lobe and cause **mediastinal shift and compression of other lung**	• Very rare • Multiloculated, thin walled cysts are present

Pulmonary Sequestrations

Pulmonary sequestrations are non-functional parts of lungs which do not communicate with rest of lung. They are most commonly located in the **left lower lobe of the lung**. Based on their location in respect to the pleura, they can be classified as intrapulmonary and extrapulmonary. Diagnosis is done by **angiography** which shows blood supply of the lesions by systemic circulation. The mainstay of treatment is **surgical excision**.

Intrapulmonary Sequestrations

This is the **most common type** of sequestration located commonly in the posterior basal segment of left lower lobe. They are supplied by the systemic circulation **(aorta)** and drain in to **pulmonary veins**. They present with cough, wheezing, haemoptysis and pneumonia.

Extrapulmonary Sequestrations

These sequestrations are most commonly located below the lower lobe of left lung. They are also supplied by systemic circulation **(aorta)**; however they drain in to the **inferior vena cava**. They may connect to **oesophagus** or **stomach** and are associated with other disorders like **bronchogenic cysts, heart defects** and **diaphragmatic hernia**. These patients are usually asymptomatic and diagnosed accidentally.

Bronchogenic Cysts

Bronchogenic cysts are caused by abnormal embryogenesis of the tracheal diverticulum of foregut. They are lined with ciliated epithelium and have cartilage in the walls. Most commonly these cysts are located in the **mediastinum (50%)** near the carina, trachea and esophagus; however **intrapulmonary locations are rare**. These cysts which are **single** and **unilocular** are most commonly located in the **right side**. These cysts **frequently get infected** and this is when they present with fever and chest pain; and if enlarged it can present with symptoms of compression of adjacent structures (esophagus – dysphagia, trachea – respiratory distress). Chest X ray shows a cyst with air-fluid level. The mainstay of treatment is surgical excision of cyst.

Macleod or Swyer-James Syndrome

Macleod syndrome is caused by ball-valve type of obstruction to the airways by bronchogenic cysts, lymphadenopathy, tumor or vascular compression. This obstruction allows air to enter lungs but does not allow to exit, which leads to **unilateral hyperinflation** of the lung or the segment involved. This should be differentiated from congenital emphysema (true emphysema) which is caused by defect in the bronchial cartilage. The patient may present with pneumonia, bronchiectasis and mediastinal shift to the opposite side. Angiography shows **pulmonary artery hypoplasia**.

CYSTIC FIBROSIS

Cystic fibrosis is an **autosomal recessive** disorder caused by mutations of the **cystic fibrosis transmembrane regulator (CFTR) gene** located in **chromosome 7**. CFTR is a pump which controls movement of salt and water through the epithelial cells of various systems.

Clinical Presentation

- **Meconium ileus** is a characteristic finding seen in newborns with cystic fibrosis.
- **Pulmonary involvement** is characterised by occlusion of the airway and an increases predisposition to **infection** with Pseudomonas, Staphylococcus and *H. influenzae*. The patient presents with productive cough, wheeze, hemoptysis and dyspnea.
- **Pancreatic insufficiency** can be seen which presents with **steatorrhea with foul smelling, bulky stools,** deficiency of fat soluble vitamins and hyperglycaemia.
- Delay in sexual development and azoospermia can be seen in males.
- Loss of chloride ion in sweat can present as hypochloremic alkalosis.

Diagnosis

- **Sweat chloride testing** — Pilocarpine induced sweating and measurement of chloride ion in the sweat is the initial diagnosis of choice. **More than 60 mEq/L** of chloride in the sweat along pulmonary or pancreatic findings or positive family history is diagnostic.

- **Nasal epithelial potential difference test** – Loss of the nasal epithelial potential difference on application of amiloride is used for diagnosis **in case sweat chloride test is normal**.
- DNA mutation for **CFTR genes(F-508)** can be done for diagnosis.

Treatment

- Bronchodilators, corticosteroids and mucolytics (human recombinant DNase and N-acetyl cysteine) are given by inhalational route for symptomatic relief.
- Antibiotic therapy is indicated for the pulmonary infections associated with cystic fibrosis.

MULTIPLE CHOICE QUESTIONS

1. A 7½-year-old girl presents with breath-lessness and fever for 6–7 days. She has non-productive cough for 6 months. X-ray chest shows hyper-lucency in the lungs and pulmonary function tests show obstructive pattern. The most probable diagnosis will be: [AIIMS Nov. 08]
   a. Lobar emphysema
   b. Bronchiolitis obliterans
   c. Follicular bronchitis
   d. Pulmonary alveolar microlithiasis

2. A 2 years old child is brought to emergency at 3 AM with fever, barking cough and stridor only while crying. The child was able to drink normally. On examination respirator rate is 36/min and tempra-ture is 39.6°C. What will be your next step?
   [AIIMS Nov. 08]
   a. Racemic epinephrine nebulization
   b. High dose dexamethasone injection
   c. Nasal wash for influenza or RS V
   d. Antibiotics and blood culture

3. A girl child with fever, cough, dyspnoea with X ray showing right lower lobe patchy consolidation, for which treatment was given. After 8 weeks symptom improved but X ray showed more dense consolida-tion involving the whole of the right lower lobe. What is the next best line of investigation?
   [AIIMS Nov. 07]
   a. Bronchoscopy
   b. Culture from nasopharynx
   c. Barium esophagogram
   d. Allergic skin test

4. Which of the following is the etiological agent most often associated with Epiglottitis in children?
   [AIIMS May 05, Nov. 04, May 94]
   a. Streptococcus pneumonae
   b. Hemophilus influenzae type b
   c. Neisseria sp
   d. Moraxella catarrhalis

5. A child with pyoderma becomes toxic and presents with respiratory distress. His chest radiograph shows patchy areas of consolidation and multiple bilateral thin walled air containing cysts. The most likely etiological agent in this case is:
   [AIIMS Nov. 03]
   a. Mycobacterium tuberculosis
   b. Staphylococcus aureus
   c. Mycobacterium avium intracellular
   d. Pneumocystis carinii

6. A 3-year-old boy is brought to the casualty by his mother with progressive shortness of breath for 1 day. The child has history of bronchial asthma. On examination, the child is blue, gasping and unresponsive. What would you like to do first?
   [AIIMS Nov. 02]
   a. Intubate
   b. Administer 100% oxygen by mask
   c. Ventilate with bag and mask
   d. Administer nebulised salbutamol

7. A month old HIV positive child following URTI developed sudden onset of breathlessness. The chest X-ray shows hyperinflation. The oxygen saturation was greater than 90%. The treatment of choice is: [AIIMS May 01]
   a. Cotrimaxozole   b. Ribavirin
   c. IV Ganciclovir   d. Nebulized acyclovir

8. A child with recent onset of URTI after 2 days presents with acute onset of breathlessness, cough and fever. All of the following can be given except:
   [AIIMS May 01]
   a. Antipyretics   b. Morphine
   c. Antibiotics   d. Oxygen inhalation

9. An 11-month-old child presents with complaints of respiratory distress. On examination there is bilateral crepitation and wheezing. Which of the following is most likely cause? [AIIMS Nov. 2000]
   a. Pneumonia
   b. Adenovirus
   c. Respiratory syncytial virus
   d. Rhinovirus

10. All are used in acute attack of asthma in a 4 year old child except: [AIIMS June 97]
    a. Theophylline   b. Corticosteroids
    c. Sedatives   d. Salbutamol

11. Following are true about bronchial cyst except:

    [AIIMS 96]

    a. Mostly mediastinal
    b. 50-70% occur in lungs
    c. Usually multiloculated
    d. Are infected quite often

12. A 3-month-old child presents with intermittent stridor. Most likely cause is: [AI 01, AIIMS Dec. 95]

    a. Laryngotracheobronchitis
    b. Laryngomalacia
    c. Respiratory obstruction
    d. Foreign body aspiration

13. Not a feature of childhood asthma is:

    [AIIMS Dec. 94]

    a. History of atopic dermatitis
    b. Raised Ig G levels
    c. Improves with age
    d. Absence of wheezing after exercise

14. In an infant with aspiration pneumonitis, the most common lung segment to be involved is:

    [AIIMS May 93]

    a. Left apical   b. Right apical
    c. Right middle   d. Right basal

15. The commonest organism causing empyema in a child under 2 years: [AIIMS 91]

    a. E.coli   b. Staphylococcus
    c. Pneumococcus   d. Klebsiella

16. A child presents raised sweat chloride levels and suspicion of cystic Fibrosis, which other test would you do to exclude the diagnosis of cystic fibrosis:

    [AI 08]

    a. Repeat sweat chloride measurements
    b. Nasal electrode potential difference
    c. Fat in stool for next 72 hours
    d. DNA analysis for delta F-508 mutation

17. A 7½ months old child with cough, mild stridor is started on oral antibiotics. The child showed initial improvement but later developed wheeze, productive cough, and mild fever. X-ray shows hyperlucency and PFT shows an obstructive curve. The most probable diagnosis is: [AI 08]

    a. Bronchiolitis obliterans
    b. Post viral syndrome
    c. Pulmonary alveolar microlithiasis
    d. Follicular bronchitis

18. Which of the statements is not true regarding Macleod's Syndrome?   [AI 07]

    a. It is not a true emphysema
    b. Occurs before 8 years of age
    c. It is unilateral emphysema
    d. The pulmonary artery on the affected side is hyperplasic
    e. It is also called Swyer-Jame's Syndrome

19. Most common mode of treatment of a 1 year old child with asthma is: [AI 07]

    a. Inhaled short acting beta 2 agonist
    b. Oral short acting theophylline
    c. Oral ketotifen
    d. Leukotriene agonist

20. A child with three days history of upper respiratory tract infection presents with stridor, which decreases on lying down postion. What is the most probable diagnosis: [AI 07]

    a. Acute epiglottitis
    b. Laryngotracheobronchiolitis
    c. Foreign body aspiration
    d. Retropharyngeal abscess

21. The most common etiological agent for acute bronchiolitis in infancy is: [AI 06]

    a. Influenza virus
    b. Para influenza virus
    c. Rhinovirus
    d. Respiratory syncytial virus

22. An infant develops cough and fever. The X-ray examination is suggestive of bronchopneumonia. All of the following viruses can be the causative agent except: [AI 04]

    a. Parainfluenza viruses
    b. Influenza virus A
    c. Respiratory syncytial virus
    d. Mumps virus

23. A 3-month-old child presents with intermittent stridor. Most likely cause is: [AI 01, AIIMS Dec. 95]

    a. Laryngotracheobronchitis
    b. Laryngomalacia
    c. Respiratory obstruction
    d. Foreign body aspiration

24. Pneumatocele is caused by.   [AI 98]

    a. Staphylococcus   b. Streptococcus
    c. E.coli   d. P. carinii

25. All are seen in asthma except: [AI 97]

    a. Cyanosis   b. Wheezing
    c. Clubbing   d. Dyspnea

26. Chandu, a one year old child should be admitted in hospital for following complaints except: [AI 97]

    a. Refusal of feed
    b. Respiratory rate of 50 per minute with chest retraction
    c. Fever 39°C
    d. Difficulty in waking

27. Immediate management of a child with foreign body inhalation is: [AI 97]

    a. IPPV
    b. Bronchoscopy
    c. Tracheostomy
    d. Exploratory thoracotomy

28. Mucoviscidosis is most commonly related to:
[AI 96]

a. Fibrocystic disease of pancreas
b. Duodenal atresia
c. Diaphragmatic hernia
d. Annular pancreas

29. Treatment of choice in bronchiolitis is: [AI 96]

a. Ribavirin   b. Amantidine
c. Vidarabine   d. Zidovudine

30. The commonest cause of bacterial pneumonia in children is: [AI 95]

a. *Streptococcus pyogenes*
b. *Hemphilus influenzae*
c. *Streptococcus pneumonae*
d. *Staphylococcus aureus*

31. The drug of choice of mycoplasma pneumonia in children is: [AI 95]

a. Tetracycline   b. Streptomycin
c. Cotrimaxozole   d. Erythromycin

32. The lung abscess in children can be caused by all except: [AI 91]

a. Pneumococcus   b. *E. histolytica*
c. Staphylococcus   d. Klebsiella

33. WHO criteria for hospital admission in pneumonia:
[PGI Dec. 08]

a. High fever
b. Nasal flaring
c. Difficulty in breathing
d. Difficulty in feeding
e. Chest indrawing

34. Features of cystic fibrosis: [PGI June 06]

a. Lung normal at birth
b. Abnormal sweat chloride tests
c. Autosomal dominant
d. Defect in chromosome 11

35. A 4 years child presents with a history of chronic left lower lobe pneumonitis. On contrast broncho-graphy, the area involved with the pneumonitis does not fill whereas the area around it does fill. The most likely diagnosis: [PGI 06]

a. Asthma
b. Pulmonary sequestration
c. Cystic fibrosis
d. Bronchopulmonary dysplasia
e. Bronchogenic cyst

36. Wheeze in children caused by: [PGI June 05, 06]

a. Foreign body
b. Gastroesophageal reflux disease
c. Bronchial asthma
d. Epiglottis
e. Laryngomalacia

37. Bronchitis in children is caused by: [PGI June 05]

a. *H. influenzae*   b. RSV
c. Mycoplasma   d. EBV
e. Influenza virus

38. Bronchiolitis in children is caused by: [PGI June 05]

a. *H. influenza*   b. RSV
c. Mycoplasma   d. EBV
e. Influenza virus

39. A 6 months old baby coming with h/o increasing difficulty in breathing of 2 days duration and on examination baby is afebrile and B/L wheeze and CXR shows B/L hyperinflation of the lungs with normal WBC count, the diagnosis is : [PGI Dec. 03]

a. Bronchiolitis   b. Asthma
c. Ch. Bronchitis   d. Pneumonia
e. FB

40. In Bronchiolitis followings is/are seen:
[PGI Dec. 02]

a. Seen in children 5 months to 3 years of age
b. Caused by *Streptococcus pneumoniae*
c. Chest X-ray shows hyperinflation bilaterally
d. Symptomatic treatment is given
e. Antibiotics should be started

41. Which of the following is/are true about bronchio-litis in children? [PGI June 01]

a. Caused by respiratory syncytial virus
b. Hyperinflation of the chest
c. Pleural effusion
d. May lead to bronchial asthma later in life
e. Lymphopenia is seen

42. Most common cause of mass in posterior media-stinum in children: [PGI June 01]

a. Rhabdosarcoma
b. Duplication cyst of oesophagus
c. Lymphoma
d. Neuroblastoma
e. Thymoma

43. True about upper airways of neonate:
[PGI Dec. 2000]

a. Cricoid is the narrowest part
b. Larynx extends from C_4 to C_6
c. Epiglottis is big and omega shaped
d. All

44. Newborn with APGAR score of 2 at 1 min. and 6 at 5 min. has respiratory distress and mediastinal shift diagnosis is: [PGI Dec. 00]

a. Congenital adenomatoid lung disease
b. Pneumothorax
c. Diaphragmatic hernia
d. Transient tachypnea of newborn
e. HMD

45. **A 4 yr old child has 'seal barking' like croupy cough. Management includes all except:** [PGI June 00]
    a. O$_2$ inhalation
    b. Antibiotic
    c. Hydration
    d. Morphine

46. **Most common cause of stridor shortly after birth:** [PGI Dec. 99]
    a. Laryngeal papilloma
    b. Laryngeal web
    c. Laryngomalacia
    d. Vocal cord palsy

47. **Child's respiratory physiology differs from adult because of:** [PGI June 99]
    a. Smaller airways
    b. Increased O$_2$ demand
    c. Decreased tidal volume
    d. Decreased residual volume

48. **Aerosolised Ribavirin is used in the treatment of bronchiolitis with:** [PGI June 98]
    a. RSV
    b. *H. influenzae*
    c. Pneumococcus
    d. Streptococcus

49. **A primi mother having 3 weeks male child, which is presenting with noisy breathing sound, child is afebrile, sleeping and feeding well and on clinical examination he is normal. Management protocol include**
    a. Begin IV antibiotics
    b. Reassure and give saline nasal drops
    c. Give racemic epinephrine
    d. Order for chest X-ray
    e. Give some decongestant

50. **In a child 1 years the commonest cause of respiratory infection with wheeze is:** [PGI 95]
    a. RSV
    b. Influenza virus
    c. Adenovirus
    d. Para influenza

51. **Acute onset of cough, stridor and dyspnea in a child is mostly due to:** [PGI 93]
    a. Foreign body
    b. Acute asthma
    c. Aspiration pneumonitis
    d. Primary complex

52. **A 4-year-old boy presented with recurrent chest infections. Sweat chloride test was done, showed values of 36 and 42. What is the next best investigation to confirm the diagnosis?**
    a. 72 hour fecal fat estimation
    b. CT chest
    c. Transepithelial nasal potential difference
    d. DMA analysis of delta F 508 mutation

53. **Pneumothorax could be a complication of:** [UPSC 2000]
    a. Staphylococcal pneumonia
    b. Pneumococcal pneumonia
    c. *Klebsiella pneumoniae*
    d. Viral pneumonia

54. **A 9-month-old infant presents with a 2 day history of fever, cough and breathlessness following an upper respiratory infection. She is febrile and has a respiratory rate of 80/min. Intercostal and subcostal retractions and extensive ronchi on auscultation. A chest X ray reveals a hyperinflated chest:** [UPSC 99]
    a. Bronchial asthma
    b. Foreign body aspiration
    c. Bacterial pneumonia
    d. Bronchiolitis

55. **Regarding bronchiolitis one of the following statements is not true:** [KCET 95]
    a. Bronchiolitis is a self-limiting viral illness secondary to respiratory syncytial virus
    b. It occurs commonly in children above 2 years
    c. Ribavirin is the drug of choice for the treatment of this condition
    d. It predisposes children for later development of asthma

56. **In a child with exercise induced asthma, which is done:**
    a. Prophylaxis with steroids
    b. Prophylaxis with beta 2 agonists
    c. Prophylaxis with theophylline
    d. Breathing exercise

57. **Child requiring repeated short acting bronchodilators and what could be next line of management:**
    a. Methylxanthines
    b. Short acting budesonide
    c. Oral prednisolone
    d. Montelukast

QUESTIONS OF OTHER EXAMINATIONS

1. **A 4-year-old child presents with history of hoarseness, croupy cough and aphonia, the child has dyspnoea with wheezing. The most probable diagnosis is:** [DPG 10]
    a. Asthmatic bronchitis
    b. Laryngeal foreign body
    c. Bronchopneumonia
    d. Retropharyngeal abscess

2. **A 3-month-old infant presents with intermittent respiratory stridor since 10 days of age. The most likely diagnosis is:** [DPG 09]
    a. Laryngomalacia
    b. Tracheoesophageal fistula
    c. Laryngotracheobronchiolitis
    d. Neoplasm

3. **If a 5-year-old child suddenly develops stridor, which one of the following would be the most likely diagnosis:** [UPSC 09]
   a. Laryngomalacia
   b. Acute laryngotracheobronchitis
   c. Foreign body aspiration
   d. Acute epiglottitis

4. **A two-year-old child is classified as having pneumonia, if the respiratory rate is more than:** [COMED 09]

   a. 30/min   b. 40/min
   c. 50/min   d. 60/min

5. **Respiratory rate in a 2-month-old to label it tachypnea is:** [DPG 08]
   a. 40   b. 50
   c. 60   d. 70

6. **A child presents with running nose, breathlessness, family history positive, most likely diagnosis is:** [UP 08]

   a. Bronchiolitis   b. Viral pneumonia
   c. Bronchial asthma   d. None

7. **Pneumatoceles often develop in children after pneumonia due to the following organism:** [COMED 07]
   a. Klebsiella
   b. Streptococcus
   c. *Staphylococcus aureus*
   d. *Hemophilus influenza*

8. **Infant with cystic fibrosis (CF) are likely to develop:** [MAHE 07]

   a. Meconium ileus
   b. Loose motions
   c. Vomiting
   d. Constipation

9. **A 2-month-old infant has had inspiratory stridor since the first month of life, but has been otherwise well. Physical examination is unremarkable except for moderate inspiratory stridor and retractions which are worse when the infant is supine or agitated and better when he is prone and quiet. The most likely cause of these findings is:** [MAHA 05]
   a. Reactive airway disease
   b. Laryngomalacia
   c. Viral croup
   d. An aspirated foreign body

10. **The correct line of management in a child who has swollen a coin is:** [TNPSC 2000]
    a. Fibreoptic endoscopy   b. Rigid endoscopy
    c. Laparotomy   d. Wait and watch

11. **Commonest sign of intrabronchial foreign body in children is:** [CUPGEE 99]
    a. Cough   b. Wheeze
    c. Dyspnea   d. Stridor

12. **Combination chemotherapy is not indicated in:** [JIPMER 95]

    a. Primary complex
    b. Acute epiglottitis
    c. Laryngotracheobronchiolitis
    d. Immunologically suppressed patients

13. **Child with which of the following throat infection needs systemic antibiotic therapy:** [Jipmer 81]
    a. Pneumococci
    b. Beta haemolytic streptococci
    c. *Staphylococcus aureus*
    d. All of the above

14. **Croup syndrome is usually caused by:** [PGI 80, AIIMS 83]
    a. Rhinovirus   b. Coxsackie A virus
    c. Coxscakie B virus   d. Para influenza

ANSWERS

MULTIPLE CHOICE QUESTIONS

1. (b) Bronchiolitis obliterans (Ref: Nelson 19th E/P1422)
Diagnosis of bronchiolitis obliterans:
- Chest X ray and CT scan shows **hyperlucency** with patchy infiltrates.
- Pulmonary function test shows **obstructive pattern.**

2. (b) High dose dexamethasone (Ref: Nelson 19th E/P1407)
Treatment of laryngotracheobronchiolitis:

Mild croup — Stridor seen on **crying**, agitation or activity i.e. no stridor at rest	• Hydration.
	• I/M dexamethasone or intra-nasal budesonide.
Moderate to severe croup — Stridor seen at rest	• Oxygenation.
	• Nebulization with epine-phrine.
	• I/M dexamethasone or intra-nasal budesonide.

3. (a) Bronchoscopy (Ref: Nelson 18th E/P1796)
- This is a case of slow resolving pneumonia. Slow resolving pneumonia is persistence of symptoms or radiologic abnormalities beyond the expected time course.
- Causes of slow resolving pneumonia are empyema, bacterial resistance, endobronchial obstruction caused by foreign body or lesions and preexisting diseases of lungs.
- The first step in case of a slow resolving pneumonia is to get another X-ray, which has been done in our case and it shows more dense consolidation.
- Among the given option the best thing to do is **bronchoscopy** to rule out endobronchial obstruction.

Also know:
- **Recurrent pneumonia** is characterised by 2 or more episodes in a single year or 3 or more episodes ever with radiological clearance of lesion in between episodes.

4. (b) *Haemophilus influenzae* type b (Ref: CPDT 19th E/P479)
- Acute epiglottitis or supraglottitis is most commonly caused by *H. influenzae*; however in patients with vaccination the common cause are *Pneumococcus, Staphylococcus aureus* and group A beta haemolytic streptococci.

5. (b) *Staphylococcus aureus* (Ref: Rudolph 22nd E/P960)
- Multiple bilateral thin walled air containing cysts are pneumatoceles.

- Pneumatoceles are characteristic features of staphylococcal pneumonia.

6. (b) Administer 100% oxygen by mask (Ref: Nelson 19th E/P772)
Treatment of acute attack of asthma:
- **Oxygen therapy** is preferred for **initial management** in an acute attack.
- Short acting β_2 agonists (salbutamol) are drug of choice for an acute attack.
- Other drugs used for treatment of acute attack are anticholinergics, oral corticosteroids, intravenous theophylline and epinephrine.

7. (b) Ribavirin (Ref: CPDT 19th E/P484)

8. (b) Morphine (Ref: CPDT 19th E/P 484)
Acute onset breathlessness, cough and fever indicates towards bronchiolitis. Bronchiolitis can be treated with:
- Bronchodilators (β_2 agonists, anticholinergics), epinephrine nebulization and corticosteroids are used for **symptomatic management.**
- Antiviral drug **ribavirin** is given by aerosol.
- Antibiotics can be used to prevent secondary bacterial infection.
- Oxygen therapy can be given in case of severe hypoxemia.
- Morphine is rather contraindicated as it can cause respiratory depression and further worsen the condition.

9. (c) Respiratory syncytial virus (Ref: CPDT 19th E/P484)
- The symptoms of respiratory distress, crepitation and wheezing in an 11 month old child indicates towards bronchiolitis.
- Bronchiolitis is most commonly caused by respiratory syncytial virus.

10. (c) Sedatives (Ref: Nelson 19th E/P772)
Treatment of acute attack of asthma:
- Oxygen therapy is preferred for initial management in an acute attack.
- **Short acting β_2 agonists (salbutamol)** are drug of choice for an acute attack.
- Other drugs used for treatment of acute attack are anticholinergics, **oral corticosteroids**, **intravenous theophylline** and epinephrine.

11. (b) and **(c)** 50–70% occur in lungs and usually multiloculated (Ref: Rudolph 22th E/P1931)

"Foregut (bronchogenic) cysts are usually single, **unilocular** and more common on the right."

- 50% of the cysts are located in the mediastinum, more commonly near the carina.
- These cysts can get infected and present with fever and chest pain.

12. **(b)** Laryngomalacia (Ref: CPDT 19th E/P477)
- **Laryngomalacia** is the most common cause of stridor in infants.
- **Laryngotracheobronchiolitis** is the most common non-infectious cause of stridor in children.

13. **(b)** Raised Ig G levels (Ref: Nelson 19th E/P760–64, CPDT 19th E/P1018–21)
- Atopic dermatitis is the strongest association seen with bronchial asthma.
- Bronchial asthma is associated with increased Ig E.
- Childhood asthma characteristically improves as the child grows.
- Exercise usually worsens asthma and increases wheezing; however in the initial stage wheezing can be decreased due to bronchodilation.

14. **(b)** Right apical (Ref: CPDT 19th E/P500)

15. **(b)** Staphylococcus (Ref: Rudolph 22th E/P960)

16. **(b)** Nasal electrode potential difference (Ref: Nelson 19th E/P1442)

    Diagnosis of cystic fibrosis:
- **Sweat chloride testing** — Pilocarpine induced sweating and measurement of chloride ion in the sweat is the initial diagnosis of choice. **More than 60 mEq/L** of chloride in the sweat along pulmonary or pancreatic findings or positive family history is diagnostic.
- **Nasal epithelial potential difference test** — Loss of the nasal epithelial potential difference on application of amiloride is used for diagnosis **in case sweat chloride test is normal**.

17. **(a)** Bronchiolitis obliterans (Ref: Nelson 19th E/P1422)
- The classical presentation of bronchiolitis obliterans in case of respiratory infection is **initial improvement followed by deterioration manifesting as fever, cough, respiratory distress, cyanosis and dyspnea.**
- Chest X-ray and CT scan shows **hyperlucency** with patchy infiltrates.
- Pulmonary function test shows **obstructive pattern.**

18. **(d)** The pulmonary artery on the affected side is hyperplastic (Ref: Nelson 19th E/P1420)
- Angiography shows **pulmonary artery hypoplasia** in the affected side.

19. **(a)** Inhaled short acting beta 2 agonist (Ref: Nelson 19th E/P772)
- **Inhaled short beta 2 agonists** are the drug of choice for an acute attack of bronchial asthma.

- **Inhaled corticosteroids** are the drug of choice for persistent bronchial asthma.

20. **(b)** Laryngotracheobronchiolitis (Ref: CPDT19th E/P478)
- The patient has a history of upper respiratory tract infection and presents with stridor.
- The most common infectious cause of stridor in children is **laryngotracheobronchiolitis.**

21. **(d)** Respiratory syncytial virus (Ref: CPDT 19th E/P484)

    Causes of bronchiolitis:
- **Respiratory syncytial virus (RSV)** — Most common cause.
- Parainfluenza virus
- Human metapneumovirus
- Influenza virus
- Adenovirus
- Mycoplasma
- Ureaplasma
- Chlamydia
- *Pneumocystis jiroveci*

22. **(d)** Mumps virus (Ref: Ghai 7th E/P352, Nelson 19th E/P1433)

    Viruses causing pneumonia:
- **Respiratory syncytial virus**
- **Influenza**
- **Parainfluenza**
- Adenovirus
- Rhinovirus
- Metapneumovirus

23. **(b)** Laryngomalacia (Ref: CPDT 19th E/P477)
- **Laryngomalacia** is the most common cause of stridor in infants.
- **Laryngotracheobronchiolitis** is the most common non-infectious cause of stridor in children.

24. **(a)** Staphylococcus (Ref: Rudolph 22nd E/P960)

25. **(c)** Clubbing (Ref: CPDT 19th E/P1019)
- The most characteristic presentation of asthma is **wheeze**; however other symptoms like cough, **cyanosis**, shortness of breath or **dyspnea** and chest tightness can also be seen.

26. **(b)** Respiratory rate of 50 per minute with chest retraction (Ref: Rudolph 22nd E/P961, Ghai 7th E/P356)

    Criterias for admission in pneumonia:
- **Chest indrawing**
- Cyanosis
- **Inability to feed**
- **Nasal flaring**
- **Temperature>38.5°C**
- Grunting
- Intermittent apnea
- **Difficulty breathing**

27. **(b)** Bronchoscopy (Ref: Rudolph 22nd E/P1953)
    * If the foreign body is located in lower respiratory tract it is removed by **rigid bronchoscopy** and if in upper respiratory tract it can be removed by **Heimlich maneuverer** or **Magill forceps.**

28. **(a)** Fibrocystic disease of pancreas (Ref: Nelson 19th E/P1449)

29. **(a)** Ribavirin (Ref: CPDT 19th E/P484)

30. **(c)** *Streptococcus pneumoniae* (Ref: Nelson 19th E/ P1433)

31. **(d)** Erythromycin (Ref: Rudolph 22nd E/P961)

32. **(b)** *E. histolytica* (Ref: CPDT 19th E/P505)
    Lung abscess can be caused by organisms like:
    * **Staphylococcus**
    * *H. influenzae*
    * **Pneumococcus**
    * **Klebsiella**
    * Group A streptococci
    * Nocardia
    * Legionella
    * Candida
    * Aspergillus.

33. **(a), (b), (c), (d)** and **(e)** (Ref: Rudolph 22nd E/P961, Ghai 7th E/P356)
    Criteria for admission in pneumonia:
    * **Chest indrawing**
    * Cyanosis
    * **Inability to feed**
    * **Nasal flaring**
    * **Temperature>38.5°C**
    * Grunting
    * Intermittent apnea
    * **Difficulty breathing.**

34. **(a)** and **(b)** Lung normal at birth and Abnormal sweat chloride test (Ref: Nelson 19th E/P1437-50)
    * At birth meconium ileus is present in 15% cases but lungs are normal.
    * Abnormal sweat chloride tests i.e. sweat chloride of >60 is diagnostic.
    * Cystic fibrosis is an AR disorder characterised by mutation of CFTR gene in chromosome 7.

35. **(b)** Pulmonary sequestration (Ref: CPDT 19th E/P492)
    * During bronchography the normal lung fills the contrast whereas area of pneumonitis does not.
    * This means that the circulation of both the areas is different.
    * Pulmonary sequestration is a non-functional part of lung with distinct blood supply and the intra-pulmonary type can present with pneumonia.
    * Hence here the answer of choice is sequestration.

36. **(a), (b), (c)** and **(e)** (Ref: Nelson 19th E/P1418)
    Causes of wheeze in children:
    * Foreign body
    * GERD
    * Laryngomalacia

* Bronchial asthma
* Lower respiratory tract infection
* Tracheoesophageal fistula
* Vascular ring
* Mediastinal mass
* Hemangioma
* Hemosiderosis
* Congenital lung defects like cysts, adenomatoid malformation
* Cystic fibrosis
* Bronchiolitis obliterans.

37. **(e)** Influenza virus (Ref: Nelson 19th E/P1415)
    * Bronchitis in children is caused by **influenza virus**, corynebacterium diphtheria and bordtella pertussis.

38. **(b), (c)** and **(e)** RSV, Mycoplasma and Influenza virus (Ref: CPDT 19th E/P484)
    Causes of bronchiolitis:
    * **Respiratory syncytial virus (RSV)** — Most common cause.
    * Parainfluenza virus
    * Human metapneumovirus
    * **Influenza virus**
    * Adenovirus
    * **Mycoplasma**
    * Chlamydia
    * Ureaplasma
    * *Pneumocystis jiroveci*

39. **(a)** Bronchiolitis (Ref: CPDT 19th E/P484)
    * Bronchiolitis usually presents with fever, sneezing and rhinorrhea followed by more severe symptoms like cough, dyspnea, tachypnea, apnea and **wheezing.**
    * Chest X-ray usually shows **hyperinflation** and patchy atelectasis.
    * **WBC count is within normal limits.**

40. **(c)** and **(d)** Chest X-ray shows hyperinflation bilaterally and Symptomatic treatment is given (Ref: CPDT 19th E/P484)
    * RSV is the most common cause of bronchiolitis.
    * Chest X ray shows hyperinflation of lungs and patchy atelectasis.
    * Bronchodilators (β_2 agonists, anticholinergics), epinephrine nebulization and corticosteroids are used for **symptomatic management**.
    * Antiviral drug **ribavirin** is given by aerosol.

41. **(a), (b),** and **(d)** Caused by respiratory syncytial virus, Hyperinflation of the chest, May lead to bronchial asthma later in life (Ref: CPDT 19th E/P484)
    * Acute bronchiolitis is most commonly caused by **respiratory syncytial virus (RSV).**
    * These children are at higher risk for development of **bronchial asthma.**
    * Chest X-ray usually shows **hyperinflation** and patchy atelectasis.
    * **WBC count is within normal limits.**

42. (c) Neuroblastoma (Ref: CPDT 19th E/P518) (See Table 1)

43. (c) Epiglottis is big and omega shaped (Ref: CPDT 19th E/P477)
- The pediatric airway is **short** and **narrow**; and larynx is more anterior than adults and extends from C_2–C_4.
- The narrowest part of pediatric airway is **subglottis** and the epiglottis is of **omega shaped.**

44. (a), (b) and **(c)** Congenital adenomatoid lung disease, Pneumothorax and Diaphragmatic hernia (Ref: Rudolph 22nd E/P1931, Ghai 7th E/P142)
- **Congenital adenomatoid lung**, diaphragmatic hernia and pneumothorax cause mediastinal shift to contralateral side due to compression by **cysts**, abdominal organs and air respectively.

45. (b) and **(d)** Antibiotic and Morphine (Ref: Rudolph 22nd E/P1951)
- Croup is characterised by a characteristic barky cough called as "a **barking seal** or dog".
- Treatment of laryngotracheobronchiolitis:

Mild croup — Stridor seen on **crying**, agitation or activity i.e. no stridor at rest	• Hydration. • I/M dexamethasone or intranasal. budesonide.
Moderate to severe croup — Stridor seen at rest	• Oxygenation. • Nebulization with epinephrine. • I/M dexamethasone or intranasal budesonide.

46. (c) Laryngomalacia (Ref: CPDT 19th E/P477)

47. (a) Smaller airways (Ref: Rudolph 22nd E/P1949)

"The pediatric airway is **shorter** and narrower and the larynx is placed more anterior than in adults."

48. (a) RSV (Ref: CPDT 19th E/P484)

49. (b) Reassure and give saline nasal drop (Ref: Ghai 7th E/P356)
- This is a clear case of no pneumonia and hence the mother needs to be reassured and child should be managed at home.

50. (a) RSV (Ref: 19th E/P484)

51. (a) Foreign body (Ref: Rudolph 22nd E/P1953)
- Most commonly children present **acutely with coughing followed by respiratory distress, aphonia, drooling and stridor.**

52. (c) Transepithelial nasal potential difference (Ref: Nelson 19th E/P1442)
Diagnosis of cystic fibrosis:
- **Sweat chloride testing** — Pilocarpine induced sweating and measurement of chloride ion in the sweat is the initial diagnosis of choice. **More than 60 mEq/L** of chloride in the sweat along pulmonary or pancreatic findings or positive family history is diagnostic.
- **Nasal epithelial potential difference test** — Loss of the nasal epithelial potential difference on application of amiloride is used for diagnosis **in case sweat chloride test is normal.**

53. (a) Staphylococcal pneumonia (Ref: Rudolph 22nd E/P960)
Staphylococcal pneumonia is associated with severe parenchymal destruction characterised by:
- **Pneumatoceles**
- **Pneumothorax**
- **Empyema**
- Microabscess
- Cavitation.

54. (d) Bronchiolitis (Ref: CPDT 19th E/P494)

55. (b) It occurs commonly in children above 2 years (Ref: CPDT 19th E/P484)

56. (b) Prophylaxis with beta 2 agonists (Ref: Nelson 19th E/P772)
Persistent asthma:
- Inhaled corticosteroids are the drug of choice for persistent asthma. Systemic corticosteroids are used for treatment of exacerbations.
- **Long acting β_2 agonists** are drug of choice for **prophylaxis of exercise induced asthma**.
- Other drugs used for persistent asthma are theophylline, omalizumab (anti Ig E Ab), leukotriene synthesis inhibitor (zileuton) and leukotriene receptor antagonists (monteleukast, zafirleukast).

57. (b) Short acting budesonide (Ref: Nelson 19th E/P772)
- Child is requiring repeated administration of bronchodilators which indicates towards persisting nature of asthma.
- For persistent asthma drug of choice is **inhaled cortoicosteroids.**

Table 1

Superiormediastinum — Area above pericardium or above line from manubrium to 4th thoracic vertebra	Anterior mediastinum — Between sternum and pericardium	Posterior mediastinum — Between pericardium and diaphragm; and 8th thoracic vertebrae.	Middle mediastinum — Between previous three mediastinum.
• Cystic hygroma • Vascular and neurogenic tumors • Thymic masses • Teratomas • Esophageal lesions • Intrathoracic thyroid pathology	• Thymic mass • Teratoma • Vascular tumors • Lymphatic mass • Pleuropericardial cyst	• **Neurogenic tumors** • Bronchogenic cysts • Thoracic meningoceles • Aortic aneurysms	• Mediastinal abscess • Lymphatic masses • Bronchogenic cysts • Pericardial cysts • Metastasis

QUESTIONS OF OTHER EXAMINATIONS

1. **(b)** Laryngeal foreign body (Ref: Rudolph 22nd E/ P1793, CPDT 19th E/P483)

2. **(a)** Laryngomalacia (Ref: CPDT 19th E/P477)

3. **(c)** Foreign body aspiration (Ref: Rudolph 22nd E/ P1953)

4. **(b)** 40/min (Ref: Park's PSM 20th E/P155)
   Tachypnea for diagnosis of pneumonia i.e. RR:
   - ≥60 in <2 months
   - ≥50 in 2–12 months
   - **≥40 in 12–60 months.**

5. **(b)** 50 (Ref: Park's PSM 20th E/P155)
   Tachypnea is defined as RR:
   - ≥60 in <2 months
   - ≥50 in 2–12 months
   - **≥40 in 12–60 months.**

6. **(c)** Bronchial asthma (Ref: CPDT 19th E/P1018)

7. **(c)** *Staphylococcus aureus* (Ref: Rudolph 22nd E/P960)

8. **(a)** Meconium ileus (Nelson 19th E/P1448)

9. **(b)** Laryngomalacia (Ref: CPDT 19th E/P477)
   - Most common cause of stridor in an infant is Laryngomalacia.
   - Stridor in Laryngomalacia characteristically worsens in supine position.

10. **(d)** Wait and watch (Ref: Rudolph 22nd E/P1793)
    - The patient has swollen a coin which might go in to the GIT or respiratory tract. In this case the patient has not presented with any acute symptoms of aspiration and hence most probably it is in the GIT.
    - So the best answer here is wait and watch.

11. **(a)** Cough (Ref: Rudolph 22nd E/P1953)

12. **(c)** Laryngotracheobronchiolitis (Ref: CPDT 19th E/ P478)

13. **(d)** All of the above (Ref: CPDT 19th E/P480)

14. **(d)** Parainfluenza (Ref: Rudolph 22nd E/P1951)
    - Croup syndrome is most commonly caused by parainfluenza type 1 virus.

10

Hematology

Hematopoesis begins in the **yolk sac** at 2nd week of gestation and continues till the 6th week. After 6th week **liver is the primary site till 2nd trimester of pregnancy** followed by bone marrow in the remaining period. Erythropoiesis is stimulated by erythropoietin produced by the liver in foetus (maternal erythropoietin cannot cross placenta), however after birth kidney is the source of erythropoietin. Granulocytopoesis is stimulated by granulocyte colony stimulating factor (G-CSF) and macrophage colony stimulating factor (M-CSF). Thrombopoesis is stimulated by thrombopoetin.

ANEMIA

A decrease in the RBC count or haemoglobin is called as anemia. In the initial phase the body tries to compensate by **increasing the cardiac output, 2-3-DPG in RBCs, right shift of oxygen dissociation curve** and **increased erythropoietin production**. However if Hb level decreases further, it results in decreased oxygen supply, which manifests as paleness, weakness, dyspnea and tachycardia. The different causes of anemia are hemoglobinopathies like sickle cell anemia and thalassemia, RBC membrane abnormality (spherocytosis, elliptocytosis, PNH), deficiency of micronutrients like iron and folic acid, metabolic abnormalities of RBC like G6PD deficiency and decreased hematopoesis (Red cell aplasia).

Hemoglobinopathies

Hemoglobin is made up of iron containing moieties called as heme which are conjugated to different polypeptides called as globin (α, β, γ, δ, ϵ, ζ or zetta). The combination of two types of polypeptides and heme results in different types of haemoglobins i.e. major adult haemoglobin or Hb A ($\alpha_2\beta_2$), minor adult haemoglobin or Hb A$_2$ ($\alpha_2\delta_2$), fetal haemoglobin or Hb F ($\alpha_2\gamma_2$), Hb Portland ($\zeta_2\gamma_2$), Gower-1 Hb ($\zeta_2\epsilon_2$) and Gower-2 Hb ($\alpha_2\epsilon_2$). Initially the foetus has predominantly **Portland, Gower-1 and Gower-2 haemoglobin till 8th week** followed by rapid rise of Hb F till the end of 2nd trimester. The initiation of Hb A synthesis begins at **24 weeks of gestation** and the **switch from Hb F to exclusive Hb A production begins at 38 weeks of gestation**. After birth the **adult values of Hb A are achieved by 1 year of age**.

Thalassemia

Thalassemia is characterised by variable **deletions** in the four α and **mutations** in two β globin genes located in chromosome 16 and 11 respectively. This results in decreased quantity of haemoglobin production and erythropoiesis.

- **β thalassemia:** Mutation of one β globin gene (heterozygous) causes thalassemia intermedia, minor, minima or HPFH syndrome, whereas mutation of both the genes (homozygous) causes thalassemia major. The most common cause is a **point mutation (missense mutation) of the intron 1 causing splicing defect**; however other genetic abnormalities like **frameshift mutation and 619 bp deletion** can be the cause. There is compensatory increase in production of α, γ and δ globulins, which results in formation of α_4 tetramers and increased amount of Hb F and Hb A$_2$.
  - ❖ **Thalassemia major or Cooley anemia:**
    - ❑ **Clinical presentation:** Since β globin is not required for foetal haemoglobin production the patients usually present after birth as the Hb A fails to rise. Apart from the features of anemia the baby presents with features of compensatory hematopoiesis in the flat bones (maxillary and frontal bone overgrowth), long bones (fractures), liver and **spleen (hepatosplenomegaly)**.

❑ **Diagnosis:** The peripheral smear shows **microcytosis, target cells, hypochromia** and reticulocytosis; however reticulocytosis is not in proportion to severity of anemia. **Increased Hb F** levels can be documented by **haemoglobin electrophoresis.**

❑ **Treatment:** Blood transfusion had been the cornerstone of thalassemia major treatment but the major drawback is hemosiderosis due to iron accumulation. If the facilities are available then bone marrow transplantation can be beneficial.

❖ **Thalassemia intermedia, minor and minima:** In thalassemia intermedia, minor and minima clinical presentations are milder than the major thalassemia; however depending on the severity of disease blood transfusion and splenectomy may be required.

❖ **Thalassemia trait:** Thalassemia trait patients are asymptomatic but **mild microcytic hypochromic anemia** can be present. It can be differentiated from iron deficiency anemia by presence of a normal red cell distribution width. Increased **Hb A$_2$ levels**(Normal Hb A$_2$ = 1.5-3.5%) of **more than 3.5%** is diagnostic of thalassemia trait. **Hb F is variable** i.e. increased in half of the patients and normal in half. The Hb levels are near normal i.e. 1-2 gm/dl less than normal. **NESTROFT** test can be done for screening of thalassemia trait.

• **α thalassemia:** Depending on the number α globin gene mutation, variable **decrease in α globin production** can be seen. There is compensatory overproduction of β and γ globulins, which can form **Bart hemoglobin (γ_4), haemoglobin H(β_4).** Since α globulin is required for Hb F formation, it is decreased and may manifest in utero.

❖ **Thalassemia trait:** Deletion of 1 gene leads to silent trait with normal hematopoesis. On the other hand deletion of 2 genes leads to trait, which presents with microcytic hypochromic anemia.

❖ **Hemoglobin H disease:** Hb H disease is caused by deletion of 3 genes. The presentation is more severe than trait with severe anemia and splenomegaly. Apart from Hb H, Bart's Hb level is also increased to more than 25%.

❖ **Hydrops fetalis:** Deletion of the all 4 genes leads to severe anemia in the foetus, which presents as hydrops fetalis. **Bart's haemoglobin** leads to foetal hypoxemia as it **doesn't release oxygen** to tissues owing to its high affinity for the same.

Sickle Cell Anemia and Trait

Sickle cell anemia is caused by **point mutation of β globin gene**, which leads to **change of glutamate to valine.** It is an **AR** condition and hence the homozygous condition (mutation of both β globin genes) presents as sickle cell anemia and heterozygous condition (mutation of one β globin gene) presents as sickle cell trait. Sickling of RBCs depend on multiple factors like:

• **Hb S concentration** — Increased Hb S concentration of >50% precipitates sickling.

• **Hb F and Hb A concentration** — Increased Hb F and Hb A (HbF > Hb A) concentration prevents polymerisation of Hb S. Since Hb F concentration is high **till 6 months of life, babies are asymptomatic till this period**.

• **Intracellular pH** — Decreased pH decreases tendency of binding of Hb to oxygen. Deoxygenation precipitates sickling.

• **RBC passing time through microvasculature** — Increase time of presence in microvascular can cause deoxygenation and sickling.

Sickle Cell Anemia

Mutation of the β globin gene leads to formation of HbS, which polymerises and changes to sickle or holly-leaf shape in deoxygenated state. On repeated oxygenation and deoxygenation the RBCs permanently become sickled shape and give rise to various pathological conditions.

• **Clinical presentation:** Since HbF prevents sickling the clinical presentation is only apparent at 6 month of age.

❖ **Hemolytic anemia** — Sickle cells are sequestered in the spleen which can lead to sever hemolytic anemia.

❖ **Cardiomegaly** — Cardiomegaly can be seen due to compensatory increase in the cardiac contraction due to anemia.

❖ **Acute infections** — Acute infections caused by encapsulated organisms like pneumococci and *H. influenzae* is a **major cause of mortality in children till 5 years**. Hence penicillin prophylaxis is advised till the child attains 5 years of age. **Salmonella is the most common cause of osteomyelitis** in children with sickle cell anemia.

❖ **Vaso-occlusion** — These malformed sickle cells are trapped in blood vessels and can present as stroke, **autosplenectomy**, hand and foot syndrome (earliest manifestation), bone infarction and **acute pain episodes (most common manifestation)**, priapism, acute chest syndrome, **pulmonary hypertension** and renal disorders (nephrotic syndrome, pyelonephritis, medullary carcinoma).

❖ **Aplastic crisis** can be seen in sickle cell anemia in case of **human parvovirus B19 infection** as it decreases the production of reticulocytes.

- **Diagnosis:**
  ❖ Neonatal screening confirms the disease by presence of abnormal haemoglobin by IEF (isoelectric focusing) and HPLC (high performance liquid chromatography).
  ❖ Hb electrophoresis shows 80–90% of **Hb S** and the rest is **Hb F and Hb A₂**; however **Hb A is absent**.
  ❖ X-ray shows **crew cut appearance of skull** and **fish mouth vertebra**.
  ❖ Peripheral smear shows reticulocytes and target cells.
  ❖ **Leucocyte count** and platelet count is **increased**.

- **Treatment:**
  ❖ **Blood transfusion** — The aim of transfusion is to keep the HbS below 30%. Most common indication for transfusion is for prevention of stroke.
  ❖ **Bone marrow transplantation** — Most common indication of bone marrow transplantation is stroke.
  ❖ **Hydroxyurea** — It increases Hb F, which decreases the sickling of RBCs.

Sickle Cell Trait

- Sickle cell trait is characterised by predominance of Hb A over Hb S, which prevents sickling. The patients have a normal life; however conditions of severe hypoxemia can cause complications like sudden death, splenic infarcts, hematuria and hyposthenuria. HPLC shows **two bands of haemoglobin** i.e. of Hb A and Hb S.

G6PD Deficiency

G6PD deficiency is an **X linked recessive** disorder characterised by NADPH deficiency. NADPH is an important component of RBCs which maintains glutathione in reduced state and hence its deficiency leads to oxidative RBC damage. **Older RBCs have relatively less G6PD** and hence are more prone to hemolysis.

- **Clinical presentation:** The infants are at risk of kernicterus due to hemolysis. Older children have episodes of hemolysis at exposure to oxidative stress caused by infection, drugs or foods like fava beans.

  Drugs causing hemolysis:

Mnemonic: **MAD FANS**
M — Methylene blue
A — Acetanilide
D — Doxorubicin, Dapsone
F — Furazolidone
A — Anti malarial drug like primaquine
N — Nalidixic acid, Nitrofurantion
S — Sulphonamides, Salicylates

- **Diagnosis:** Periods of hemolysis are characterised by decrease in haemoglobin and increase in bilirubin and reticulocyte count. Peripheral smear shows **"Bite cells"** or blister cells, Heinz bodies and some spherocytes.
- **Treatment:** The most important part of treatment is to avoid the above mentioned drugs and fava beans.

Iron Deficiency Anemia

Iron stores of the newborn are sufficient for erythropoiesis till 9 months of age and hence anemia due to iron deficiency is uncommon before this period. However it can be seen in this period in case baby has prematurity, small for gestational age and perinatal blood loss. **Iron is absorbed from duodenum** and factors that can hinder absorption are cow milk feeding, infection with hookworm and *H. pylori*. **Cow milk has more iron than breast milk** but is poorly absorbed and it can also induce colitis that can further decrease iron absorption.

Clinical Presentation

Iron deficiency can present with pallor, fatigue, pagophagia or pica (eating of inedible substances like clay), irritability, **decreased alertness** and attention; and delayed motor development.

Diagnosis

- Peripheral smear shows **microcytic and hypochromic RBCs;** anisocytosis and **target cells.**
- **Serum ferritin** is the **best indicator of iron status** as it reflects iron status of both liver and reticuloendothelial system. **Serum ferritin level** is the earliest to decrease and a **low ferritin level** i.e. <10-15 ng/ml absolutely indicates iron deficiency and hence is the **most specific and sensitive test.**
- Serum iron and **serum transferrin saturation**(<15%) are also decreased but **total iron binding capacity** and serum transferrin receptor(>8.5 mg/L) **is increased.**
- **Red cell distribution width (RDW) is elevated.**
- Bone marrow shows **erythroid hyperplasia** and decreased iron content. The **iron content of bone marrow is decreased earlier than serum iron.**

Treatment

Oral iron supplement in the form of sulphate, gluconate and fumarate salts is given at a dose of 6 mg/kg/day and **continued 8 weeks after Hb levels are normalised.** The **dose of iron** can be calculated by a formula i.e. **3 × weight in k.g × Hb deficit in gm/dl.** The **earliest response to iron therapy is increase in reticulocyte count** within 3–5 days and **maximises in 5–7 days.** This follows **increase in Hb** at a rate of 0.5 gm/dl/24 hours in the **2nd week.**

Megaloblastic Anemia

Megaloblastic anemia is caused by deficiency of Vitamin B_{12} and folic acid.

- **Vitamin B_{12}** deficiency is primarily caused by **malabsorption.** Vitamin B_{12} is absorbed from the terminal ileum and hence its absorption can be decreased in conditions like Crohn disease, **bacterial overgrowth syndrome** caused by ileocaecal valve incompetence and **blind loop syndrome,** chronic pancreatitis and infestation with fish tapeworm.
- Folic acid deficiency is primarily caused by insufficient dietary intake and increased demand during rapid growth in infancy and chronic hemolysis. It can also be caused by group of drugs like anticonvulsants (phenobarbitone, phenytoin, valproate, and primidone), antifolate (sulphonamides, methotrexate, pyrimethamine, proguanil, dapsone, trimethoprim, PAS) and inhibitors of DNA synthesis (pyrimidine and purine analogues, hydroxyurea, acyclovir). Celiac sprue and chronic diarrhoea can also precipitate folate deficiency.

Clinical Presentation

The symptoms of megaloblastic anemia range from typical symptoms of anemia like pallor and jaundice to neurological symptoms like paraesthesia, hypotonia and seizures. The tongue has a smooth surface and **red beefy appearance.**

Diagnosis

- Peripheral smear shows macrocytes and **hypersegmented neutrophils.**
- MCV and MCHC are increased.
- Serum vitamin B_{12} and folic acid levels are decreased; however RBC folic acid is a better predictor of folic acid deficiency.
- Methylmalonic acid is increased in vitamin B_{12} deficiency.
- Homocystinemia is seen in both B_{12} and folic acid deficiency.

Treatment

Treatment comprises of dealing with the underlying disorder and supplementing folic acid and vitamin $B1_{12}$. The exact cause of megaloblastic anemia should be evaluated as treatment with only folic acid can improve anemic picture but worsen neuropathic features.

RBC Membrane Disorders

Hereditary Spherocytosis

Hereditary spherocytosis is an AD condition caused by frame shift mutation of various RBC proteins like ankyrin, spectrin, band 3 and band 4.2. This leads to **loss of some part of the RBC membrane with some cytoplasm** and it assumes a shape to accommodate maximum volume i.e. sphere. This spheroid RBC which is inflexible undergoes sequestration in the spleen.

- **Clinical presentation:** The patient presents with anemia, pallor, jaundice and splenomegaly. Gallstones are frequently seen in case of spherocytosis. Patients are at high risk of **parvovirus infection and resultant aplastic crisis.**
- **Diagnosis:**
  - ❖ **MCV is normal** and **MCHC is increased.**
  - ❖ Peripheral smear shows spherocytes and reticulocytes.
  - ❖ **Osmotic fragility test (pink test)** — Osmotic fragility is increased if there is a relative decrease in the RBC membrane circumference as compared to the RBC volume. It is **increased** in hereditary spherocytosis but is not specific as it can be positive in other conditions with spherocytes like haemolytic anemia. Osmotic fragility is decreased in thalassemia, iron deficiency anemia and splenomegaly.
- **Treatment:** Splenectomy is the mainstay of treatment. Folic acid is advised prophylactically to maintain an effective erythropoiesis.

DISORDERS OF THROMBOCYTES

Platelet count normally ranges from 150×10^9 to 450×10^9 and any value lesser than the former one is called as thrombocytopenia. **The most common cause of acute thrombocytopenia in children is ITP.** The other causes are DIC, Kasabach-Merritt syndrome, **Wiskott-Aldrich syndrome**, congenital platelet dysfunction (Bernard soulier syndrome, Glanzmann thrombasthenia), TAR syndrome and acute leukemias.

Idiopathic Thrombocytopenic Purpura

ITP is an acute **immune mediated** accelerated destruction of thrombocytes caused by **antiplatelet antibodies**. There is always a **history of viral infection** (EBV, HIV, rubella, varicella, measles, parvovirus, and influenza) prior to the onset of disease. The **most common age group** affected is **children from 2 to 5 years.**

Clinical Features

The classical presentation is **sudden onset of petechiae and purpura** in a previously normal child. Bleeding from gums and mucous membranes, epistaxis and haemorrhage in to organs can also be seen. **Splenomegaly is usually not seen** and if present leukaemia should be considered. Most of the cases i.e. around **80% resolve spontaneously** and only the rest **20% persist** for more than 6 months to become **chronic.** The **risk factors for chronicity** are **female sex**, age> 10 years and presence of other autoantibodies.

Diagnosis

- Platelet count is severely decreased to $<20 \times 10^9$ and **bleeding time is prolonged.**
- Peripheral smear shows larger platelets.
- Bone marrow shows **increase in megakaryocyte number.**
- **Antiplatelet antibodies** can be demonstrated in the serum.

Treatment

- **Prednisolone** is used for a brief period of 2–3 weeks in mild to moderate cases of bleeding.
- IVIG is the **drug of choice** for severe cases of bleeding and also in **neonatal ITP**.
- Anti-Rho D Ig can be given for Rh+ patients.
- Splenectomy is indicated for long standing (> 1 year) and resistant cases.
- **Platelet transfusion is contraindicated** as they will also be destroyed by the antibodies.

Kasabach-Merritt Syndrome

Kaposiform hemangioendotheliomas in **newborn** can cause **platelet sequestration** followed by **thrombocytopenia, consumptive coagulopathy** and microangiopathic haemolytic anemia. Heart failure can be seen in case of arteriovenous malformations. The lesions are treated by drugs (corticosteroids, alpha interferon and vincristine), laser photocoagulation and radiation. Surgery is usually not indicated due to risk of haemorrhage.

Platelet Dysfunction

Congenital Platelet Dysfunction

Blood vessel injury causes vasoconstriction and the platelet VWF receptor binds to the **VWF present on the endothelial matrix** of blood vessels. Following this adhesion platelets are activated and they release factors like ADP and thromboxane A_2 which cause aggregation of platelets. Further fibrinogen also binds to GP IIb-IIIa receptors of platelets and continues aggregation. After aggregation the platelets form a **temporary hemostatic plug**. Congenital defect in VWF receptor (Bernard-Soulier syndrome) and GP IIb-IIIa receptor (Glanzmann thrombasthenia) can lead to thrombocytopenia and its symptoms (petechiae, purpura) shortly after birth. Platelet dysfunction can also be seen due to absence of ADP in platelet granules (storage pool disease, Quebec platelet disorder, Hermansky-Pudlak syndrome, **Wiskott-Aldrich syndrome**, Chediac-Higashi syndrome) and α granules of platelet (grey platelet syndrome).

- **Bernard soulier syndrome and Glanzmann thrombasthenia:**

Bernard soulier syndrome	*Glanzmann thrombasthenia*
- It is an AR disorder.	- It is an AR disorder.
- Caused by defect of VWF or GP Ib receptor.	- Caused by defect of GP IIb-IIIa receptors.
- **Thrombocytopenia** is seen and **bleeding time is prolonged. PT and aPTT** are normal.	- **Thrombocytopenia** is seen and **bleeding time is prolonged. PT and aPTT** are normal.
- Despite of severe thrombocytopenia, **bleeding is not seen in newborns.**	- **Newborns** present with generalised purpura and **bleeding from the umbilical stump**. Older children present with nose bleeds, easy bruising and menorrhagia.
- **Platelet aggregation in response to ristocetin is absent;** however is **present with other agonists like ADP,** epinephrine, **collagen,** and thrombin.	- Platelet aggregation is seen only in response to ristocetin.
- Platelets are of large size.	- Platelets are of normal size.
- **Desmopressin** is used to treat acute bleeding episode. **Platelet transfusion** is done to maintain homeostasis. In case of resistance due to antiplatelet antibody production, **recombinant factor VIIa** is given.	- **Desmopressin** is used to treat acute bleeding episode. **Platelet transfusion** is done to maintain homeostasis. In case of resistance due to antiplatelet antibody production, **recombinant factor VIIa** is given.

- **Wiskott Aldrich syndrome:**
  ❖ Wiskott-Aldrich syndrome is an X-linked recessive disorder characterised caused by mutation in the Wiskott-Aldrich syndrome protein (WASP) gene in chromosome 11.
  ❖ The WASP is required for anchoring the membrane receptors to the cytoskeletal elements and plays an integral role in regulating the cytoskeletal architecture of both platelets and T lymphocytes in response to receptor-mediated cell signalling.
  ❖ The presenting symptoms are —
    ❑ **Thrombocytopenia**
    ❑ **Eczema**
    ❑ **Recurrent infections caused by immunodeficiency characterised by T lymphocyte depletion and decreased Ig M.**
  ❖ There is progressive depletion of lymphocytes in the blood and lymphnodes, however thymus is usually normal.
  ❖ Antibody production in response to antigens is blunted. There is decreased Ig M production; however Ig G production is normal. The levels of Ig A and E is increased.
  ❖ Bone marrow transplantation is the treatment of choice.

Acquired Platelet Dysfunction

Platelet dysfunction can be acquired by medical conditions like uremia, cirrhosis, sepsis, myeloproliferative disorders, congenital heart disease and viral infections; and drugs like **NSAIDs**, synthetic penicillins and sodium valproate.

Disorders of Coagulation

The temporary hemostatic plug formed by platelet aggregation is consolidated in to definitive clot by fibrin. The process of fibrin formation is a sequential activation of various clotting factors in two pathways i.e. extrinsic and intrinsic pathways. Both the pathways follow different routes to activate factor X. Activated factor X along with phospholipase, factor V and calcium convert prothrombin (factor II) to thrombin (factor IIa). Finally thrombin converts fibrinogen (factor I) to fibrin (factor Ia) which forms the definitive clot.

- The extrinsic pathway is activated by tissue thromboplastin which activates factor VII and subsequently factor IX and **X are activated**.
- The intrinsic pathway is activated by HMW kininogen and kallikrein which activates factor XII and subsequently factor XI and IX are activated. Factor IX along with factor VIII **activate factor X**.

Prothrombin time (PT) is used to diagnose the defect in **extrinsic pathway** and is prolonged in deficiency of **factor VII. Activated partial thromboplastin time (aPTT)** is used to diagnose the defect in **intrinsic pathway** and is prolonged in deficiency of **factors XII, XI, IX and VIII.** Both PT and aPTT are prolonged in deficiency of factors X, V, II and I.

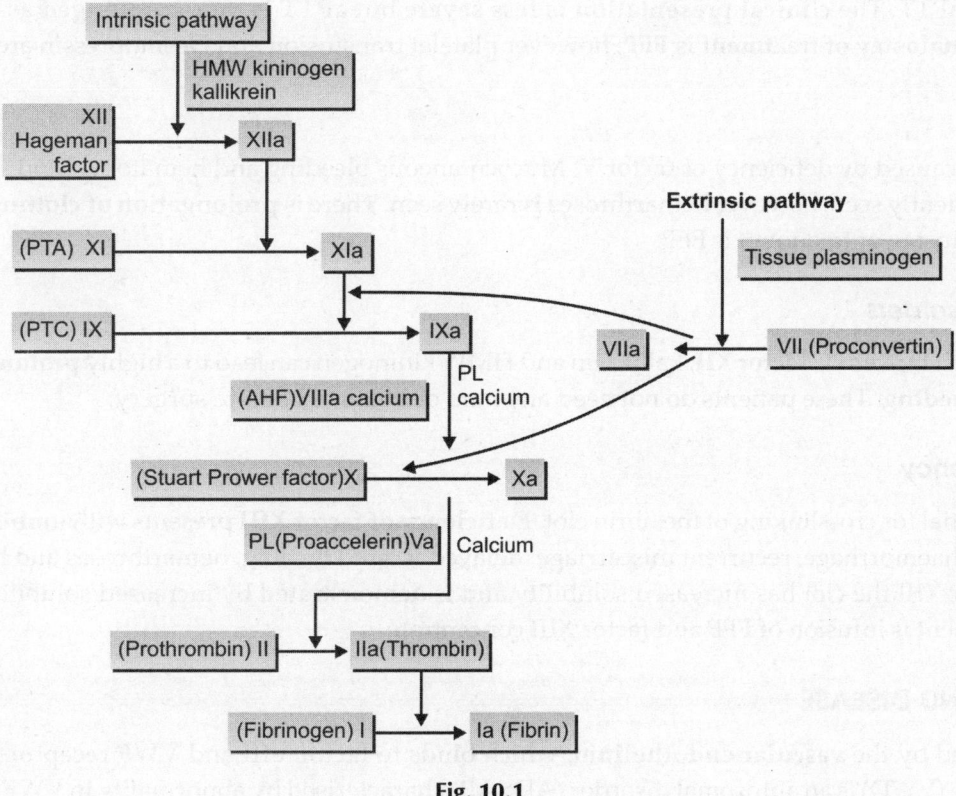

Fig. 10.1

Hemophilia A

Hemophilia A or classic hemophilia is an X linked recessive disorder (males are affected, females are carrier) caused by deficiency of factor VIII. The normal level of **factor VIII** is 0.5–1.5 U/ml (50–150%) and has a **half-life of 8–12 hours.** The **disease manifests when the level of factor VIII falls below 40%** and can be classified as mild (5–40%), moderate (1–5%) and severe (<1%).

- **Clinical presentation:** The patients have episodes of bleeding in skin, mucous membrane, **joints (hemophilic arthropathy)**, muscles (compartment syndrome) and organs. The earliest joint to be involved is **ankle joint.** Arthropathy is caused by iron deposition in the joints and it is called as **"target"** joint. Intracranial haemorrhage is the most common cause of death.
- **Diagnosis:** Factor VIII deficiency causes **prolongation of clotting time and aPTT.** Bleeding time and PT is normal.
- **Treatment:**
  - ❖ **Recombinant factor VIII** is the mainstay of treatment; however antibodies can be developed against factor VIII and decreases its effect. Anti-factor VIII antibodies can be detected by **Bethesda assay.**
  - ❖ **Desmopressin** can be given in mild cases. It acts by releasing factor VIII from the endothelium of blood vessels.

❖ **Antifibrinolytic therapy** in the form of **epsilon aminocaproic acid** and **tranexemic acid** is indicated for treatment of **epistaxis, oral bleeding** and bleeding associated with **tooth extraction.**

Hemophilia B

Hemophilia B or Christmas disease is caused by deficiency of factor IX. The half-life of factor IX is 20-22 hours. It is associated with prolonged clotting time and aPTT. The mainstay of treatment is recombinant factor IX. The clinical presentation is similar to hemophilia A.

Hemophilia C

Hemophilia C is caused by deficiency of factor XI. Factor XI has a half-life of > 48 hours. It is associated with prolonged clotting time and aPTT. The **clinical presentation is less severe** but **aPTT is more prolonged** as compared to other hemophilias. The **mainstay of treatment is FFP**; however platelet transfusion and Desmopressin are also used.

Parahemophilia

Parahemophilia is caused by deficiency of **factor V**. Mucocutaneous bleeding and hematomas and severe menorrhagia in females are frequently seen; however hemarthroses is rarely seen. There is **prolongation of clotting time** and **both PT and aPTT.** The mainstay of treatment is FFP.

Non-bleeding Disorders

Deficiency of contact factors i.e. **factor XII**, kallikrein and HMW kininogen can lead to a highly **prolonged aPTT** but there is **no history of bleeding**. These patients do not need any kind of treatment before surgery.

Factor XIII Deficiency

Factor XIII is essential for crosslinking of the fibrin clot. **Deficiency of factor XIII** presents with **umbilical bleeding after birth**, intracranial haemorrhage, recurrent miscarriage, delayed wound healing, hemarthroses and hematoma. Because of decreased factor XIII the clot has increased solubility and is demonstrated by increased solubility in 5 M urea. The mainstay of treatment is infusion of FFP and factor XIII concentrate.

VON-WILLEBRAND DISEASE

VWF is synthesised by the **vascular endothelium**, which binds to factor VIII and VWF receptors on platelets. Von-Willebrand disease (VWD) is an autosomal disorder (AD>AR) characterised by abnormality in VWF. The most common cause is partial deficiency of VWF and is called as type 1 VWD. The other types are type 2 (defect in VWF) and type 3 (complete absence of VWF). Acquired VWF disorders can be seen with hypothyroidism, Wilms tumor, SLE, cardiac and renal disease.

Clinical Presentation

Patients may present with history of prolonged bleeding, epistaxis, bruising episodes and menorrhagia in females.

Diagnosis

- Bleeding time and APTT are prolonged.
- Factor VIII is decreased.
- Aggregation of platelets in response to agonists like collagen and ristocetin is decreased.

Treatment

The mainstay of treatment is **desmopressin** during bleeding episodes; however tachyphylaxis is seen because of depletion of endothelial VWF. In case of resistance VWF should be replaced.

MULTIPLE CHOICE QUESTIONS

1. **Kostmann's syndrome-treatment is:**
   [AIIMS Nov. 09]
   a. Antithymocte globulin + cyclosporine
   b. Antithymocyte globulin + cyclosporine + GM-CSF
   c. G-CSF
   d. GM-CSF

2. **Absent thumb, radial deviation of wrist, bowing of forearm with thrombocytopenia. Which investigation need not be done?** [AIIMS May 08]
   a. Echocardiography
   b. Bone marrow examination
   c. Platelet count
   d. Karyotyping

3. **A 5-year-old boy comes with overnight petechial spots. 2 weeks back he had history of abdominal pain and no hepatosplenomegaly. Diagnosis is:**
   [AIIMS May 07]
   a. Acute lymphatic leukemia
   b. Aplastic anemia
   c. Idiopathic thrombocytopenic purpura
   d. Acute viral infection

4. **In beta thalassemia the most common gene mutation is:** [AIIMS Nov. 06]
   a. Intron 1 inversion   b. Intron 22
   c. 619 bp deletion   d. 3.7 bp deletion

5. **Which organ is primary site of hematopoesis in the foetus before midpregnancy:** [AIIMS May 06]
   a. Bone   b. Liver
   c. Spleen   d. Lung

6. **All of the following are true of β thalassemia major, except:** [AIIMS May 06]
   a. Splenomegaly
   b. Target cells on peripheral smear
   c. Microcytic hypochromic anemia
   d. Increased osmotic fragility

7. **Which of the following hemoglobin (Hb) estimation will be diagnostically helpful in a case of beta thalassemia trait?** [AIIMS May 06]
   a. Hb-F   b. Hb1-C
   c. Hb-A2   d. Hb-H

8. **When does switchover from fetal to adult hemoglobin synthesis begin:**
   [AIIMS Nov. 04, Nov. 05, May 05]
   a. 14 weeks gestation   b. 30 weeks gestation
   c. 36 weeks gestation   d. 7-10 days postnatal

9. **Which of the following is generally not seen in idiopathic thrombocytopenic purpura (ITP)?**
   [AIIMS Nov. 04]
   a. More common in females
   b. Petechiae, ecchymosis and bleeding

c. Palpable splenomegaly
d. Increased megakaryocytes in bone marrow

10. **A child underwent a tonsillectomy at 6 years of age with no complications. He underwent a preoperative screening for bleeding at the age of 12 years before an elective laparotomy, and was found to have a prolonged partial thromboplastin time but normal prothrombin time. There was no family history of bleeding. The patient is likely to have:**
    [AIIMS Nov. 04]
    a. Acquired VitK deficiency
    b. Acquired liver disease
    c. FactorXIIdeficiency
    d. Mild hemophilia A

11. **A child died soon after birth. On examination there was hepatosplenomegaly and edema all over body. Most probable diagnosis in:** [AIIMS May 02]
    a. β-thalassemia
    b. α-thalassemia
    c. Hereditary spherocytosis
    d. ABO incompatibility/sickle cell anemia

12. **Sickle cell trait patient do not have manifestations as that of sickle cell disease because:**
    [AIIMS Nov. 01]
    a. 50% HbS is required for occurrence of sickling
    b. Hb A prevents sickling
    c. 50% sickles
    d. Hb A prevents polymerisation of Hb S

13. **In beta thalassemia there is:** [AIIMS May 01]
    a. Increased beta chain, decreased alpha chain
    b. Decreased in beta chain, increase in alpha chain
    c. Decrease in beta chain, decrease in alpha chain
    d. Increase in beta chain, increase in alpha chain

14. **Thrombocytopenia in a new born baby can be caused by:** [AIIMS Nov. 1999]
    a. ABO incompatibility
    b. Isoimmune thrombocytopenia
    c. Autoimmune thrombocytopenia
    d. SLE

15. **A patient has ecchymosis and petechiae all over the body with no hepatosplenomegaly. All are true except:** [AIIMS Nov. 99]
    a. Increased megakaryocytes in bone narrow.
    b. Bleeding into the joints
    c. Decreased platelet in blood
    d. Disease resolves itself in 80% of Pt. in 2–6 weeks

16. **Commonest presentation of sickle cell anemia:**
    [AIIMS Nov. 98]
    a. Priapism   b. Bone pain
    c. Fever   d. Splenomegaly

17. **Feature of foetal RBC in adult:** [AIIMS June 98]
    a. Alkali denaturation resistant
    b. Small in size
    c. Has more 2, 3 DGP level
    d. More iron than adult RBC

18. **All are true regarding foetal RBCs except:**
    [AIIMS Dec. 97]
    a. Elevated 2, 3 DGP
    b. Decrease carbonic anhydrase activity
    c. Decreased life span
    d. High RBC volume

19. **Cause of ITP is:** [AIIMS Feb. 97]
    a. Vasculitis
    b. Antibody to vascular epithelium
    c. Antibody to platelets
    d. Antibody to clotting factors

20. **The earliest sign of iron deficiency anemia:**
    [AIIMS Feb. 97]
    a. Increase in iron binding capacity
    b. Decrease in serum ferritin level
    c. Decrease in serum iron level
    d. All of the above

21. **von Willebrands disease all are true except:**
    [AIIMS 97]
    a. Factor VIII c deficiency
    b. B.T prolonged
    c. Normal ristocetin test
    d. Defective aggregation

22. **Megaloblastic anemia may be caused by all of the following except:** [AIIMS 96, AI 98]
    a. Phenytoin   b. Methotrexate
    c. Pyrimethamine   d. Amoxicillin

23. **Drug of choice in neonatal ITP is:** [AIIMS 91]
    a. Platelet transfusion   b. Prednisolone
    c. Dexamethasone   d. Gammaglobulin

24. **All are true for sickle cell anemia, except:**
    [AIIMS May 94]
    a. Pulmonary arterial hypertension
    b. Fish vertebra
    c. Leukopenia
    d. Increased size of heart

25. **Crew haircut appearance on X-ray skull and Gandy gamma bodies are seen in:** [AIIMS Nov. 93]
    a. G6PD deficiency
    b. Hodgkin's lymphoma
    c. Hereditary spherocytosis
    d. Sickle cell anemia

26. **The haemoglobin to appear first in the foetus is:**
    [AIIMS 83]
    a. Hb A   b. Hb A_2
    c. Hb F   d. Hb Gower's

27. **A patient on aspirin will show the following finding?**
    [AI 07]
    a. Prolonged BT   b. Prolonged PT
    c. Prolonged APTT   d. Prolonged CT

28. **Which of the following findings is diagnostic of iron deficiency anemia:** [AI 07]
    a. Increased TIBC, decreased serum ferritin
    b. Decreased TIBC, decreased serum ferritin
    c. Increased TIBC, increased serum ferritin
    d. Decreased TIBC, increased serum ferritin

29. **Megaloblastic anemia due to folic acid deficiency is commonly due to:** [AI 06]
    a. Inadequate dietary intake
    b. Defective intestinal absorption
    c. Absence of folic acid binding protein in serum
    d. Absence of glutamic acid in the intestine

30. **The earliest indicator of response after starting iron in a 6 years old girl with iron deficiency is:** [AI 06]
    a. Increased reticulocyte count
    b. Increased hemoglobin
    c. Increased ferritin
    d. Increased serum iron

31. **Diagnosis of beta thalassemia is established by:**
    [AI 05]
    a. NESTROFT Test
    b. Hb A1, C estimation
    c. Hb electrophoresis
    d. Target cells in peripheral smear

32. **Bart's hydrops fetalis is lethal because:** [AI 05]
    a. Hb Bart's cannot bind oxygen
    b. The excess α-globin form insoluble precipitates
    c. Hb Bart's cannot release oxygen to fetal tissues
    d. Microcytic red cells become trapped in the placenta

33. **The coagulation profile in a 13-years old girl with menorrhagia having von Willebrands disease is:**
    [AI 05]
    a. Isolated prolonged PTT with a normal PT
    b. Isolated prolonged PT with a normal PTT
    c. Prolongation of both PT and PTT
    d. Prolongation of thrombin time

34. **All of the following statements are true about sickle cell disease except:** [AI 04]
    a. Patient may require frequent blood transfusions
    b. Acute infection is the most common cause of mortality before 3 years of age
    c. There is positive correlation between conc. Hb S and polymerisation of Hb S
    d. Patient present early in life before 6 months of life

35. **A nine months old boy of Sindhi parents presented to you with complaints of progressive lethargy, irritability and pallor since 6 months of age. Examination revealed severe pallor. Investigation showed Hb-3.8 mg%; MCV-58 fl; MCH-19.4 pg/cell.**

Blood film shows osmotic fragility is normal (target cells and normoblasts). X-ray skull shows expansion of erythmoid marrow. Which of the following is the most likely diagnosis?   [AI 04]

a. Iron deficiency anemia
b. Acute lymphoblastic anemia
c. Hemoglobin D disease
d. Hereditary spherocytosis

36. Most sensitive and specific test for diagnosis of iron deficiency is: [AI 03]

a. Serum iron level
b. Serum ferritin levels
c. Serum transferrin receptor populations
d. Transferrin saturation

37. The primary defect which leads to sickle cell anemia is: [AI 03]

a. An abnormality in porphyrin part of hemoglobin
b. Replacement of glutamate by valine in β-chain of HbA
c. A nonsence mutation in the (β-chain of HbA
d. Substitution of valine by glutamate in the a-chain of HbA

38. Best test for assessment of iron status is: [AI 01]

a. Transferrin   b. Ferritin
c. Serum iron   d. Hemoglobin

39. Which of the following is not seen on haemoglobin electrophoresis in sickle cell anemia?   [AI 01]

a. Hb A   b. Hb A_2
c. Hb F   d. Hb S

40. A child aged 2 years presents with nonspecific symptoms suggestive of anemia. On peripheral blood smear target cells are seen. He has hypochromic microcytic picture and Hb of 6 gm%. He also has a positive family history. Next investigation of choice is: [AI 01]

a. Hb electrophoresis   b. Coomb's test
c. Liver function tests   d. Osmatic fragility test

41. Which is not seen in iron deficiency anemia?   [AI 2000]

a. Hypersegmented neutrophils
b. Microcytosis precedes hypochromia
c. MCHC< 50%
d. Commonest cause of anemia in India

42. Megaloblastic anemia in blind loop syndrome is due to: [AI 99]

a: Vitamin B_{12} malabsorption
b. Bacterial overgrowth
c. Frequent diarrhoea
d. Decrease iron intake

43. Major source of von Willebrand factor (VWF) is: [AI 98]

a. Erythrocytes   b. Neutrophils
c. Endothelial cells   d. Monocytes

44. Primaquine may cause hemolysis in: [AI 98]

a. G6PD deficiency
b. NADP deficiency
c. Methemoglobin deficiency
d. Crabb's disease

45. Hemophilia A have the following diagnostic features except?   [AI 97]

a. Factor VIII   b. PTT
c. PT   d. Normal BT

46. Which of the following is not seen in a chronic case of sickle cell anemia?   [AI 96]

a. Hepatomegaly
b. Pulmonary hypertension
c. Cardiomegaly
d. Splenomegaly

47. Kasabach-Merritt syndrome, true about A/E: [PGI Nov. 09]

a. Platelet sequestration
b. Infantile hemangioma
c. Consumption coagulopathy
d. Portwine hemangioma
e. Thrombocytosis

48. MCV in infant of 1 month of age is: [PGI Nov. 09]

a. 76–80   b. 80–100
c. 90–100   d. 101–125
e. 125–135

49. True about iron deficiency anemia in children: [PGI June 09]

a. Iron absorption from terminal ileum
b. Cow milk contains less iron than breast milk
c. Serum ferritin depletes first
d. Decreased alertness
e. Decreased red cell distribution width (RDW)

50. Characteristic lab findings of hemophilia A are: [PGI June 06]

a. Increase PT
b. Increase aPTT
c. X-linked recessive
d. Presence of 30% of factor level express the disease
e. Increased bleeding time

51. Regarding G6PD deficiency true are: [PGI June 06]

a. Autosomal dominant
b. Bite cell (+)
c. Protects against kalaazar
d. Enzyme level directly proportional to age of RBC
e. Sex preponderance

52. Which of the following is true about oral therapy for iron deficiency anemia?   [PGI Dec. 05]

a. In 300 mg elemental iron given 100 mg get absorbed
b. Reticulocytosis appears in one to 2 weeks and then peaks in 3–4 weeks

c. Response to treatment seen in 4 weeks

d. Decrease in absorption with improvement of symptoms

e. Stop the treatment after normalising the Hb

53. True about iron deficiency anemia: [PGI June 05]

a. Microcytic hypochromic anemia

b. Decreased TIBC

c. Increased ferritin

d. Bone marrow iron decreased earlier than serum iron

54. True about acute ITP: [PGI June 05]

a. More common in female

b. Specific antiplatelet antibodies detected

c. Viral infection predisposes as seen after vaccination

d. 80% cases transforms to chronic

e. Disease resolves itself in 80% of Pt. in 2-6 week

55. β-thalasemia trait; true about: [PGI June 04]

a. ↑ HbF   b. ↑ HbA$_2$

c. Microcytosis   d. Severe anemia

56. Platelet function defect is seen in: [PGI June 03]

a. Glanzmann syndrome

b. Bernard soulier syndrome

c. Wiskott Aldrich syndrome

d. von Willebrand disease

e. Weber Christian disease

57. Platelet function assessed by: [PGI Dec. 02]

a. Platelet adhesion   b. BT

c. CT   d. PTT

e. ↓^{ed} TLC

58. Mutation leading to sickle cell anemia:

[PGI June 01]

a. Crossover mutation

b. Frame shift

c. Deletion

d. Nondysjunction

e. Point mutation

59. Thalassemia occurs due to which mutations:

[PGI Dec. 2000]

a. Missense   b. Splicing

c. Transition   d. Frame-shift

e. Truncation

60. Hb A 2 concentration in thalassemia trait is:

[PGI June 99]

a. 1   b. 1-2.5

c. 2.5-3.5   d. >3.5

61. Salmonellosis is most common in: [PGI June 98]

a. Sickle cell anemia   b. Thalassemia

c. Hemophilia   d. Cystic fibrosis

62. Which enzyme deficiency causes hemolytic anemia? [PGI 98]

a. G6PD   b. Aldolase

c. Isomerase d. Enolase

63. In sickle cell trait, number of bands found in Hb:

[PGI June 98]

a. 2   b. 1

c. 4   d. 5

64. Following are the findings in sickle cell anemia except: [PGI June 98]

a. Fish vertebra

b. Enlarged heart

c. Splenomegaly usually seen

d. Leucocytosis

65. Defect leading to thalassemia lies in: [PGI Dec. 97]

a. Haemoglobin

b. Osmotic fragility

c. RBC membrane

d. Platelets

66. Glanzmans disease is: [PGI 96]

a. Congenital defects of platelets

b. Congenital defects of RBC

c. Defect of neutrophils

d. Clotting factor deficiency

67. In α-thalassemia: [PGI 92]

a. Excess α chain

b. No α chain

c. Excess β chain

d. No β chain

68. Megaloblastic anemia develop in: [PGI 88]

a. Sideroblastic anemia

b. Thalassemia

c. Infants fed on goat milk

d. Vitamin C deficiency

69. Aminocaproic acid would be recommended for a hemophilic child with: [PGI 79]

a. Epistaxis

b. Hematuria

c. Oral bleeding

d. Hemarthroses

70. In thrombasthenia there is a defect in: [Jipmer 91]

a. Platelet aggregation

b. Platelet adhesion

c. Decreased ADP release

d. Disordered platelet secretion

71. The following laboratory determinants is abnormally prolonged in ITP:

a. APTT

b. Prothrombin time

c. Bleeding time

d. Clotting time

72. Which does not cause hemolysis in G6PD deficiency?

a. Oestrogen   b. Salicylates

c. Primaquine   d. Nitrofurantion

QUESTIONS OF OTHER EXAMINATIONS

1. Constitutional pancytopenia can be seen in following except: [Maharashtra 10]
   a. Fanconi anemia
   b. Diamond-Blackfan syndrome
   c. Dyskeratosis congenita
   d. Schwachman Diamond syndrome

2. The following are the features of β thalassemia major except: [UPSC 09]
   a. Bone marrow hyperplasia
   b. Hair-on-end appearance
   c. Splenomegaly
   d. Increased osmotic fragility

3. Fetal erythropoiesis first occurs at what week of gestation?   [COMED 08]
   a. 6   b. 10
   c. 12   d. 14

4. Which of the following is not associated with a high reticulocyte count?   [UPSC 07]
   a. Acute bleed
   b. Hemolytic anemia
   c. Megaloblastic anemia
   d. Response to treatment in nutrition deficiency anemia

5. A 10-year-old boy presents with mucosal bleeding of 1 week duration. The investigation of choice that would be most useful in him are: [COMED 06]
   a. Prothrombin time
   b. Clotting time
   c. Partial thromboplastin time
   d. Platelet count

6. What is the definitive finding of G6PD?   [Manipal 06]
   a. Bite cells
   b. Intravascular hemolysis
   c. Splenomegaly
   d. Hemoglobinuria

7. Hemoglobin with zetta 2 and gamma 2 chains are seen in which of the following?   [APPG 06]
   a. Gower 1   b. Gower 2
   c. Portland Hb   d. Fetal Hb

8. Quinine induced thrombocytopenia is: [Jipmer 04]
   a. Antibody mediated
   b. Dose related toxicity
   c. Idiosyncratic reaction
   d. Inhibits production of platelets

9. Fetal Hb is replaced by adult Hb completely at: [TN 99]
   a. At birth   b. 2 months
   c. 4 months   d. 6 months

10. % of Hb F found in a 6 month old infant is: [Kerala 97]
    a. 10   b. 30
    c. 50   d. 60

11. Macrocytosis is seen in all of the following disorders, except: [UP 97]
    a. Hypothyroidism
    b. Thalassemia major
    c. Folic acid deficiency
    d. B_{12} deficiency

12. A child who bleeds from gum and has swollen knee-probably due to: [AMU 95]
    a. Hemophilia
    b. ITP
    c. Scurvy
    d. Trauma

13. Fanconi's anemia is a: [Jipmer 03]
    a. Constitutional anemia
    b. Hemolytic anemia
    c. Iron deficiency anemia
    d. Autoimmune anemia

14. A 6-month-old baby with sever pallor and hepatosplenomegaly. Similar history with the sibling. Investigation of choice:
    a. Bone marrow biopsy
    b. Hb electrophoresis
    c. Hb estimation
    d. Platelet count

15. Adult haemoglobin consists of which of the following tetramer of chains?
    a. $2\alpha + 2\beta$ b. $2\alpha + 2\delta$
    c. $2\beta + 2\gamma$ d. $2\alpha + 2\gamma$

ANSWERS

MULTIPLE CHOICE QUESTIONS

1. (c) G-CSF (Ref: Nelson 19th E/P721)
Kostmann's syndrome:
- Kostmann's syndrome or severe congenital neutropenia is an autosomal condition caused by mutation of elastase gene of neutrophils. This leads to accelerated apoptosis and death of the myeloid precursors.
- Absolute neutrophil count is decreased but monocytes and eosinophils are increased.
- The patients present with recurrent pyogenic infections, anemia of chronic inflammation.
- AML can be seen in these patients.
- G-CSF is the drug of choice.

2. (a) Echocardiography (Ref: CPDT 19th E/P804-05)
Fanconi anemia: Fanconi anemia is an AR disorder caused by defective DNA repair.
- **Clinical presentation:**
  - ❖ Pancytopenia is eventually seen but the **earliest finding is thrombocytopenia** and associated findings like petechiae and purpura.
  - ❖ Skeletal anomalies like **hypoplasia or absence of radius and thumb** can be seen.
  - ❖ Pigmentation abnormalities like **café-au-lait spots** can be seen.
  - ❖ Other anomalies like horse-shoe kidney, microcephaly, microopthalmia and hypogenitalism can be seen.
- **Diagnosis:**
  - ❖ Chromosome breakage in lymphocyte confirms the diagnosis.
  - ❖ Peripheral smear shows macrocytes and Hb F levels are increased.
  - ❖ **Bone marrow** examination shows **hypoplastic picture.**
  - ❖ **Platelet count** is decreased.
- **Treatment**
  - ❖ Treatment of choice is bone marrow transplantation.
  - ❖ Blood transfusion is required.
  - ❖ Drugs like oxymetholone and androgen can be used.

3. (c) Idiopathic thrombocytopenic purpura (Ref: Nelson 19th E/P1670)
- Sudden acute onset of petechial spots indicates towards thrombocytopenia.
- History of abdominal pain 2 weeks back indicate towards some viral infection.
- Acute thrombocytopenia (without hepatosplenomegaly) is most commonly caused in children by ITP.

4. (a) Intron 1 inversion (Ref:Sachdeva Hemoglobinopathies P19)
- The most common cause is a **point mutation (missense mutation) of the intron 1 causing splicing defect**; however other genetic abnormalities like **frameshift mutation and 619 bp deletion**.

5. (b) Liver (Ref: Rudolph 22nd E/P1538)
Hematopoesis:

2–6 weeks	Yolk sac
6–24 weeks	Liver
After 24 weeks	Bone marrow

6. (d) Increased osmotic fragility (Ref: Rudolph 22nd E/P1565)
- Peripheral smear in thalassemia shows microcytes, hypochromia, reticulocytes and target cells.
- Extramedularry hematopoesis can lead to enlargement of spleen and liver.
- Increased osmotic fragility is seen in spherocytosis.

7. (c) Hb-A_2 (Ref: Rudolph 22nd E/P 1565)
- An elevated Hb A_2 level of more than 3.5% is seen in thalassemia trait.
- Hb F can be increased in 50% of patients but is normal in rest. Hence it cannot be used for diagnosis.

8. (c) 36 weeks (Ref: Rudolph 22nd E/P1539)
- The switch from fetal to adult haemoglobin synthesis occurs at 38 weeks of gestation; however the adult values of adult haemoglobin are reached only by 1 year of age.

9. (c) Palpable splenomegaly is seen (Ref: Nelson 19th E/P1670)
- Splenomegaly is rarely seen in ITP.

10. (c) Factor XII deficiency (Ref: Nelson 19th E/P1660-61)
- In this case there is prolongation of aPTT without any history of bleeding. This hints towards deficiency of contact factors like **factor XII**, kallekrein and HMW kininogen.

11. (b) α-thalassemia (Ref: Rudolph 22nd E/P1564)
- This is a case of hydrops fetalis which is caused by deletion of all the four α genes and results in α thalassemia major.

12. (a) 50% Hb S is required for occurrence of sickling
Factors affecting sickling of RBCs:
- **Hb S concentration** — Increased Hb S concentration of >50% precipitates sickling.
- **Hb F and Hb A concentration** — Increased Hb F and Hb A (HbF > Hb A) concentration prevents polymerisation of Hb S.

- **Intracellular pH** — Decreased pH decreases tendency of binding of Hb to oxygen. Deoxygenation precipitates sickling.
- **RBC passing time through microvasculature** — Increase time of presence in microvascular can cause deoxygenation and sickling.

13. (b) Decrease in beta chain, increase in alpha chain (Ref: Rudolph 22nd E/P1564)
- Mutation of one β globin gene leads to **decreased production of beta globin**. There is compensatory **increase in production of α, γ and δ globulins**, which results in formation of α_4 tetramers and increased amount of Hb F and Hb A_2.

14. (b) Isoimmune thrombocytopenia (Ref: Nelson 18th E/P2087)
- Isoimmune thrombocytopenia is characterised by development of maternal antibodies against foetal platelets.

15. (b) Bleeding in to joints (Ref: Nelson 19th E/P1657)
- Bleeding in to joints or hemarthroses is a hallmark feature of haemophilia but not seen in ITP.

16. (b) Bone pain (Ref: Rudolph 22nd E/P1559)
- Acute painful episodes seen due to bone infarction are the hallmark of sickle cell anemia.

17. (a) Alkali denaturation resistant (Nelson 19th E/P1602)
   Features of foetal RBC:
- Hb F is **resistant to denaturation by strong alkali** which is used to differentiate foetal RBCs from the maternal RBCs by **Klieihauer-Betke test**.
- Foetal RBC has **lesser 2,3 DGB** which allows Hb F to bind more avidly with oxygen and extract from maternal circulation.
- Despite of high Hb F binding to oxygen, the delivery to tissues is unaffected because of **high total Hb concentration in the foetal RBC.**
- **Foetal RBC is larger** as compared to adult RBC.
- The lifespan of foetal RBC in the newborn period is around **90 days** as compared to the normal 120 days.

18. (a) Elevated 2, 3 DGP (Ref: Rudolph 22nd E/P1540)
- Foetal RBC has **lesser 2, 3 DGB** which allows Hb F to bind more avidly with oxygen and extract from maternal circulation.

19. (c) Antibody to platelets (Ref: Nelson 19th E/P1670)

20. (b) Decrease in serum ferritin level (Ref: Rudolph 22nd E/P1547)

21. (c) Normal ristocetin test (Ref: CPDT 19th E/P839)

22. (d) Amoxicillin (Ref: CPDT 19th E/P812)

23. (d) Gammaglobulin (Ref: Rudolph 22nd E/P1584)
- IVIG is drug of choice for neonatal ITP.

24. (c) Leukopenia (Ref: Rudolph 22nd E/P1558)
- Sickle cell anemia is associated with **increased leucocyte and platelet count** even without infection.

25. (d) Sickle cell anemia (Ref: Robbins 7th E/P630)

26. (d) Hb Gower's (Ref: Rudolph 22nd E/P1539)

Hemoglobin synthesis:

Till 8 weeks	Hb Portland, **Hb Gower** 1 and 2
8-38 weeks	Hb F
At 38 weeks	**Exclusive switch to Hb A synthesis**

27. (a) Prolonged BT (Ref: CPDT 19th E/P835)
- Aspirin causes thromboxane A_2 deficiency and decreases the aggregation of platelets.
- This results in prolonged bleeding time.

28. (a) Increased TIBC, decreased serum ferritin (Ref: CPDT 19th E/P811)
- Iron deficiency anemia is characterised by increased TIBC and decreased serum ferritin.

29. (a) Inadequate dietary intake (Ref: CPDT 19th E/P812)
- Folic acid deficiency is primarily due to insufficient intake and increased demand.
- Vitamin B_{12} deficiency is primarily due to malabsorption.

30. (a) Increased reticulocyte count (Ref:CPDT 19th E/P811)
- The earliest finding after iron therapy is increase in reticulocyte count after 3–5 days.
- Maximum increase in reticulocyte count is seen between 5–7 days.

31. (c) Hb electrophoresis (Ref: Rudolph 22nd E/P1565)
- Diagnosis of beta thalassemia is done by increased fetal haemoglobin found by Hb electrophoresis.

32. (c) Hb Bart's cannot release oxygen to fetal tissues (Ref: Rudolph 22nd E/P1564)
- Bart's hydrops fetalis is caused by deletion of all 4 α genes.
- This leads to higher production of Hb Bart's which has high affinity for oxygen and causes fetal hypoxemia.

33. (a) Isolated prolonged PTT with a normal PT (Ref: CPDT 19th E/P839)
- VWD is characterised by deficiency of VWF and factor VIII.
- VWF deficiency causes **increased bleeding time.**
- Factor VIII deficiency causes **prolonged aPTT.**

34. (d) Patient present early in life before 6 months of life (Ref: CPDT 19th E/P818)
- Patients **rarely present before 6 months** due to abundance of Hb F which inhibits polymerisation of Hb S.

35. (a) Iron deficiency anemia (Ref: CPDT 19th E/P811)
- This is a case of microcytic, hypochromic anemia along with erythroid marrow hyperplasia.

- Lethargy, irritability and pallor along with the above findings indicate towards iron deficiency anemia.

36. (b) Serum ferritin levels (Ref: Rudolph 22nd E/P1547)
- A low serum ferritin level invariably indicates iron deficiency and hence is the most specific and sensitive test for iron deficiency anemia.

37. (b) Replacement of glutamate by valine in β chain of Hb A (Ref: Rudolph 22nd E/P1557)
- Sickle cell anemia is caused by **point mutation of β globin gene**, which leads to **change of glutamate to valine.**

38. (b) Ferritin (Ref: Rudolph 22nd E/P1547)
- Serum ferritin level indicates the amount of iron present in both liver and reticuloendothelial system and hence is the best assessment of iron status.

39. (a) Hb A (Ref: CPDT 19th E/P819)
- Hb electrophoresis shows 80–90% of **Hb S** and the rest is **Hb F** and **Hb A₂**; however **Hb A is absent.**

40. (a) Hb electrophoresis (Ref: Rudolph 22nd E/P1565)
- A low Hb of 6 gm%, microcytic and hypochromic RBCs and target cell indicates towards thalassemia major.
- Thalassemia major is diagnosed by elevated Hb F in Hb electrophoresis.

41. (a) Hypersegmented neutrophils (Ref: CPDT 19th E/P812)
- Hypersegmented neutrophils are seen in megaloblastic anemia.

42. (b) Bacterial overgrowth (Ref: Nelson 19th E/P1262)
Blind/stagnant loop syndrome (Bacterial overgrowth syndrome):
- It is characterised by increase in bacterias in the small intestine which deconjugate the bile salts (steatorrhea), **bind to vitamin B₁₂ (decrease absorption)** and decrease disaccharidase activity.
- The cause is usually incomplete obstruction owing to congenital lesions like malrotation with duodenal bands, duodenal webs, diverticulum and intestinal duplication. Acquired lesions of inflammatory bowel disease and surgical procedures can also be attributed.
- **Metronidazole** is the drug of choice.

43. (c) Endothelial cells (Ref: CPDT 19th E/P838)

44. (a) G6PD deficiency (Ref: CPDT 19Th E/P822)

45. (c) PT (Ref: CPDT 19th E/P835)
- Hemophilia is characterise by **deficiency of factor VIII.**

- PTT and clotting time are prolonged.
- PT and bleeding time are normal.

46. (c) Splenomegaly (Ref: Rudolph 22nd E/P1558-60)

47. (d) and **(e)** Portwine hemangioma and Thrombocytosis (Ref: Nelson 19th E/P1968)
- **Kaposiform hemangioendotheliomas** in **newborn** can cause **platelet sequestration** followed by **thrombocytopenia, consumptive coagulopathy** and microangiopathic haemolytic anemia.
- Heart failure can be seen in case of arteriovenous malformations.
- The lesions are treated by drugs (corticosteroids, alpha interferon and vincristine), laser photocoagulation and radiation. Surgery is usually not indicated due to risk of haemorrhage.

48. (c) 80–100 (Ref: Ghai 7th E/P298)

Age	MCV Values
Birth	98–108
1 month	**85–104**
2 month	77–96
3–6 months	74–91
6 months–2 years	70–78
2–6 years	75–81
6–12 years	77–86

49. (c) and **(d)** Serum ferritin depletes first and Decreased alertness (Ref: Rudolph 22nd E/P1546–47)
Kindly refer text for details.

50. (b), (c) and **(d)** Increase aPTT, X-linked recessive and Presence of 30% of factor level express the disease (Ref: CPDT 19th E/P835-37)
- Factor VIII deficiency is characterised by **prolonga-tion in clotting time and aPTT. PT and bleeding time are normal.**
- Hemophilia A is an **X linked recessive disorder.**
- The disease manifests when factor VIII level falls below 40%. So 30% of factor VIII will manifest the disease.

51. (b), (d) and **(e)** (Ref: CPDT 19th E/P821–22)
Kindly refer text for details.

52. (d) Decrease in absorption with improvement of symptoms (Ref: Rudolph 22nd E/P1548)
- Oral iron supplement in the form of sulphate, gluconate and fumarate salts is given at a dose of 6 mg/kg/day and **continued 8 weeks after Hb levels are normalised**.
- The **earliest response to iron therapy is increase in reticulocyte count** within 3–5 days and maximises in 5–7 days.
- This follows **increase in Hb** at a rate of 0.5 gm/dl/24 hours in the **2nd week**.

- Only 10% of the iron given by oral route is absorbed i.e. out of 300 mg only 30 mg will be absorbed.
- The normalisation of body iron store relatively decreases the iron absorption.

53. **(a)** and **(d)** Microcytic hypochromic anemia and Bone marrow iron decreased earlier than serum iron (Ref: Rudolph 22nd E/P1546–47)

Kindly refer text for details.

54. **(b)**, **(c)** and **(d)** Specific antiplatelet antibodies detected, Viral infection predisposes as seen after vaccination and Disease resolves itself in 80% of Pt. in 2-6 week (Ref: Nelson 19th E/P1670)

- Chronic ITP is more common in female but not acute ITP.
- Only 20% cases of ITP transform in to chronic state.

55. **(a)**, **(b)** and **(c)** ↑ HbF, ↑ HbA$_2$, Microcytosis (Ref: Rudolph 22nd E/P1565)

- Thalassemia trait is characterised by consistent elevation of Hb A$_2$ and Hb F levels are elevated in 50% cases and normal in other 50%.
- The Hb level is just 1–2 gm/dl lower than normal i.e. mild anemia.

56. **(a)**, **(b)** and **(c)** Glanzmann syndrome, Bernard soulier syndrome and Wiskott Aldrich syndrome (Ref: CPDT 19th E/P834–35)

Platelet function defect can be seen in:

- **Glanzmann thrombasthenia**
- **Bernard soulier syndrome**
- Storage pool disease
- Quebec platelet disease
- Hermansky-Pudlak syndrome
- Chediac-Higashi syndrome
- **Wiskott-Aldrich syndrome**
- Grey platelet syndrome.

57. **(a)** and **(b)** Platelet adhesion and BT (Ref: CPDT 19th E/P 830)

Platelet function assessment:

- **PFA-100** — This is a test to measure the **platelet adhesion-aggregation** in response to agonist combination like collagen-epinephrine or collagen-ADP.
- **Bleeding time** — The usual bleeding time is 4–8 minutes. Bleeding for a longer time suggests platelet defects.

58. **(e)** Point mutation (Ref: Rudolph 22nd E/P1557)

- Sickle cell anemia is caused by **point mutation of β globin gene**, which leads to **change of glutamate to valine**.

59. **(a)**, **(b)** and **(d)** Missense, Splicing and Frame-shift (Ref: Sachdeva Hemoglobinopathies P19)

- The most common cause is a **point mutation (missense mutation) of the intron 1 causing splicing defect**; however other genetic abnormalities like **frameshift mutation and 619 bp deletion**.

60. **(d)** >3.5 (Ref: Rudolph 22nd E/P1565)

"The normal level of Hb A$_2$ is 1.5% to 3.5% and Hb A$_2$ > 3.5% is consistent with β thalassemia trait."

61. **(a)** Sickle cell anemia (Ref: Rudolph 22nd E/P1559)

62. **(a)** G6PD (Ref: CPDT 19th E/P821)

- Enzyme deficiencies that can cause hemolysis are **G6PD** and **pyruvate kinase.**

63. **(a)** 2 (Ref: Rudolph 22nd E/P1560)

- Sickle cell trait is characterised by predominance of Hb A over Hb S. HPLC demonstrates bands of HB A and Hb S i.e. 2 bands.

64. **(c)** Splenomegaly is usually seen (Ref: Rudolph 22nd E/P1559)

- Usually recurrent splenic infarction leads to autosplenectomy; however splenomegaly can be seen in initial stages.

65. **(a)** Haemoglobin (Ref: Rudolph 22nd E/P1564)

- Thalassemia is a genetic disorder of globin synthesis, which leads to defect in haemoglobin.

66. **(a)** Congenital defects in platelets (Ref: Nelson 19th E/P1674)

Kindly refer text for details.

67. **(b)** No α chain (Ref: Rudolph 22nd E/P1563)

68. **(c)** Infants fed on goat milk (Ref: CPDT 19th E/P812)

"**Folic acid deficiency** due to dietary deficiency alone is rare but occurs in severely malnourished infants and has been reported in **infants fed goat milk** not fortified with folic acid."

69. **(a)** and **(c)** Epistaxis and Oral bleeding (Ref: Nelson 19th E/P1659)

70. **(a)** Platelet aggregation (Ref: Nelson 19th E/P1674)

- Glanzmann thrombasthenia is caused by defect in GP IIb-IIIa which results in defective aggregation in response to fibrinogen.

71. **(c)** Bleeding time (Ref: Nelson 19th E/P1670)

- ITP is characterised by thrombocytopenia which **prolongs the bleeding time.**

72. **(a)** Oestrogen (Ref: CPDT 19th E/P822)

QUESTIONS OF OTHER EXAMINATIONS

1. (b) Diamond-Blackfan syndrome (Ref: Nelson 19th E/P1642)

Causes of constitutional pancytopenia:
- **Fanconi anemia** — Most common
- **Dyskeratosis congenita**
- **Schwachman Diamond syndrome**
- Amegakaryocytic thrombocytopenia
- Reticular dysgenesis.

2. (d) Increased osmotic fragility (Ref: Rudolph 22nd E/P1564)

3. (a) 6 (Ref: Rudolph 22nd E/P1538)
- Hematopoesis begins in the **yolk sac** at 2nd week of gestation and continues till the 6th week.

4. (c) Megaloblastic anemia (Ref: CPDT 19th E/P812)
- Reticulocytes are increased in anemia because of rapid compensatory proliferation of erythrocytes.
- However reticulocyte count will not be increased in megaloblastic anemia because **deficiency of folic acid will inhibit RBC proliferation** as folic acid is essential for DNA replication.

5. (d) Platelet count (Ref: CPDT 830)

"Excessive mucosal bleeding is suggestive of a **platelet disorder**, von Willebrand disease, dysfibrinogenemia or vasculitis."

6. (a) Bite cells (Ref: CPDT 19th E/P822)
- Peripheral smear in G6PD deficiency shows **"Bite cells"** or blister cells, Heinz bodies and some spherocytes.

7. (c) Portland Hb (Ref: Nelson 19th E/P1602)

Hemoglobin type	Chains
Hb A	$\alpha_2\beta_2$
Hb A$_2$	$\alpha_2\delta_2$
Hb F	$\alpha_2\gamma_2$
Hb Portland	$\zeta_2\gamma_2$ i.e. zetta2 gamma2
Gower-1 Hb	$\zeta_2\varepsilon_2$
Gower-2 Hb	$\alpha_2\varepsilon_2$

8. (a) Antibody mediated (Ref: Rudolph 22nd E/P1584)

"The most common drugs causing thrombocytopenia are heparin, **quinine/quinidine**, sulfa derivatives, gold and valproic acid. Thrombocytopenia results from either binding of drug to the platelet followed by **binding of antidrug antibody** or by direct binding of a drug and antidrug complex to the platelet surface."

9. (d) 6 months (Ref: Rudolph 22nd E/P1539)

"Consequently the proportion of Hb F falls to less than 20% by 4 months of age and **less than 2% at 1 year of age**, which is the normal proportion in older children and adults."

- The correct answer is 1 Year but here the best answer is 6 months.

10. (a) 10% (Ref: Rudolph 22nd E/P1539)

"Consequently the proportion of Hb F falls to **less than 20% by 4 months of age** and **less than 2% at 1 year of age**, which is the normal proportion in older children and adults."

11. (b) Thalassemia major (Ref: CPDT 19th E/P817)

12. (a) Hemophilia (Ref: CPDT 19th E/P837)

13. (a) Constitutional anemia (Ref: Nelson 19th E/P1642)

14. (b) Hb electrophoresis (Ref: Rudolph 22nd E/P 1564)
- Presence of pallor and hepatosplenomegaly at 6 month of age indicates towards thalassemia major, which can be diagnosed by Hb electrophoresis.

15. (a) $2\alpha + 2\beta$ (Ref: Nelson 19th E/P1602)

Endocrinology

11

HYPOTHALAMUS AND PITUITARY DISORDERS

The hypothalamus secretes the releasing hormones like GHRH, CRH, TRH and GnRH which are agonists at receptors on the hormone secreting cells in pituitary i.e. at somatotrophs, corticotrophs, thyrotrophs and gonadotrophs respectively. Activation of these cells leads to secretion of respective hormones from the pituitary like GH, ACTH, TSH, LH and FSH. The hormonal disorders of pituitary can be classified based on deficiency (hypopituitarism) and abundance (hyperpituitarism) of the above mentioned hormones.

Hypopituitarism

The term hypopituitarism means isolated deficiency of growth hormone (GH) or combined deficiency of all hormones.

Growth Hormone Deficiency

Growth hormone deficiency can be due to congenital factors (mutation of GHRH receptor gene, GH gene and BTK gene on X chromosome) or acquired factors (CNS infections, histiocytosis, radiation, craniopharyngioma and germinoma).

- **Clinical presentation:** Neonates with congenital hypopituitarism have normal birth weight and a near normal length which is followed by a prolonged physiological jaundice. The other findings of growth hormone deficiency are **hypoglycemia**, seizures, **micropenis**, saddle nose, cold sensitivity, delayed puberty, **delayed dentition** with overcrowding of teeth, **delayed bone age**, **delayed closure of epiphysis**, **proportionate growth retardation** and **increased fat content in the body** with decreased muscle mass.
- **Diagnosis:** Growth hormone deficiency in children is diagnosed if the serum **GH value is <10 ng/mL.**
- **Treatment:** The drugs that can be used for treatment of GH deficiency are GHRH analogue (sermorelin), GH analogue (somatrem, somatropin) and IGF I analogue (mecasermin).
  - ❖ GH shows maximum effect during 1st year of treatment.
  - ❖ GH is stopped if the desired height is gained, growth rate decreases to <1 inch/year and a bone age of >14 years in girls and >16 years in boys is achieved.

Hyperpituitarism

Primary hyperpituitarism in children is usually seen because of pituitary adenoma. Pituitary adenomas secreting GH also have increased prolactin levels as the cells in adenoma are mammosomatrophs, however the other anterior pituitary hormones are decreased.

- **Clinical presentation:** Growth hormone excess in children present as gigantism but in adults as acromegaly. The features of gigantism and acromegaly overlap. Apart from accelerated growth, gigantism may present with additional features of adenoma like headache, features of optic nerve compression and symptoms of deficiency of other pituitary hormones. Acromegalic features like macroglossia, broad nose, carpal tunnel syndrome, kyphosis and raised intracranial tension can be seen; however **fatigue and weakness** are the earliest features.

- **Diagnosis: Failure of Oral glucose challenge test** confirms the diagnosis. Patient is given oral glucose and if the GH level does not fall below 5 ng/ml, it confirms the diagnosis.
- **Treatment:**
  - ❖ Surgical removal of adenoma by transsphenoid approach is preferred if tumor has not spread.
  - ❖ In other cases radiation and medical management is preferred. Drugs that are given are somatostatin analogues (octreotide, lanreotide and paseriotide), GH receptor inhibitor (pegvisomant) and bromocriptine (if both GH and prolactin are increased).

ADRENAL CORTEX DISORDERS

Adrenal Cortex Physiology

The adrenal cortex is controlled by the hypothalamopituitary axis. Hypothalamus secretes CRH (corticotrophin releasing hormone) which acts on the corticotroph cells of pituitary and increases release of ACTH predominantly in the **early morning hours**. ACTH is a melanopeptide which acts on various melanocortin receptors like MC1 receptors (Increased ACTH causes hyperpigmentation by acting on MC1) on melanocytes and MC2 in the adrenal glands. Activation of MC2 receptors in adrenals leads to uptake of cholesterol (precursor of adrenal steroids) by the mitochondria and subsequently aldosterone, cortisol and sex hormones are synthesised in the glomerular, fasciculate and reticular zones respectively.

Adrenal Cortex Hormone Synthesis

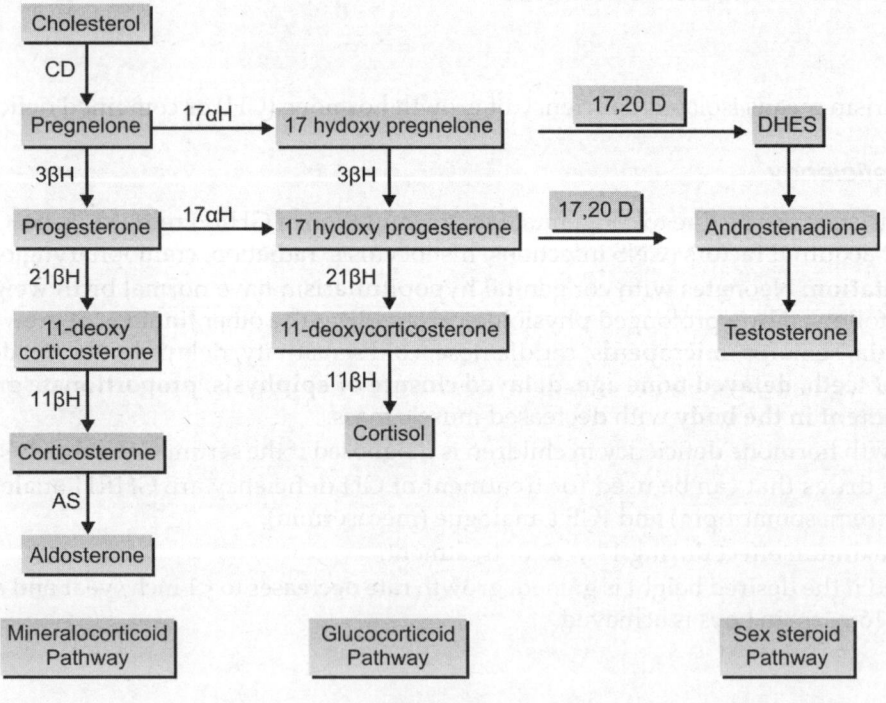

Fig. 11.1

Note: **CD** — cholesterol desmolase, **17, 20 D** — 17, 20 desmolase, **3βH** — 3 beta hydroxysteroid dehydrogenase, **21βH** — 21 beta hydroxylase, **11βH** — 11 beta hydroxylase, **17αH** — 17 alpha hydroxylase, **AS** — aldosterone synthase

Adrenal Insufficiency

Adrenal insufficiency can be caused by a wide range of disorders like congenital adrenal hyperplasia, Addison disease, Waterhouse-Frederickson syndrome and CNS tumors.

- **Clinical presentation:** The patients present with GIT symptoms (nausea, vomiting, and diarrhoea), symptoms of salt wasting (hypotension and dehydration), increased pigmentation in primary adrenal insufficiency; and both fever and hypothermia can be seen.

- **Diagnosis:**
  - ❖ Chest X-ray shows a **small heart.**
  - ❖ ACTH stimulation test — ACTH is given to the patient and after 1 hour, plasma aldosterone and cortisol is measured. If both are increased then it is a case of central adrenal insufficiency and if no change is seen then it is primary adrenal insufficiency.
- **Treatment:**
  - ❖ Acute insufficiency is treated initially with **hydrocortisone** and IV fluids (5% glucose with NS). When the patient can accept oral medication, **fludrocortisone** is started.
  - ❖ Chronic insufficiency is treated with both hydrocortisone and fludrocortisone.

Congenital Adrenal Insufficiency

CAH is an autosomal recessive disorder which can be caused by deficiency of Cholesterol desmolase, 3-beta hydroxysteroid dehydrogenase, 21 beta hydroxylase, 11 beta hydroxylase and 17 alpha hydroxylase. However **21 beta hydroxylase is the most common cause** seen in almost 90% cases.

- **3-beta hydroxysteroid dehydrogenase deficiency:** Deficiency of 3βHD leads to abolition of the glucocorticoid and mineralocorticoid pathway but partial potentiation of the sex steroid pathway increasing DHES.
  - ❖ Glucocorticoid and mineralocorticoid deficiency presents with symptoms of adrenal insufficiency.
  - ❖ DHES is increased but androstenadione and testosterone is decreased —
    - ❑ **Males** — Decreased androstenadione and testosterone leads to **ambiguous genitalia (pseudo-hermaphroditism).**
    - ❑ **Females** — Increased DHES causes mild **virilisation.**
- **17 α hydroxylase deficiency:** Deficiency of 17α hydroxylase leads to potentiation of mineralocorticoid pathway but the glucocorticoid and sex steroid pathways are compromised.
  - ❖ Increased amount of aldosterone leads to **hypernatremia, hypertension** and **hypokalemia.** Glucocorticoid deficiency is compensated by corticosterone excess, which has glucocorticoid property.
  - ❖ All forms of sex steroid hormones are decreased:
    - ❑ **Males** — Decreased sex hormones leads to incomplete development of genitalia i.e. **pseudo-hermaphroditism.**
    - ❑ **Females** — Usually females are normal.
- **21 β hydroxylase deficiency:** Deficiency of 21β hydroxylase leads to partial abolition of the mineralocorticoid and glucocorticoid pathways but the sex steroid pathway is completely potentiated. This can present clinically in two forms i.e. classical and non-classical.
  - ❖ **Classical form** — Classical form or salt wasting form is associated with decrease in glucocorticoids and mineralocorticoids, whereas sex steroids are increased.
    - ❑ Decreased aldosterone leads to **hyponatremia, hypotension** and **hyperkalemia.** Decreased cortisol can cause **hypoglycemia.**
    - ❑ DHES, androstenadione and testosterone is increased —
      - – **Males** — Increased sex hormones cause **precocious puberty,** virilisation and rapid growth.
      - – **Females** — Increased sex hormones cause **ambiguous genitalia(pseudohermaphroditism), virilisation** and rapid growth.
    - ❑ If there is history of 21 hydroxylase deficiency, prenatal diagnosis can be done by DNA analysis of **chorionic villous sample** obtained in late 1st or 2nd trimester. Once diagnosis is confirmed **dexamethasone** should be started **at 6 weeks of gestation,** which would normalise the sex hormone pathway.
    - ❑ Since 21 hydroxylase deficiency accounts for 90% of cases of CAH, newborn screening can be done for increased level of **17-hydroxyprogesterone** in blood obtained by heel-stick.

❖ **Non-classical form:**

❑ **Non-classical form or simple virilising form of CAH** is associated with normal levels of glucocorticoids and mineralocorticoids with selective increase in sex steroids.

❑ Hence these patients present only with symptoms of increased DHES, androstenadione and testosterone:

– **Males** — Increased sex hormones cause **precocious puberty**, virilisation and rapid growth.

– **Females** — Increased sex hormones cause **ambiguous genitalia(pseudohermaphroditism), virilisation** and rapid growth.

• **11β hydroxylase deficiency:** Deficiency of 11β hydroxylase leads to partial abolition of the mineralocorticoid and glucocorticoid pathways but the sex steroid pathway is potentiated.

❖ Aldosterone is decreased but increased DOCA can compensate for it and even cause **hypernatremia, hypokalemia** and **hypertension.**

❖ DHES, androstenadione and testosterone is increased.

❑ **Males** — **Precocious puberty** and virilisation is seen.

❑ **Females** — Increased sex hormones cause virilisation and **ambiguous genitalia (pseudohermaphroditism).**

Summary of CAH

Enzyme deficiency	Effect on sexual development in males	Effect on sexual development in females	Electrolyte imbalance
17 alpha hydroxylase — Decreased testosterone and increased aldosterone	Pseudohermaphroditism	Normal	Hypernatremia Hypokalemia
3 beta hydroxylase — Increased DHES, decreased testosterone and aldosterone	Pseudohermaphroditism	Virilisation	Hyponatremia Hyperkalemia
21 beta hydroxylase(Classical type) — Increased testosterone and decreased aldosterone	Precocious puberty Virilisation	Pseudohermaphroditism Virilisation	Hyponatremia Hyperkalemia
21 beta hydroxylase(Non-classical/ simple virilising type) — Increased testosterone and normal aldosterone	Precocious puberty Virilisation	Pseudohermaphroditism Virilisation	Not seen
11 beta hydroxylase — Increased testosterone and DOCA	Precocious puberty	Pseudohermaphroditism	Hypernatremia Hypokalemia

GONADAL DISORDERS

Gonadal Development

The gonadal development of both sexes takes place at the end of **5th gestational week** from the **genital ridge.** The different factors like WT1 and SF1 stimulate the genital ridge, which differentiates in to bipotential gonad. Further the products of SRY gene and; WNT4 and RSPO1 genes differentiate bipotential gonad in to testes and ovary respectively.

If testes is developed then the leydig cells secrete testosterone which causes development of Wolffian duct (precursor of male reproductive organs), male external genitalia and virilisation; and sertoli cells secrete anti mullerian hormone (AMH) which inhibits the mullerian duct (precursor of female reproductive organs). But if ovary is developed then testicular pathway is abolished i.e. AMH is not secreted and by default mullerian duct develops in to female reproductive organs and female external genitalia is developed.

Embryology of Gonadal Development

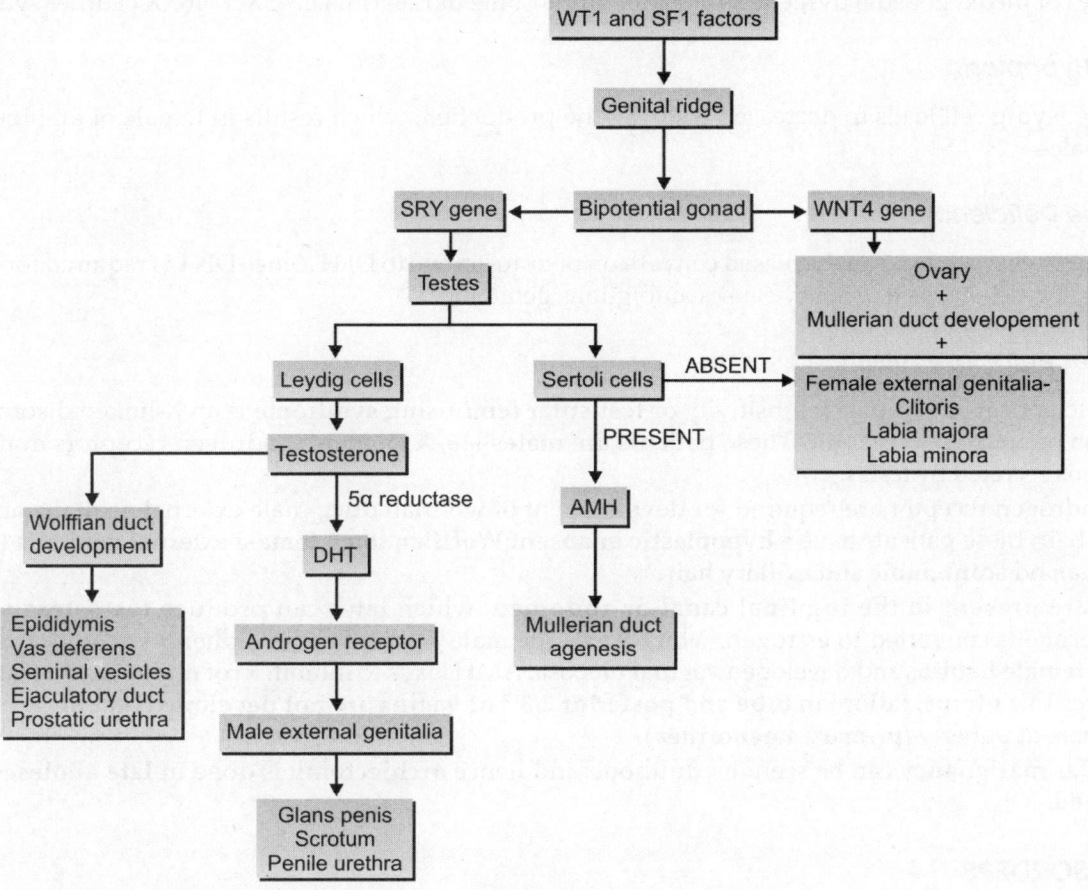

Fig. 11.2

Gonadal Development Disorders

Abnormality in any step of the gonadal development can present with ambiguous genitalia. There can be mutation of WT1 gene, SRY gene translocation to X chromosome, gonadal dysgenesis (testis and ovary), leydig cell hypoplasia, 5α reductase deficiency and androgen receptor insensitivity.

WT1 and SF1 Gene Mutation

Mutation of WT1 gene leads to various syndromes like Denys-Drash syndrome, Frasier syndrome and WAGAR syndrome, which are associated with dysgenic testis and ambiguous genitalia. SF1 gene mutation can lead to gonadal dysgenesis and adrenal insufficiency.

SRY Gene Translocation to X Chromosome

SRY gene translocation on X chromosome leads to masculinization and ambiguous genitalia in a female.

Gonadal Dysgenesis

Embryological development of gonads can be altered by various causes and depending on the cause and presentation it can be either pure or mixed gonadal dysgenesis.

- **Pure gonadal dysgenesis:** It is defined as the complete dysgenesis of gonads but the external and internal genitalia is normal. SRY gene mutation or deletion causes **Swyer syndrome (XY gonadal dysgenesis)** which leads to complete dysgenesis of testis and in absence of testosterone and AMH, the external genitalia (female type) and mullerian duct is developed.

- **Mixed gonadal dysgenesis:** It is characterised by asymmetrical dysgenesis of gonads and depending on the asymmetry the genitalia can widely vary from male to female; however mostly **ambiguous genitalia is seen.** Examples of mixed gonadal dysgenesis are sex chromosome mosaicism i.e. 45XO/46XX (Turner syndrome).

Leydig Cell Hypoplasia

Hypoplasia of leydig cell leads to decreased testosterone production, which results in female or ambiguous external genitalia in males.

5α Reductase Deficiency

Deficiency of 5α reductase leads to decreased conversion of testosterone to DHT. Since DHT is required for development of male external genitalia; its deficiency causes ambiguous genitalia.

Androgen Receptor Insensitivity

- Complete androgen receptor insensitivity or **testicular feminising syndrome** is an X-linked disorder caused by mutation of androgen receptor. These patients are **males (46, XY)** whose androgen receptors don't respond to androgens secreted by testes.
- Since androgen receptor are required for development of wolffian duct, male external genitalia and; pubic and axillary hair; these patients have a **hypoplastic or absent Wolffian duct, female external genitalia (anterior 1/3ʳᵈ of vagina)** and **scant pubic and axillary hair.**
- **Testes are present in the inguinal canal or abdomen,** which later can produce **testosterone and AMH.** Testosterone is converted to estrogen, which gives the male a typical female phenotype with well-developed breasts, **female habitus** and developed vaginal mucosa. AMH leads to inhibition of mullerian duct and the related structures like **uterus, fallopian tube and posterior 2/3ʳᵈ of vagina are not developed** and these patients fail to menstruate at puberty (**primary amenorrhea**).
- **Testicular malignancy** can be seen in adulthood and hence **orchiectomy** is done in **late adolescence or early adulthood.**

PUBERTY DISORDERS

Female Puberty Disorders

- **Precocious puberty in females:** In females precocious puberty is defined as onset of secondary sexual characteristics before 8 years of age. Increase in GnRH release from the CNS due to conditions like **hypothalamic hamartoma,** CNS tumours and trauma, hydrocephalus, **CNS irradiation** can cause central precocious puberty. Peripheral precocious puberty is caused by disorders like tumors of ovary, CAH, adrenal tumors, ovarian cysts, **McCune-Albright syndrome** and **hypothyroidism** (Increased TSH acts on LH receptors).
  - ❖ **Hypothalamic hamartoma:**
    - ❑ Hypothalamic hamartoma is congenital presence of ectopic neural tissue releasing gonadotropin releasing hormone.
    - ❑ It is characterised by **rapidly progressive sexual precocity** associated with **unnatural crying or laughing** (gelastic seizures).
    - ❑ **MRI** is the diagnostic method of choice, which shows a small pedunculated mass or a sessile mass, which remains static in size over years.
    - ❑ Treatment is usually done with GnRh agonists. Surgical management is not preferred, except in case of refractory seizures.
  - ❖ **McCune-Albright syndrome:** McCune-Albright syndrome is characterised by over functioning of stimulatory GPCRs like LH, FSH, TSH and ACTH receptors. This results in over-activity of the organs on which these receptors are located.
    - ❑ LH and FSH receptor — **Precocious puberty**
    - ❑ TSH receptor — **Hyperthyroidism**
    - ❑ ACTH receptor — **Cushing syndrome**
    - ❑ Other abnormalities that can be seen are **growth hormone excess, skeletal dysplasia (bone cysts)** and **cutaneous pigmentation.**

Mnemonic (Males+Females): **MATURE CHILD**
M — McCune-Albright syndrome
A — Adrenal tumors
T — Teratoma
U — Use of estrogen
R — Radiation
E — Encephalitis
C — Cyst of ovary, craniopharyngioma, choriocarcinoma
H — Hypothalamic hamartoma, hypothyroidism
I — Idiopathic
L — Leydig cell tumor
D — Deficiency of 11 and 21 hydroxylase

Note: Hypothyroidism can cause both precocious and delayed puberty.

- **Delayed puberty in females:** Puberty is said to be delayed in females if signs of puberty are absent by 13 years or menarche is not attained by 16 years of age (bone age). The **most common cause of delayed puberty in females is constitutional growth delay**; however growth delay due to **hypothyroidism** and growth hormone deficiency can also delay puberty. Puberty can also be delayed by primary ovarian failure in gonadal dysgenesis (**Turner syndrome**), autoimmune ovarian failure, chemo-radiation and galactosemia. Decreased GnRH secretion can delay puberty in cases like **Kallman syndrome**, **hypopituitarism**, CNS tumors, cystic fibrosis, sickle cell disease, **malabsorption due to chronic GIT diseases**, **anorexia and bulimia nervosa**, gaucher disease and infections like AIDS. Miscellaneous causes like **chronic diseases**, hyperprolactinemia and heavy exercise have also been associated.

Mnemonic (Males + Females): **LATE PICKINGS**
L — Laurence-Moon-Biedel syndrome
A — Autoimmune oophoritis, AIDS
T — Turner syndrome
E — Enteric malabsorption
P — Prader-Willi syndrome
I — Increased TSH (Hypothyroidism)
C — Constitutional, Cystic fibrosis, Chronic diseases
K — Klinefelter syndrome, Kallman syndrome
I — Increased prolactin (Hyperprolactinemia)
N — Noonan syndrome
G — Galactosemia, Gaucher disease
S — Sickle cell disease

Male Puberty Disorders

The first sign of puberty in males is **testis growth** and some other changes like thinning and pigmentation of scrotum followed by penis growth and finally pubarche.

- **Precocious puberty in males:** In males precocious puberty is defined as appearance of secondary sexual characters before the age of 9 years. The different causes are CAH (deficiency of 11 hydroxylase and 21 hydroxylase), adrenal tumors, leydig cell tumors, tumors secreting HCG like hepatoblastoma and teratomas; and **McCune-Albright syndrome.**
- **Delayed puberty in males:** In males delayed puberty is characterised by absence of secondary sexual characteristics by 14 years of age. The **most common cause of delayed puberty is constitutional growth delay**; however other causes of growth delay like **hypothyroidism** and growth hormone deficiency can also delay puberty. Testicular failure (Hypergonadotrophic hypogonadism) due to **infection (mumps orchitis), Klinefelter syndrome, radiation**, trauma and tumor can delay puberty in males. Decreased GnRH secretion (Hypogonadotrophic hypogonadism) due to **Kallman syndrome**, CNS disorders like infection, trauma, tumours; Prader-Willi syndrome and **Laurence-Moon syndrome** may also delay puberty.
  - ❖ **Laurence-Moon syndrome:**
    - ❏ It is an AR disorder of **hypogonadotrophic hypogonadism**, which is characterised by mental retardation, **obesity, Polydactyly**, retinitis pigmentosa and **hypogonadism.**

Mnemonic: **MOON**
M — Mental retardation
O — Obesity, Ovary and testis hypofunction
O — Ocular abnormality (Retinitis pigmentosa)
N — Number of fingers is increased (Polydactyly)

Cryptorchidism

- Cryptorchidism is defined as failure of descent of testis in to the scrotum. The most common genetic abnormality associated is Klinefelter syndrome. It is most commonly seen on the **right side** and is frequently **unilateral**.
- Incidence is higher in premature babies (30%) but decreases to 4% in term babies and 0.3% by the time babies are of 1 year age.
- It is associated with **infertility** and **testicular neoplasia** that can be seen in both the descended and undescended testis.
- **Surgical orchidopexy** is the treatment of choice if the testis fails to descent by the age of 1 year. The most preferred age of surgical intervention is between **6 months to 1 year**, as after 1 year the incidence of neoplasia and infertility increases.

Rudolph 22nd E/P1747

"Most recent studies have suggested that the number of germ cells in a cryptorchid testes is decreased after the 7th month of age when compared to controls, favouring orchidopexy between 6 and 12 months of age, compared with the previous practice of undergoing surgery between ages 1 and 2 years."

- Medical management is less preferred; however testosterone and HCG can be tried.

THYROID

The physiological function of the thyroid gland is to trap iodine and synthesise T$_3$ and T$_4$ hormones. The daily required amount of iodine for infants is **30 µg/kg** and children is **90–120 µg/kg**. Thyroid secretes more T$_4$ as compared to T$_3$; however the **potency of T$_3$ is more than T$_4$.** The function of thyroid hormones is mostly to assist in metabolic pathways and causes lipolysis, protein breakdown, carbohydrate absorption, LDL receptor formation and increased oxygen consumption. It helps in muscle and skeletal growth; CNS development and has positive inotropic and chronotropic effect on heart. Pathological conditions associated with increased (**hyperthyroidism**) or decreased (**hypothyroidism**) thyroid hormones will potentiate or inhibit the above mentioned effects respectively.

Hypothyroidism

Hypothyroidism can be present from birth (congenital) or can be acquired later due to various causes.

Congenital Hypothyroidism

Congenital hypothyroidism can be caused by iodine deficiency (endemic goitre), abnormalities in development of thyroid (thyroid dysgenesis) and thyroxin synthesis; and presence of maternal anti-thyrotropin antibodies (transient hypothyroidism). **Iodine deficiency** is the most common cause of congenital hypothyroidism and goitre is mostly associated. Thyroxin synthesis can be inhibited by abnormality in uptake of iodine by mutation of sodium iodide symporter and **pendrin** gene (located in thyroid and **cochlea**); and organification and coupling defect by mutation of TPO. Mutation of **Pendrin gene (SL26A4)** located in **chromosome 7** leads to **Pendred syndrome** which is characterised by **bilateral sensorineural deafness, goitre** and **hypothyroidism.**

- **Clinical presentation:** Most of the neonates are asymptomatic at birth due to presence of maternal thyroid hormones. Very often the first clinical sign is **prolongation of physiological jaundice**. The other findings can be a macroglossia **(large protruded tongue), thin eyebrows**, hypotonia, constipation, **umbilical hernia, nonpitting edema**, macrocytic anemia, cardiomegaly, **large fontanels** and dry skin. As the child grows there can be delay in development, dentition, **bone age** and **puberty**; and pseudohypertrophy of muscles can be seen.
- **Diagnosis:** Since the neonates are asymptomatic at birth screening of all the newborns is essential for diagnosis of hypothyroidism. TSH is estimated either in the cord blood at the time of birth or in baby's blood obtained from heel prick after 2 days of birth (in 1st 48 hours of birth false positive result can be seen). In Asian countries like **India** most patients do not turn up for screening after 2 days, hence **cord blood analysis at birth is the preferred approach.**
- **Treatment: Levothyroxine** at a dose of 10–15 µg/kg is the drug of choice.

Acquired Juvenile Hypothyroidism

Acquired hypothyroidism in children can be caused by thyroiditis, iodine deficiency, medications, nephropathic cystinosis, langerhans cell histiocytosis, radiation and hepatic hemangiomas. Iodine deficiency is the most common cause of acquired hypothyroidism also. Girls are more commonly affected than boys.

- **Clinical presentation:** The earliest sign of hypothyroidism is **growth retardation** which is characterised by **short extremities** with broad hands and short fingers. Other findings are **mental retardation, generalised weakness (most common), paraesthesia**, goitre, constipation, weight gain, **epiphyseal breaking**, cold intolerance, yellow skin (sclera is white), nonpitting edema, dry skin, alopecia, bradycardia, **umbilical hernia**, transient deafness, menorrhagia and amenorrhea;and pseudohypertrophy of muscles. **Puberty can be delayed**; however precocious puberty can also be seen due to overactivity of TSH on LH receptors.

  Iodine deficient areas have increased prevalence of endemic goitre and cretinism. Cretinism is the most severe form of iodine deficiency and is characterised by **goitre, mental retardation, deafness**, gait abnormality, **growth retardation** and delayed puberty. It is prevented and treated by iodinated poppy seed oil injection. Iodine deficiency is the most common cause of mental retardation that can be prevented.

Mnemonic: **HYPOTHYROIDISM**
H — Hair loss
Y — Yellow skin
P — Puberty delayed or precocious
O — Obesity
T — Transient deafness, Tongue protrusion
H — Hernia (umbilical)
Y — Yellow baby (prolonged physiological jaundice)
R — Retardation of growth
O — Ossification centre breakage (epiphysis)
I — Intellectual deficit
D — Dry skin
I — Intolerance to cold
S — Short limbs
M — Menstrual abnormalities (Menorrhagia and amenorrhea)

- **Diagnosis:** The TSH level is increased and; T_4 levels and T_3 resin uptake is decreased. Cardiomegaly, epiphyseal breaking and intersutural or **wormian bones** can be seen in X-ray.
- **Treatment: Levothyroxine** is the drug of choice.

Hyperthyroidism

The most common cause of hyperthyroidism in children is **Graves disease** and minority of cases can be caused by TSH receptor mutation with constitutive activity (activation without TSH), McCune-Albright syndrome, Plummer disease (toxic nodular goitre), thyroiditis, thyroid cancer and acute iodine overdose.

- **Clinical presentation:** The peak age of presentation is **adolescence** and is **more common in girls**. The earliest finding is **emotional disturbance** which may be followed by poor school performance, tremor, increased appetite, exophthalmos, moist skin, CVS abnormalities (tachycardia, atrial fibrillation, mitral regurgitation) and heat intolerance.

  Congenital hypothyroidism is caused by activation of the TSH receptors in the neonate by the maternal TSH receptor antibodies. The baby is usually hyperactive along with other findings like microcephaly, ventriculomegaly, hepatosplenomegaly, jaundice, **accelerated bone age, goitre, triangular face** and **cranial syntosis.** Prematurity and IUGR are frequently associated with congenital hypothyroidism
- **Diagnosis:** Hyperthyroidism can be confirmed by increased serum T_4 and T_3.The diagnosis of Graves disease is confirmed by elevated levels of TSRAb (TSH Receptor Stimulating Antibody).
- **Treatment:** Anti-thyroid drugs propylthiouracil and methimazole can be used for treatment; however **methimazole is the drug of choice** in children.

DIABETES MELLITUS

Diabetes mellitus can be classified as insulin dependent diabetes mellitus (IDDM), noninsulin dependent diabetes mellitus (NIDDM) and maturity onset diabetes mellitus (MODY).

Classification

- **IDDM:** IDDM is the **most common type of DM** encountered in **children**. It is usually caused by autoimmune destruction of β islet cells of the pancreas. There is genetic association related to inheritance of **HLA DR3 and HLA DR4 genes.** IDDM can be associated with other autoimmune conditions like **autoimmune Hashimoto's thyroiditis**, celiac disease and **Addison's disease**.
- **NIDDM:** NIDDM is usually seen after the 4th decade; however for the last 2 decades there has been a rise in the prevalence of NIDDM in children due to increasing obesity. It is a **polygenic disorder** which can be caused by multiple factors like genetic and environmental factors.
- **MODY:** MODY is an **AD inherited** form of DM, seen in **at least 3 generations before age of 25 years**, which is characterised by defect in insulin secretion. It is caused by mutation in the glucokinase gene.

Clinical Presentation

DM presents classically with symptoms of polyuria, polydipsia, hyperphagia and weight loss. NIDDM which is associated with insulin resistance is characterised by increased serum insulin. This insulin can cause hyperpigmentation of neck and armpits called as **acanthosis nigricans**.

Diagnosis

- The criteria for diagnosis of DM are increased fasting blood sugar (>126 mg/dl), random blood sugar (>200 mg/dl) and blood sugar >200 mg/dl 2 hours after glucose load of **1.75 g/kg to a maximum amount of 75 g (glucose challenge test)**.
- **Glycosylated haemoglobin (HbA$_{1C}$)** levels determine the blood glucose status over the last 3 months. The pediatric ranges of normal HbA$_{1C}$ decreases with age i.e. for >5 years is 7.5–8.5%, 6–11 years is <8% and 12–19 years is <7.5%. However the normal value of HbA$_{1C}$ in **adults is less than 6.5**.

Treatment

- **IDDM:** IDDM is treated by a mixture of rapid acting insulin and long acting insulin.
- **NIDDM:** NIDDM needs a multidirectional approach in the form of oral hypoglycemic agents, diet modification and exercise.

Complications

- **Acute complications:**
  - ❖ **Hypoglycemia:** The blood sugar level of less than 60 mg/dl is considered as hypoglycemia. The presenting symptoms are sweating, palpitation, drowsiness and behavioural changes. For mild to moderate hypoglycemia **sweet products** like sugar, juice or glucose powder can be given. In case of severe hypoglycemia **glucagon** should be given at a dose of 30 units for children below 5 years and 50 units for children older than 5 years.
  - ❖ **Diabetic ketoacidosis:** Ketoacidosis is most commonly caused by missing the dose of insulin. Glucose is not metabolised and glycosuria results in loss of fluids (dehydration). Further increased ketone bodies, loss of sodium, potassium and phosphate; and decreased bicarbonate can be seen. The **fluid loss (dehydration)** is best treated by **normal saline** followed by half saline. Acidosis is effectively treated by insulin which is given at a dose of 0.1 U/kg/hour. After blood glucose level is below 250 mg/dl, 5% dextrose is added. Potassium is replaced in the form of both acetate and chloride. Bicarbonate is usually not used to correct acidosis, though it is decreased.
- **Chronic complications:**
  - ❖ **Diabetic retinopathy:** Diabetic retinopathy is characterised by various changes like microaneurysms, vasculogenesis and exudates in the retina. Cataract can be seen because of accumulation of **sorbitol** in lens. **Prophylactic fundus examination** should be done immediately after diagnosis of NIDDM and **after 3–5 years in IDDM**.
  - ❖ **Diabetic nephropathy:** Glycation of the proteins in kidneys result in thickening of glomerular basement membrane. Gradually there is microalbuminuria and hypertension.
  - ❖ **Diabetic neuropathy:** Both peripheral and autonomic nervous system can be involved.

CALCIUM DISORDERS

Calcium level in the blood is usually maintained by the action of parathyroid hormone (PTH), calcitonin and calcitriol (active form of vitamin D). PTH increases absorption of calcium and excretion of phosphate by acting on the PTH receptors. Calcitonin decreases both calcium and phosphate levels by incorporation in to the bones. Calcitriol increases the level of calcium and phosphate by increasing absorption in intestine and renal tubules.

Hormone	Effect on serum calcium and phosphate
PTH	Increases calcium Decreases phosphate
Calcitonin	Decreases calcium Decreases phosphate
Calcitriol	Increases calcium Increases phosphate

Hypocalcemia

The serum calcium is normally between **8.9–10.2 mg/dl**; however symptomatic hypocalcemia is seen after serum calcium falls below **7.5 mg/dl**. The calcium levels can be decreased because of decreased PTH levels (hypoparathyroidism) or PTH receptor mutations (pseudohypoparathyroidism and pseudopseudohypoparathyroidism).

Hypocalcemia presents with symptoms of tetany like carpopedal spasm, laryngospasm, twitching of muscles, numbness and muscle cramps. Other findings that can be seen are photophobia, diarrhoea and raised intracranial tension. **Chvostek sign** (facial muscle spasm on tapping of face in front of ear) and **Trousseau's sign** (inflation of sphygmomanometer causes flexion of wrist and hyperextension of fingers) are characteristic of hypocalcemia. Acute symptomatic hypocalcemia is treated by calcium gluconate or calcium chloride by intravenous route.

Hypoparathyroidism

Hypoparathyroidism can be caused by aplasia of parathyroid gland (Degeorge syndrome), HDR syndrome (Hypoparathyroidism, deafness and renal anomaly), Mendelian pattern of hypoparathyroidism (X linked recessive, AD and AR), autoimmune parathyroid destruction (autoimmune polyglandular disease I) and accidental surgical removal of parathyroid gland during thyroid surgery. The PTH level is low along with decreased calcium and increased phosphate.

Pseudohypoparathyroidism

Pseudohypoparathyroidism is caused by mutation of the maternal PTH receptor gene. This results in decreased calcium and increased phosphate level but the PTH level is also increased.

Pseudopseudohypoparathyroidism

Pseudopseudohypoparathyroidism is characterised by the mutation of paternal PTH receptor gene. But the calcium and phosphorous levels are normal along with a slightly elevated PTH level. Both pseudohypoparathyroidism and pseudopseudohypoparathyroidism are associated with **Albright hereditary osteodystrophy**, which is characterised by short fourth metacarpal, mental retardation, delayed dentition and a round face.

Hypercalcemia

Hypercalcemia is characterised by a serum calcium level of more than 11 mg/dl. The different hypercalcemic states are hyperparathyroidism, idiopathic hypercalcemia of infancy and familial hypocalciuric hypercalcemia.

Hypercalcemia presents with hypotonia, hypertension, polyuria, constipation, anorexia, depression, band keratopathy, hyperreflexia, short QT intervals, pancreatitis and peptic ulcer. Symptomatic hypercalcemia is treated with furosemide, glucocorticoids, calcitonin and bisphosphonates.

Hyperparathyroidism

The most common cause of hyperparathyroidism in children is a benign adenoma. Other causes are multiple endocrine neoplasia I and II; and jaw tumor syndrome.

Hereditary Hypocalciuric Hypercalcemia

It is an AD condition caused by mutation of calcium sensing receptors (CASR) in the renal tubules and parathyroid gland. This results in increased PTH secretion followed by hypercalcemia, hypophosphatemia and hypocalciuria; however patient is asymptomatic and treatment is not required. Magnesium levels can be both increased and decreased.

Idiopathic Hypercalcemia of Infancy (Williams Syndrome)

Williams syndrome is caused by abnormal metabolism of vitamin D. It is associated with elastin gene mutation and FISH may be used for diagnosis. The associated features are **elfin facies**, **mental retardation**, **supravalvular aortic stenosis** and **motor deficits**. It is treated by restriction of calcium and vitamin D; however it **spontaneously resolves by the age of 4 years.**

MULTIPLE CHOICE QUESTIONS

1. **A 10-month-old baby previously normal, suddenly becomes distress in his crib. The external appearance of genitalia was normal, except hyperpigmentation. Blood glucose showed a level of 30 mg%. What is the most probable diagnosis?**
   [AIIMS May 10, 9; AI 11]
   a. 21 hydroxylase deficiency
   b. Hyperinsulinism
   c. Familial glucocorticoid deficiency
   d. Cushing's syndrome

2. **A 3 month old male child with normal genitalia presents to the emergency department with severe dehydration, hyperkalemia and hyponatremia. The measurement blood levels of which of the following will be helpful?** [AIIMS May 09]
   a. 17-hydroxyprogesterone
   b. Renin
   c. Cortisol
   d. Aldosterone

3. **A 5-year-old girl presents with hypertension and virilisation. There is also finding of hypokalemia what is the diagnosis:** [AIIMS May 07]
   a. 21-hydroxylase deficiency
   b. 3-β hydroxy steroid deficiency
   c. 11-β hydroxylase deficiency
   d. Conn's disease

4. **16 years old girl with primary amenorrhea attends OPD. She has normal sexual development and normal breast but with absent pubic and axillary hair. Examination shows B/L inguinal hernias. USG shows absent uterus and blind vagina. Diagnosis will be:** [AIIMS May 07]
   a. Turner syndrome
   b. Mullerian agenesis
   c. Star syndrome
   d. Androgen insensitivity syndrome

5. **Orchidopexy is done in cases of undescended testes at the age of:** [AIIMS Nov. 06]
   a. Neonate   b. 1–2 years
   c. 5 years   d. Puberty

6. **A 6 month old boy weighing 3.2 kg presents with recurrent vomiting and polyuria. Investigations show blood urea 60 mg/dl, creatinine 0.7 mg/dl, calcium 12.8 mg/dl, phosphate 3 mg/dl, pH 7.45, bicarbonate 25 mEq/L and PTH 140 pg/ml (normal <60 pg/ml). Daily urinary calcium excretion is reduced. Ultrasound abdomen shows bilateral nephrocalcinosis. The most likely diagnosis is:**
   [AIIMS Nov. 05]
   a. Bartter syndrome
   b. Mutation of calcium sensing receptors
   c. Pseudo-pseudohypoparathyroidism
   d. Parathyroid adenoma

7. **A 9-year-old boy presents with growth retardation and propensity to hypoglycemia. Physical examination reveals short stature, micropenis, increased fat and high-pitched voice. The skeletal survey reveals bone age of 5 years. Which of the following is most appropriate diagnosis:** [AIIMS Nov. 04]
   a. Malabsorption
   b. Growth hormone deficiency
   c. Adrenal tumor
   d. Thyroxin deficiency

8. **A baby girl presents with bilateral inguinal masses, thought to be hernias but are found to be testes in the inguinal canals. Which karyotype would you expect to find in the child:** [AIIMS Nov. 04]
   a. 46, XX   b. 46, XY
   c. 46, XXY   d. 47, XXY

9. **Injection of glucagon is effective for management of persistent hypoglycemia in all except:**
   [AIIMS May 04]
   a. Large for date baby
   b. Galactosemia
   c. Infant of diabetic mother
   d. Nesidioblastosis

10. **'Weak giants' are produced by:** [AIIMS May 04]
    a. Thyroid adenomas
    b. Thyroid carcinomas

c. Parathyroid adenomas

d. Pituitary adenomas

11. **A 8-day-old breast fed baby presents with vomiting, poor feeding and loose stooled. On examination the heart rate is 190/minute, blood pressure 50/30 mm Hg, respiratory rate 72 breaths/minute and capillary refill time of 4 seconds. Investigations show hemoglobin level of 15g/DL. Na-12mEq/L, K-6.8mEq/L, Cl-81mEq/L, bicarbonate 15mEq/L, Urea 30 mg/dL, creatinine 0.6 mg/dL. The most likely diagnosis is:** [AIIMS Nov. 03]

    a. Congenital adrenal hyperplasia

    b. Acute tubular necrosis

    c. Congenital hypertrophic pyloric stenosis

    d. Galactosemia

12. **In neonatal screening program for detection of congenital hypothyroidism, the ideal place and time to collect the blood sample for TSH estimation is :** [AIIMS May 03]

    a. Cord blood at time of birth

    b. Heal pad blood at the time of birth

    c. Heal pad blood on 4 day of birth

    d. Peripheral venous blood on 28 day

13. **A 3-year-old boy is detected to have bilateral renal calculi. Metabolic evaluation confirms the presence of marked hypercalciuria with normal blood levels of calcium, magnesium, phosphate, uric acid and creatinine. A diagnosis of idiopathic hypercalciuria is made. The dietary management includes all except:** [AIIMS May 03]

    a. Increased water intake

    b. Low sodium diet

    c. Reduced calcium intake

    d. Avoid meat proteins

14. **Blood specimen for neonatal thyroid screening is obtained on:** [AI 05; AIIMS May 03]

    a. Cord blood   b. 24 hours after birth

    c. 48 hours after birth d. 72 hours after birth

15. **8 years old child presents with lethargy multiple epiphyseal breaks, wormian bones with growth retardation and mental retardation Diagnosis is?** [AIIMS Nov. 01]

    a. Rickets   b. Hypothyroidism

    c. Scurvy   d. Hypoparathyroidism

16. **In India the commonest cause of Juvenile Onset of Diabetes mellitus:** [AIIMS May 01]

    a. IDDM

    b. Fibrocalcific pancreaticopathy

    c. Mody

    d. Gall stones

17. **Short stature, secondary to growth hormone deficiency is associated with:** [AIIMS Dec. 95]

    a. Normal body proportion

    b. Low birth weight

c. Normal epiphyseal development

d. Height age equal to skeletal age

18. **Prophylactic gonadectomy is done in:** [AIIMS Dec. 97]

    a. Testicular feminising syndrome

    b. Klinefelter syndrome

    c. Kallman's syndrome

    d. Down's syndrome

19. **All of the following can cause precocious puberty in males except:** [AIIMS Dec. 95]

    a. 17 alpha hydroxylase deficiency

    b. 21 beta hydroxylase deficiency

    c. 11 beta hydroxylase deficiency

    d. None of the above

20 **Late onset puberty in male is defined as:** [AIIMS May 94]

    a. Puberty onset after 16 years

    b. Puberty onset after 17 years

    c. Puberty onset after 18 years

    d. Puberty onset after 21 years

21. **Treatment of choice in childhood thyrotoxicosis:** [AIIMS 92]

    a. Radioiodine   b. Lugols iodine

    c. Carbimazole   d. Surgery

22. **Characteristic features of growth hormone deficiency include all of the following except:** [AIIMS 83]

    a. Short stature since birth

    b. Symptomatic hypoglycemia

    c. Delayed tooth eruption

    d. Sexual infantilism

23. **ACTH secretion is highest during:** [PGI Dec. 99]

    a. Noon   b. Evening

    c. Morning   d. Night

24. **A baby presents with tetany. First thing to be done is administration of:**

    a. Diazepam   b. Vitamin D

    c. Calcium gluconate   d. Calcitonin

25. **The following is true about Nesidioblastosis except:** [AI 11]

    a. Presents with hypoglycemic attacks

    b. More common in adults than in children

    c. Histology shows hyperplasia of islet cells

    d. Diazoxide is used for treatment

26. **A 7-year-old boy underwent neurosurgery for craniopharyngioma following which pituitary functions were lost. Which of the following hormone should be replaced first?** [AI 11]

    a. Hydrocortisone

    b. Thyroxine

    c. Growth hormone

    d. Prolactin

27. A five-years-old boy has precocious puberty BP130/80. Estimation of which of the following will help in diagnosis? [AI 09]
    a. 17-Hydroxyprogesterone
    b. 11-Deoxycortisol
    c. Aldosterone
    d. DOCA

28. All of the following statements about androgen insensitivity syndrome are true except: [AI 08]
    a. It is an X linked disorder
    b. XY genotype is present
    c. Affected individuals have female phenotype
    d. Abundant pubic hairs are present

29. Most common cause of delayed puberty in males is: [AI 08]
    a. Kallamann syndrome   b. Klinefelter syndrome
    c. Constitutional   d. Prader-willi syndrome

30. Which of the following statements about 21 alpha hydroxylase deficiency is false: [AI 08]
    a. Most common cause of Congenital Adrenal Hyperplasia (CAH) in children
    b. Affected females present with ambiguous genitalia
    c. Affected males present with precocious puberty
    d. Hypokalemic alkalosis is seen

31. Blood specimen for neonatal thyroid screening is obtained on: [AI 05; AIIMS May 03]
    a. Cord blood   b. 24 hours after birth
    c. 48 hours after birth d. 72 hours after birth

32. Which one of the following drugs is used for fetal therapy of congenital adrenal hyperplasia? [AI 05]
    a. Hydrocortisone   b. Prednisolone
    c. Flurocortisone   d. Dexamethasone

33. A 21 years woman presents with complaints of primary amenorrhea. Her height is 153 cms, weight is 51 kg. She has well developed breasts. She has no pubic or axillary hair and no hirsutism. Which of the following is the most probable diagnosis: [AI 04]
    a. Turner syndrome
    b. Stein-Leventhal syndrome
    c. Premature ovarian failure
    d. Complete androgen insensitivity syndrome

34. Unilateral undescended testes is ideally operated around: [AI 04]
    a. 2 months of age   b. 6 months of age
    c. 12 months of age   d. 24 months of age

35. A 10-years-old boy has a fracture of femur. Biochemical evaluation revealed Hb 11.5 gm/dL and ESR 18 mm first hour. Serum calcium 12.8 mg/dL, serum phosphorus 2.3 mg/dL, alkaline phosphate 28 KA units and blood urea 32 mg/dL. Which of the following is the most probable diagnosis in his case? [AI 04]
    a. Nutritional rickets   b. Renal rickets
    c. Hyperparathyroidism d. Skeletal dysplasia

36. A 1-month-old baby presents with frequent vomiting and failure to thrive. There are features of moderate dehydration. Blood sodium is 122 mEq/L and potassium is 6.1mEq/L. The most likely diagnosis is: [AI 03, 02]
    a. Gitelman syndrome
    b. Bartter syndrome
    c. 21-hydroxylase deficiency
    d. 11-β hydroxylase deficiency

37. The most common cause of ambiguous genitalia in newborn is: [AI 02]
    a. 21-hydroxylase deficiency
    b. 11β-hydroxylase deficiency
    c. 17α-hydroxylase deficiency
    d. 3β-hydroxysteroid deficiency

38. A 10-day-old male pseudohermaphrodite child with 46 XY karyotype presents with BP of 110/80 mmHg. Most likely enzyme deficiency is: [AI 01]
    a. 21 hydroxylase   b. 17 hydroxylase
    c. 11 hydroxylase   d. 3-beta hydroxylase

39. A female has previous child with congenital adrenal hyperplasia. In the present pregnancy, steroid therapy should be started: [AI 2000]
    a. After karyotyping
    b. At the time of delivery
    c. Before conception
    d. As soon as pregnancy is diagnosed

40. The diagnosis of a patient presenting with familial polyostiosis, precocious puberty and pigmentation is: [AI 95]
    a. Tuberous sclerosis
    b. McCune-Albright syndrome
    c. Klinefelter syndrome
    d. SLE

41. Pseudohermaphroditism in a female child is most commonly due to: [AI 94]
    a. 21-Hydroxylase deficiency
    b. 17-hydroxylase deficiency
    c. 11-hydroxylase deficiency
    d. 3-hydroxylase deficiency

42. Deficiency of growth hormone leads to: [AI 89]
    a. Delayed fusion of epiphysis
    b. Proportionate dwarfism
    c. Acromegaly
    d. Mental retardation

43. Commonest feature of hypothyroidism in children: [AI 89]
    a. Cataract   b. Recurrent seizures
    c. Cold extremities   d. Laryngospasms

44. The most effective correction of acidosis in diabetic ketoacidosis is: [AI 81]
    a. IV bicarbonate   b. IV saline
    c. IV insulin   d. Oral bicarbonate

45. **Oral glucose tolerance test in children is done with:** [PGI Dec. 07]
    a. 1.5 gm/kg
    b. 1.75 gm/kg
    c. 2 gm/kg
    d. 2.5 gm/kg
    e. 75 gm as an adult

46. **Male pseudohermaphroditism is seen in:** [PGI Dec. 07]
    a. 5-a reductase deficiency
    b. 21 hydroxylase deficiency
    c. 17 hydroxylase deficiency
    d. Gonadal dysgenesis

47. **In children with type I DM when is ophthalmologic evaluation indicated:** [PGI June 06]
    a. At the time of diagnosis
    b. After 1 year
    c. After 2 years
    d. After 5 years
    e. After 10 years

48. **Common presentations of Juvenile Hypothyroidism:** [PGI June 06]
    a. Growth retardation
    b. Mental retardation within 2 years
    c. Delayed puberty
    d. Umbilical Hernia
    e. Moist skin

49. **Delayed puberty seen in:** [PGI Dec. 06]
    a. Chronic disease
    b. Hypothyroidism
    c. Turner's syndrome
    d. Malabsorption syndrome

50. **True about pandered syndrome:** [PGI Dec. 04]
    a. Diffuse colloid goiter
    b. Nodular goiter
    c. Mental retardation
    d. B/L sensory neural deafness
    e. Normal cochlea

51. **True statement about testicular feminising syndrome:** [PGI June 04]
    a. Absent uterus
    b. Absent vagina
    c. Chromosome pattern 47 XY
    d. Absent ovary

52. **Testicular feminizing syndrome is characterised by:** [PGI June 03]
    a. 47 XX
    b. 47 XY
    c. Ambiguous genitalia
    d. Female genitalia
    e. Mullerian derivatives present

53. **Precocious puberty is seen in:** [PGI Dec. 02]
    a. Hypothyroidism
    b. CNS irradiation
    c. MC cune-Albright syndrome
    d. Turner's syndrome
    e. Congenital adrenal hypoplasia

54. **Pendred's syndrome is:** [PGI June 02]
    a. Consistently associated with deafness
    b. Hypothyroidism is seen
    c. Mutation in connection coding gene
    d. Mutation in chromosome 21 causing receptor defect

55. **True of testicular feminization syndrome is:** [PGI June 02]
    a. Testes are present
    b. Female habitus
    c. XY genotype
    d. Secondary amenorrhea
    e. Uterus present

56. **Which is false in congenital hypopituitarism?**
    a. Growth hormone level<7 ng/ml
    b. Hypoglycemia
    c. Baby small at birth
    d. Delayed puberty

57. **Which of the following is true in cretinism:** [PGI Dec. 01]
    a. Goitre present at birth
    b. Can be diagnosed by serum T4 levels
    c. Prolonged physiological jaundice present
    d. Common in iodine deficiency endemic areas
    e. Delayed skeletal development

58. **Salt losing hydroxylase deficiency is characterised by:** [PGI June 01]
    a. Hyponatremia
    b. Hyperkalemia
    c. Hypoglycemia
    d. Hypocalcemia

59. **A boy with undescended testis, your concern to ask for operation is due to:** [PGI 01]
    a. Cosmetic reasons
    b. Infertility
    c. Risk of malignancy
    d. Impotence

60. **Delayed puberty in children is associated with:** [PGI June 00]
    a. Poliomyelitis
    b. Hypothyroidism
    c. Hypopituitarism
    d. Anorexia nervosa

61. **Congenital adrenal hyperplasia is associated with:** [PGI Dec. 00]
    a. Hypoglycemia
    b. Hyponatremia
    c. Hypokalemia
    d. Hyperkalemia

62. **First sign of puberty in girls:** [PGI Dec. 99]
    a. Pubearche
    b. Thelarche
    c. Growth spurt
    d. Menarche

63. **Hyperglycemia occurs after what % of beta cell mass is destroyed:** [PGI 78, UPSC 83]
    a. 40%
    b. 60%
    c. 80%
    d. 90%

QUESTIONS OF OTHER EXAMINATIONS

1. **A one week old male newborn suddenly presents with lethargy, poor oral intake and features of shock. Investigations reveal hyperkalemia, hyponatremia and hypoglycemia. What is the most likely diagnosis?** [UPSC 10]
   a. SIADH
   b. Gram negative sepsis
   c. Congenital adrenal hyperplasia
   d. Phenylketonuria

2. **Most common type of congenital adrenal hyperplasia?** [Maharastra 10]
   a. 21-hydroxylase deficiency
   b. 11-beta hydroxylase deficiency
   c. 3-hydroxylase deficiency
   d. 17-alpha hydroxylase deficiency

3. **Sexual ambiguity may be seen in which of the following conditions?** [COMED 09]
   a. Androgen insensitivity
   b. Pure gonadal dysgenesis
   c. Sawyer syndrome
   d. Mixed gonadal dysgenesis

4. **A newborn baby presents with shock, hyperkalemia and hypoglycemia. What is the most likely diagnosis?** [UPSC 09]
   a. Septicemia
   b. Inborn errors of metabolism
   c. Diabetes mellitus
   d. Congenital adrenal hyperplasia

5. **Features of Laurence-Moon-Biedl syndrome are:** [Manipal 09]
   a. Hypogonadism   b. Obesity
   c. Polydactyly   d. All of the above

6. **The features of neonatal hypothyroidism include all except:** [DPG 09]
   a. Triangular facies with craniosyntosis
   b. Congestive cardiac failure
   c. Advanced osseous maturation
   d. Goitre is rare

7. **Association of sexual precocity, multiple cystic bone lesions and endocrinopathies are seen in:** [COMED 08]
   a. Mc-Cune-Albright syndrome
   b. Granulosa cell tumor
   c. Androblastoma
   d. Hepatoblastoma

8. **The immediate treatment of a 10 kg weight infant presented with tetany is:** [UP 07]
   a. IV Diazepam
   b. IV calcium gluconate with cardiac monitoring
   c. IV slow phenobarbitone
   d. Wait and watch

9. **Features of hypothyroidism in infancy include the following except:** [UPSC 06]
   a. Premature closure of posterior fontanel
   b. Coarse facies
   c. Umbilical hernia
   d. Constipation

10. **Clinical features of hypothyroidism in a newborn are all except:** [MAHE 05, DPG 09]
    a. Sluggishness+++
    b. Large tongue
    c. Large posterior fontanel
    d. Mental retardation

11. **Adrenal hyperplasia due to 21 hydroxylase deficiency is treated with low dose of:** [Kerela 04]
    a. Androgen   b. Estrogen
    c. Cortisone   d. Antiandrogen

12. **A 6 month old infant is brought with a history of constipation and excessive sleepiness. On examination, he is lethargic, has periorbital puffiness, large tongue and umbilical hernia. The investigation which will help diagnose the condition is:** [UPSC 02]
    a. T4 TSH assay
    b. Karyotyping
    c. Rectal mucosal biopsy
    d. Knee X ray

13. **Infant with no social smile, no eyebrows, protruded tongue. Diagnosis:** [TN 99]
    a. Cretinism   b. Down's syndrome
    c. Mucopolysaccharidosis d. Rickets

14. **Which of the following is seen in 95% of patients with diabetes mellitus:** [TN 95]
    a. HLA B27   b. HLA B3–B4
    c. HLA DR3–DR4   d. HLA A3

15. **Dehydration in ketoacidosis is best treated with:** [TN 91]
    a. Isolyte P   b. Isolyte M
    c. Normal saline   d. Molar 1/6 lactate

16. **Minimum amount of carbohydrate required to prevent ketonuria in a case of diabetes is about:** [DNB 90, 91]
    a. 50 gm/daily   b. 25gm/daily
    c. 100 gm/daily   d. 150 gm/daily

17. **Estimation of glycosylated haemoglobin gives in assessment of the blood glucose level in the previous........weeks:** [Kerala 89]
    a. 1   b. 2
    c. 8   d. 10

18. **Which one of the following statements about non-insulin dependent diabetes mellitus (NIDDM) is NOT true:**
    a. Circulating islet cell antibodies are usually found
    b. There is no HLA association
    c. Ketosis is rare
    d. Relative resistance to insulin is present

ANSWERS

1. (c) Familial glucocorticoid deficiency (Ref: Rudolph 22nd E/P2054)

Familial glucocorticoid deficiency

- FGD is an AR condition caused by **mutation of the ACTH receptor.**
- Mineralocorticoids are secreted normally as it is controlled by the RAAS system but there is deficiency of glucocorticoids.
- The baby presents with **hyperpigmentation** as ACTH level is increased. Other findings are **hypoglycemia**, lethargy, pallor and seizures.

2. (a) 17-hydroxyprogesterone (Ref: Rudolph 22nd E/P2048–50)

- This is a case of a male child with **normal genitalia**, **hyponatremia** and **hyperkalemia**.
- Decreased aldosterone secretion (**hyponatremia and hyperkalemia**) and increased testosterone secretion (virilisation and **normal genitalia in males**) is seen with 21-hydroxylase deficiency.
- 21-hydroxylase deficiency will lead to accumulation of **17-hydroxyprogesterone**.

3. (c) 11-b hydroxylase deficiency (Ref: Rudolph 22nd E/P2048–52)

This is the case of a female with **hypertension, virilisation and hypokalemia**. Now let us analyse each option.

- 21-hydroxylase deficiency is characterised by decreased aldosterone, which causes **hyponatremia**, **hyperkalemia** and **hypotension**. Increased testo-sterone can cause **virilisation** and pseudo-hermaphroditism in females.
- 11-hydroxylase deficiency is characterised by increased DOCA, which can cause **hypernatremia, hypertension** and **hypokalemia**. Increased testo-sterone can cause **virilisation** and pseudo-hermaphroditism in females.
- 3-β hydroxy steroid deficiency is characterised by decreased aldosterone which causes **hyponatremia**, **hyperkalemia** and **hypotension**. Increased DHES can cause **virilisation** in females.
- Conn's syndrome is characterised by increased aldosterone which causes **hypernatremia, hypertension** and **hypokalemia** but there is **no virilisation**.

4. (d) Androgen insensitivity syndrome (Ref: Rudolph 22nd E/P2067)

Kindly refer text for details.

5. (b) 1–2 years (Ref: Rudolph 22nd E/P1747)

- Though the best age for orchidopexy currently is between 6 months and 1 year, the earlier guidelines were in favour of 1–2 years. Hence the best answer is 1–2 years.

6. (b) Mutation of calcium sensing receptors (Ref: CPDT 19th E/P932)

- The findings in this case are hypocalciuria, hypercalcemia, normal phosphorous level and increased PTH level.
- These findings are consistent with hereditary hypocalciuric hypercalcemia, which is caused by mutation of calcium sensing receptors in kidney and parathyroid gland.

7. (b) Growth hormone deficiency (Ref: Nelson 19th E/P1850)

Growth hormone deficiency: Growth hormone deficiency presents with —

- **Hypoglycemia**
- **Micropenis**
- Saddle nose
- Cold sensitivity
- Delayed puberty, **delayed dentition** with overcrowding of teeth, **delayed bone age**, **delayed closure of epiphysis**
- **Proportionate growth retardation**
- **Increased fat content in the body**
- Decreased muscle mass.

8. (b) 46, XY (Ref: Rudolph 22nd E/P2067)

- This is a case of androgen insensitivity syndrome, which is caused by mutation of androgen receptors in a **male foetus (46, XY).**

9. (b) Galactosemia (Ref: Nelson 19th E/P475–76)

- Glucagon surge is seen just after birth which maintains blood sugar level by glycogenolysis and gluconeogenesis in the liver. In large for date baby and infant of diabetic mother the glucagon surge is blunted and hence glucagon can be used to maintain euglycemia.
- Galactosemia is associated with liver dysfunction and hence glucagon cannot effectively potentiate glycogenolysis and gluconeogenesis.

10. (d) Pituitary adenomas (Ref: Nelson 19th E/P1859)

- **Pituitary adenomas**, specifically which consists of somatotroph cells is characterised by growth hormone excess but other hormones are decreased.
- Growth hormone excess presents as **gigantism** but the **patient is weak** and in fact fatigue is the earliest presentation.

11. **(a)** Congenital adrenal hyperplasia (Ref: Rudolph 22nd E/P2048)

This is a case with hypotension, hyponatremia and hyperkalemia. Now let us analyse each option.
- Congenital adrenal hyperplasia — In 21-hydroxylase deficiency decreased mineralocorticoids leads to **hyponatremia, hypotension and hyperkalemia.**
- Acute tubular necrosis — It is associated with hypertension and hyperkalemia.
- Congenital hypertrophic pyloric stenosis — It is associated with hypokalemia.
- Galactosemia — Vomiting is seen which can cause hypokalemia and hypoglycemia is seen.

12. **(a)** Cord blood at time of birth (Ref: Gregory TFT P53)
- TSH is estimated either in the cord blood at the time of birth or in baby's blood obtained from heel prick after 2 days of birth (in 1st 48 hours of birth false positive result can be seen).
- In Asian countries like **India** most patients do not turn up for screening after 2 days, hence **cord blood analysis at birth is the preferred approach**.

13. **(c)** Reduced calcium intake (Ref: Nelson 19th E/P1748)

Idiopathic hypercalciuria:
- Idiopathic hypercalciuria is an AD disease characterised by hypercalciuria, hematuria, dysuria and abdominal pain. Renal calculus is usually not seen; however can be seen in long standing cases.
- It is diagnosed by 24 hour urinary calcium excretion of more than 4 mg/kg.
- Thiazides, potassium citrate and **sodium restriction are recommended**; however **calcium restriction is contraindicated as calcium is required for growth and development.**

14. **(a)** Cord blood (Ref: Gregory TFT P53)
- TSH is estimated either in the cord blood at the time of birth or in baby's blood obtained from heel prick after 2 days of birth (in 1st 48 hours of birth false positive result can be seen).
- In Asian countries like **India** most patients do not turn up for screening after 2 days, hence **cord blood analysis at birth is the preferred approach**.

15. **(b)** Hypothyroidism (Ref: CPDT 19th E/P923)
- Lethargy, epiphyseal breaks, wormian bones, growth retardation and mental retardation can be seen in hypothyroidism.

16. **(b)** Fibrocalcific Pancreaticopathy (Ref: Ref: API 6th E/P994)

17. **(a)** Normal body proportion (Ref: Nelson 19th E/P1850)

18. **(a)** Testicular feminising syndrome (Ref: Rudolph 22nd E/P2067)
- Testicular feminising syndrome or androgen insensitivity syndrome is associated with risk of malignancy, which is seen before adulthood.

- Hence orchiectomy is advised in late adolescence or early adulthood.

19. **(a)** 17 alpha hydroxylase deficiency (Ref: Rudolph 22nd E/P2048–52)
Kindly refer text for details.

20. **(a)** Puberty onset after 16 years (Ref: Rudolph 22nd E/P2082)
- Puberty is said to be delayed if secondary sexual characters appear **after 14 years in male** and **after 13 years in female**.

21. **(c)** Carbimazole (Ref: CPDT 19th E/P925)

22. **(a)** Short stature since birth (Ref: Nelson 19th E/P1850)
- Hypoglycemia, delayed teeth eruption and sexual infantilism (micropenis) can be seen due to growth hormone deficiency.
- Baby's length at birth is usually normal.

23. **(c)** Morning (Ref: CPDT 19th E/P940)
- Maximum ACTH is secreted during the early morning hours.

24. **(c)** Calcium gluconate (Ref: CPDT 19th E/P930)
- Acute tetany is best treated by intravenous administration of calcium gluconate or calcium citrate.

25. **(b)** More common in adults than in children (Ref: Ernest Pathology of pancreas/P178)

Nesidioblastosis (Hyperinsulinemic hypoglycemia):
- Nesidioblastosis is characterised by **diffuse or focal islet cell hyperplasia** of the pancreas.
- It presents usually in the **infancy** with **postprandial hypoglycemia** and fasting hypoglycemia is unusual.
- Surgery is advised and depending on the type of hyperplasia, **neartotal or partial pancreatectomy** is advised.
- Medical management is required to maintain euglycemia and **diazoxide** is the standard drug used in Nesidioblastosis. Longer acting somatostatin analogues like **octreotide** can also be used.

26. **(a)** Hydrocortisone (Rudolph 22nd E/P2020)
- Craniopharyngioma is the most common neoplasm causing hypopituitarism.
- After surgery all pituitary functions are lost and the first and earliest intervention should be replacement of the hormone required for maintain most vital functions i.e. glucocorticoids.

27. **Normal blood pressure range in children**

Age	B.P
1–3 months	75/50
4–12 months	84/65
1–8 years	95/65
9–14 years	105/65

- So clearly this is a boy with **hypertension** and **precocious puberty.**
- Hypertension and precocious puberty in males can be seen due to increased DOCA and testosterone, which is seen due to deficiency of 11β hydroxylase.
- Look at the diagram of adrenal hormone synthesis and it will be clear that deficiency of 11β hydroxylase will lead to accumulation of **11 deoxycortisol.**

28. **(d)** Abundant pubic hairs are present (Ref: Rudolph 22nd E/P2067)
    - Pubic and axillary hairs are characteristically sparse in androgen insensitivity syndrome, as androgens cannot act on receptors.

29. **(c)** Constitutional (Ref: CPDT 19th E/P937)
    - Most common cause of delayed puberty both in males and females is constitutional growth delay.

30. **(d)** Hypokalemic alkalosis is seen (Ref: Rudolph 22nd E/P2048)
    21β hydroxylase deficiency: Deficiency of 21β hydroxylase leads to partial abolition of the mineralocorticoid and glucocorticoid pathways but the sex steroid pathway is completely potentiated. This is the **most common form of CAH** accounting for almost 90% cases.
    - Decreased aldosterone leads to hyponatremia, hypotension and **hyperkalemia**. Decreased cortisol can cause hypoglycemia.
    - DHES, androstenadione and testosterone is increased.
      - ❖ **Males** — Increased sex hormones cause **precocious puberty**, virilisation and rapid growth.
      - ❖ **Females** — Increased sex hormones cause **ambiguous genitalia** (pseudohermaphroditism), virilisation and rapid growth.

31. **(a)** Cord blood (Ref: Gregory TFT P53)
    - TSH is estimated either in the cord blood at the time of birth or in baby's blood obtained from heel prick after 2 days of birth (in 1st 48 hours of birth false positive result can be seen).
    - In Asian countries like **India** most patients do not turn up for screening after 2 days, hence **cord blood analysis at birth is the preferred approach.**

32. **(d)** Dexamethasone (Ref: Nelson 19th E/P1912)
    - Dexamethasone is the preferred drug for foetal therapy in CAH.

33. **(d)** Complete androgen insensitivity syndrome (Ref: Rudolph 22nd E/P2067)
    Kindly refer text for details.

34. **(b)** 6 months of age (Ref: Rudolph 22nd E/P1747)
    - Since the number of germ cell in cryptorchid testes start decreasing after 7 months, the best age for orchidopexy is **6 months of age.**

35. **(c)** Hyperparathyroidism (Ref: CPDT 19th E/P932)
    - This is a case of fracture associated with hypercalcemia and hypophosphatemia. So the disgnosis is hyperparathyroidism.
    - In case of rickets both calcium and phosphorous is decreased.

Hormone	Effect on serum calcium and phosphate
PTH	Increases calcium Decreases phosphate
Calcitonin	Decreases calcium Decreases phosphate
Calcitriol	Increases calcium Increases phosphate

36. **(c)** 21-hydroxylase deficiency (Ref: Rudolph 22nd E/P2048–50)
    This is a case with nausea and vomiting along with **hyponatremia** and **hyperkalemia**. Now let us try each of these options.
    - Gitelman and Bartter syndrome is characterised by **hypokalemic metabolic alkalosis**.
    - 21-hydroxylase deficiency is characterised by decreased aldosterone, which causes **hyponatremia**, **hyperkalemia** and hypotension.
    - 11-hydroxylase deficiency is characterised by increased DOCA, which can cause **hypernatremia** and **hypokalemia**.

37. **(a)** 21-hydroxylase deficiency (Ref: Rudolph 22nd E/P2048–50)
    - **21-hydroxylase deficiency** is the **most common form of CAH** i.e. 90% cases and it can cause **ambiguous genitalia in females**.

38. **(b)** 17 hydroxylase (Ref: Rudolph 22nd E/P2048)
    - This is a case of a **male with pseudohermaphroditism**, which is caused by decreased production of sex hormones.
    - **17-hydroxylase deficiency** causes decreased sex hormone production which results in **male pseudo-hermaphroditism.**
    - Deficiency of 21-hydroxylase, 11-hydroxylase and 3-beta hydroxylase can lead to increased sex hormone production and female pseudohermaphroditism.

39. **(d)** As soon as pregnancy is diagnosed (Ref: Nelson 19th E/P1912)
    - Dexamethasone should be started at **6 weeks of fetal life or as soon as pregnancy is confirmed**.
    - Chorionic villous sampling is done to confirm the sex. If the foetus is of female sex then therapy is continued.

40. (b) McCune-Albright syndrome (Ref: Nelson 19th E/ P1867)

Kindly refer text for details.

41. (a) 21-hydroxylase deficiency (Rudolph 22nd E/ P2048–50)

CAH and pseudohermaphroditism:

- **Males** — 17-hydroxylase and 3-hydroxylase deficiency can cause pseudohermaphroditism in males.
- **Females — 21-hydroxylase** and 11 hydroxylase deficiency can cause **pseudohermaphroditism in females.** However **21-hydroxylase deficiency is the most common cause of CAH.**

42. (a) and (b) Delayed fusion of epiphysis and Proportionate dwarfism (Ref: Nelson 19th E/P1850)

43. (c) Cold extremities (Ref: CPDT 19th E/P923)

44. (c) IV insulin (Ref: CPDT 19th E/P954)

45. (b) and (e) 1.75 gm/kg and 75 gm as an adult (Ref: CPDT 19th E/P950)

Criteria for diagnosis of DM:

- Fasting blood sugar >126 mg/dl
- Random blood sugar >200 mg/dl
- Blood sugar >200 mg/dl 2 hours after glucose load of **1.75 g/kg to a maximum amount of 75 g (glucose challenge test).**

46. (a), (c) and (d) (Ref: Rudolph 19th E/P2048–52, 2067–68)

Kindly refer text for details.

47. (d) After 5 years (Ref: Nelson 19th E/P1966)

- **Prophylactic fundus examination** should be done immediately after diagnosis of NIDDM and **after 3–5 years in IDDM.**

48. (a), (b), (c) and (d) Growth retardation, Mental retardation within 2 years, Delayed puberty and Umbilical hernia (Ref: CPDT 19th E/P922–23)

Clinical presentation of hypothyroidism:

Mnemonic: **HYPOTHYROIDISM**
H — Hair loss
Y — Yellow skin
P — **Puberty delayed** or precocious
O — Obesity
T — Transient deafness
H — **Hernia (umbilical)**
Y — Yellow baby (prolonged physiological jaundice)
R — **Retardation of growth**
O — Ossification center breakage (epiphysis)
I — **Intellectual deficit**
D — **Dry skin**
I — Intolerance to cold
S — Short limbs
M — Menstrual abnormalities (Menorrhagia and amenorrhea)

49. ALL (Ref: Rudolph 22nd E/P2083)

Kindly refer text for details.

50. (a), (b), (c) and (d) Diffuse colloid goitre, Nodular goitre, Mental retardation and B/L sensory neural deafness (Ref: Nelson 19th E/P1873)

- Pendrin is a transport protein located in thyroid and **cochlea.**
- Mutation of gene encoding pendrin can lead to Pendred syndrome, which is characterised by **goitre, mental retardation and sensory neural deafness.**

51. (a), and (d) Absent uterus and Absent ovary (Ref: Rudolph 22nd E/P2067)

- Patient of a testicular feminising syndrome is a male with **46 XY genotype** and hence testes are present and **ovaries are absent.**
- Mullerian duct is inhibited by the AMH secreted by testes and hence **uterus**, fallopian tubes, posterior 2/3rd of vagina is absent. However the **anterior 1/3rd of vagina is present**.

52. (d) Female genitalia (Ref: Rudolph 22nd E/P2067)

- Patient is a male with 46 XY genotype, however phenotypical appearance is that of a male with presence of anterior 1/3rd of vagina and well developed breasts.
- Mullerian derivatives are absent as AMH is synthesised by the testes.

53. (b), (c) and (e) CNS irradiation, MC cune-Albright syndrome, Congenital adrenal hypoplasia (Ref: CPDT 19th E/P935)

Kindly refer text for details.

54. (b) Hypothyroidism is seen (Ref: Nelson 19th E/P1873)

- Mutation of **Pendrin gene (SL26A4)** located in **chromosome 7** leads to **Pendred syndrome** which is characterised by **sensorineural deafness**, **goitre** and **hypothyroidism**.

55. (a), (b) and (c) Testes are present, Female habitus and XY genotype (Ref: Rudolph 22nd E/P2067)

Kindly refer text for details.

56. (c) Baby small at birth (Ref: Nelson 19th E/P1850)

57. (b), (c), (d) and (e) Can be diagnosed by serum T4 levels, Prolonged physiological jaundice present, Common in iodine deficiency endemic areas, Delayed skeletal development(Ref: Danninson's Endemic cretinism)

Kindly refer text for details.

58. (a), (b) and (c) Hyponatremia, Hyperkalemia, Hypoglycemia (Ref: Rudolph 22nd E/P 2048)

- Salt loosing hydroxylase (21 hydroxylase deficiency) results in mineralocorticoid deficiency (hyponatremia and hyperkalemia) and glucocorticoid deficiency (hypoglycemia).

59. (b) and **(c)** Infertility and Risk of malignancy (Rudolph 22nd E/P1747)
Kindly refer text for details.

60. (b), (c) and **(d)** Hypothyroidism, Hypopituitarism, Anorexia nervosa (Ref: Rudolph 22nd E/P2083)
Kindly refer text for details.

61. (a), (b), (c) and **(d)** Hypoglycemia, Hyponatremia, Hypokalemia and Hyperkalemia (Ref: Rudolph 22nd E/P2049)
Kindly refer text for details.

62. (b) Thelarche (Ref: CPDT 19th E/P936)

- The first pubertal sign in female is thelarche followed by pubarche and menarche.

63. (d) 90% (Ref: CPDT 19th E/P949)

"The damage occurs gradually – over months and years in most people – and symptoms do not appear until about **90%** of the pancreatic islet cells have been destroyed."

QUESTIONS OF OTHER EXAMINATIONS

1. (c) Congenital adrenal hyperplasia (Ref: Rudolph 22nd E/P2048–50)

- Hyperkalemia and hyponatremia indicates towards mineralocorticoid deficiency and hypoglycemia towards glucocorticoid deficiency.
- Combination of this can be seen due to deficiency of 21 hydoxylase deficiency type of congenital adrenal hyperplasia.

2. (a) 21-hydroxylase deficiency (Ref: Rudolph 22nd E/P2048)

- 21-hydroxylase deficiency accounts for almost 90% cases of congenital adrenal hyperplasia.

3. (d) Mixed gonadal dysgenesis (Ref: Rudolph 22nd E/P2068–69)

- Mixed gonadal dysgenesis is commonly associated with ambiguous genitalia e.g. Turner syndrome.
- Androgen insensitivity is associated with female type external genitalia.
- Swyer syndrome which is a XY type of pure gonadal dysgenesis caused by SRY gene mutation or deletion is characterised by normal external and internal genitalia.

4. (d) Congenital adrenal hyperplasia (Ref: Rudolph 22nd E/P2048–50)

- Hyperkalemia and shock (hyponatremia) indicates towards mineralocorticoid deficiency and hypoglycemia towards glucocorticoid deficiency.
- Combination of this can be seen due to deficiency of 21 hydroxylase deficiency type of congenital adrenal hyperplasia.

5. (c) All of the above (Ref: Rudolph 22nd E/P2084)
Laurence-Moon syndrome:

- It is an AR disorder of **hypogonadotrophic hypogonadism**, which is characterised by mental retardation, **obesity, polydactyly**, retinitis pigmentosa and **hypogonadism.**

Mnemonic: **MOON**
M — Mental retardation
O — Obesity, Ovary and testis hypofunction
O — Ocular abnormality – Retinitis pigmentosa
N — Number of fingers is increased (Polydactyly)

6. (d) Goitre is rare (Ref: Nelson 19th E/P1886)

7. (a) McCune-Albright syndrome (Ref: Nelson 19th E/P1867)
Kindly refer text for details.

8. (b) IV calcium gluconate with cardiac monitoring (Ref: Nelson 19th E/P930)

- Acute tetany is treated by IV calcium gluconate at a dose of 10 mg/kg; however the dose should not exceed 50 mg/min to prevent cardiac arrhythmia.

9. (a) Premature closure of posterior fontanel (Ref: CPDT 19th E/P922–23)

- Hypothyroidism is associated with delayed closure of fontanels.

10. (d) Mental retardation (Ref: CPDT 19th E/P922)

- Mental retardation is not seen at birth, rather seen later as child starts growing.

11. (c) Cortisone (Ref: CPDT 19th E/P944)

- CAH is treated with **hydrocortisone** to suppress adrenal function and **fludrocortisone** to maintain electrolyte balance.

12. (a) T4 TSH assay (Ref CPDT 19th E/P923)

- Clearly this is a case of hypothyroidism which can be diagnosed by elevated THS and decreased T4 levels in serum.

13. (a) Cretinism (Ref: CPDT 19th E/P923)

14. (c) HLA DR3-DR4 (Ref: Nelson 19th E/P1949)

15. (c) Normal saline (Ref: CPDT 19th E/P954)

16. (c) 100 gm/daily (Ref:Anssi H Manninen: Metabolic Effects of the Very-Low-Carbohydrate Diets: Misunderstood "Villains" of Human Metabolism)

"According to the American Heart Association (AHA) Nutrition Committee, *Some popular high-protein/low-carbohydrate diets limit carbohydrates to 10 to 20 g/d, which is one fifth of the minimum 100 g/day that is necessary to prevent loss of lean muscle tissue*. Clearly, this is an incorrect statement since **catabolism of lean body mass is reduced by ketone bodies** (possibly through suppression of the activity of the branched-chain 2-oxo acid dehydrogenase), which and probably explains the preservation of lean tissue observed during very-low-carbohydrate diets."

17. (d) 10 (Ref: CPDT 19th E/P953)

"HbA$_{1C}$ reflects the frequency of elevated blood sugar level over the previous 3 months."

18. (a) Circulating islet cell antibodies are usually found (Ref: Nelson 19th E/P1951)

Autoimmune mechanism is a cause of insulin dependent diabetes mellitus.

12

Genetic and Genetic Disorders

Genetics is the branch which deals with the physiological and pathological aspect of genes located in the chromosomes. The genetic disorders can be because of abnormality in the genes or the chromosomes.

CHROMOSOME DISORDERS

There are 23 pairs of chromosome i.e. 22 pairs of autosomes and 1 pair of sex chromosome. Each chromosome has a short arm (p or petite) and a long arm (q). Depending on the variability of length of both arms, chromosomes can be classified as **metacentric** (p = q), **submetacentric** (p < q) and **acrocentric** (p <<<< q or absent p). Chromosome related diseases can be caused by change in number and structure of chromosomes, mosaicism, uniparental disomy and chromosome fragility.

Chromosome Number Disorders

The number of chromosomes in a germ cell is 23 (haploid). After fertilization normally it becomes 23 pairs or 46 (diploid). Disease occurs when there is a change in chromosome number, which can be euploidy (exact multiple of 23 e.g. 69) or aneuploidy (not a multiple of 23). **Most common chromosomal number disorders are aneuploidies like trisomy** of chromosome 21 (Down syndrome), 13 (Patau syndrome) and 18 (Edwards syndrome).

Down Syndrome

Down syndrome is the **most common form of trisomy as well as chromosomal disorder** which is caused by **maternal meiotic nondisjunction** of chromosome 21 **(trisomy 21)** in 95% cases. Rest 5% cases are caused by **translocation between chromosomes 13, 14, 15 and 21 e.g. t(13q,15q) and t(21q, 21q); and mosaicism.** There is a **100% risk of Down's syndrome in t(21q, 21q),** whereas in **other translocations the risk is lesser i.e. 1 in 8.** The most important predisposing factor for Down syndrome is **maternal age more than 35 years.**

- **Clinical findings:**
  - ❖ The baby can be born with generalised **hypotonia**, microcephaly, **brachycephaly**, **simian crease**, pelvic dysplasia, congenital cataracts and **brushfield spots on iris.**
  - ❖ A characteristic facies with upslanting palpebral fissures or **mangoloid slant**, epicanthal folds, midface hypoplasia and small pinnae can be seen.
  - ❖ Limb abnormalities that can be seen are short and broad hands, hypoplasia and curving of 5th finger towards 4th i.e. **clinodactyly** and gap between great and first toe i.e. **sandal gap.**
  - ❖ Infections are more commonly seen in children with Down syndrome and specifically **pulmonary infections are a major cause of death.**
  - ❖ **Transient leukemia or myeloproliferative syndrome** can be seen with Down syndrome. ALL and AML both are seen; however **ALL is more common** as in case of general population.
  - ❖ Down syndrome can also be associated with disorders of CVS (ASD, **VSD**, PDA and TOF), GIT (**esophageal and duodenal atresias;** Hirsprung's disease and celiac disease), reproductive system (delayed sexual development and sterility), thyroid (Hashimoto thyroiditis, **hypothyroidism** and hyperthyroidism) and CNS (**MR and Alzheimer's disease**).

Mnemonic: Chinese**BATSMAN**
Chinese — Clinodactyly
B — Brushfield spots on iris, Brachycephaly
A — ALL>AML, Alzheimer's disease
T — Thyroid disorders, Transient myeloproliferative syndrome
S — Sandal gap, Simian crease, Septal defects (ASD, VSD)
M — Mental retardation, Mongolian slant
A — Atresia of duodenum and esophagus
N— No tone or hypotonia

- **Diagnosis:**
  - ❖ Prenatal diagnosis should be done and if positive, **abortion should be advised**. Diagnosis can be done by chromosomal analysis of amniocentesis or chorionic villous sample and USG, which shows **nuchal fold thickening, absent nasal bone**, short femur and other systemic congenital anomalies.
  - ❖ **Triple screening test** can also be done for diagnosis, which involves a **low maternal serum α fetoprotein** and **unconjugated estriol;** and **high HCG**. The other maternal markers for diagnosis of Down syndrome are an increased serum inhibin A and **decreased serum PAPPA** (pregnancy associated plasma proteins).

Patau Syndrome

- Patau syndrome or **trisomy 13** is more common in females.
- The babies present with failure to thrive, growth retardation, apnoeic spells, seizures,deafness and a characteristic facies with bulbous nose and low set malformed ears. Other abnormalities associated are **midline cleft lip, cleft palate, scalp defects, microcephaly, polydactyly** or syndactyly and hypoplastic or absent ribs.
- Disorders of CNS (holoprosencephaly and arrhinencephaly), CVS (VSD) and eye (**microopthalmia**, colobomas and hypertelorism) can be seen.

Edward Syndrome

- Edward syndrome or trisomy 18 is more common in females.
- The baby usually small for gestational age (SGA) and has **hypertonicity**. Micrognathia, microcephaly and prominent occiput can be associated.
- Disorders of CVS (VSD and PDA), CNS (microcephaly and MR) and kidney can be seen.
- Limb defects like overlapping of fingers and **rockerbottom feet;** and skeletal abnormalities like short sternum and narrow hips can be seen.

Sex Chromosome Disorders

The sex chromosome disorders that are commonly seen are Turner syndrome (45 XO) and Klinefelter syndrome (46 XXY).

Turner Syndrome

Turner syndrome is caused by **monosomy of sex chromosome i.e. an X chromosome is absent in females (45XO)**. 95% of foetuses are aborted in 2nd trimester with hydrops and cystic hygroma; and only 5% are born live.

- **Clinical presentation:**
  - ❖ The baby is born with low birth weight and decreased length. Later she can develop a **short stature**, low posterior hairline, **webbed neck**, rotated ears, **lymphedema of hands and feet**; and a triangular face.
  - ❖ The dysgenesis of gonads(**streak ovaries**) causes decreased female hormones and secondarily **amenorrhea**, infertility and lack of secondary sexual characteristics (**sexual infantilism**) are seen.
  - ❖ Skeletal abnormalities like **short fourth metacarpals** and metatarsals; **a shield chest with wide spaced nipples**, cubitus valgus, scoliosis and an **increased carrying angle at elbow** can be seen.
  - ❖ CVS defects that can be associated are **bicuspid aortic valve** in 50% cases and **coarctation of aorta** in 20% cases.

❖ Disorders of kidney (**horse shoe kidney**, ureteropelvic junction obstruction and single kidney), GIT (Inflammatory bowel disease and GIT bleeding due to mesenteric vascular malformation), thyroid (Hashimoto thyroiditis and hypothyroidism) and ear (recurrent otitis media in 75% cases and hearing loss) can be associated.

Mnemonic: **Short CABINS**
Short – Short 4th metacarpal and short stature
C — Coarctation of aorta
A — Amenorrhea
B — Bicuspid aortic valve
I — Increased carrying angle at elbow
N — Neck is webbed and nipples are wide
S — Sexual infantilism

- **Treatment :**
  ❖ Estrogen replacement is given for development of secondary sexual characteristics and normal menstruation.
  ❖ Growth hormone can be given for treatment of short stature.

Klinefelter Syndrome

Klinefelter syndrome is the most common sex chromosome abnormality caused by an extra X chromosome in the males (**47 XXY**). Both maternal and paternal X chromosomes are responsible equally i.e. 50% cases each and advanced age of parents is a contributing factor.

- **Clinical presentation:**
  ❖ The baby is born with a normal male phenotype and usually presents after puberty when signs of puberty do not appear.
  ❖ The male has a normal external genitalia but there is **microorchidism** and decreased testosterone level which results in **azoospermia and sterility**; decreased libido, **decreased facial and pubic hair**; and gynaecomastia.
  ❖ Unlike Turner syndrome, the male in Kleinfelter syndrome is **tall with long arms and legs**.
  ❖ A **normal to borderline IQ** can be seen and most patients complete schooling.
- **Treatment:** Testosterone replacement therapy is given for alleviation of symptoms seen due to its deficiency.

Chromosome Structure Disorders

The different structural abnormalities that can be seen in chromosome structure are deletion, microdeletion, duplication, inversion, ring chromosome, translocation and insertion.

Deletion

Deletion describes the absence of part of a normal chromosome. The common deletions that can be seen are of chromosomes 1p (1p36 deletion syndrome), 4p (Wolf-Hirschhon syndrome) and 5p (cri du chat syndrome).

Microdeletion

Microdeletion disorders, also called as contiguous gene disorders are characterised by small chromosome deletions. The common microdeletion that can be seen are of chromosome 7 (Williams's syndrome), 17(Miller-Dieker syndrome and Smith-Magenis syndrome) and 22 (Velocardiofacial syndrome).

- **William's syndrome:**
  ❖ William's syndrome is caused by microdeletion in chromosome 7 and since these are new deletions, parents are unaffected.
  ❖ The younger children usually have **mental retardation** and older children have an **outgoing "cocktail party" personality.**
  ❖ In infants a typical facies with periorbital fullness, broad nasal bridge, anteverted nares, long philtrum, open mouth, and full cheeks can be seen. Older children have an elongated face and thicker lips.
  ❖ The most common CVS defect seen is **supravalvular aortic stenosis.**
  ❖ Hypercalcemia is seen in most cases; however resolves spontaneously.

Duplication

Duplication refers to the presence of an extra copy of a segment of chromosome. The **duplication of chromosome 22q11** (chromosome no 22, band 11) results in partial trisomy of chromosome 22 at band 11 and causes **cat eye syndrome**.

Mosaicism

Mosaicism is characterised by presence of two or more different numbers or arrangements of chromosome in a same person. Example of Down syndrome with mosaicism is the presence of chromosomes with trisomy 21 (47 XX+21) along with normal chromosomes (46XX). The different disorders that can be seen because of mosaicism are Pallister-Killian syndrome and hypomelanosis of Ito. Mosaicism is a disorder is associated with milder symptoms and skin pigmentation. In place of lymphocytes, fibroblasts are used for cytogenetic studies in mosaics.

Uniparental Disomy

Homologous pair of chromosomes are derived from both the parents i.e. one from each. Uniparental disomy is a condition in which both pair of homologues chromosomes are derived from a single parent. The disorders which are associated with uniparental disomy are **Prader-Willi syndrome**, **Angelman syndrome**, Beckwith-Widemann syndrome and cystic fibrosis.

Chromosome Fragility

Chromosome fragility is caused by various DNA repair defects. The disorders associated are **Bloom syndrome**, **Fanconi syndrome** and **ataxia-telangiectasia.**

MENDELIAN DISORDERS

Mendelian disorders are based on the principles of segregation and independent assertion. The genes (alleles) are always in pairs; however each gamete receives only one gene (segregation). These genes in the gametes are paired independently during fertilisation (independent assertion). Depending on the phenotypic expression of the genes or alleles the Mendelian disorders can be either dominant or recessive.

Autosomal Dominant Disorders

AD disorders manifest in heterozygous state in which mutation of only one copy of gene is sufficient for disease. In this condition at least one parent is affected and both males and females are equally affected and transmit the disease. **When one of the parents is affected there is 50% chance of transmission. AD inheritance is responsible for the maximum number of Mendelian disorders**.

The various AD disorders are mostly related with structural abnormality of proteins. Diseases that can be transmitted by AD inheritance are **Huntington disease, neurofibromatosis, myotonic dystrophy, tuberous sclerosis, polycystic kidney disease**, AIP, familial hypercholesterolemia, **Marfan syndrome, Ehlers-Danlos syndrome**, osteogenesis imperfecta, achondroplasia, MODY(maturity onset diabetes of the young),** familial polyposis coli, **hereditary spherocytosis, von Willebrand disease, retinoblastoma**, CHARGE syndrome, Noonan syndrome, Cornelia de Lange syndrome and Treacher Collins syndrome.

Mnemonic: **DOMINANT FATHER**
D — Dystrophia myotonica
O — Osteogenesis imperfecta
M — Marfan syndrome, MODY
I — Intermittent porphyria
N — Noonan syndrome
A — Achondroplasia
N — Neurofibromatosis
T — Treacher-Collins syndrome
F — Familial polyposis coli and Familial hypercholesterolemia
A — Adhesion defect of platelet i.e. von Willebrand disease
T — Tuberous sclerosis
H — Huntington disease, Hereditary spherocytosis
E — Ehlers-Danlos syndrome
R — Retinoblastoma, Renal polycystic disease

Autosomal Recessive Disorders

AR disorders manifest only in homozygous state i.e. mutation of both the genes or alleles of the pair is a must for the manifestation of disease. Parents having trait (heterozygous i.e. one affected gene) do not manifest, but there is **25%** chances of disease in the siblings. AR disorders are frequently associated with enzyme deficiency (metabolic disorders). The different disorders having AR transmission are **hemochromatosis, Wilson disease (hepatolenticular degeneration)**, lysosomal storage disease, α_1 antitrypsin deficiency, glycogen storage diseases, **homocystinuria**, galactosemia, **phenylketonuria, sickle cell anemia**, thalassemia, CAH, alkaptonuria, **Fredrich's ataxia**, spinal muscular atrophy, **cystic fibrosis, albinism** and Smith-Lemeli-Opitz syndrome.

Mnemonic: **RECESSING HALF**
R—Rotor syndrome
E—Enzyme deficiency disease like Phenylketonuria
C—CAH, Cystic fibrosis
E—Endocardial fibroelastosis
S—Sickle cell anaemia
S—Spinal muscular atrophy
I—Iron storage disease (hemochromatosis)
N—Niemann Pick disease
G—Galactosemia
H—Homocystinuria, Hepatolenticular degeneration
A—Alkaptonuria, Albinism
L—Lysosomal storage disease
F—Fredrich's ataxia

X Linked Disorders

Sex chromosome disorders are usually of X chromosome and not Y, because mutation of genes on Y chromosome leads to abnormality in spermatogenesis and hence males are infertile. X linked recessive disorders are more common than X linked dominant ones.

X Linked Recessive Disorders

X linked recessive disorders are characterised by mutation of gene or allele on X chromosome. Normally the Y chromosome does not have the second gene of the pair because it is not homologous to X. Hence **males are affected (xY) and all daughters are carriers (xX) but none of the sons are affected (XY)**. On the other hand the second gene is present in the homologous X chromosome in females. Hence **heterozygous females are carrier or mildly affected and have 50% chance that each daughter will be carrier and 50% chance that each son will be affected**.

The disorders which are transmitted by X linked recessive inheritance are **fragile X syndrome, Duchenne muscular dystrophy, G6PD deficiency**, agammaglobulinemia, Wiskott-Aldrich syndrome, **haemophilia**, chronic granulomatous disease, diabetes insipidus, Lesch-Nyhan syndrome, congenital aqueductal stenosis, ocular albinism, **colour blindness**, complete androgen insensitivity, **kinky hair syndrome (Menkes disease), Fabry disease** and adrenoleucodystrophy.

Mnemonic: **X LINKED Fabulous WOMAN**
X—Fragile X syndrome
L—Lesch-Nyhan syndrome
I—Insensitivity to androgen (complete)
N—Nephrogenic diabetes insipidus
K—Kinky hair syndrome
E—hEmophilia
D—Deficiency of G6PD
Fabulous—Fabry disease
W—Wiskott-Aldrich syndrome
O—Ocular albinism
M—Muscle dystrophy (Duchenne and Becker)
A—Agammaglobulinemia, Adrenoleucodystrophy
N—Non communicating hydrocephalus due to congenital aqueductal stenosis

X Linked Dominant Disorders

In X linked dominant disorders both males and females can be affected. Male can transfer the disease to all daughters but no son is affected. Heterozygous female can transfer the disease to 50% of her children i.e. both son and daughters. The disorders associated with X linked dominant inheritance are incontinentia pigmenti, **vitamin D resistant rickets (hypophosphatemic)**, focal dermal hypoplasia and orofaciodigital syndrome.

NON MENDELIAN DISORDERS

Non Mendelian disorders can be seen because of abnormality in genomic imprinting, genetic anticipation and mitochondrial DNA.

Genomic Imprinting Disorders

Normally genes are inherited in pairs i.e. one from the maternal and another from paternal chromosomes. Inactivation of these genes in ovum or sperm before fertilization by methylation or acetylation is called as **genomic imprinting**. The **expression of the gene inactivation strictly depends on the parent of origin e.g. inactivation of 15q11 in ovum causes Angelman syndrome whereas in sperm causes Prader-Willi syndrome**. Disorders of imprinting can also be seen because of **uniparental disomy** when both the genes are inherited from one parent. The disorders that can be seen because of imprinting are **Prader-Willi syndrome**, **Angelman syndrome** and **Beckwith-Wiedmann syndrome**.

Prader-Willi Syndrome

- Prader willi syndrome is caused most commonly by **genomic imprinting** i.e. inactivation of **paternal gene of 15q11** chromosome. The least common cause is **maternal disomy** i.e. if both the genes of 15q11 chromosome are derived from the mother.
- The baby is born with hypotonia and a characteristic facies i.e. almond-shaped eyes and strabismus. **Growth hormone deficiency** can lead to short stature, obesity, hypogenitalism, small hands and feet.
- There is compensatory **increase in Ghrelin levels** due to decrease in GH. Ghrelin is secreted by the stomach>arcuate nucleus of hypothalamus, which stimulates growth hormone releasing hormone (GHRH) receptor in the somatotroph cells of pituitary and increases GH release.
- Hypogonadotrophic hypogonadism, due to impaired GnRH secretion can be seen which is associated with **decreased LH and FSH release**.
- Obsessive hyperphagia and DM can be commonly seen

Angelman Syndrome

- Angelman syndrome is most commonly caused by genomic imprinting i.e. inactivation of the **maternal gene of 15q11** chromosome. **Paternal disomy** is the least common cause, in which both the genes of 15q11 chromosome are derived from father (**paternal disomy**).
- It is associated with severe mental retardation, prognathism, seizures, developmental delay, puppet gait and paroxysmal laughter (happy puppets) and tongue thrusting.
- Hypogonadotrophic hypogonadism, due to impaired GnRH secretion can be seen, which is associated with **decreased LH and FSH release**.

Beckwith-Wiedemann Syndrome

Beckwith-Wiedemann syndrome can be caused if the maternal gene for IGF2 in 11p15 chromosome is inactivated (maternal imprinting) or if both the genes for IGF2 in 11p15 chromosome are derived from father (paternal uniparental disomy). It is associated with macrosomia, macroglossia, omphalocele, hypertelorism, hypoglycemia caused by hyperinsulinemia, cleft palate and Wilms tumor.

Genetic Anticipation Disorders

Genetic anticipation is characterised by **worsening and early presentation of symptoms in the subsequent generations**. It is usually associated with trinucleotide repeats and the symptoms worsen due to increase in the number of repeats with each generation. For example in **myotonic dystrophy which is caused by CTG trinucleotide repeat**, a person with

35-49 repeats is asymptomatic. However because of anticipation there can be increase in CTG repeats in the siblings and they can manifest the disease. Disorders associated with anticipation are spinal cerebellar atrophy, Hutington disease, myotonic dystrophy, Fredrich's ataxia and fragile X syndrome.

Mitochondrial Inheritance Disorders

Mitochondrial DNA is found in the cytoplasm and since after fertilization only oocyte cytoplasm is retained, mitochondrial disorders are **maternally inherited**. Both normal and abnormal mitochondrial DNA is present in the cytoplasm and the amount of the later decides the severity of disorder. Since mitochondria is required for ATP generation, mitochondrial disorders primarily affect the **CNS** (hypotonia, developmental delay, convulsions) and **skeletal muscles** (myopathy), which are highest consumer of ATP.

MULTIFACTORIAL OR POLYGENIC INHERITANCE DISORDERS

Polygenic disorders are characterised by multiple contributing factors like multiple gene mutations and environmental factors. The different polygenic disorders are hypertension, stroke, thrombophlebitis, alcoholism, neural tube defect, cleft lip and palate; and Hirschsprung disease.

MULTIPLE CHOICE QUESTIONS

1. **Maternal disomy of chromosome 15 is seen in:**
   [AIIMS Nov. 10]
   a. Prader-Willi syndrome
   b. Klinefelter syndrome
   c. Angelman syndrome
   d. Turner's syndrome

2. **Turner syndrome is maximally associated with:**
   [AIIMS May 08]
   a. Horseshoe kidney
   b. Coarctation of aorta
   c. VSD
   d. ASD

3. **A baby presenting with multiple deformities, cleft lip, cleft palate, microcephaly, small eyes, scalp defect and polydactyly, seen in which syndrome:**
   [AIIMS Nov. 06, May 08]
   a. Trisomy 13   b. Trisomy 18
   c. Trisomy 21   d. Monosomy 2

4. **Single gene defect causing multiple unrelated problems:**   [AIIMS Nov. 06]
   a. Pleotropism   b. Pseudo dominance
   c. Penetrance   d. Anticipation

5. **Which of the following is an example of disorders of sex chromosomes?**   [AIIMS May 06]
   a. Marfan's syndrome
   b. Testicular feminization syndrome
   c. Klinefelter syndrome
   d. Down syndrome

6. **Which of the following diseases is an autosomal dominant disorder:**   [AIIMS May 2005]
   a. Hemochromatosis
   b. Phenylketonuria
   c. Maturity onset diabetes of the young
   d. G6PD deficiency

7. **The chances of having an unaffected baby, when both parents have achondroplasia, are:**
   [AI 05, AIIMS May 04]
   a. 0%   b. 25%
   c. 50%   d. 100%

8. **The following statements regarding Turner syndrome are true except:**   [AIIMS May 2003]
   a. Occurrence of Turner syndrome is influenced by maternal age
   b. Most patients have primary amenorrhea
   c. Most patients have short stature
   d. Edema of feet and hand is an important feature during infancy

9. **Common ocular manifestation in trisomy 13 is:**
   [AIIMS 03]
   a. Capillary hemangioma
   b. Bilateral micropthalmos
   c. Neurofibroma
   d. Dermoid cyst

10. **Triple test for diagnosis of Down syndrome includes all of the following except:**
    [AI 99, AIIMS 03]
    a. β-hCG
    b. α-Fetoprotein
    c. Serum HPL level
    d. Serum estriol level

11. **In turner syndrome which of the following is not seen:**   [AIIMS June 2000]
    a. Short stature   b. Widely spaced nipple
    c. Webbed neck   d. Mental retardation

12. **Commonest cause of intestinal obstruction in Down syndrome is:**   [AIIMS June 2000]
    a. Colonic atresia   b. Intestinal atresia
    c. Duodenal atresia   d. Oesophageal atresia

13. A 35 years old lady has chromosomal translocation 21/21. The risk of Down syndrome in the child is: [AIIMS June 99]
    a. 100%   b. 0%
    c. 10%   d. 50%

14. Which one of the following is an autosomal dominant disorder?   [AIIMS 96]
    a. Duchenne's muscular dystrophy
    b. Fragile X syndrome
    c. Fanconi anemia
    d. Hutingtons chorea

15. Most common chromosomal syndrome is: [AIIMS Dec. 94]
    a. Fragile X syndrome   b. Trisomy 17
    c. Trisomy 21   d. Trisomy 13

16. A parent is homozygous and a parent heterozygous for an autosomal recessive gene. What will be the outcome?   [AIIMS May 94]
    a. 75% children affected
    b. No child affected, but all are carriers
    c. 50% children affected, rest are carriers
    d. 25% children affected, rest are carriers

17. All are true about XO chromosomal pattern except: [AIIMS 94]
    a. All are hermaphrodites
    b. Gonadal dysgenesis
    c. Webbed neck
    d. Mental retardation

18. Which condition is autosomal dominant?   [AIIMS Nov. 93]
    a. Hemophilia A
    b. Duchenne muscular dystrophy
    c. Wilson's disease
    d. Adult polycystic kidney disease

19. All are common in Down syndrome, except: [AIIMS May 93]
    a. Simian crease
    b. Clinodactyly
    c. Mother's age> 35 years
    d. Respiratory tract infections uncommon

20. Down's syndrome most commonly occurs due to?   [AI 2010]
    a. Reciprocal translocation
    b. Nondisjunction in maternal meiosis
    c. Translocation defect
    d. Nondisjunction in paternal meiosis

21. A Down syndrome patient is posted for surgery, the necessary preoperative investigation to be done is: [AI 08]
    a. Echocardiography   b. CT brain
    c. X-ray cervical spine d. USG abdomen

22. All of the following conditions have autosomal dominant inheritance except: [AI 07]
    a. Fabry disease
    b. Marfan's syndrome
    c. Osteogenesis imperfecta
    d. Ehlers Danlos syndrome

23. In an Autosomal Recessive (AR) disorder, one parent is normal and the other is carrier and the child is also affected. What is the reason?   [AI 07]
    a. Germ line mosaicism   b. Genomic imprinting
    c. Penetration   d. Uniparental disomy

24. Cat eye syndrome is: [AI 07]
    a. Partial trisomy 18   b. Partial trisomy 13
    c. Partial trisomy 21   d. Partial trisomy 22

25. A child with a small head, minor anomalies of the face including a thin upper lip, growth delay, and developmental disability can have all of the following, except: [AI 06]
    a. A chromosomal syndrome
    b. A teratogenic syndrome
    c. A mendelian syndrome
    d. A polygenic syndrome

26. An affected male infant born to normal parents could be an example of all of the following, except: [AI 06]
    a. An Autosomal dominant disorder
    b. An Autosomal recessive disorder
    c. A polygenic disorder
    d. A vertically transmitted disorder

27. In family, the father has widely spaced eyes, increased facial hair and deafness. One of the three children has deafness with similar facial features. The mother is normal. Which one of the following is least likely pattern of inheritance in this case?   [AI 06]
    a. Autosomal dominant   b. Autosomal recessive
    c. X-linked dominant   d. X-linked recessive

28. All of the following may occur in Down's syndrome except: [AI 06]
    a. Hypothyroidism
    b. Undescended testis
    c. Ventricular septal defect
    d. Brushfield's spots

29. Differential expression of same gene depending on parent of origin is referred to as: [AI 05, 06]
    a. Genomic imprinting   b. Mosaicism
    c. Anticipation   d. Nonpenetrance

30. The chances of having an unaffected baby, when both parents have achondroplasia, are: [AI 05, AIIMS May 04]
    a. 0%   b. 25%
    c. 50%   d. 100%

31. All of the following are features of Down syndrome except: [AI 05]
    a. Increased PAPPA
    b. Increased free beta HCG levels

c. Absent nasal bone

d. Abnormal ductus venous flow velocity

32. **Kinky hair disease is disorder where an affected child has peculiar white stubby hair, does not grow, brain degeneration is seen and dies by age of two years. Mrs A is hesitant about having children because her two sisters had sons who had died from kinky hair disease. Her mother's brother also died of the same condition. Which of the following is the possible mode of inheritance in her family:** [AI 04]
   a. X-linked recessive
   b. X-linked dominant
   c. Autosomal recessive
   d. Autosomal dominant

33. **Webbing of neck, increased carrying angle, low posterior hairline and short fourth metacarpal are characteristics of:** [AI 04]
   a. Klinefelter syndrome
   b. Turner syndrome
   c. Cri du chat syndrome
   d. Noonan syndrome

34. **Males who are sexually underdeveloped with rudimentary testes and prostate glands, sparse pubic and facial hairs, long arms and legs and large hands and feet are likely to have the chromosome complement of:** [AI 04]
   a. 45XXY
   b. 46XY
   c. 46XXY
   d. 46X

35. **A nineteen year old female with short stature, wide spread nipples and primary amenorrhea most likely has karyotype of:** [AI 03]
   a. 47 XX+ 18
   b. 46XXY
   c. 47XXY
   d. 45XO

36. **An albino girl gets married to a normal boy, What are the chances of their having an affected child and what are the chances of their children being carriers?** [AI 03]
   a. None affected, all carriers
   b. All normal
   c. 50% carriers
   d. 50% affected, 50% carriers

37. **Transient myeloproliferative disorder of the newborn is seen in association with:** [AI 03]
   a. Turner syndrome
   b. Down's syndrome
   c. Neurofibromatosis
   d. Ataxia telangiectasia

38. **Which of the following is an autosomal dominant disorder?** [AI 02]
   a. Cystic fibrosis
   b. Hereditary sp herocytosis
   c. Sickle cell anaemia
   d. G6PD deficiency

39. **Which of the following is autosomal dominant?** [AI 2000]
   a. Retinoblastoma
   b. Ataxia telangiectasia
   c. Bloom's syndrome
   d. Xeroderma pigmentosa

40. **Most common group of diseases following mendelian inheritance are:** [AI 99]
   a. Autosomal dominant
   b. Autosomal recessive

c. X-linked dominant

d. X-linked recessive

41. **Fragile X-syndrome is characterized by all of the following features except:** [AI 99]
   a. Long face
   b. Large ear
   c. Large-nose
   d. Large-testis

42. **Triple test for diagnosis of Down's syndrome includes all of the following except:** [AI 99, AIIMS 03]
   a. β-HCG
   b. α-Fetoprotein
   c. Serum HPL level
   d. Serum estriol level

43. **Increased nuchal fold thickness is a feature of:** [AI 99]
   a. Paul-Bunnel syndrome
   b. De-Pan syndrome
   c. Down's syndrome
   d. Cri du chat syndrome

44. **Which one of the following is autosomal recessive?** [AI 98]
   a. Homocystinuria
   b. G6PD deficiency
   c. Myotonic dystrophy
   d. Otospongiosis

45. **All of the following are X linked except:** [AI 98]
   a. G6PD deficiency
   b. Hemophilia A
   c. Von-Willebrands disease
   d. Fragile X syndrome

46. **True in Klinefelter's syndrome:** [AI 98]
   a. Short stature
   b. Pituitary adenoma
   c. Subnormal intelligence
   d. Breast adenoma

47. **All of the following are features of Down's syndrome except:** [AI 94]
   a. Brushfield's spots in iris
   b. Simian crease
   c. Mental retardation
   d. Hypertonicity

48. **For a normal husband and wife the first child was diagnosed to have cystic fibrosis. What is the percentage of chances for the second child be affected:** [PGI June 06]
   a. 25
   b. 50
   c. 0
   d. 75
   e. 100

49. **In Down syndrome:** [PGI 06]
   a. Sandal gap
   b. Antimongolian slant
   c. Clinodactyly
   d. Hypotonia

50. **A patient with short stature, sexual infantilism and congenital anomalies with chromosomal abnormalities 'XO'. Diagnosis is:** [PGI June 04]
   a. Turner's syndrome
   b. Klinefelter syndrome
   c. Testicular feminization syndrome
   d. Gonadal agenesis
   e. Gonadal dysgenesis

51. True about Down syndrome are all except:

[PGI June 04]

a. Predisposed to acute leukemias

b. Associated with congenital heart diseases

c. Increased risk of CNS tumors

d. Early onset of Alzheimer's disease

e. Increased risk of infections

52. Infant with Down syndrome have all except:

[PGI June 03]

a. VSD   b. Duodenal atresia

c. Leukemia   d. Normal intelligence

e. Delayed skeletal maturation

53. Down syndrome is associated with: [PGI Dec. 02]

a. Congenital heart disease

b. ALL

c. Early onset Alzheimer's disease

d. CNS tumors

e. Infection

54. True about Turner syndrome: [PGI June 02]

a. Primary amenorrhea   b. 45 XO

c. Short stature patient   d. Puberty usually late

e. Streak ovaries

55. Klinefelter's syndrome is associated with:

[PGI June 02]

a. XXY genotype   b. Male habitus

c. Infertility   d. Azoospermia

e. Barr body absent

56. Mutation leading to sickle cell anemia:

[PGI June 01[

a. Crossover mutation   b. Frameshift

c. Deletion   d. Nondisjunction

e. Point mutation

57. Single gene autosomal recessive disease is:

[PGI June 99]

a. Wilson's disease   b. Tuberous sclerosis

c. Hutington's disease   d. Schizophrenia

58. Atavism means child resembles with his:

a. Father   b. Siblings

c. Grandparents   d. Neighbour

QUESTIONS OF OTHER EXAMINATIONS

1. Which of the following is a distinguishing feature of Edward's syndrome?   [UPSC 07]

a. Hypotonia   b. Hypertelorism

c. Holoprosencephaly   d. Rocker bottom feet

2. The following are autosomal dominant disorders except: [COMED 07]

a. Myotonic dystrophy   b. Von Willebrand disease

c. Hemochromatosis   d. Marfan's syndrome

3. Which of the following is autosomal dominant type of genetic disorder?   [UPSC 07]

a. Colour blindness   b. Haemophilia

c. Phenylketonuria   d. Tuberous sclerosis

4. The chromosomal disorder in Patau syndrome is:

[UP 07]

a. Chromosome 21   b. Chromosome 18

c. Chromosome 13   d. Chromosome 45x/46xx

5. Which one of the following is not true about Noonan syndrome?   [COMED 06]

a. Affects males and females

b. Short stature

c. Chromosomal abnormality

d. Congenital heart disease-ASD

6. Down syndrome predisposes to......... cancer:

[MAHE 05]

a. AML   b. CML

c. ALL   d. CLL

7. In Down syndrome the shape of the head is:

[MAHE 05]

a. Oxycephalic   b. Scapocephalic

c. Brachicephalic   d. Plagiocephalic

8. Which one of the following neurological conditions is not inherited in autosomal dominant pattern?

[UPSC 05]

a. Neurofibromatosis   b. Fredrich's ataxia

c. Marfan's syndrome

9. A 4-year-old baby is having large face, large jaw, large ear and microorchidism is: [AMU 05]

a. Mccune Albright syndrome

b. Down syndrome

c. Cri du chat syndrome

d. Fragile X syndrome

10. All of the following are chromosomal breakage syndromes except: [Karnataka 04]

a. Fanconi's anaemia   b. Ehler-Danlos syndrome

c. Bloom syndrome   d. Ataxia teleangectasia

11. Which is X linked dominant condition?

[Manipal 04]

a. Phosphate diabetes   b. Hemophilia

c. Gaucher disease   d. Cystic fibrosis

12. Glucose-6-phosphayte dehydrogenase deficiency is: [UPSC 95]

a. Autosomal recessive   b. Autosomal dominant

c. Sex-linked recessive   d. Sex-linked dominant

ANSWERS

MULTIPLE CHOICE QUESTIONS

1. (a) Prader-Willi syndrome (Ref: CPDT 19th E/P995)
Prader willi syndrome can be caused by 2 process:
- **Genomic imprinting** — If the **paternal gene of 15q11** chromosome is inactivated.
- **Maternal disomy** — If both the genes of 15q11 chromosome are derived from the mother.

2. (b) Coarctation of aorta (Ref: Rudolph 22nd E/P696)
- Bicuspid aortic valve is seen in 50% and coarctation of aorta is seen in 50% of patients of Turner syndrome.

3. (a) Trisomy 13 (Ref: Nelson 19th E/P384)
Kindly refer text for details on Trisomy 13 or Patau syndrome.

4. (a) Pleotropism (Ref:The genetic basis of common diseases P7)
- **Pleotropism** is a feature of Mendelian disorders when a **single gene defect can lead to multiple effects.**
- Example is Marfan syndrome where a single gene mutation causes disorders of multiple organs.

5. (c) Klinefelter's syndrome (Ref: CPDT 19th E/P1002)
- Sex chromosome disorders are **Turner syndrome** and **Klinefelter syndrome.**

6. (c) Maturity onset diabetes of the young (Robins 8th E/P181)

7. (b) 25% (Ref: Robins 7th E/P171)
- Achondroplasia is an autosomal dominant disorder.
- If both the parents are affected i.e. Aa and Aa; then the children will be AA, Aa, Aa and aa. Hence as you can see the chances of having an affected baby is 75% (AA, Aa and Aa) and unaffected is 25% (aa).

8. (a) Occurrence of Turner syndrome is influenced by maternal age (Ref: CPDT 19th E/P1002)
- Maternal age is a risk factor in Down syndrome and both maternal and paternal age are risk factor in Klinefelter syndrome.
- Turner syndrome is not associated with increased maternal age.

9. (b) Bilateral micropthalmos (Ref: Nelson 19th E/P384)
- Ocular manifestations seen in trisomy 13 are **micro-opthalmia**, colobomas (hole or defect on the iris) and hypertelorism.

10. (c) Serum HPL level (Ref: Nelson 19th E/P386)

11. (d) Mental retardation (Ref: Nelson 19th E/P1933)
- Short stature, wide spaced nipple and webbed neck are typically and commonly seen in Turner syndrome.

- Mental retardation is not typical of Turner syndrome as it is rarely seen if the patient is having 2 sets of chromosome i.e. 46X, rX (ring chromosome) along with the 45X.

12. (c) Duodenal atresia (Ref: Rudolph 22nd E/P692)

"Obstructive gastrointestinal lesions including **duodenal atresia** and Hirschsprung disease occur in about 5% of infants with Down syndrome."

13. (a) 100% (Ref: Nair's The high risk newborn/P350)
Recurrence risk of Down syndrome in translocations:

Translocation type	Risk in percentage
De novo inherited	1%
t(13, 21), t(21, 22) in a case of normal father and carrier mother	10–15%
t(13, 21), t(21, 22) in a case of carrier father and normal mother	5%
t(21, 21)	**100%**

14. (a) Hutingtons chorea (Ref: Robins 7th E/P171)

15. (c) Down syndrome (Ref: Rudolph 22nd E/P692)

"**Down syndrome** is caused by trisomy 21 and is the **most common autosomal chromosome abnormality** in humans."

16. (c) 50% (Ref: CPDT 19th E/P991)
- In autosomal recessive mode of inheritance both the genes should be defective for manifestation of disease.
- In this case one parent is homozygous (affected) i.e. both gene are defective (AA) and one is heterozygous (carrier) i.e. only 1 gene is defective (Aa).
- Hence the outcome will be **50% carriers i.e. Aa,Aa and 50% affected i.e. AA and AA.**

17. (a) All are hermaphrodites (Ref: CPDT 19th E/P1002)
- XO chromosomal pattern is seen in Turner syndrome.
- Gonadal dysgenesis and webbed neck can be seen with Turner syndrome.
- Mental retardation is usually not seen but can be associated in a mosaic variant when another set of chromosome are present i.e. 45XO and 46X, rX (ring chromosome).

18. (d) Adult polycystic kidney disease(Ref: Robbins 8th E/P141)

19. (d) Respiratory tract infections uncommon(Ref: Rudolph 22nd E/P692)
- Simian crease and clinodactyly are features of Down syndrome.

- Mother's age of more than 35 years is a risk factor for Down syndrome.
- Respiratory tract infections are common in Down syndrome and in fact are a leading cause of mortality.

20. (b) Nondisjunction in maternal meiosis (Ref: Nelson 19th E/P384)

Etiology of trisomies:
- Normally oocytes are held in midprophase of meiosis 1 from birth till ovulation.
- Aging results in breakdown of chiasmata that keeps paired chromosome aligned.
- Now during ovulation nondisjunction occurs which results in trisomies.

21. (a) Echocardiography (Ref: Nelson 19th E/P384)
- Down syndrome is associated with congenital heart defects like ASD, VSD, PDA and TOF. Hence echo-cardiography should be done prior to surgery to rule out these defects.

22. (a) Fabry disease (Ref: Robins 7th E/P151)
- Fabry disease has a X linked recessive pattern of inheritance.
- Autosomal dominant disorders are associated with abnormal protein formation as in the case of Marfan's syndrome (fibrillin 1), osteogenesis imperfecta (type 1 collagen) and Ehlers Danlos syndrome (collagen).

23. (d) Uniparental disomy (Ref: CPDT 19th E/P986)
- Uniparental disomy is a condition in which the offspring gets both copies of a chromosome from one parent.
- It can be seen in AR disease cystic fibrosis, when one parent is a carrier and other is normal.

24. (d) Partial trisomy 22 (Ref: Nelson essentials of paediatrics)
- Cat eye syndrome is caused by interstitial duplication of chromosome 22q11.
- Colobomas of iris gives typical appearance to the eye and hence the name cat eye syndrome.
- Other features of cat eye syndrome are:
  ❖ Mild mental retardation
  ❖ Behavioural abnormalities
  ❖ Ocular hypertelorism
  ❖ Downward slanting palpebral fissures
  ❖ Micrognathia
  ❖ Auricular pits/tags
  ❖ Anal atresia with rectovestibular fistula
  ❖ Renal agenesis
  ❖ Colobomas of iris.

25. (d) A polygenic syndrome (Ref: CPDT 19th E/P 993-94)
- **Polygenic disorders** are characterised by multiple contributing factors like multiple gene mutations and environmental factors.

- The different polygenic disorders are hypertension, stroke, thrombophlebitis, alcoholism, neural tube defect, cleft lip and palate; and Hirschsprung disease.

26. (a) An autosomal dominant disorder (Ref: CPDT 19th E/P990)

Autosomal dominant inheritance:
- Dominant inheritance is characterised by vertical transmission i.e. the disease passes from one generation to next in a vertical manner. Hence in AD transmission one of the parents is affected and transfers the disease to offsprings.
- AD inheritance can be differentiated from X linked dominant inheritance by the fact that the later does not have any male to male transmission.

27. (d) X linked recessive (Ref: CPDT 19th E/P992)
- First of all let us collect the facts in the question:
  1. Male is affected and has transmitted the disease to offspring
  2. Female is unaffected
- Now let us analyse the different modes of transmission by using the facts mentioned above
  1. **AD** — In this mode any parent can transfer the disease (father in this case) and if 1 parent is affected then 50% of offsprings will be affected i.e. 2 out of 4. Here they have 3 children out of which 1 is affected. There is a possibility that the 4th might get affected. So AD transmission is a possibility.
  2. **AR** — In this mode of inheritance though parents are carrier and usually normal, some may manifest the disease. The chance of the transmission is 25% i.e. 1 in 4 children will be affected. Hence this is also a possibility.
  3. **X linked recessive** – In this mode if male is affected (as in this case) then all daughters are carrier and none of his sons are affected. In this case one child has manifested the disease. Hence X linked recessive mode of inheritance is least likely.
  4. **X linked dominant** — In this mode if male is affected then all daughters and no son is affected. Hence this is also a possibility.

28. (b) Undescended testis (Ref: Nelson 19th E/P384)
- Thyroid disorders, VSD and brushfield spots on iris can be seen in Down syndrome.
- Delayed sexual development and sterility can be seen in males; however undescended testis is not associated.

29. (a) Genomic imprinting (Ref: CPDT 19th E/P995)

"The term imprinting refers to the process by which preferential **transcription of certain genes** takes place, **depending on the parental origin**, that is, which homolog (maternal or paternal) the gene is located on."

30. (b) 25% (Ref: Robins 7th E/P171)
- Achondroplasia is an autosomal dominant disorder.
- If both the parents are affected i.e. Aa and Aa; then the children will be AA, Aa, Aa and aa. Hence as you can see the chances of having an affected baby is 75% (AA, Aa and Aa) and unaffected is 25% (aa).
- **Now the chances for each baby to beaffected is25% (AA)**, carrier is 50% (Aa, Aa) and normal is 25% (aa).

31. (a) Increased PAPPA (Ref: Ghai 7th E/P614)
Kindly refer text for details on diagnosis of Down syndrome.

32. (a) X-linked recessive (Ref: CPDT 19th E/P992)
- Kinky hair disease has AR pattern of inheritance.
- Now if the disease name is not given, still answer can be derived. The pattern given in question states that only males are affected (sons of his sisters and brother of his mother).
- In the text it has been mentioned that in X-linked recessive pattern of inheritance only males are affected but females are normal because of the presence of a normal X chromosome (Xx).
- Hence by that way also the answer is X-linked recessive inheritance.

33. (b) Turner syndrome (Ref: CPDT 19th E/P2012)
Kindly refer text for details on presentation of Turner syndrome.

34. (c) 46 XXY (Ref: CPDT 19th E/P1002)
This is clearly a case of Klinefelter syndrome:
- The male has a normal external genitalia but there is **microorchidism** and decreased testosterone level which results in **azoospermia and sterility**; decreased libido, **decreased facial and pubic hair**; and gynaecomastia.
- Unlike Turner syndrome, the male in Kleinfelter syndrome is **tall with long arms and legs**.
- Klinefelter syndrome is caused by the presence of an extra X chromosome in males i.e. **46XXY**.

35. (d) 45 XO (Ref: CPDT 19th E/P2012)
- Short stature, widespread nipples and amenorrhea are seen in Turner syndrome.
- Turner syndrome is caused by absence of an X chromosome in females and gives the typical genotype i.e. 45 XO.

36. (a) Non affected, all carriers (Ref: CPDT 19th E/P991)
- Albinism has AR pattern of inheritance. In the given case female is affected (AA) and male is normal (aa).
- Hence the outcome will be aA, aA, aA and aA. So as you can see **all of the offsprings are homozygous and will be carrier.**

37. (b) Down syndrome (Ref: Nelson 19th E/P1697)

Down syndrome and leukemia:
- Acute leukemia is 14 times more seen in patients with Down syndrome. ALL is more commonly seen than AML.
- Transient leukemia or myeloproliferative syndrome can also be seen, which is characterised by anemia, thrombocytopenia, leucocytosis, blasts in peripheral circulation and hepatosplenomegaly.

38. (b) Hereditary spherocytosis (Ref: Robins 8th E/P141)
39. (a) Retinoblastoma (Ref: Robins 8th E/P141)
40. (a) Autosomal dominant (Ref: Robins 7th E/P171)
41. (c) Large nose (Ref: CPDT 19th E/P1010)
Fragile X syndrome:
- Fragile sites are present on the chromosomes which tend to break. Fragile X syndrome, an X linked recessive disorder is caused by mutation of the FMR1 gene, which results in CGG trinucleotide repeat.
- This is the most common inherited cause of MR in males.
- The babies are born with **long face, large ears, prominent jaws and large testicles (microorchidism).**

42. (c) Serum HPL level (Ref: Nelson 19th E/P386)
Triple test for diagnosis of Down syndrome:
- Decreased α-Fetoprotein
- Decreased **serum oestriol level**
- Increased β-HCG.

43. (c) Down syndrome (Ref: Nelson 19th E/P395)
- Prenatal USG finding in Down syndrome is **increased nuchal fold thickness**, absent nasal bone and a short femur.

44. (a) Homocystinuria (Ref: Robins 7th E/P171)
- Usually enzyme deficiency disorders like homocystinuria have AR inheritance.

45. (c) von Willebrands disease (Ref: Robins 7th E/P171)
46. (c) Subnormal intelligence (Ref: CPDT 19th E/P1002)
- Short stature is seen in Turner syndrome but patient of Klinefelter syndrome is typically tall with long arms and legs.
- **IQ** in patients of Klinefelter syndrome varies from **normal to borderline (subnormal)**.
- Gynaecomastia can be seen but breast adenoma is not seen.

47. (d) Hypertonicity (Ref: Nelson 19th E/P384)
- Brushfield spot on iris, simian crease and mental retardation are seen in Down syndrome.
- Hypertonicity is not seen in Down syndrome; rather hypotonicity is seen.

48. (a) 25% (Ref: CPDT 19th E/P 991)
- Cystic fibrosis has autosomal recessive inheritance. In AR inheritance for manifestation both the genes should be mutated i.e. homozygous (AA).
- As normally seen with AR inheritance, here also parents are normal i.e. they are carrier or heterozygous (Aa and Aa).

49. **(a)**, **(c)** and **(d)** Sandal gap, Clinodactyly and Hypotonia (Ref: Nelson 19th E/P384)

    Kindly refer text for details on presentation of Down syndrome.

50. **(a)** Turner's syndrome (Ref: CPDT 19th E/P1002)
    - Turner syndrome is caused by absence of an X chromosome in a female and gives the typical genotype i.e. 45XO.

51. **(c)** CNS tumors (Ref: CPDT 19th E/P1001)

    Kindly refer text for details on presentation of Down syndrome.

52. **(d)** and **(e)** Normal intelligence and Delayed skeletal maturation (Ref: Nelson 19th E/P384)

    Kindly refer text for details on presentation of Down syndrome.

53. **(a)**, **(b)**, **(c)** and **(e)** Congenital heart disease, ALL, Early onset Alzheimer's disease and Infection (Ref: CPDT 19th E/P1001)
    - Congenital heart diseases, leukemias (ALL>AML), Alzheimer's disease are well associated with Down syndrome.

- Infections are commonly seen in patients of Down syndrome and specifically pulmonary infection is a major cause of mortality.

54. All (Ref: CPDT 19th E/P1002)
    - Turner syndrome is caused by absence of an X chromosome in females and gives the typical genotype i.e. 45XO.
    - Ovaries are atrophied (streak ovary) and female hormones are not produced which results in amenorrhea and delayed puberty.
    - Short stature is typically seen in Turner syndrome.

55. **(a)**, **(b)**, **(c)** and **(d)** XXY genotype, Male habitus, Infertility and Azoospermia (Ref: CPDT 19th E/P1002)
    - In Klinefelter syndrome the patient is a **male** with an extra X chromosome i.e. **46 XXY genotype**.
    - **Infertility** and **azoospermia** can be seen as testosterone level is decreased in Klinefelter syndrome because of testicular atrophy.

56. **(e)** Point mutation (Robins 8th E/P647)

57. **(a)** Wilson's disease (Ref: Robbins 8th E/P142)

58. **(c)** Grandparents (Ref: Redei Genetics P84)
    - Atavism is the recurrence of expression of traits of ancestors beyond grandparents.

QUESTIONS OF OTHER EXAMINATIONS

1. **(d)** Rocker bottom feet (Ref: CPDT 19th E/1001)
   - Limb defects like overlapping of fingers and **rocker-bottom feet**, and skeletal abnormalities like short sternum and narrow hips can be seen.

2. **(c)** Hemochromatosis (Ref: Robins 8th E/P141)

3. **(d)** Tuberous sclerosis (Ref: Robins 8th E/P141)

4. **(c)** Chromosome 13 (Ref: Nelson 19th E/P384)

Trisomy 13	**Patau syndrome**
Trisomy 18	Edward syndrome
Trisomy 21	Down syndrome

5. **(c)** Chromosomal abnormality (Ref: Nelson 19th E/P1925)

   Noonan syndrome:
   - It is an **autosomal dominant disorder(Mendelian disorder)** caused by mutation of tyrosine phosphatase gene on chromosome no 12.
   - **Both males and females can be affected** and phenotypically resemble Turner syndrome to a greater extent.
   - The salient features of Noonan syndrome are:
     ❖ **Short stature**, webbed neck, epicanthal folds and cubitus valgus are common features seen in both Turner and Noonan syndrome.
     ❖ Skeletal abnormalities like pectus carinatum and excavatum, clinodactyly; and vertebral anomalies can be seen.
     ❖ CVS abnormalities like **ASD**, HOCM and pulmonary stenosis can be seen.

   ❖ A characteristic facies with hypertelorism, downward slanted palpebral fissures, ptosis and micrognathia is seen.
   ❖ Other abnormalities like hernias, hepatosplenomegaly, ALL and CML can be associated.

6. **(c)** ALL (Ref: Nelson 19th E/P384)
   - Leukemias are 10-12 times more commonly seen in patients of Down syndrome.
   - However the prevalence of subtypes i.e. ALL and AML is same as that seen in normal population.
   - In children ALL is seen in 77% and AML is seen in 11% of patients.

7. **(c)** Brachycephalic (Ref: CPDT 19th E/P1001)

   Kindly refer text for details on presentation of Down syndrome.

8. **(b)** Fredrich's ataxia (Ref: Robins 8th E/P141)

9. **(d)** Fragile X syndrome (Ref:CPDT 19th E/P1010)

   Fragile X syndrome:
   - Fragile sites are present on the chromosomes which tend to break. Fragile X syndrome, an X linked recessive disorder is caused by mutation of the FMR1 gene, which results in CGG trinucleotide repeat.
   - This is the most common inherited cause of MR in males.
   - The babies are born with **long face, large ears, prominent jaws and large testicles (microorchidism).**

10. **(b)** Ehler-Danlos syndrome (Ref: Robins 8th E/P168)

11. **(a)** Phosphate diabetes (Ref: Robins 8th E/P142)

12. **(c)** Sex-linked recessive (Ref: Robins 8th E/P142)

13

Metabolic Disorders

DISORDERS OF CARBOHYDRATE METABOLISM

Carbohydrates are the most important source of energy for our body. Glucose is the most important monosaccharide for ATP generation which can be derived from food, other monosaccharides like galactose (milk and milk products) and fructose (fruits and vegetables); and from degradation of the storage polysaccharide glycogen. Deficiencies in enzymes involved in metabolism of these products can lead to disorders like galactosemia, fructose intolerance and glycogen storage disease.

Glycogen Storage Disease

Cyclic AMP dependent protein kinase activates muscle and liver **phosphorylase kinase** which subsequently activate muscle and liver **phosphorylase** respectively. These **phosphorylase** and **debranching enzyme** are responsible for conversion of glycogen to glucose-1-phosphate and further glucose-1-phosphate is converted to glucose-6-phosphate. Glucose-6-phosphate is converted to glucose and fructose-6-phosphate with the help of **glucose-6-phosphatase** and isomerase respectively. Further fructose-6-phosphate is converted to fructose 1-6-biphosphate with the help of **phospho-fructokinase**. The defect in these various enzymes responsible for glycogen metabolism leads to accumulation of glycogen in the liver and/or muscle. Based on this they can be classified as liver and muscle glycogen storage diseases (GSD).

Glycogenesis, Glycogenolysis and GSD

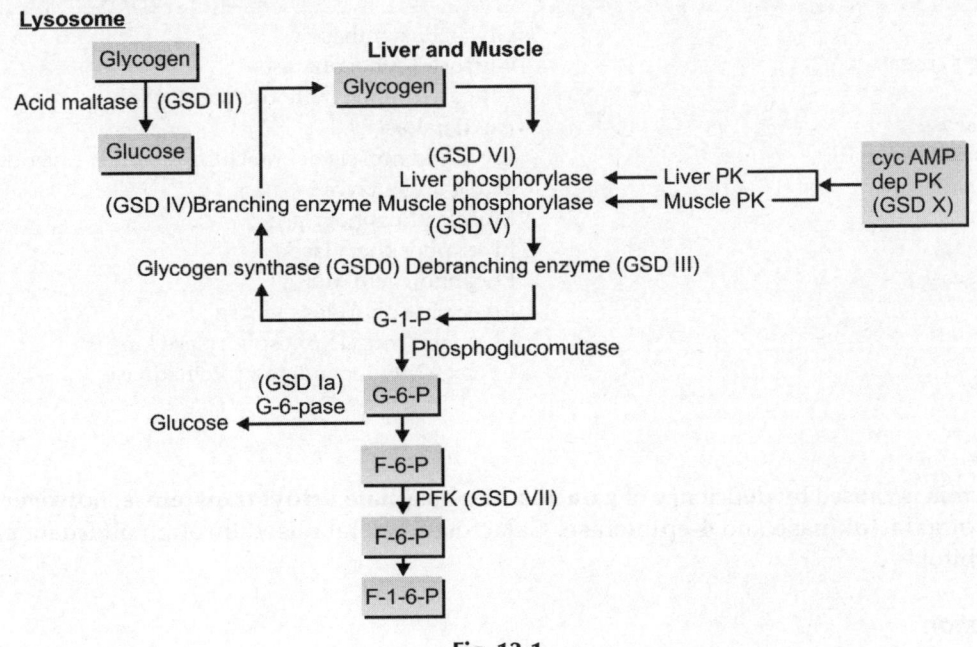

Fig. 13.1

Liver GSD

GSD affecting liver are **von Gierke's disease**, **Type IIIa or Cori's disease**, Andersen's disease, **Her's disease** and Type X disease. The common findings in these disorders are fasting **hypoglycemia** and **hepatomegaly.**

- **Type Ia GSD or von Gierke's disease** is caused by deficiency of **glucose-6-phosphatase**. The specific findings are hyperuricemia, hyperlipidemia, lactic acidosis, platelet adhesion and aggregation defect, PCOD, growth retardation, hepatic adenomas, renal disorders with an enlarged kidney and pulmonary hypertension. **Type Ib GSD** is caused by defective glucose-6-phosphate transporter. Apart from the features of type Ia, **neutropenia** is also seen in type Ib. Diagnosis is based on the laboratory findings as well as test that demonstrates **no rise in glucose level after administration of glucagon or epinephrine** because of **defective glycogenolysis and gluconeogenesis.**

- **Type IIIa or Cori's disease** is caused by deficiency of both liver and muscle debranching enzyme. The specific features are hyperlipidemia, growth retardation, splenomegaly, PCOD, myopathy, hepatocellular carcinoma, and hepatic adenomas. Type IIIb is caused by deficiency of only liver debranching enzyme and presents with only hepatic features.

- **Type IV or Andersen's disease** is caused by deficiency of branching enzyme. The most common presentation is progressive liver cirrhosis, hepatosplenomegaly and failure to thrive. Some patients may have neuromuscular type of presentation with hypotonia, myopathy and cardiomyopathy.

- **Type VI or Her's disease** is caused by deficiency of liver phosphorylase. The characteristic findings are growth retardation, hyperlipidemia and hyperkeratosis.

- **Type IX GSD** is caused by deficiency of cyclic AMP dependent phosphorylase kinase.

Muscle GSD

GSD affecting muscles are Pompe's disease, McArdle's disease and Tarui's disease:

- **Pompe's disease** is caused by deficiency of lysosomal enzyme glucosidase that breaks glycogen. The accumulation of lysosomal glycogen in cardiac and smooth muscle presents as hypertrophic cardiomyopathy; skeletal muscle weakness and atrophy, hypotonia, floppy infant and **hepatomegaly**. Chest X-ray shows cardiomegaly and ECG shows **tall QRS complex** and short PR interval.

- **McArdle** and Tarui disease is caused by deficiency of muscle phosphorylase and phosphofructokinase respectively. These disorders are characterised by **exercise intolerance**, **muscle cramps** and **myoglobinuria**.

Types of GSD

Name and type of glycogenoses	Enzyme deficiency
Type o	Glycogen synthase
Type Ia- von Gierke's disease	Glucose-6-phosphatase
Type Ib	Glucose-6-phosphate transporter
Type II-Pompe's disease	Acid maltase
Type IIIa-Cori's disease, Type IIIb	Liver and muscle debranching enzyme, Liver debranching enzyme
Type IV-Andersen's disease	Branching enzyme
Type V-McArdle's disease	Muscle phosphorylase
Type VI-Her's disease	Liver phosphorylase
Type VII-Tarui's disease	Phosphofructokinase
Type VIII	Liver phosphorylase kinase
Type IX	Liver and muscle phosphyrylase kinase
Type X	Cyclic AMP dependent protein kinase

Galactosemia

Classical galactosemia is caused by deficiency of **galactose-1-phosphate uridyl transferase**; however it can also be seen due to deficiency of **galactokinase** and **4-epimerase**. Galactose is metabolised through alternate pathway by aldose reductase in to sorbitol.

Clinical Presentation

- In classical type galactose-1-phosphate is accumulated in liver and kidney causing **hepatomegaly**, **cirrhosis** and **Fanconi syndrome.**

- The neonates characteristically present with **vomiting** and **jaundice** after milk feeding.
- Sorbitol gets accumulated in lens and can cause **cataract.**
- **Mental retardation**, tremor, **seizures** and ataxia can also be seen.
- Most common cause of death is **sepsis caused by E. coli.**

Diagnosis

Beutler test: It demonstrates deficiency of galactose-1-phosphate uridyl transferase deficiency in RBCs.

Treatment

A galactose free diet is advised along with monitoring of galactose-1-phosphate levels in RBC and calcium supplementation.

Fructose Intolerance

Fructose intolerance is caused by deficiency of **fructose-1-phosphate aldolase deficiency**. After fructose ingestion the patient presents with vomiting and jaundice. Further the patient can develop hepatomegaly and growth retardation. **Intravenous fructose loading test** shows **hypoglycaemia** and **hypophosphatemia**; and demonstration of reduced fructose-1-phosphate aldolase in liver can confirm the diagnosis. The treatment consists of dietary fructose restriction.

DISORDERS OF AMINO ACID METABOLISM

Phenylketonuria

Classical phenylketonuria is caused by deficiency of **phenylalanine hydroxylase** which leads to increased phenylalanine in the body and phenyl ketones in urine; and **decreased tyrosine**. Milder form of phenylketonuria can be caused by deficiency of **dihyrdopterin reductase** that produces **tetrahydrobiopterin (BH$_4$)**, a cofactor of phenylalanine hydroxylase.

Clinical Presentation

- The babies are normal at birth but may present with **vomiting**. Gradually later **mental retardation** and growth retardation may develop. The other findings are **rash**, hypertonia, **seizures**, microcephaly, **exaggerated deep tendon reflexes**, wide spaced teeth, **enamel hypoplasia** and hyperactivity.
- The babies are of **light complexion with blue iris** due to decreased tyrosine.
- Phenyl ketones in the urine give it a **musty or mousy odour.**
- Pregnant females with increased phenylalanine can have babies with **mental retardation, microcephaly** and **congenital heart diseases.**

Diagnosis

- Neonatal screening for phenylketonuria should be done. The conventional method of screening is **Guthrie test** (bacterial inhibition assay); however now a days better tests like **fluorometry** and **tandem mass spectrometry** is used.
- **Ferric chloride test**: If phenylketons are present in the urine addition of ferric chloride changes it to **green colour.**

Treatment

- Various formulas with **limited phenylalanine** should be used for feeding.
- **Tetrahydrobiopterin** can be used for replacement in milder forms of phenylketonuria.

Disorders of Branched Chain Amino and Organic Acid Meatabolism

Valine, leucine and isoleucine are branched chain amino acids. They are metabolised by an enzyme complex of branched chain α ketoacid dehydrogenase (α ketoacid decarboxylase, dihydrolipoyl dehydrogenase and transacylase) along with thiamine (vitamin B1). This is followed by carboxylation with carboxylases (Propionyl Co A carboxylase and 3-methylcrotonyl Co A carboxylase) along with biotin. Carboxylases are activated by holocarboxylase synthetase and biotin is synthesised by biotinidase. The errors of metabolism of these aminoacids are maple syrup urine disease and **organic acidurias** like isovaleric, propionic, methylmalonyl and 3-methylglutaconic acidurias. The organic acidurias have common finding of **metabolic acidosis**, **mental retardation** and **hyperammonemia**.

Metabolism of Branched Chain Amino Acids

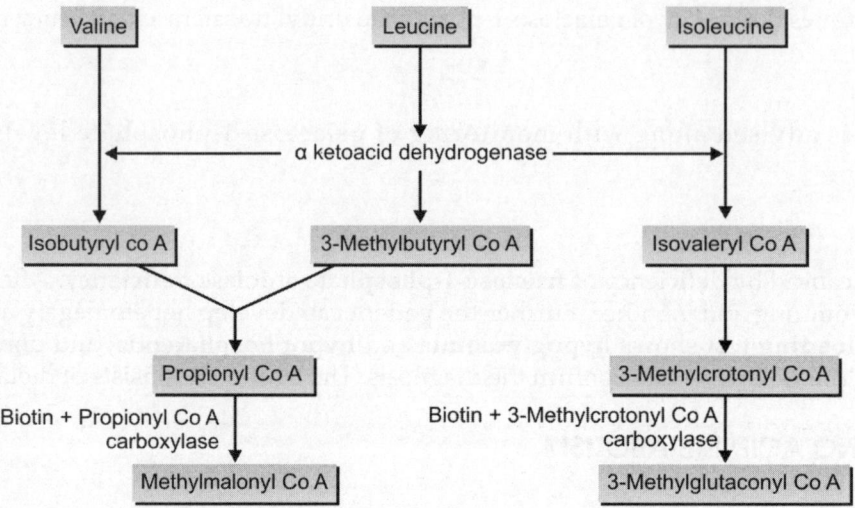

Fig. 13.2

Maple Syrup Urine Disease

Maple syrup urine disease or branched chain ketonaciduria is caused by deficiency of **branched chain ketoacid dehydrogenase complex** (α **ketoacid decarboxylase**, dihydrolipoyl dehydrogenase and transacylase).

- **Clinical presentation:**
  - ❖ Feeding difficulties and vomiting are the initial symptoms followed by hypertonicity, muscular rigidity with opisthotonos and convulsions.
  - ❖ Hypoglycaemia is seen but correction does not improve the symptoms.
- **Diagnosis:**
  - ❖ Urine has a peculiar smell of maple syrup and hence the name of the disease.
  - ❖ Increased branched chain ketoacids i.e. **leucine, isoleucine and valine** can be documented in blood and **urine**. Alanine level in the blood is decreased.
  - ❖ Ketoacids in urine can be detected by 2, 4-dinitrophenylhydrazine and **ferric chloride**. The former forms a yellow precipitate in the urine whereas the later causes **blue discolouration of urine**.
- **Treatment:**
  - ❖ Acute symptoms are treated by dialysis.
  - ❖ On long term basis limited branched chain amino acid diet is advised.

Multiple Carboxylase Deficiency

Deficiency of holocarboxylase synthetase or biotinidase causes deficiency of all carboxylases and hence the name multiple carboxylase deficiency.

- **Clinical presentation:**
  - ❖ Holocarboxylase deficiency presents with **metabolic acidosis**, feeding difficulty and vomiting followed by hypotonia, seizures, developmental delay and immunodeficiency. An erythematous rash with exfoliation and alopecia can be seen. The urine has a peculiar smell of **tomcat urine.**
  - ❖ Biotinidase deficiency is characterised by not only the above mentioned symptoms but also symptoms of biotin deficiency like dermatitis, alopecia, ataxia, seizures and sensorineural hearing loss.
- **Diagnosis:** Diagnosis is established by documenting the enzyme deficiency in serum.
- **Treatment:** The mainstay of treatment is administration of **biotin.**

Alcaptonuria

Alcaptonuria is caused by deficiency of **homogentisic acid oxidase,** which results in accumulation of homogentisic acid. Polymerisation of homogentisic acid and its accumulation in various locations gives specific presentation like ochronosis and arthritis. **Ochronosis** is the dark spots seen on the ear cartilage and sclera. **Large joints** are involved and the **arthritis** is characterised by **narrow joint spaces** and **calcified intervertebral discs**. Heart if involved presents with calcification and inflammation of valves. The **urine characteristically turns to black colour on standing**. Only drug used for treatment is **nitisinone** which inhibits production of homogentisic acid.

Aminoacid Transport Disorders

The amino acids are absorbed by various transporters across the membrane in intestine and renal tubules. Mutations in genes encoding these pumps can lead to loss of various amino acids and cause disorders like cystinuria, Hartnup's disease and lysinuric protein intolerance.

Cystinuria

Cystinuria is characterised by excretion of cysteine and dibasic aminoacids in urine. Accumulation of **cysteine in the renal tubule** leads to **recurrent radiopaque renal stones** and related symptoms like abdominal and low back pain, hematuria and pyuria. Diagnosis is established by a positive nitroprusside test. The mainstay of treatment is hydration and alkalisation of urine to dissolve the renal stones. D-penicillamine is the second line treatment.

Hartnup Disease

Hartnup disease is characterised by **massive loss (20 times) of aminoacids** like **alanine, serine, threonine, valine, leucine, isoleucine, phenylalanine, tyrosine, tryptophan, histidine, citrulline, asparagine and glutamine in the urine**; however the plasma concentration is decreased. The patients present with symptoms of niacin deficiency like dermatitis, cerebellar ataxia and muscle pain.

LYSOSOMAL STORAGE DISORDERS

Lysosomal storage disorders are caused by absence of different enzymes responsible for breakdown of glycosphingolipids. Accumulation of these lipids in the CNS causes neurodegeneration and in visceral organs causes **hepatomegaly, splenomegaly** and; **pulmonary** and **bone infiltrations**. All are AR disorders except Fabry disease which is X linked disorder. The diagnosis of these disorders is established by demonstration of the enzyme deficiency in leucocytes or cultured fibroblasts.

Gangliosidosis

- **GM1 gangliosidosis:** This is caused by deficiency of β galactosidase. Apart from the usual features angiokeratoma, macular cherry red spot and a typical facies (low set ears, frontal bossing, and long philtrum) can be seen.
- **GM2 gangliosidosis:** This includes two disorders named Taysachs disease and Sandhoff disease. Taysachs disease is caused by deficiency of β hexoaminidase A. Sandhoff disease is caused by deficiency of both hexoaminidase A and B. These patient presents with retinal cherry red spot, hyperacusis, macrocephaly and seizures.

Gaucher Disease

Gaucher disease is caused by deficiency of **glucocerebrosidase** which leads to accumulation of **glucocerebroside** in reticuloendothelial system. Bone marrow infiltration is the prominent finding and presents with anemia, thrombocytopenia, bone pain, pathological fractures, Erlenmeyer flask deformity of distal femur, osteolytic lesions and osteosclerosis. **Gaucher cells** present in the reticuloendothelial system are **positive for PAS.** Treatment is advised in the form of **enzyme replacement** therapy i.e. imiglucerase (recombinant β glucosidase).

Niemann-Pick disease

Niemann-Pick disease is caused by deficiency of **sphingomyelinase** which leads to accumulation of **sphingomyelin**. Type A is characterised by CNS involvement and in type B lungs are involved. **Childhood cholelithiasis** can be seen with Niemann-Pick disease.

Fabry Disease

Fabry disease is caused by deficiency of α galactosidase A. The patients present with angiokeratomas and neuropathic pain. Lipid inclusions with **"Maltese crosses"** are seen in urinary sediment.

Metachromatic Leucodystrophy

Metachromatic leucodystrophy is caused by deficiency of aryl sulfatase A. The patient presents with symptoms of white matter degeneration and demyelination like genu recurvatum, **decreased deep tendon reflexes**, muscle wasting, **optic atrophy** and myoclonic seizures. Metachromatic bodies in CNS are positive for **PAS** and **alcian blue**.

Krabbe Disease

Krabbe disease is caused by deficiency of galactocerebrocidase. The patient presents with optic atrophy, opisthotonos and seizures. CT scan of brain shows **density in thalamus** and cortex and periventricular white matter.

Farber Disease

Farber disease is caused by deficiency of ceramidase. These patients have typically joint involvement causing swelling and nodule formation.

Wolman Disease

Wolman disease is caused by deficiency of acid lipase. The most characteristic finding is **adrenal calcification** along with other common findings like hyperlipidemia, **abdominal distention** and **hepatosplenomegaly.**

DISORDERS OF WATER SOLUBLE VITAMINS

Vitamin B$_{12}$ Disorders

Vitamin B$_{12}$ or cobalamin is required for conversion of homocysteine to methionine by methionine synthase and methylmalonyl Co A to succinyl Co A by methylmalonyl Co A mutase. Thus abnormality in cobalamin can lead to accumulation of **homocysteine (non-classical homocystinuria)** and **methylmalonyl Co A (methylmalonyl aciduria).**

Vitamin B$_6$ Disorders

Vitamin B$_6$ or pyridoxine is dephosphorylated by alkaline phosphatase in the intestine before absorption. After absorption pyridoxine is phosphorylated by pyridoxal kinase to pyridoxine phosphate, which is further oxidised to pyridoxal phosphate (active form). The errors in metabolism of pyridoxine can lead to pyridoxine dependent states like vannillacetic aciduria, hypophosphatasia (alkaline phosphatase deficiency), **classical homocystinuria** (cystathione β synthase deficiency), **xanthurenic aciduria, cystathionuria,** X linked sideroblastic anemia and gyrate atrophy of choroids.

MULTIPLE CHOICE QUESTIONS

1. **A child presents with hepatosplenomegaly, abdominal distention, jaundice, anaemia and adrenal calcification. Which of the following is the diagnosis?** [AIIMS May 09, 10]
   a. Adrenal haemorrhage b. Wolman's disease
   c. Pheochromocytoma d. Addison's disease

2. **Macrocephaly is seen in which of the following syndromes?** [AIIMS May 08]
   a. Metachromatic leukodystrophy
   b. Adrenoleukodystrophy
   c. Canavan's disease
   d. Krabbe's disease

3. **Deep white matter lesion with bilateral deep bright thalamic appearance is suggestive of:** [AIIMS Nov. 07]
   a. Alexander disease
   b. Canavan's diseases
   c. Krabbe's disease
   d. Metachromatic leukodystrophy

4. **For which of the following diseases is enzyme replacement therapy available?** [AI 04, AIIMS May 06, Nov. 03]
   a. Albinism
   b. Neimann-Pick disease

c. Metachromatic leukodystrophy

d. Gaucher's disease

5. **Deficiency of enzyme α ketoacid decarboxylase leading to a block in the metabolism of branch chain amino acids is observed in:** [AIIMS May 05]

a. Maple syrup urine disease

b. Hartnup's disease

c. Alkaptonuria

d. Phenylketonuria

6. **Coarse facies, hepatosplenomegaly and tall QRS on ECG are characteristic feature of:** [AIIMS Nov. 01]

a. Glycogen storage disease type II

b. Hurler's disease

c. Hunters disease

d. Hemochromatosis

7. **Child of Vasanthi was weaned from breast milk on the 5th day and was given sugarcane juice the child developed hypoglycemia and hepatomegaly Biochemical examination showed hypophosphatemia and reducing substances in urine. The child is probably suffering from which of the following enzyme deficiencies?** [AIIMS Nov. 00]

a. Fructokinase

b. Aldolase B

c. Glucose 6 Phosphatase

d. Beta galactosidase

8. **A 5 day old child presents with intractable seizures. He had rashes all over the body. Blood examination showed hyperammonemia and lactic acidosis. The probable diagnosis is:** [AIIMS 2K]

a. Organic aciduria

b. Mitochondrial encephalopathy with lactic aciduria

c. Phenylketonuria

d. Urea cycle enzyme deficiency

9. **A child of phenylketonuric mother may develop:** [AIIMS June 99]

a. Microcephaly, mental retardation, congenital heart disease

b. Mental retardation, cataract, congenital heart disease

c. Hydrocephalus, cataract

d. Microcephaly, cataract, renal dysplasia

10. **An 8 days old child presents with yellow sclera, whitish stool and turmeric colour urine on 3rd day of septicemia on broad spectrum antibiotics, the likely diagnosis is:** [AIIMS June 98]

a. Galactosidase deficiency

b. Ammonia toxicity

c. Galactose 1-4 phosphatase uridyl transferase deficiency

d. Glucose 6 phosphatase deficiency

11. **Childhood cholelithiasis is seen in:** [AIIMS June 98]

a. Hurler syndrome

b. Mucopolysaccharidosis

c. Niemann Pick's disease

d. Autoimmune hepatitis

12. **A child with increased conjugated bilirubin develops seizures and cataract the probable diagnosis is:** [AIIMS Sep. 96]

a. Tyrosinemia

b. Fructosemia

c. Galactosemia

d. Glycogen storage disorder

13. **Which of the following inborn errors of metabolism is associated with mental retardation?** [AIIMS 83]

a. Alkaptonuria b. Homocystinuria

c. Pentosuria d. Glactosemia

14. **Cystinuria is characterised by:** [AIIMS 83]

a. Generalised aminoaciduria

b. Systemic acidosis

c. Deposition of cysteine crystals in renal tubule cells

d. Recurrent urinary calculi

15. **A child presents with hepatomegaly and hypoglycemia. There is no improvement of blood sugar even after administration of epinephrine. What is the likely diagnosis?** [AI 10]

a. von Gierke's disease b. Anderson's disease

c. Pompe's disease d. Mc Ardle's disease

16. **A child presents with massive hepatomegaly and hypoglycemia. There is no improvement in blood glucose on administration of Glucagon. The probable diagnosis is:** [AI 09]

a. von Gierke disease b. McArdle disease

c. Cori's disease d. Forbe's disease

17. **Treatment of multiple carboxylase deficiency:** [AI 07]

a. Biotin b. Pyridoxine

c. Thiamine d. Folic acid

18. **A child has microcephaly, blue eyes, fair skin, and mental retardation, ferric chloride test is positive. What is the likely diagnosis?** [AI 07]

a. Phenylketonuria (PKU)

b. Homocystinuria

c. Tyrosinosis

d. Alkaptonuria

19. **Darkening of urine on standing is associated with:** [AI 07]

a. Alkaptonuria b. Cystinuria

c. Fabry's disease d. Tyrosinemia

20. **For which of the following diseases is enzyme replacement therapy available:** [AI 04, AIIMS May 06, Nov. 03]

a. Albinism

b. Neimann-Pick disease

c. Metachromatic leukodystrophy

d. Gaucher's disease

21. An infant presents with history of seizures and skin rashes. Investigations show metabolic acidosis increased blood ketone levels. This child is likely to be suffering from: [AI 02]
    a. Propionic aciduria
    b. Urea cyclic disorder
    c. Phenylketonuria
    d. Multiple carboxylase deficiency

22. True statement regarding a 3 week old child with Phenyl-ketonuria is all, except: [AI 00]
    a. Provocative protein meal tests helps in the diagnosis.
    b. Tyrosine becomes an Essential amino-acid in diet.
    c. Serum Phenylalanine is increased and urinary Phenyl Pyruvate level is elevated.
    d. Phenylalanine should be completely stopped in diet

23. Enzyme deficient in phenylketonuria: [AI 99]
    a. Tyrosinase
    b. Phenylalanine hydroxylase
    c. Tyrosine transaminase
    d. Homogentisic oxidase

24. All are liver glycogenoses except: [AI 97]
    a. von Gierke's disease b. Her's disease
    c. Type III glycogenoses d. Pompe's disease

25. Child with recurrent hypoglycaemic attacks and hepatomegaly is likely to have: [AI 93]
    a. von Gierke's disease b. Neonatal diabetes
    c. Neonatal hepatitis   d. Galactosemia

26. Glucose-6-phosphatase deficiency is seen in: [AI 92]
    a. Pompe's disease   b. von Gierke's disease
    c. Mc Ardle's syndrome d. Down syndrome

27. True about Gaucher's disease: [PGI 2010]
    a. PAS positive cells
    b. Oil Red O-He cells
    c. Deficiency of acid Sphingomyelinase
    d. Deficiency of Glucocerebrosidase
    e. Gaucher cells are present

28. PKU is a congenital aminoacid metabolic disorder. In one of the following rare variants of PKU dihydrobiopterin synthesis is affected. The enzyme deficient is: [PGI June 08]
    a. Histidine decarboxylase
    b. Phenylalanine hydroxylase
    c. Dihydropterin reductase
    d. Tyrosine deficiency

29. True regarding galactosemia: [PGI Dec. 01]
    a. Mental retardation occurs
    b. Absent disaccharidase in intestine
    c. Defect in epimerase
    d. Defect in galactose 1 phosphate uridyl transferase

30. An infant has hepatomegaly, hypoglycemia, hyperlipidemia, acidosis and normal structured glycogen deposition in liver. What is the diagnosis? [PGI June 01]
    a. Her's disease
    b. Von Gierke's disease
    c. Cori's disease
    d. Anderson's disease
    e. Pompe's disease

31. Glycogen storage diseases include all of the following except: [PGI 01]
    a. von Gierke's disease
    b. Fabry's disease
    c. Mc Ardle's disease
    d. Fragile syndrome
    e. Krabbe disease

32. In a patient, muscle cramps on exercise, +ve myoglobulinemia, the disorder is: [PGI June 98]
    a. Pompe's disease
    b. Myotonic congenital
    c. Myotonic dystrophy
    d. Mc Ardle's disease

33. Mousy odour urine is seen in: [PGI Dec. 97]
    a. Maple syrup urine   b. Phenylketonuria
    c. Isovaleric acid uria d. Cystinuria

34. In phenylketonuria FeCl₃ test with urine gives .... colour: [PGI 97]
    a. Green   b. Blue
    c. Red   d. Purple

35. In maple syrup urine disease FeCl₃ test with urine gives .... colour: [PGI 97]
    a. Green   b. Black
    c. Blue   d. Red

36. Pompe's disease is due to deficiency of which enzyme? [PGI 97]
    a. Branching enzyme
    b. Glucose 6 phosphatase
    c. Acid maltase deficiency
    d. Muscle phosphorylase

37. Muscles are not involved in which glycogen storage disease? [APPG 08, PGI 97]
    a. I   b. II
    c. III   d. IV

38. The tissue with highest glycogen content (mg/100 mg): [PGI 88]
    a. Liver   b. Muscle
    c. Kidneys   d. Testes

39. In maple syrup urine disease the amino acids excreted in urine are: [PGI 87]
    a. Leucine   b. Isoleucine
    c. Valine   d. a, b and c
    e. Arginine

40. Large doses of pyridoxine are of value in some cases of: [PGI 87]
    a. Phenylketonuria
    b. Homocystinuria
    c. Nonketotic hyperglycaemia
    d. Ketotic hyperglycaemia

41. In Hartnup's disease .... is excreted in urine: [PGI 86]
    a. Ornithine
    b. Glycine
    c. Tryptophan
    d. Phenylalanine
    e. Cysteine

42. Von Gierke's disease is due to deficiency of: [PGI 85]
    a. Glu-6-phosphatase
    b. Glu-1-phosphatase
    c. Branching enzyme
    d. Myophosphorylase
    e. Glu-1-6-diphisphatase

43. Guthrie test can be used for the diagnosis of: [UPSC 10]
    a. Tyrosinemia
    b. Galactosemia
    c. Alkaptonuria
    d. Phenylketonuria

44. Which of the following is not a feature of phenylketonuria? [UPSC 04]
    a. Severe mental retardation
    b. Reduced tendon reflexes
    c. Enamel hypoplasia
    d. Vomiting in early infancy

45. In phenylketonuria, the treatment of choice is?
    a. Limit intake of substrate for the enzyme
    b. Provide the deficient aminoacid
    c. Correct the enzyme defect
    d. Symptomatic management

QUESTIONS OF OTHER EXAMINATIONS

1. Massive aminoaciduria without a corresponding increase in plasma amino acid level is characteristic of which one of the following diseases? [UPSC 08]
   a. Homocystinuria
   b. Hartnup disease
   c. Tyrosinemia
   d. Maple syrup urine disease

2. Muscles are not involved in which glycogen storage disease? [APPG 08, PGI 97]
   a. I
   b. II
   c. III
   d. IV

3. Which of the following is not a pyridoxine dependent disorder? [UPSC 07]
   a. Homocystinuria
   b. Methylmalonic academia
   c. Cystathionuria
   d. Xanthurenic aciduria

4. All are seen in metachromatic leucodystrophy except: [TN 03]
   a. Mental retardation
   b. Optic atrophy
   c. Decerebrate posture
   d. Exaggerated tendon reflex

5. Which of the following is false about alkaptonuria? [Jharkhand 03]
   a. Genitourinary system not involved
   b. Homogentisic oxidase deficiency
   c. Black urine
   d. Calcification in vertebral bodies

6. Andersen disease is due to deficiency of: [TN 97]
   a. Debranching enzyme
   b. Branching enzyme
   c. Myophosphorylase
   d. Acid maltase

7. Enzyme deficiency in glycogen storage disease type five is: [Kerala 94]
   a. Glu-6-phosphatase
   b. Acid maltase
   c. Debranching enzyme
   d. Myophosphorylase deficiency

8. Arthritis occurs in: [Kerala 97]
   a. Alkaptonuria
   b. Cystinosis
   c. Maple syrup diseases
   d. Homocystinuria

9. Accumulation of increased amount of sphingomyelin in liver and spleen is found in: [KCET 97]
   a. Gaucher's disease
   b. Niemann-Pick disease
   c. Obstructive jaundice
   d. Von Gierke's disease

10. In Gaucher's disease there is accumulation of .... inside cells: [TN 95]
    a. Galactosidases
    b. Sphingomyeline
    c. Glucosidases
    d. Cerebrosidases

11. Enzyme deficiency in alkaptonuria is: [Kerala 94]
    a. Tyrosine hydroxylase
    b. Homogentisic acid oxidase
    c. Cystathionine synthase
    d. Phenylalanine hydroxylase

12. Maple syrup urine disease is due to deficiency of: [TN 91]
    a. Decarboxylation
    b. Dehydroxylation
    c. Transamination
    d. Deamination

13. In alkaptonuria the urine contains: [NIMHANS 86]
    a. Homogentisic acid
    b. Phenylalanine
    c. Ketones
    d. Acetate
    e. None of the above

14. McArdles disease is due to deficiency of: [Jipmer 86]
    a. Glu-1-phosphatase
    b. Glu-1-6-diphosphatase
    c. Glu-6-phosphatase
    d. Myophosphorylase

ANSWERS

MULTIPLE CHOICE QUESTIONS

1. (b) Wolman's disease (Ref: Nelson 19th E/P467)
- Hepatosplenomegaly is a common feature of lysosomal storage disorders. Among all the disorders adrenal calcification is highly characteristic of Wolman's disease.

2. (c) Canavan's disease (Ref: Rudolph 22nd E/P2260)
Leukodystrophies:
- **Alexandar disease** — It is caused by deficiency of aspartoacylase. The patient presents with macrocephaly, hypotonia and poor head control. CT scan shows extensive white matter lesions with pre-dominant involvement of frontal lobe.
- **Canavan disease** — It is caused by deficiency of aspartoacylase. The patient presents with triad of macrocephaly, hypotonia and poor head control.
- **Krabbe disease or globoid cell leukodystrophy**— It is caused by deficiency of galactocerebrocidase. The presenting features are optic atrophy, opisthotonos and seizures. CT scan shows increased density in thalamus, brainstem, caudate nucleus, corona radiate and periventricular and capsular white matter.
- **Metachromatic leukodystrophy** — It is caused by deficiency of aryl sulfatase A. The presenting are features genu recurvatum, decreased deep tendon reflexes, muscle wasting, optic atrophy and seizures. CT scan shows diffuse symmetric lesions of white matter.
- **Pelizaeus-Merzbacher disease** — It is caused by deficiency of myelin proteolipid protein. The patient presents with nystagmus, ataxia and cognitive dysfunction.

3. (c) Krabbe's disease (Ref: Rudolph 22nd E/P2262)
CT scan findings of leukodystrophies:
- **Krabbe's disease** — Increased density in brainstem, thalamus, caudate nuclei, corona radiate, cerebellar cortex and periventricular and capsular white mater.
- **Alexandar disease** — Symmetric white matter lesions with predominant involvement of frontal lobe.
- **Metachromatic leukodystrophy** — Cerebellar white mater lesions.
- **Canavan disease** — Diffuse symmetric white mater lesions.

4. (d) Gaucher's disease (Ref: Nelson 19th E/P464)
- Treatment is advised in the form of **enzyme replacement** therapy i.e. imiglucerase (recombinant β glucosidase).

5. (a) Maple syrup urine disease (Ref: Nelson 19th E/P409)
- Maple syrup urine disease or branched chain ketonaciduria is caused by deficiency of **branched chain ketoacid dehydrogenase complex** (α **ketoacid decarboxylase**, dihydrolipoyl dehydrogenase and transacylase).

6. (a) Glycogen storage disease type II (Ref: Nelson 19th E/P474)
- Type II GSD or Pompe's disease is characterised by tall QRS complex and short PR intervals in ECG.
- Other features are hypertrophic cardiomyopathy; skeletal muscle weakness and atrophy, hypotonia, floppy infant and **hepatomegaly.**

7. (b) Aldolase B (Ref: CPDT 19th E/P963)
- The patient developed hypoglycaemia and hepatomegaly after taking fructose present in sugarcane juice.
- Further hypophosphatemia and reducing substances in urine confirms the diagnosis of fructose intolerance.
- Fructose intolerance is caused by deficiency of aldolase.

8. (a) Organic aciduria (Ref: Rudolph 22nd E/P565–67)
- The errors of branched chain amino and organic acid metabolism are maple syrup urine disease and **organic acidurias** like isovaleric, propionic, methylmalonyl and 3-methylglutaconic acidurias.
- The organic acidurias have common finding of **metabolic acidosis**, **mental retardation** and **hyperammonemia.**

9. (a) Microcephaly, mental retardation, congenital heart disease (Ref: Nelson 19th E/P400)
- Pregnant with increased phenylalanine can have babies with **mental retardation**, **microcephaly** and **congenital heart diseases.**

10. (c) Galactose 1–4 phosphate uridyl transferase deficiency (Ref: CPDT 19th E/P962)
- The symptoms of jaundice and septicaemia in a 8 year old child point towards galactosemia.
- Galactosemia is caused by deficiency of galactose 1-4-phosphate uridyl transferase deficiency.

11. (c) Niemann-Pick's disease (Ref: Ghai 7th E/P293)

12. (c) Galactosemia (Ref: CPDT 19th E/P962)

13. (b) and **(d)** Homocystinuria and Galactosemia (Ref: CPDT 19th E/P962)

14. (d) Recurrent urinary calculi (Ref: Rudolph 22nd E/P579)

15. (a) von Gierke's disease (Ref: Nelson 19th E/P470)
- Administration of glucagon or epinephrine causes no increase in blood glucose level in Von Gierke's disease.

16. (a) von Gierke disease (Ref: Nelson 19th E/P471)
- Administration of glucagon or epinephrine causes no increase in blood glucose level in Von Gierke's disease.

17. (a) Biotin (Ref: CPDT 19th E/P972)
- **Oral biotin** can reverse all the symptoms of multiple carboxylase deficiency.

18. (a) Phenylketonuria (Ref: Nelson 19th E/P399)
- The babies are normal at birth but gradually **mental retardation** and growth retardation may develop.
- The babies are of **light complexion with blue iris** due to decreased tyrosine.
- Phenylketons in the urine can be detected by **ferric chloride test.**

19. (a) Alkaptonuria (Ref: Nelson 19th E/P404)

20. (d) Gaucher's disease (Ref: Nelson 19th E/P464)
- Treatment for Gaucher's disease is advised in the form of **enzyme replacement** therapy i.e. imiglucerase (recombinant β glucosidase).

21. (d) Multiple carboxylase deficiency (Ref: CPDT 19th E/P972)
- Holocarboxylase deficiency presents with **metabolic acidosis**, feeding difficulty and vomiting followed by hypotonia, **seizures**, developmental delay and immunodeficiency.
- An **erythematous rash** with exfoliation and alopecia can be seen.

22. (d) Phenylalanine should be completely stopped in diet (Ref: Rudolph 22nd E/P561–62)
- Phenylalanine is converted to tyrosine by phenylalanine hydroxylase. Hence in phenylketonuria since endogenous production of tyrosine is affected, body completely depends on exogenous tyrosine and it becomes an essential aminoacid.
- Phenylalanine is metabolised by alternate pathway to phenylpyruvate, phenyllactic acid, phenylacetic acid and phenylacetylglutamine.
- Treatment comprises of giving phenylalanine restricted diet i.e. its administration should be decreased but not completely abolished.

23. (b) Phenylalanine hydroxylase (Ref: Nelson 19th E/P399)

24. (d) Pompe's disease (Ref: Nelson 19th E/P474)
- **Pompe's disease** or type II GSD caused by deficiency of lysosomal glucosidase is a **muscle glycogenoses.**

25. (a) von Gierke's disease (Ref: Nelson 19th E/P470)

26. (b) von Gierke's disease (Ref: Nelson 19th E/P470)

27. (a), (d) and **(e)** PAS positive cells, deficiency of glucocerebrosidase and Gaucher cell are present (Ref: Nelson 19th E/P464)
- Gaucher disease is caused by deficiency of **glucocerebrosidase.**
- **Gaucher cells** present in the reticuloendothelial system are **positive for PAS.**

28. (c) Dihydropterin reductase (Ref: Nelson 19th E/P399)
- Milder form of phenylketonuria can be caused by deficiency of **dihyrdopterin reductase** that produces **tetrahydrobiopterin (BH$_4$)**, a cofactor of phenyl-alanine hydroxylase

29. (a), (c) and **(d)** Mental retardation occurs, Defect in epimerase, Defect in galactose 1 phosphate uridyl transferase (Ref: CPDT 19th E/P962)
- CNS features like mental retardation, tremor and ataxia is seen.
- Classical galactosemia is caused by deficiency of galactose-1-phosphate uridyltransferase; however epimerase and galactokinase deficiency can also be attributed.

30. (b) von Gierke's disease (Ref: Nelson 19th E/P470)
- Though von Gierke's, Her's, Anderson's and Cori's disease all of them can present with the symptoms mentioned in the question, only in Von Gierke's normal structure glycogen is deposited. Since von Gierke's disease is caused by deficiency of glucose-6-phosphatase the metabolism of glucagon is unaffected.
- Her's disease, Anderson's disease and Cori's disease are caused by deficiency of liver phosphorylase, branching enzyme and debranching enzyme respectively. These are enzymes responsible for degradation of glycogen and hence in their absence the products of glycogen metabolism will be accumulated and not normal structure glycogen.

31. (a) and **(c)** von Gierke's disease and Mc Ardle's disease (Ref: Nelson 19th E/P470)

32. (d) Mc Ardle's disease (Ref: Nelson 19th E/P474)
- **McArdle** and Tarui disease is caused by deficiency of muscle phosphorylase and phosphofructokinase respectively.
- These disorders are characterised by **exercise intolerance**, **muscle cramps** and **myoglobinuria**.

33. (b) Phenylketonuria (Ref: Nelson 19th E/P400)

34. (a) Green (Ref: Nelson 19th E/P400)

35. (c) Blue (Ref: Nelson 19th E/P409)
- Ketoacids in urine can be detected by 2, 4-dinitrophenylhydrazine and **ferric chloride**. The former forms a yellow precipitate in the urine whereas the later causes **blue discolouration of urine.**

36. (b) Acid maltase (Ref: Nelson 19th E/P470)

37. **(a)** I (Ref: Nelson 19th E/P470)
38. **(a)** Liver (Ref: Nelson 19th E/P469)
   - The amount of glycogen present per mg of tissue is maximum in liver; however overall maximum glycogen is seen in muscles due to more weight as compared to liver.
39. **(a), (b), (c)** and **(d)** Leucine, Isoleucine, Valine and a, b and c (Ref: Nelson 19th E/P409)
40. **(b)** Homocystinuria (Ref: Rudolph 22nd E/P593)
41. **(c)** and **(d)** Tryptophan and Phenylalanine (Ref: CPDT 22nd E/P580)
   - Hartnup disease is characterised by **massive loss (20 times) of aminoacids** like alanine, serine, threonine, valine, leucine, isoleucine, **phenylalanine,** tyrosine, **tryptophan,** histidine, citrulline, aspargine and glutamine in the urine.

42. **(a)** Glu-6-phosphatase (Ref: Nelson 19th E/P470)
43. **(d)** Phenylketonuria (Ref: Nelson 19th E/P400)
   - Neonatal screening for phenylketonuria should be done.
   - The conventional method of screening is **Guthrie test** (bacterial inhibition assay); however now a days better tests like **fluorometry** and **tandem mass spectrometry** is used.
44. **(b)** Reduced tendon reflexes (Ref: Nelson 19th E/ P399–400)
   - Tendon reflexes are exaggerated and not depressed.
45. **(a)** Limit the intake of substrate for the enzyme (Ref: Nelson 19th E/P400)
   - The mainstay of treatment of phenylketonuria is administration of phenylalanine restricted diet.

QUESTIONS OF OTHER EXAMINATIONS

1. **(b)** Hartnup disease (Ref: CPDT 22nd E/P580)
   - Hartnup disease is characterised by massive aminoaciduria i.e. 20 times of normal excretion; however plasma concentration is decreased.
2. **(a)** I (Ref: Nelson 19th E/P470)
3. **(b)** Methylmalonyl academia (Ref: Rudolph 22nd E/ P593)
   - The errors in metabolism of pyridoxine can lead to pyridoxine dependent states like vannillacetic aciduria, hypophosphatasia (alkaline phosphatase deficiency), **classical homocystinuria** (cystathione β synthase deficiency), **xanthurenic aciduria, cystathionuria,** X linked sideroblastic anemia and gyrate atrophy of choroids
4. **(d)** Exaggerated tendon reflex (Ref: Nelson 19th E/ P466)
   - The patient presents with symptoms of white matter degeneration and demyelination like genu recurvatum, **decreased deep tendon reflexes,** muscle wasting, **optic atrophy** and myoclonic seizures.
5. **(a)** Genitourinary system is not involved (Ref: Nelson 19th E/P404)
6. **(b)** Branching enzyme (Ref: Nelson 19th E/P470)
7. **(d)** Myophosphorylase (Nelson 19th E/P470)
8. **(a)** Alkaptonuria (Ref: Nelson 19th E/P404)
9. **(b)** Niemann-Pick disease (Ref: Nelson 19th E/P464)
10. **(d)** Cerebrosidases (Ref: Rudolph 22nd E/P2252) Gaucher disease is caused by deficiency of **lysosomal hydroxylase** and **glucocerebrosidase** or acid β **glucosidase** which leads to accumulation of **glucosylceramide or glucocerebroside.**
11. **(b)** Homogentisic oxidase (Ref: Nelson 19th E/P403)
12. **(a)** Decarboxylation (Ref: Nelson 19th E/P409)
13. **(a)** Homogentisic acid (Ref: Nelson 19th E/P404)
14. **(d)** Myophosphorylase (Ref: Nelson 19th E/P470)

Fluid and Electrolytes

PHYSIOLOGY OF FLUID AND ELECTROLYTES

- Around 60 – 80% of body weight is contributed by total body water (TBW).
- The total body water is further divided in to various compartments.

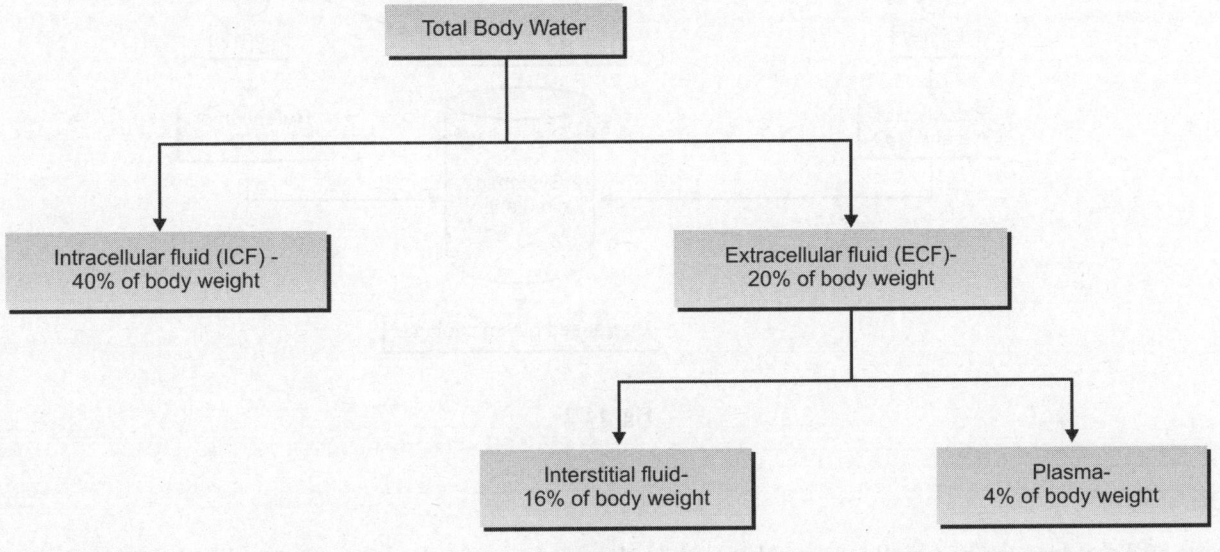

Fig. 14.1

- Electrolytes (e.g. Na, Cl) are molecules that dissociate in water to cataion (Na^+) and anion (Cl^-) which do not reassociate due to net charge on water molecules and behave as osmotically active particles. Na^+, Cl^-, HCO_3^- regulate the ECF volume whereas K^+ and its coupled anions such as PO_4^- regulate the ICF volume.
- ECF and ICF volume keeps on changing to adapt to the concentration of osmotically active particles by movement of water through cell membrane.
- A systematic involvement of various organs and their products regulate the amount of water and electrolytes in human body.
- Imbalance of fluid and electrolytes can lead to conditions like dehydration — intracellular, extracellular and dyselectrolytemia. In acute conditions it can lead to hypovolemic shock and death, while if chronic it can lead to impairment of growth and development in children.

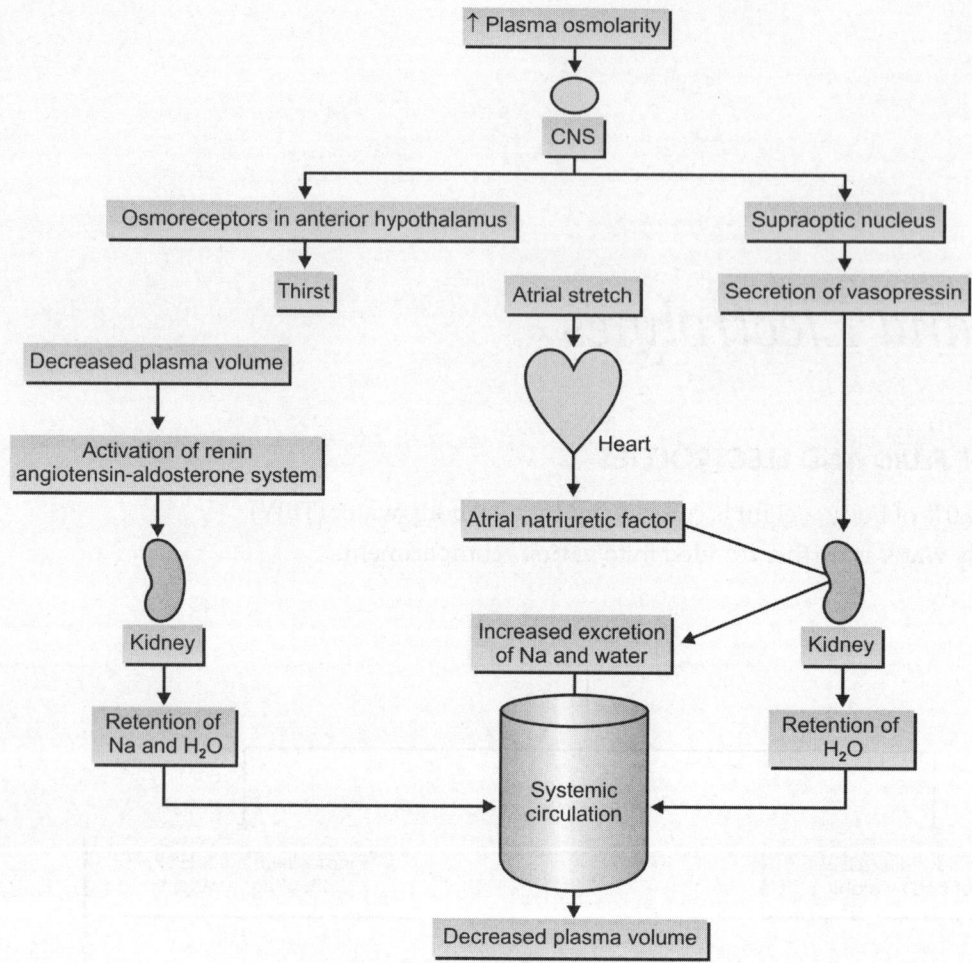

Fig. 14.2

DEHYDRATION

The infants and children are especially vulnerable to dehydration because of various factors like larger body surface area that contributes to increased evaporation of fluid, decreased ability to independently access water, that can lead to fluid deprivation and decreased ability of kidney to concentrate urine. Dehydration can be managed by following three basic steps i.e. estimation of the severity of dehydration, finding the type of dehydration and accordingly plan to replenish the amount of water and electrolytes in a proper time frame.

Severity of Dehydration

Mild dehydration (3 – 5%)	*Moderate dehydration (6 – 10%)*	*Severe dehydration (11 – 15%)*
No signs of dehydration History of • Vomiting/diarrhea • Normal urine output	Signs of dehydration • Tenting of skins • Sunken eyes and fontanel • Drylips and mouths. • History of reduced urine output • Increased thirst is present • Slight lethargy	In addition there can be other signs of CVS incompetence • Mottling of skin • Tachycardia • Hypotension Neurological changes: • Extreme irritability • Coma
Skin pinch goes back immediately	**Skin pinch goes back slowly (less than 2 seconds)**	**Skin pinch goes back very slowly (More than 2 seconds)**

Types of Dehydration

Isotonic dehydration	Hypotonic dehydration	Hypertonic dehydration
• Water and sodium loss is equal to plasma tonicity. • Serum sodium — 135 – 145 m mol/L. • **ECF volume is decreased and ICF is normal.**	• Sodium loss is greater than water loss. • Serum sodium — <135 mmol/L. • Hyponatremia leads to movement of fluid in to cells and cause **increase in ICF and decreased ECF.**	• Water loss is greater than sodium loss. • **Serum sodium — >145 mmol/L.** • Hypernatremia leads to **movement of fluid in to extracellular space** and causes **decrease in ICF** and **normal ECF.** • **Normal ECF may mask the symptoms of dehydration and the treatment** may be delayed.

Treatment of Dehydration

Mild dehydration	Moderate dehydration	Severe dehydration
• **Oral rehydration solution** • **Home available fluids**	• 75 ml/kg of ORS in first four hours as replacement therapy. • Once signs of dehydration have disappeared, the baby can be given replacement ORS as per need e.g. 10–20 ml/kg ORS for each liquid stool.	• ORS is given until IV line is inserted. • Dose of IV fluids: ❖ Baby <12 months — **30 ml/kg in 1st hour** and 70ml/kg in 5 hours. ❖ Baby 1 – 5 years — 30ml/kg in 30 minutes and 70 ml/kg in 2.5 hours. ❖ Best IV fluid is **Ringer's lactate.** ❖ Ideal fluid is Ringer's lactate with 5% dextrose. ❖ **Normal saline** can also be used (0.9%).

- In isotonic dehydration replacement can be rapid, where as **in hypotonic and hypertonic dehydration replacement has to be gradual** or else can lead to neurologic abnormalities.
- Brain cells accommodate to **hypertonicity** by producing intracellular idiogenic osmoles like taurine, glycine, glutamine, sorbitol and inositol. Hence **rapid correction will lead to cellular swelling, osmotic demyelination syndrome, cerebral edema and increased ICT.**
- Composition of Oral Rehydration Solutions (Rudolph 22nd E/P1680):

Component	Standard WHO ORS	Reduced osmolarity WHO ORS	Pedialyte	Gastrolyte
Na (mmol/L)	90	74	45	50
K (mmol/L)	20	20	20	20
Cl (mmol/L)	80	65	35	52
Citrate or HCO_3 (mmol/L)	30	30	30	18
Glucose (mmol/L)/mg/dL	20/1.11	13.5/0.75	25/1.40	20/1.10

DYSELECTROLYTEMIA

Hypernatremia

Hypernatremia is defined as a serum sodium concentration more than **150mEq/L**. It is common in preterm and ELBW infants. Most common cause of hypernatremia is **dehydration** usually due to less water intake (loss of total body water). Other significant cause in preterm infants is bolus infusion of normal saline to treat low B.P (Gain in total body sodium).

Clinical Presentation

- In acute hypernatremia symptoms develop when serum sodium level is more than **158 mmol/L**.
- Mild to moderate hypernatremia can cause fever, **irritability, lethargy, weakness** and **patency of ductus arteriosus** especially when it is caused by bolus normal saline infusion which leads to transient hypervolemia.
- Severe hypernatremia can lead to shift of fluid from ICF (Brain cells) to ECF (Interstitium and cerebral veins). Flooding of cerebral veins can lead to **intracerebral and subarachnoid hemorrhage**, which can cause **seizures, coma and death**.
- There is a strong correlation between **cerebral palsy** and H/O neonatal **hypernatremia**.

Diagnosis

- The ECF volume correlates well with body weight, which can be useful to diagnose the cause of hypernatremia instantly. Increased body weight indicates sodium gain and decreased body weight indicates loss of body water.
- On pinching abdominal skin has a **doughy feeling** due to movement of fluid from intracellular space to extra-cellular space.
- **Hypoglycemia** and **hypocalcemia** may be seen in routine investigations.

Management

- In mild to moderate hypernatremia correction of sodium level should be gradual at a rate **0.3mmol/L/hr (8mmol/L/hr)** to avoid osmotic neurologic side effects.
- In severe hypernatremia with seizures serum sodium can be rapidly reduced to **3 – 4 mmol/L**.

Hyponatremia

Hyponatremia is defined as a serum sodium concentration less than 130 mEq/L. It is even more common than hypernatremia in extremely small preterm infants. The usual cause is high intravenous infusion in early days of neonate to prevent dehydration(Gain of total body water). Late hyponatremia is usually a cause of diuretic use (Loss of body sodium).

Clinical Presentation

Hyponatremia leads to movement of fluid from ECS (Plasma) to ICS (Brain cells) which results in swelling and damage to brain. This can subsequently present as headache, irritability, lethargy, **muscle cramps**, **seizures**, disorientation, agitation, anorexia, nausea and even death due to cerebral edema and brain herniation.

Diagnosis of Hyponatremia

The primary aim is to know the ECF status.

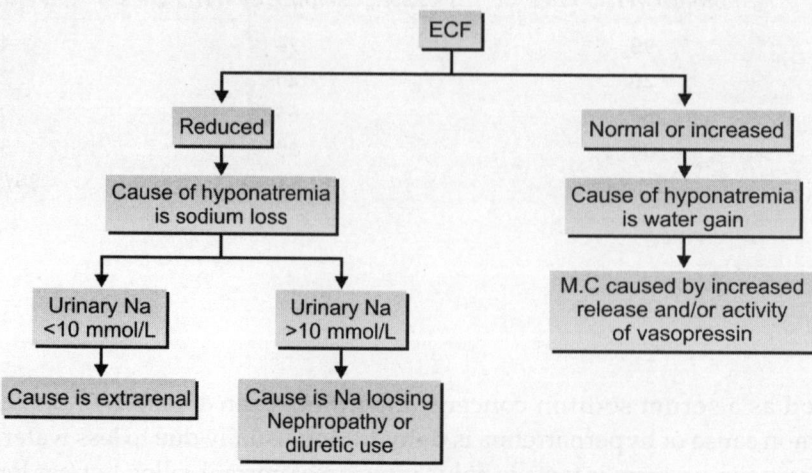

Fig. 14.3

Treatment

- Hyponatremia with symptoms is corrected by administrating **3% NaCl**. In mild cases it should be corrected at a 0.3 mmol/L/hr and in severe cases it can be rapidly corrected to 4 – 5 mmol/L.
- Rapid correction of hyponatremia should be avoided as it can lead to **osmotic demyelination syndrome, hemorrhage or cerebral edema.**

SHOCK

Shock is an acute syndrome characterized by inability of the body to supply sufficient amount of oxygen and nutrients and meet the metabolic demand of body. Various pathological conditions can lead to shock and can be named as the types of shock. **Hypovolemic shock** (Due to **dehydration** or hemorrhage) and septic shock account for the most common cause of shock in children. Other types are cardiogenic shock (Due to congenital heart diseases, cardiomyopathy or myocarditis) and distributive shock (Due to redistribution of blood from vital to nonvital organs).

Pathophysiology of Shock

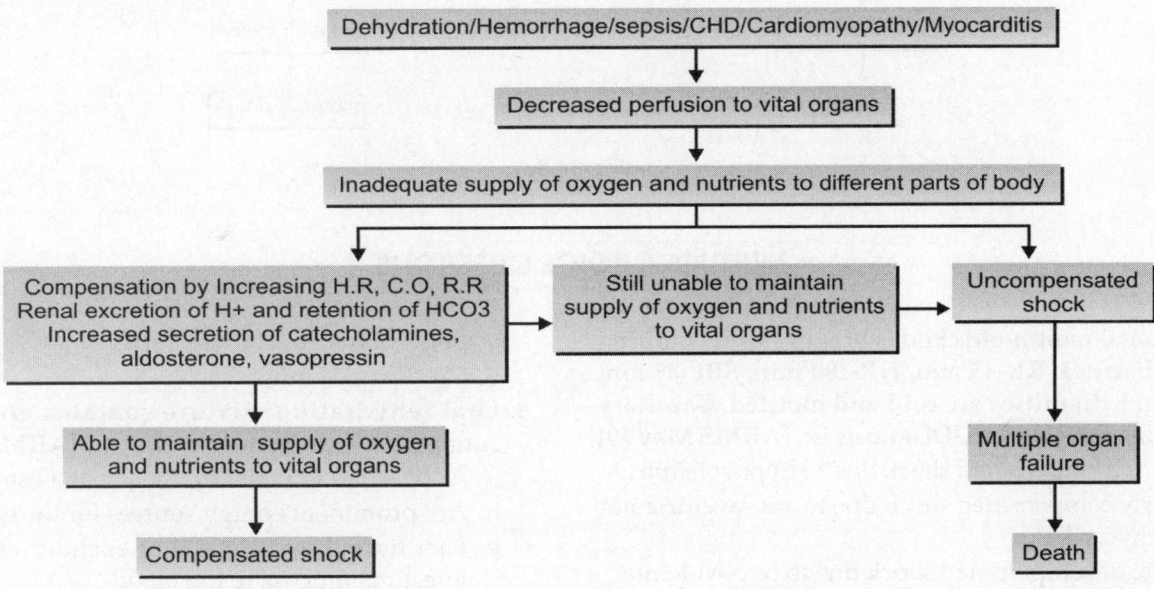

Fig. 14.4

Clinical Presentation

- **Tachycardia** is the earliest indicator of shock.
- **Narrowing of pulse pressure** is the earliest finding of shock due to decreased systolic B.P and increased diastolic B.P.
- Capillary refill (rate of refill after pressure over soft tissue or nail bed for 3 seconds) is delayed due to decreased blood supply.

Compensated shock	Uncompensated shock
• **Slightly delayed capillary refill time i.e. 2–3 seconds**	• **Significant decrease in capillary refill time**
• **Mild tachypnea**	• **Marked tachypnea**
• **Tachycardia**	• **Marked tachycardia**
• Mild irritability	• Agitation, confusion and stupor
• Cold extremities	• Cold extremities with mottling
• B.P usually normal	• Hypotension and oliguria

Management

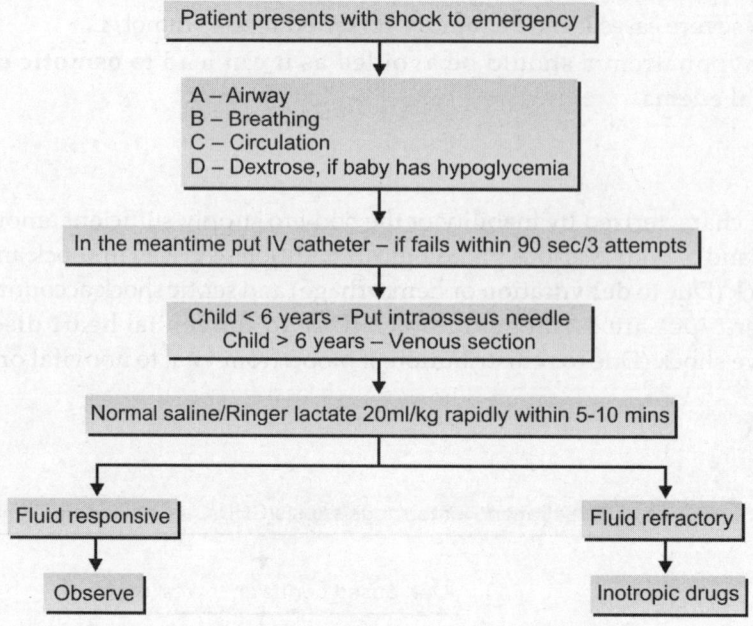

Patient presents with shock to emergency

A – Airway
B – Breathing
C – Circulation
D – Dextrose, if baby has hypoglycemia

In the meantime put IV catheter – if fails within 90 sec/3 attempts

Child < 6 years - Put intraosseus needle
Child > 6 years – Venous section

Normal saline/Ringer lactate 20ml/kg rapidly within 5-10 mins

Fluid responsive   Fluid refractory

Observe   Inotropic drugs

Fig. 14.5

MULTIPLE CHOICE QUESTIONS

1. An alert 6-month-old child is brought with vomiting and diarrhea. RR-45/min, HR-180/min, SBP-85 mm of Hg. Extremities are cold and mottled. Capillary refilling time is 4 secs. Diagnosis is: [AIIMS May 10]
a. Early compensated shock due to hypovolemia
b. Early compensated shock due to supraventricular tachycardia
c. Late decompensated shock due to hypovolemia
d. Late decompensated shock due to supra ventricular tachycardia

2. Most sensitive indicator of intravascular volume depletion in infant is: [AIIMS May 2010]
a. Stroke volume   b. Heart rate
c. Cardiac output   d. Blood pressure

3. Which of the following would be the plasma osmolality of child with plasma Na+ 125 mEq/L, glucose of 108 mg/dl, and blood urea nitrogen (BUN) of l40 mg/dl? [AIIMS May 05, Nov. 03]
a. 360 mOsm/kg   b. 306 mOsm/kg
c. 312 mOsm/kg   d. 318 mOsm/kg

4. A child presents with diarrhea and peripheral circulatory failure. The arterial pH is 7.0, PCO2 15 mm Hg, and PO₂ 76 mm Hg. What will be the most appropriate therapy:
[AIIMS Nov. 05; Nov. 04; May 01]
a. Sodium bicarbonate infusion
b. Bolus of Ringers lactate

c. Bolus of hydroxyethyl starch
d. 5% Dextrose infusion

5. Oral rehydration mixture contains glucose and sodium because both of them: [AIIMS Nov. 04]
a. Are needed to maintain the plasma osmolality
b. Are prominent energy sources for the body
c. Facilitate the transport of each other from the intestinal mucosa to the blood
d. Are required for the activation of sodium potassium ATPase

6. In Pediatric advanced life support, interosseous access for drug/fluid administration is recommended for pediatric age of: [AIIMS Nov. 02]
a. < 1 year age   b. < 5 years age
c. < 6 years age   d. Any age

7. A 6 month child having severe dehydration comes to casualty with weak pulse and unrecordable BP. Repeated attempt in gaining IV access has failed — The next best step is: [AIIMS May 01]
a. Try again
b. Jugular vein catheterization
c. Intraosseus IV fluids
d. Venous section

8. A girl of 8 years suffering from vomiting and diarrhea for last 2 days when pinched on abdomen, skin goes within seconds, she is most likely to be suffering from: [AIIMS June 00]

a. No dehydration

b. Some dehydration

c. Severe dehydration

d. Skin turgor cannot be commented

9. **In a patient who has diarrhea and vomiting with inadequate water intake is suffering from:**

[AIIMS June 00]

a. Intracellular dehydration with hypernatremia

b. Intracellular dehydration with hyponatremia

c. Extracellular dehydration with hyponatremia

d. Extracellular dehydration with hypernatremia

10. **A breast fed child presents with hypernatremia (Serum sodium > 170 mEq/L). His urine sodium is 70 mEq/L. Which of the following is the most likely cause?** [AIIMS Nov. 00]

a. Diabetes insipidus

b. Acute necrosis

c. Severe dehydration

d. Excessive intake of sodium

11. **A child had repeated vomiting and developed metabolic alkalosis. The treatment given is:**

[AIIMS June 99]

a. Ringer lactate

b. IV normal saline and potassium

c. ORS

d. IV normal saline

12. **The sodium content of ReSoMal (rehydration solution for malnourished children) is:** [AI 06]

a. 90 mmol/L

b. 60 mmol/L

c. 45 mmol/L

d. 30 mmol/L

13. **The requirement of potassium in a child is:** [AI 06]

a. 1–2 mEq/kg/24 hours

b. 4–7 mEq/kg

c. 10–12 mEq/kg

d. 13–14 mEq/kg

14. **A 5-year-old boy passed 18 loose stools in last 24 hours and vomited twice in last 4 hours. He is irritable but drinking fluids. The optional therapy for this child is:** [AI 03]

a. Intravenous fluids

b. Oral rehydration therapy

c. Intravenous fluid initially for 4 hours followed by oral fluids

d. Plain water ad libitum

15. **Kallu 2-year-child weighing 6.7 Kg presents in the casualty with history of vomiting and diarrhea for last 2 days. On examination skin pinch over the ant. abdominal wall go quickly to its original position. Interpretation of skin-pinch test in this child will be:** [AI 02]

a. No dehydration

b. Some dehydration

c. Severe dehydration

d. Skin pinch cannot be evaluated in this child

16. **True about ORS:** [PGI Dec. 00; Dec. 06]

a. Na^+ = 90 mEq/L   b. K^+ = 30 mEq/L

c. Cl^- – 20 mEq/L   d. HCO_3 = 40 mEq/L

e. Glucose = 111 gm

17. **WHO ORS, composition are (mmol):** [PGI June 04]

a. Glucose – 111   b. K^+ – 80

c. Na^+ – 20   d. Cl^- – 30

e. Total osmolarity –311

18. **Hypernatremic dehydration is characterized by:**

[PGI Dec. 03]

a. Serum sodium > 150 mmol/L

b. Signs of dehydration are minimal

c. ECF volume ↓ed

d. Rapid correction is required

e. Shift of water from ECF to ICF

19. **WHO ORS contains:** [PGI June 02]

a. Sodium chloride 2.5 g

b. Potassium chloride 1.5 g

c. Glucose 20 g

d. Sucrose 10 g

e. Potassium bicarbonate 2.5 g

20. **Composition of ORS, which of the following is correct:** [PGI Dec. 02]

a. Na^+ 90 mEq/L   b. HCO_3 – 10 mEq/L

c. K^+ 20 mEq/L   d. Cl^- 5 mEq/L

e. Osmolarity – 310

21. **The composition of ORS recommended by WHO is:**

[PGI Dec. 01]

a. 3.5 g NaCl

b. 4.5 g NaCl

c. 2.9 g sodium-potassium citrate

d. 2.8 g sodium bicarbonate

e. 1.5 g potassium chloride

22. **Most dangerous dehydration is:** [PGI June 98]

a. Hyponatremic   b. Hypernatremic

c. Isonatremic   d. Non-diarrheal cause

ANSWERS

1. **(a)** Early compensated shock due to hypovolemia (Ref: Rudolph 22nd E/P388, Nelson 18th E/P 416, Ghai 7th E/P697)

"The signs of early shock include **tachycardia, mild tachypnea, slightly delayed capillary refill (>2–3 seconds), orthostatic changes in blood pressure or pulse and mild irritability.**"

- Normal R.R varies according to age and so is the borderline of tachypnea.
  Rudolph 22nd E/P1920

Age	R.R which is tachypnea
<6 months	>59
6 – 11 months	>52
1 – 2 years	>42

Rudolph 22nd E/P185
- "In the first ten minutes of birth the average heart rate is 160 beats per minute. Thereafter the average is 120–130 beats per minute (range- **90–175 BPM**).
- The given patients HR is 180 — Mild increase
  RR is 45 — Mild increase
Capillary refill time is   4 sec — Slight increase
- Thus the current baby can be labeled as having early compensated shock.
Kindly refer text for details of compensated and uncompensated shock.

2. **(b)** Heart rate (Ref: Ghai 7th E/P697)

"Unexplained **tachycardia** may be an earliest indicator of shock."

For details of shock please refer text.

3. **(b)** 306 mOsm/kg (Ref: Ganong 21st E/P6)
Osmolality can be calculated by the formula,
      $2(Na^+) + 0.055(glucose) + 0.36(BUN)$
Putting the values in the question,
      $2(125) + 0.055(108) + 0.36(140) = $ **306.**

4. **(b)** Bolus of Ringer's lactate (Ref: Harrison 17th E/P290)
A Ph of 7.0 and peripheral circulatory failure are sufficient to diagnose it as a case of lactic acidosis.

"An increase in plasma L-lactate may be secondary to **poor tissue perfusion** (type A)–Circulatory insufficiency or aerobic disorders (type B)."
"The **underlying condition** that disrupts lactate metabolism must **first be corrected**; tissue perfusion must be restored when inadequate. **Alkali therapy** is generally advocated for acute severe academia (**pH<7.15**) to improve cardiac function and lactate utilization."

- In this case of lactic acidosis the primary cause is poor tissue perfusion due to circulatory failure. Hence the first thing to be done is to improve tissue perfusion by giving bolus Ringers lactate. As far as bicarbonate is concerned it is also indicated as the pH is 7, but it is to be dealt after increasing the tissue perfusion.

5. **(c)** Facilitate the transport of each other from the intestinal mucosa (Ref: Ganong 28th E/P460)

"**Glucose** and galactose are absorbed by **sodium** dependent process. They are carried by same transport protein SGLT 1, and compete with each other for **intestinal absorption**."

6. **(c)** <6 years age (Ref: Rudolph 22nd E/P404)

"If IV line is not available in life threatening emergency, **intraosseous access** should be attained as rapidly as possible, especially in children **under 6 years of age**."

Intraosseus infusion:

Indications	Benefits	Side-effects
• Emergent vascular access	• Attained rapidly and reliably	• Osteomyelitis
• Cardiac arrest		• Compartment syndrome
• Decompensated shock		• Fracture
		• Soft tissue necrosis

7. **(c)** Intraosseus IV fluids (Ref: Rudolph 22nd E/P389, Nelson 18th E/P 416)

"If not possible to insert an intravenous catheter in to a peripheral vein within **90 sec** or within **3 attempts**, an **intraosseus needle** should be administered to administer fluid."

For details of management of shock kindly see text.

8. **(b)** or **(c)** Some dehydration or Severe dehydration (Ref: Ghai 7th E/P264, Rudolph 22nd E/P1679)
- No dehydration can be easily ruled out as the skin pinch goes back immediately and skin turgor can be commented here as it is not a case of under-nutrition or obesity.
- Skin turgor within seconds, is not sufficient to distinguish between some and severe dehydration as within seconds doesn't mean any specific time period.
For details of dehydration please refer text.

9. (c) Extracellular dehydration with hyponatremia (Rudolph 22nd E/P1678, Ghai 7th E/P261)
- The extracellular fluid consists of mainly Na^+, Cl^-, HCO_3^- ions.
- Diarrhea and vomiting leads to loss of extracellular fluid and hence hyponatremia is unavoidable.
- Thus the given patient in the given circumstances is suffering from Extracellular dehydration with hyponatremia.

10. (d) Excessive intake of sodium (Ref: Rudolph 22nd E/ P1680–81, Ghai 7th E/P52)
- Hypernatremia can be either due to loss of body water or gain in total body sodium.
- An increase in urinary Na i.e. more than 10 mEq/L as well as increase in serum Na i.e. more than 150mEq/L suggests total gain in body sodium.
- Let us rule out other options:
  ❖ In diabetic insipidus due to loss of body water there will be hypernatremia but urinary Na will be low i.e. less than 10 mEq/L.
  ❖ In acute necrosis there will be salt wasting nephropathy, i.e. urinary sodium will be high but it will lead to hyponatremia due to loss in total body sodium.
  ❖ In severe dehydration due to compensatory mechanism body will try to retain sodium and hence urinary sodium will be decreased.

11. (b) IV normal saline and potassium (Ref: Nelson 22nd E/P305)

"Most children with metabolic alkalosis have 1 of the chloride responsive etiologies. In these situations, addition of sufficient amount of **sodium chloride and potassium chloride** to correct the volume deficit and the potassium deficit is necessary to correct the metabolic alkalosis."

12. (c) 45 mmol/L (Ref: Ghai 6th E/P106)
- ReSoMal is rehydration solution for severely malnourished child.
- Components of ReSoMal:

Component	nMol/L
Glucose	125
Chloride	70
Sodium	45
Potassium	40
Citrate	7
Magnesium	3
Zinc	0.3
Copper	0.045
Total osmolarity	300

- As you can see relatively small amount of Na and cl and more amount of glucose and K is given is justified by the fact that the malnourished child develops hypernatremia, hypokalemia and hypoglycemia.

13. (a) 1–2 mEq/kg/24 hours (Ref: Nelson 18th E/P279)

"Potassium is plentiful in food. Dietary consumption varies considerably though **1–2 mEq/kg** is the recommended intake."

14. (b) Oral rehydration therapy (Ref: Rudolph 22nd E/ P 1680, Ghai 7th E/P 264–65)

"Mild to moderate dehydration can usually be treated with small, frequent administration of **ORS**."

In this case only history of vomiting and loose stools is given along with irritability and drinking fluids. Hence we can put the child in mild to moderate category of dehydration.
Note: Even in severe dehydration in emergency while putting IV line if the baby is accepting orally **ORS** is to be given.

15. (d) Skin pinch cannot be evaluated in this child (Ref:Ghai 7th E/P 264)

"The **skin pinch** is less useful in infants or children with **marasmus or kwashiorkor** or obese children."

- Formula for weight of a child weight between 1 and 6 year is Age (in years) × 2 + 8. Putting the age of child in formula the normal weight of the child should be, $2 \times 2 + 8 = $ **12 kg.**
- The given baby is approximately half of the normal weight. Thus invariably he is suffering from PEM and skin pinch cannot be determined.

16. (a) and (e) Na^+ = 90 mEq/L and Glucose = 111 gm (Ref: Rudolph 22nd E/P1680)
Kindly see text for details about constituents of ORS.

17. (a) Glucose 111 (Ref: Rudolph 22nd E/P1680, Table 466–4)
Normal amount of glucose in WHO ORS is 1.11 mg/dL or 111mg/L.
Kindly see text for details about composition of various ORS.

18. (a) and (b) Serum sodium >150 mmol/L and Signs of dehydration are minimal(Ref: Rudolph 22nd E/P 1681–82, Ghai 7th E/P261)
- Hypernatremia is characterized by serum sodium more than **150 mmol/L.**
- Signs of dehydration are masked by the extravasation of fluid **from intracellular compartment to extracellular compartment**, thereby **normalizing the ECF volume.**
- Rapid correction can lead to neurologic complications like **cellular swelling, osmotic demyelination syndrome, cerebral edema and increased ICT.**

19. (b) Potassium chloride 1.5 gm (Ref: Park's PSM 20th E/P197)

Reduced osmolarity ORS	Grams/L
NaCl	2.6
Glucose	13.5
KCl	1.5
Trisodium citrate	2.9
Total	245

20. (a) and **(b)** Na$^+$ 90 mEq/L and K$^+$ 20 mEq/L (Ref: Rudolph 22nd E/P1680)

Kindly refer text for details on ORS.

21. (c) and **(e)** 2.9 g sodium-potasium citrate and 1.5 gm Potassium chloride a (Ref: Park's PSM 20th E/P197)

Reduced osmolarity ORS	Grams/L
NaCl	2.6
Glucose	13.5
KCl	1.5
Trisodium citrate	2.9
Total	245

22. (b) Hypernatremic (Ref: Rudolph 22nd E/P 1680, Ghai 7th E/P261)
- Hypernatremia leads to **movement of fluid in to extracellular space** and causes **decrease in ICF** and **normal ECF.**
- **Normal ECF may mask the symptoms of dehydration and the treatment** may be delayed.
- Hence it is most dangerous one.

Neoplastic Disorders

The most common cancer in children is **acute lymphoblastic leukemia(ALL)** followed by CNS tumors. In infants the most common malignant tumor is **neuroblastoma** and benign tumor is **hemangioma**. In fetus and newborns the most common tumor is **sacrococcygeal teratoma**.

NEOPLASTIC DISORDERS OF WHITE BLOOD CELLS

The neoplasms of WBCs can be classified as lymphoid neoplasms, myeloid neoplasms and neoplasms of histiocytes.

Lymphoid Neoplasms

Lymphoid neoplasms are tumors of B cells, T cells and natural killer cells. The precursor B cell and T cell neoplasm is **acute lymphoblastic leukemia (ALL)**. The peripheral B cell neoplasms are CLL and various lymphomas (mantle cell, follicular, marginal zone), hairy cell leukemia and Burkitt lymphoma. The peripheral T cell neoplasms also present as various lymphomas and leukemias.

Development of Lymphoid Cell Lineage

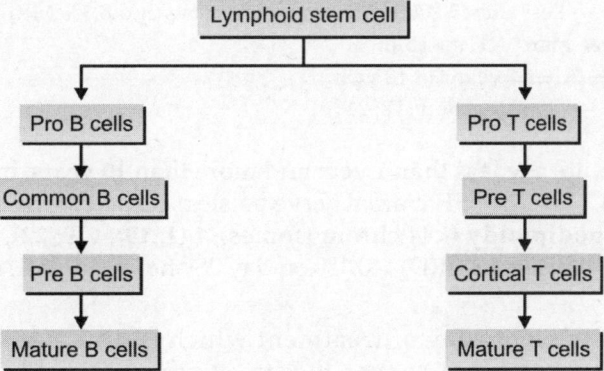

Note: **B cell ALL is more common** than T cell ALL. **Pro B ALL** is most common in **infants**. Most common precursor of ALL is **common B cells**.

Acute Lymphoblastic Leukemia (ALL)

ALL is tumor of immature B and T cells which are also called as lymphoblast. According to FAB's morphological classification lymphoblast can be of 3 types i.e. L1, L2 and L3. L1 blasts are the most common type followed by L2. **L3 blasts** which are the least common type **are derived from mature B cells**. ALL L3 is also called as Burkitt leukemia which has a poor prognosis.

15

- **Clinical presentation:**
  - ❖ Increased proliferation of immature B and T cells in bone marrow decreases the mature leucocytes; erythroid and platelet precursors are compromised resulting in anemia and thrombocytopenia.
  - ❖ **Intermittent fever is** a common finding caused by compensatory increase in cytokine production and opportunistic infections.
  - ❖ **Bone pain** can be seen due to bone marrow infiltration.
  - ❖ Extramedullary hematopoesis can result in **hepatomegaly**, **splenomegaly** and **lymphadenopathy**.
  - ❖ **Mediastinal mass** is usually a **feature of T cell ALL** caused by lymphadenopathy or thymic infiltration. It can cause **superior vena cava syndrome** and **respiratory distress.**
  - ❖ Leukemic infiltration of the testes and CNS can be seen.
- **Diagnosis:**
  - ❖ Bone marrow is hypercellular and lymphoblast cells are seen. **More than 25% blast cells** in the bone marrow, even without other features **is diagnostic of ALL**. Macrophages engulfing the lymphoid cells give a **starry sky appearance.**
  - ❖ Peripheral smear shows **tear drop RBCs.**
  - ❖ Uric acid and LDH are increased.
  - ❖ X-ray of chest shows **mediastinal widening** and anterior mediastinal mass. X-ray of long bone shows features of **osteoporosis, periosteal elevation and new bone formation** caused by leukemic cells infiltration, **growth arrest lines (metaphyseal translucent lines)** and compression of vertebral bodies.
- **Prognosis:** There are various features which determine the outcome of disease and responsiveness to treatment; however the single most important prognostic factor of the disease is treatment, without which the disease is fatal.
  - ❖ The good prognostic factors are an age of **1-10 years, female sex,** L1 type ALL, **WBC count of <50,000/µl,** presence of **hyperploidy (>51 chromosomes), trisomies (4, 17, 10), t (12; 21)** or TEL-AML1 translocation, < 5% blasts on day 14 of induction, minimal residual disease (MRD) < 0.1% on day 28 and early pre B cell ALL which have CD 10 (common ALL antigen, CALLA) on their membrane.

> Mnemonic: **Good Females Tried Less Hyper-man AT 1221**
>
> **Good** — Good prognosis
> **Females** — Females
> **Tried** — Trisomy 4, 17, 10
> **Less** — Less than 50,000 leucocytes, 5% blasts and 0.1% MRD
> **Hyper-man** — Hyperploidy
> **AT** — After 1 year Till 10 year
> **1221** — Translocation (12; 21)

  - ❖ The bad prognostic factors are **age less than 1 year and more than 10 years,** male sex, L2 and L3 type ALL, CNS involvement (> 5 WBC/µl, blasts in CSF, cranial nerve palsies), testicular involvement, **mediastinal mass,** WBC count of > 100,000/µl, **hypodiploidy (<44 chromosomes), t (1; 19), t (9; 22), t (4; 11),** > 5% blasts on day 14 of induction, minimal residual disease (MRD) > 0.1% on day 28 and; **pre B cell,** mature B cell and T cell **ALL.**
- **Treatment:**
  - ❖ Medical management is the mainstay of treatment which is divided in to three phases i.e. induction, consolidation and maintenance. Anticancer therapy with **prednisolone, vincristine,** daunorubicin, **L-asparginase,** 6-mercaptopurine and **methotrexate** are used for induction and consolidation. Maintenance phase is administration of these drugs at regular intervals. Maintenance therapy for **prophylaxis of CNS complications** consists of **intrathecal methotrexate or a combination of methotrexate, cytarabine and dexamethasone.**
  - ❖ Bone marrow transplantation can be done but is less preferred than medical management.
  - ❖ **Intensive chemotherapy** along with **bone marrow transplantation** has significantly **increased the survival and decreased the relapse rate** in patients of ALL in recent years.

Myeloid Neoplasms

Myeloid neoplasms are relatively less commonly seen in children. They can be classified as acute myeloid leukemia (AML), myelodysplastic syndrome and myeloproliferative disorders (CML, JMML). AML accounts for 20% cases of childhood leukemia.

Acute Myeloid Leukemia

AML is a tumor of progenitor cells of bone marrow i.e. myeloblasts, which leads to accumulation of blasts and suppression of hematopoesis. Increase incidence of AML is associated with **Down syndrome**, **Klinefelter syndrome**, **Turner syndrome**, congenital bone marrow failure (Diamond-Blackfan anemia, Kostmann syndrome), DNA repair defect (Fanconi anemia, **Bloom syndrome, and ataxia telangiectasia**), neurofibromatosis 1, Wiskott-Aldrich syndrome, Li-Fraumeni syndrome, radiation and drugs (alkylating agents and topoisomerase II inhibitors). Alkylating agents associated AML develops earlier and has poorer prognosis than with topoisomerase II inhibitors. FAB classification of AML includes 8 subtypes i.e. M0-M7.

Classification of AML

AML subtype	Genetic abnormality	Associated features
M0 — Minimally differentiated AML	Inv 3q, t (3; 3)	MPO –ve.
M1 — AML without maturation	>3% blasts are	MPO +ve.
M2 — AML with maturation	T (8; 21), t (6; 9)	• **Chloromas.** • Aurer rods are present. • Blasts are **MPO +ve.**
M3 — Promyelocytic leukemia	t (15; 17)	• DIC, Low leucocyte count. • Most curable form of AML. • Auer rods are most common and blasts are called as faggot cells. • Promyelocytes are **MPO and NSE +ve.**
M4 — Myelomonoblastic leukemia	11q abnormalities, inv 3, t (3; 3), t(6; 9)	• Hyperleucocytosis causing CNS, skin and gum involvement. • Myeloblasts are **MPO +ve** and mono-blasts are **NSE +ve.**
M5 — Monoblastic leukemia	11q abnormalities, t (9; 11), t (8; 16)	• Hyperleucocytosis causing CNS, skin and gum involvement. • Monoblasts are **NSE +ve.**
M6 — Erythroleukemia		
M7 — Megakaryoblastic leukemia	t (1; 22)	• Most common AML in Down syndrome. • Most common type in infants.

Note: **Myeloblasts** are positive for **myeloperoxidase (MPO)** and **monoblasts** are positive for **nonspecific esterase (NSE).**

- **Clinical features:**
  - ❖ Proliferation of myeloblasts leads to ineffective hematopoesis. The most common finding is **neutropenia** followed by anemia and thrombocytopenia.
  - ❖ Extramedullary leukemic presentations are subcutaneous nodules (**blueberry muffins**), **blue-grey coloured rash, gingival bleeding** and CNS involvement (raised ICT, cranial nerve palsies-**M.C is 7th nerve palsy**).
  - ❖ **Chloromas** (Myeloblastomas or granulocytic sarcomas) are solid tumors of myeloid cells seen in bones, CNS and soft tissue of head and neck. These are more common with the **M2 subtype.**
  - ❖ Extramedularry hematopoetic features like hepatomegaly, splenomegaly and lymphadenopathy are rarely seen.
  - ❖ **Disseminated intravascular coagulation** is common with **M3 subtype**; however it can also be seen with M4 and M5 subtype.
- **Diagnosis:**
  - ❖ Bone marrow is hypercellular and **>30% myeloblasts** confirmed by presence of **myeloperoxidase(MPO)** establishes the diagnosis of AML.
  - ❖ Complete blood count shows leukopenia, anemia and thrombocytopenia. Leucocytosis is seen in M4-5 subtype.
- **Prognosis:** There are various factors which decide the outcome of disease and response to treatment —
  - ❖ Good prognostic factors are **t (8; 21), inversion 16, t (15; 17)**, CEBPα gene mutation, NPM mutations and association of Down syndrome.
  - ❖ Bad prognostic factors are **monosomy 7**, monosomy 5, deletion of 5q, FLT3 gene duplication and abnormalities of 11q chromosome.

- **Treatment:**
  - ❖ Remission is achieved by induction with anticancer drugs like daunorubicin, cytarabine and etoposide. **All trans retinoic acid** and **arsenic trioxide** is used for treatment of **promyelocytic leukemia (PML).**
  - ❖ Following remission consolidation can achieved either by bone marrow transplantation or by continuing the anticancer drug for 6-9 months.
  - ❖ CNS relapse treatment by **intrathecal methotrexate or a combination of methotrexate and cytarabine** is advocated by some protocols; however the response is poor as compared to ALL CNS relapse.
  - ❖ **Supportive care: Hyperleukocytosis** i.e. WBC count >100,000/μl can cause hyperviscosity associated thrombosis and haemorrhage which can damage organs like CNS, kidney and lungs. Treatment is **started with hydration (IV fluids without potassium)** and leukophoresis. After this induction chemotherapy should be started and rapid destruction of cells can cause tumor lysis syndrome. Tumor lysis syndrome should be treated with **alkalinisation of urine (IV sodium bicarbonate)** and **allopurinol.**

Juvenile Myelomonocytic Leukemia

Juvenile myelomonocytic leukemia or Juvenile CML is associated with neurofibromatosis 1 and monosomy 7, deletion of long arm of 7th chromosome. Most common age group affected is less than 2 years. The baby presents with hepatosplenomegaly, **lymphadenopathy**, xanthomas, café au lait spots and rashes. Investigations of blood show anemia, **thrombocytopenia**, leucocytosis, absolute monocytosis and **high Hb F.** The treatment of choice is **hematopoetic stem cell transplantation (HSCT).**

Histiocyte Neoplasms

Histiocyte neoplasms are proliferative disorder of macrophages and dendritic cells. There are three classes of histiocytosis i.e. class I (Langerhans cell histiocytosis), class II (Hemophagocytic lymphohistiocytosis) and class III (Acute monocytic leukemia, true malignant histiocytosis).

Langerhans Cell Histiocytosis

Langerhans cell histiocytosis or histiocytosis X is a reactive proliferation of the dendritic cells. The different syndromes included are eosinophilic granuloma, Hand-Schuller-Christian disease and Letterer-Siwe disease. **Eosinophilic granuloma** is a **localised disease** characterised by not only proliferation of histiocytes but also other cells and predominantly eosinophils. **Hand-Schuller-Christian disease** is characterised by triad of **calvarine bone defects, diabetes insipidus** and **exophthalmos. Letterer-Siwe disease** is characterised by involvement at **multiple foci and organs.**

- **Clinical presentation:**
  - ❖ Incidence of LCH is evenly distributed among adults and children i.e. 50% in both. It is commonly seen in children of 1–2 year age group.
  - ❖ Localised disease is characterised by **osteolytic bony lesions** which is **most common presentation.** Most common bone involved is **skull** and mastoid involvement can lead to **chronic ear discharge.**
  - ❖ **Seborrheic dermatitis** of the scalp and diaper area (**diaper rash**) is seen.
  - ❖ Bone marrow dysfunction can cause **pancytopenia** and compensatory extramedullary hematopoesis can lead to **hepatomegaly** and **splenomegaly.**
  - ❖ Cystic lesions in the lung (**honeycomb lung**) can be seen and these lesions if rupture can cause pneumothorax.
  - ❖ Pituitary involvement can lead to hormonal disorders like **diabetes insipidus** and **growth hormone deficiency.**
- **Diagnosis:** The definitive diagnostic procedure is biopsy of the lesions and demonstrations of **histiocytes (antigen presenting cells).** These cells are **CD1a, s-100 positive** and **MHC II (HLA-DR)** positive and have **bierbeck granules** of **tennis racket shape.**
- **Treatment:**
  - ❖ Localised lesions are treated with intralesional corticosteroids, radiation and curettage.
  - ❖ Multifocal diseases are treated with agents like vinblastine or etoposide with prednisolone.
  - ❖ Refractory cases can be treated with stem cell transplantation and drugs like **cladribine**, interferon α and etarncept.

CNS TUMORS

Brain tumors are the **most common solid neoplasms in children**. The most common location of CNS tumors is **infratentorial**; however it follows an unusual pattern according to age i.e. infratentorial in age group of 1-10 years and supratentorial in <1 year and > 10 years. The CNS tumors which are commonly seen in children are astrocytomas, medulloblastoma, germ cell tumors, choroid plexus tumor and craniopharyngioma. Overall **astrocytomas** are the most common tumors and the **juvenile pilocytic astrocytoma** being the leading one; however in infants i.e. children <1year **choroid plexus tumors** are most common. **Craniopharyngiomas** are the most common tumor of supratentorial area. **Supratentorial tumors (choroid plexus tumor, craniopharyngioma)** usually present with behavioural changes due to raised ICP and signs of focal involvement like motor weakness, partial seizures, speech disorders and sensation abnormality depending on the location of the tumor. **Infratentorial tumors (astrocytoma, medulloblastoma, ependymoma)** present with features of cerebellar involvement in the form of ataxia and nystagmus. Hydrocephalus, raised ICP and its features like **papilledema**, headache, nausea and vomiting is seen. Papilledema is usually not seen in infants due to open sutures.

Astrocytoma

Astrocytomas are primarily tumor of **posterior fossa** which can be classified as low grade astrocytomas (juvenile pilocytic astrocytoma, fibrillary infiltrating astrocytoma) and high grade astrocytomas (anaplastic astrocytoma, glioblastoma multiforme). **P53 mutation** is associated with astrocytoma.

Low Grade Astrocytomas

Low grade astrocytomas are most common in **first two decades i.e. children and young adults. Juvenile pilocytic astrocytoma** (grade I) is the most common type of astrocytoma, which is most commonly located in the **cerebellum**. The diagnosis is confirmed by the presence of **Rosenthal fibres** in the specimen. **Fibrillary infiltrating astrocytoma** is the second most common type which is characterised by infiltration of neoplastic tissue in to CNS tissue. These are brain tumors with **best outcome** after resection followed by radiotherapy and chemotherapy.

High Grade Astrocytomas

Anaplastic astrocytoma (grade III) is the most common form followed by glioblastoma multiforme (grade IV). **Oligodendrogliomas** are infiltrating brain tumors of **cerebral cortex** characterised by calcification.

Medulloblastoma

Medulloblastoma (grade IV) is the most common type of PNET located in the **posterior fossa**. It arises from **midline cerebellar vermis** and extends in to 4th ventricle causing hydrocephalus. **17p deletion** is associated with medulloblastoma. **Males** are more commonly affected than females. Medulloblastoma staging done by **Chang** is the basis for prognosis.The histopathological analysis of specimen shows blue round cells which have **Homer Wright rosettes** and are positive for **synaptophysin**. Extracranial metastasis can be seen with medulloblastoma. Surgery is the mainstay of treatment followed radiotherapy and chemotherapy.

Choroid Plexus Tumor

Most common CNS tumor in infants is choroid plexus tumor. These are supratentorial tumors which present with the characteristic symptoms. They are associated with Li-Fraumeni syndrome and simian virus 40 infection.

Ependymoma

Ependymoma (grade II) is a tumor arising from the ependymal lining of ventricles. These are the **posterior fossa tumor** which is usually noninvasive.

Craniopharyngioma

Craniopharyngiomas (grade I) are neoplastic proliferation of the remnants of primordial craniopharyngeal duct (**rathke's pouch**) in pituitary. They are solid tumor with **cysts** and **calcification** located in the suprasellar region. It presents with symptoms of compression of hypothalamopituitary axis (short stature is common) and **optic tract (visual field defect, optic atrophy)**; and hydrocephalus. Complete resection of the tumor was earlier preferred but owing to its complications now partial resection with radiotherapy is more preferred.

NEUROBLASTOMA

Neuroblastoma is a tumor of sympathetic nervous system arising from pluripotent sympathetic cells of neural crest. It is the **most common solid tumor of children** and **most common malignancy of infants**. Males are more commonly affected than females. Increased incidence of neuroblastoma is seen with neurofibromatosis 1, central congenital hypoventilation syndrome and Hirschsprung disease.

Clinical Presentation

- Most common site of involvement is **adrenal gland** followed by paravertebral ganglia of the abdomen, pelvis, **mediastinum** and **neck**. Most common presentation is an abdominal **mass** that **frequently crosses the midline** and **displaces the kidney downwards without compressing the collecting system**. Midline tumors can invade **esophagus** and **trachea**. Involvement of the cervical ganglions can present as **Horner syndrome**. Paraspinal tumors can **invade spinal cord** and cause compression.

- At the time of diagnosis more than **50%** cases have already metastasised. Metastasis is commonly seen in **long bones** and **skull** which may present with **bone pain**, **sutural separation**, **orbital proptosis** and periorbital ecchymosis. Other common sites of metastasis are liver, lymphnodes and skin but **lungs are seldom involved**. Some infants with even metastatic disease may **regress spontaneously without any treatment.**

- Paraneoplastic syndromes are commonly associated with neuroblastoma. **Vasoactive intestinal peptide (VIP) syndrome** is characterised by **secretory diarrhoea**. **Opsomyoclonus-myoclonus-ataxia syndrome** is characterised by myoclonic jerks and ataxia. **Increased catecholamine** secretions can cause hypertension, tachycardia, **sweating** and **flushing.**

Diagnosis

- **Computer tomography** is the imaging modality of choice for abdominal neuroblastoma which shows **calcification** and **haemorrhage.**

- **MRI** is more preferred for **paraspinal neuroblastoma** and **MIBG** is preferred for evaluation of **metastasis.**

- Histopathological analysis shows **small round cells**. **Shimda** classification of the histopathological changes is used for evaluating the prognosis.

- Increased tumor markers of catecholamine metabolism like **homovanillic acid (HVA)** and **vanillylmandelic acid (VMA)** are seen in urine.

Prognosis

- Good prognostic factors are age<1year at the time of diagnosis, stage 1 and 2 of disease and **hyperdiploidy**.

- Bad prognostic factors are age>1 year at the time of diagnosis, stage 3 and 4 of disease, **MYCN proto-oncogene amplification, Trk-A overexpression**, **deletion of 1p**, allelic loss of 11q and 14q; and gain of 17q.

Treatment

- **Surgery** is the mainstay of treatment for **early stage disease** i.e. stage 1 and 2.

- For **late stages** i.e. stage 3 and 4 **surgery** is usually combined with **chemotherapy** (cisplatin, cyclophosphamide, etoposide, and doxorubicin) and **radiotherapy**.

WILMS TUMOR

Wilms tumor or nephroblastoma is the second most common abdominal tumor. The three classical component of Wilms tumor are epithelium, blastema and stroma. It is associated with **deletion of 11p chromosome** containing WT1 gene, imprinting loss of IGF2, mutation of β catenin gene and loss of heterozygosity of 1p and 16q. Increased incidence of Wilms tumor is seen with WAGAR syndrome (Wilms tumor, Aniridia, **Genitourinary abnormalities** and mental retardation), Denys-Drash syndrome, Frasier syndrome, **Beckwith-Widemann syndrome** (large organs, e.g. **macroglossia, hypoglycemia**), Simpson-Golabi-Behmel syndrome, Sotos syndrome, Perlman syndrome, **hemihypertrophy**, genitourinary anomalies (**horse-shoe kidney**, duplication of collecting system, cryptorchidism, hypospadias) neurofibromatosis, sporadic **aniridia** and von Wilebrand disease.

Clinical Presentation

- Wilms tumor is a well-defined solid mass that **compresses the parenchyma and collecting system.** The most common presentation is that of an **abdominal mass** which usually **does not cross the midline**. The other common findings are constipation, abdominal pain and vomiting whereas fever, hematuria, hypertension and anemia are less common.
- Tumor can **extend in to IVC** followed by heart and lungs till **aorta.**
- Most commonly Wilms tumor is **unilateral** but bilateral tumors are common at younger age and associated with syndromes.
- **Metastasis** is commonly seen in **lungs** and **seldom in liver**; however the **clear cell sarcoma** variant of Wilms tumor commonly **metastasises to the bones.**

Prognosis

There are various prognostic factors; however **tumor stage** at the time of diagnosis is the **best prognostic indicator**.

- Good prognostic factors are early stage disease i.e. stage I and II, favourable histology, age< 2 years and tumor<500 grams.
- Poor prognostic factors are anaplastic histology characterised by huge hyperchromatic nuclei and hyperdiploidy, age>2 years, tumor>500 grams, late stage disease (III and IV), loss of heterozygosity of 1p and 16q and; renal vessel and capsule invasion.

Diagnosis and Staging

- USG shows presence of a well-defined mass that is clearly separated from the rest of kidney with a pseudocapsule. **IVC invasion** can also be seen in USG.
- CT scan shows stretching and splaying of renal parenchyma (**beak sign**) and signs of **tumor necrosis** and fat deposition. **Calcification** is very **rarely seen.**
- Staging of Wilms tumor are of two types based on the time of staging in relation to surgery and chemotherapy. **NWTS (National Wilms Tumor Study)** staging is based on the principle that **first surgery and staging** is done followed by chemotherapy. SIOP **(International Society Of Pediatric Oncology)** staging is based on the principle that **first chemotherapy** is given followed by surgery and staging.

Differential Diagnosis

The most important differential diagnosis of Wilms tumor is neuroblastoma:

Neuroblastoma	Wilms Tumor
- Arises from **adrenal gland** most commonly and **displaces kidney downwards without affecting the collecting system.** - Ill-defined mass which **crosses the midline.** - Midline mass can compress **trachea** and **esophagus** and paraspinal mass can invade **spinal cord.** - **Lungs** are the **least common** site of **metastasis.** - CT scan shows **calcification.**	- Arises in the **kidney** and **compresses the parenchyma and collecting system.** - Well-defined mass that **does not cross the midline.** - Extends in to **IVC** → heart →lungs →**aorta.** - **Lungs** are the **most common** site of **metastasis.** - CT scan shows **tumor necrosis** and **haemorrhage.**

Treatment

- Surgical removal of the tumor is the mainstay of treatment. An **open anterior surgical approach** is used to explore the abdomen for spread of disease to other organs and both the kidneys. This is followed by **nephrectomy** i.e. an en-block resection of the tumor.
- Chemotherapy is given in all stages. For stage I and II **vincristine** and **actinomycin D** is used whereas for stage III and IV **doxorubicin** is also added to the regimen.
- **Radiation therapy** is reserved for the advanced stages i.e. stage III and IV which should be started **within 10 days of surgery.**

RETINOBLASTOMA

Retinoblastoma is the most common primary intraocular tumor in children. Most of the cases i.e. 60% are acquired. The remaining **40% are hereditary** and caused by inactivation of both alleles of **tumor suppressor gene (RB1)** located on **chromosome 13**. The risk of transmitting the disorder to offspring is 50%. Retinoblastomas are **unilateral** in most of the cases but bilateral disease can be seen in 25% cases.

Clinical Presentation

- Most common presentation of retinoblastoma is **leucokoria (white pupil)** and the earliest presentation is strabismus.
- Retinoblastoma arises from the inner layer of retina and its overgrowth can lead to vitreous seeding and retinal detachment. Due to insufficient blood supply caused by tumor growth ultimately **necrosis** and **calcification occurs**.
- Trilateral retinoblastoma syndrome is characterised by association of neuroectodermal tumor of the pineal gland.
- Increased incidence of osteosarcoma, soft tissue sarcoma and malignant melanoma can be seen in cases of hereditary retinoblastoma.

Diagnosis

Most of the cases are diagnosed before 3 years of age.
- Ophthalmoscopy under general anaesthesia is the mainstay of diagnosis.
- CT scan demonstrates the presence of calcification.
- MRI is preferred for diagnosis to rule out trilateral retinoblastoma syndrome. CT and MRI can also quantify the extraocular spread of tumor.

Treatment

- The treatment of choice is chemotherapy (carboplatin, vincristine, etoposide) for reduction of tumor size followed by laser photocoagulation for small tumor or cryotherapy for large tumors.
- Enucleation is done only for tumors with no possibility of vision restoration.
- Radioterapy is reserved for treatment resistant cases.

MULTIPLE CHOICE QUESTIONS

1. Chang staging is used for: [AIIMS May 2010]
   a. Retinoblastoma   b. Medulloblastoma
   c. Ewing's sarcoma   d. Rhabdomyosarcoma
2. **Which of the following childhood tumors show extracranial metastasis?** [AIIMS May 2010]
   a. Glioblastomamultiforme
   b. Medulloblastoma
   c. Choroid plexus carcinoma
   d. Ependymoblastoma
3. **The poor prognostic factor associated with ALL in children is:** [AIIMS Nov. 09]
   a. Total leucocyte count 4000-100,000
   b. Age less than 2 years
   c. Testicular involvement
   d. Blast in peripheral smear
4. **Pilocytic astrocytoma false is:** [AIIMS May 09]
   a. Spreads to posterior fossa
   b. Seen at eighty years of age
   c. Best prognosis among allintracranial neoplasms.
   d. Surgery and radiation therapy used for treatment

5. **Which of the following drugs is used for the treatment of refractory histiocytosis:** [AIIMS Nov. 08]
   a. High dose methotrexate
   b. High dose cytarabine
   c. Cladribine
   d. Fludarabine
6. **All of the following are good prognostic factor for ALL except:** [AIIMS Nov. 08]
   a. Age of onset between 2 and 8 years
   b. Initial WBC count less than 50000
   c. Hyperdiploidy
   d. t (9 : 22), t (8 : 14), t (4 : 11)
7. **Most common site of histiocytosis is:** [AIIMS May 07]
   a. Bone   b. Skin
   c. Lung   d. Liver
8. **AML with worst prognosis:** [AIIMS May 07]
   a. 8/21 translocation
   b. Inversion 16
   c. Normal cytogenetics
   d. Monosomy 7

9. Arsenic is used in the management of:
   [AIIMS May 07]
   a. Acute promyelocytic leukaemia
   b. ALL
   c. CML
   d. Transient myeloproliferative disorder

10. A 17-year-old boy presented with TLC of 138 × 10⁹/L with 80% blasts on the peripheral smear. Chest X-ray demonstrated a large mediastinal mass. Immunophenotyping of this patients blasts would most likely demonstrate: [AIIMS May 2006]
   a. No surface antigen (Null phenotype)
   b. An immature T cell phenotype (Tdt/CD34/CD37)
   c. Myeloid markers, such as CD13, CD33 and CD15
   d. B cell markers such as CD19, CD20 AND CD22

11. A 15-year-old boy presented with one day history of bleeding gum, subconjunctival bleed and purpuric rash. Investigations revealed following results: Hb-6.4 gm/gl; TLC-26500/mm³; prothrombin time-20 sec with a control of 13 sec; partial thromboplastin time-50 sec; and fibrinogen 10 mg/dl. Peripheral smear was suggestive of acute myeloblastic leukemia. Which of the following is the most likely?   [AIIMS May 06]
   a. Myeloblastic leukaemia without maturation
   b. Myeloblastic leukaemia with maturation
   c. Promyelocytic leukaemia
   d. Myelomonocytic leukaemia

12. In PML, all of the following are seen except: [AI 07]
   a. Retinoic acid is used in treatment
   b. 15/17 translocation may be seen
   c. CD 15/34 both seen in same cell
   d. Associated with disseminated intravascular coagulation

13. Which of the following is the most common inherited malignancy?   [AIIMS May 05]
   a. Infant leukemia
   b. Retinoblastoma
   c. Wilm's tumor
   d. Neuroblastoma

14. A 7-year-old boy with left renal mass had bone pain and was detected to have bone metastatic deposits. The most likely renal tumor is: [AIIMS Nov. 04]
   a. Favorable histology Wilms tumor
   b. Renal cell carcinoma
   c. Clear cell sarcoma
   d. Rhabdoid tumor

15. A 2-year-old child presents with scattered lesions in the skull. Biopsy revealed Langerhans giant cells. The most commonly associated is marker with this condition will be: [AIIMS 05]
   a. CD 1a   b. CD 57
   c. CD 3   d. CD 68

16. A 2-year-old child comes with discharge, Seborrheic dermatitis, polyuria and hepato-splenomegaly. Which of the following is the most likely diagnosis: [AIIMS May 04]
   a. Leukemia
   b. Lymphoma
   c. Langerhans's cell histiocytosis
   d. Germ cell tumor

17. A 6-year-old boy has been complaining of headache, ignoring to see objects on the sides for four months. On examination he is not mentally retarded, his grades at school are good, and visual accuity is diminished in both eyes. Visual charting showed significant field defect. CT scan of head showed suprasellar mas with calcification. Which of the following is the most probable diagnosis?   [AIIMS May 04]
   a. Astrocytoma   b. Craniopharyngioma
   c. Pituitary adenoma   d. Meningioma

18. A one-year-old boy presented with hepato-spleno-megaly and delayed milestones. The liver biopsy and bone marrow biopsy revealed presence of histocytes with PAS positive. Electron microscopic examination of these histicytes is most likely to reveal the presence of: [AIIMS 03]
   a. Birbeck granules in the cytoplasm
   b. Myelin figures in the cytoplasm
   c. Parallel rays of tubular structures in lysosomes
   d. Electron dense deposit in the mitochondria

19. A 10-year-old child presented with headache, vomiting, gait instability and diplopia. On examination he had papilledema and gait ataxia. The most probable diagnosis is: [AIIMS Nov. 02]
   a. Hydrocephalus
   b. Brain stem tumor
   c. Suprasellar tumor
   d. Midline posterior fossa tumor

20. Poor prognostic indicator of ALL is:
   [AIIMS May 02]
   a. Female sex
   b. Leukocyte count < 50,000
   c. Age greater than 1 year
   d. Hypodiploidy

21. Neuroblastoma differs from Wilms tumor radio-logically by all except: [AIIMS June 01]
   a. Calcification
   b. Aorta and IVC are not eroded but pushed aside
   c. Same location
   d. Intraspinal extension of tumor

22. A 10-year-old boy presents with midline swelling arising from cerebellum. The diagnosis is :
   [AIIMS Dec. 98]
   a. Astrocytoma
   b. Glioblastoma multiforme

c. Ependymoma

d. Medulloblastoma

23. **Most common urinary bladder tumor in children is:**
[AIIMS June 97]

a. Hemangioma

b. Rhabdomyosarcoma

c. Transitional cell carcinoma

d. Squamous cell carcinoma

24. **Increased fetal haemoglobin is seen in:** [AIIMS 97]

a. Juvenile CML

b. Congenital red cell aplasia

c. Hereditary spherocytosis

d. AML

25. **Which is the commonest abdominal mass in neonate?** [AI 94, 96, AIIMS Feb. 97]

a. Wilm's tumor

b. Polycystic kidney disease

c. Neuroblastoma

d. Rhabdomyosarcoma

26. **Most common supratentorial tumor in children is:**
[AIIMS Sep. 96]

a. Craniopharyngioma   b. Astrocytoma

c. Glioma   d. Meningioma

27. **Suprasellar cystic mass in children is:**
[AIIMS May 95]

a. Medulloblastoma   b. Craniopharyngioma

c. Meningioma   d. Secondaries

28. **Which is not a tumor of the first decade of life?**
[DPG 10, AIIMS 92]

a. Rhabdomyosarcoma   b. Neuroblastoma

c. Ameloblastoma   d. Retinoblastoma

29. **Which of the following is poor prognostic factor in a child with ALL?** [AI 11]

a. Age 2–8 years

b. Total leucocyte count <50,000

c. t (9; 22), t (4;11), t (1;19)

d. Absent blasts in peripheral smear

30. **A child with acute myeloid leukaemia presents with hyperleukocytosis. Treatment includes all of the following except:** [AI 09]

a. IV fluid

b. Allopurinol

c. Alkalinisation

d. Immediately start induction therapy

31. **Which of the following statements about neuro-blastoma is not true?** [AI 09]

a. Most common extracranial solid tumor in child-hood

b. >50% present with metastasis at the time of diagnosis

c. Lung metastasis are common

d. Often encase aorta and its branches at the time of diagnosis

32. **Which of the following is Post-chemotherapy based staging system in Wilms tumor?** [AI 09]

a. National Wilms tumor staging system (NWTS)

b. International society of pediatric oncology (SIOP)

c. AJCC TNM

d. Chadwick

33. **Poor prognosis in AML is seen in which cytogenetic abnormality:** [AI 08]

a. Monosomy 7

b. No cytogenetic abnormality

c. t (15; 17)

d. Inv. 16

34. **Which of the following statements about cerebellar astrocytomas in pediatric age group is False:** [AI 08]

a. These are usually Low grade tumors

b. These tumors have a good prognosis

c. These are more commonly seen of the 1st and 2nd decades

d. These tumors are more common in females

35. **Non specific esterase is positive in all the categories of AML except:** [AI 07]

a. M3   b. M4

c. M5   d. M6

36. **Most common tumor in children is:** [AI 07]

a. Leukemia   b. Lymphoma

c. Neuroblastoma   d. Wilm's tumor

37. **All of the following is associated with good prognosis in childhood leukemia except:** [AI 07]

a. Hyperdiploidy   b. Female sex

c. Precursor B cell ALL d. t (12; 21) translocation

38. **ALL L$_3$ morphology is a malignancy arising from which cell lineage:** [AI 07]

a. Mature B cell

b. Precursor B cell

c. Immature T cell

d. Mixed B cell and T cell

39. **The ideal timing of radiotherapy for Wilms tumor after surgery is:** [AI 06]

a. Within 10 days

b. Within 2 weeks

c. Within 2 months

d. Any time after surgery

40. **The most important determinant of prognosis in Wilms tumor:** [AI 06]

a. Stage of the disease

b. Loss of heterozygosity of chromosome Ip

c. Histology

d. Age less than one year at presentation

41. **A malignant tumor of childhood, that metastasizes to bones most often, is:** [AI 06, 02]

a. Wilm's tumor

b. Neuroblastoma

c. Adrenal gland tumors

d. Granulose cell tumor of ovary

42. The most common malignant neoplasm of infancy is: [AI 05]
    a. Malignant teratoma   b. Neuroblastoma
    c. Wilm's tumor   d. Hepatoblastoma

43. The most common presentation of a child with Wilms' tumor is: [AI 05]
    a. As asymptomatic abdominal mass
    b. Hematuria
    c. Hypertension
    d. Hemoptysis due to pulmonary secondary

44. To which of the following events is 'good' outcome in neuroblastoma associated: [AI 04]
    a. Diploidy
    b. N-myc amplification
    c. Chromosome Ip depletion
    d. Trk A expression

45. A 5-year-old child presents with history of fever off and on for past 2 weeks and petechial spots all over the body and increasing pallor for past 1 month. Examination reveals splenomegaly of 2 cm below costal margin. The most likely diagnosis is: [AI 04]
    a. Acute leukemia
    b. Idiopathic thrombocytopenic purpura
    c. Hypersplenism
    d. Aplastic anemia

46. All of the following are poor prognostic factors for acute myeloid leukemias except: [AI 03]
    a. Age more than 60 years
    b. Leucocyte count more than 100,000/µl
    c. Secondary leukemia
    d. Presence of t (8; 21)

47. Transient myeloproliferative disorder of the newborn is seen in association with: [AI 03]
    a. Turner syndrome   b. Down syndrome
    c. Neurofibromatosis   d. Ataxia telangiectasia

48. A child presents with seborrheic dermatitis, lytic skull lesions, ear discharge and hepato-splenomegaly; likely diagnosis: [AI 01]
    a. Leukemia   b. Lymphoma
    c. Histiocytosis X   d. Multiple myeloma

49. True statement regarding Brain Tumor in children is: [AI 00]
    a. Mostly is infra-tentorial
    b. Papilledema is rare
    c. Is the most common tumor in children
    d. Hydrocephalus is rare

50. Common posterior-cranial fossa tumors include all of the following except: [AI 99]
    a. Medulloblastoma
    b. Oligodendroglioma
    c. Ependydoma
    d. Cystic astrocytoma

51. Most common malignancy in children is: [AI 99]
    a. Retinoblastoma
    b. Lymphoma and leukemia
    c. Wilm's tumor
    d. Neuroblastoma

52. Most common presentation of neuroblastoma is: [AI 98]
    a. Lytic lesion in skull with suture diasthesis
    b. Lung metastasis
    c. Renal invasion
    d. Secondaries in brain

53. Which of the following types of leukemia is administered prophylactic methotrexate for CNS prophylaxis? [AI 97]
    a. Diffuse histiocytic leukemia
    b. Lymphoblastic leukemia
    c. Promyelocytic leukemia
    d. CML

54. Most common cause of suprasellar enlargement with calcification in children is: [AI 97]
    a. Craniopharyngioma
    b. Astrocytoma
    c. Meningioma
    d. Secondaries

55. Most common posterior fossa tumor in children is: [AI 97]
    a. Medulloblastoma
    b. Glioblastoma multiforme
    c. Astrocytoma
    d. Meningioma

56. Tumor associated with best prognosis in children is: [AI 97, 94]
    a. Medulloblastoma
    b. Ependymoma
    c. Cerebellar astrocytoma
    d. Glioblastoma multiforme

57. The most common intracranial tumor in children is: [AI 96]
    a. Glioma
    b. Ependymoma
    c. Meningioma
    d. Lymphangioma

58. Which of the following presents as mediastinal enlargement? [AI 95]
    a. Promyelocytic leukemia
    b. CML
    c. ALL
    d. Diffuse histiocytic lymphoma

59. L-asparginase is particularly used in which type of leukemia: [AI 94-95]
    a. ALL   b. AML
    c. CLL   d. CML

60. **All of the following are features of juvenile CML except:** [AI 94]
   a. Thrombocytopenia
   b. Fetal Hb is increased
   c. Philadelphia chromosome is positive
   d. Lymphadenopathy

61. **Wilms tumor is associated with all of the following except:** [AI 94]
   a. Aniridia
   b. Beckwith syndrome
   c. Polycystic kidney
   d. Hemihypertrophy

62. **A 1-year-old child presents with a swelling in the left flank with episodes of flushing, diarrhoea, sweating and bone pain. The diagnosis is:** [AI 94]
   a. Neuroblastoma
   b. Wilm's tumor
   c. Medulloblastoma
   d. Pheochromocytoma

63. **Which is the commonest abdominal mass in neonate?** [AI 94, 96, AIIMS Feb. 97]
   a. Wilm's tumor
   b. Polycystic kidney disease
   c. Neuroblastoma
   d. Rhabdomyosarcoma

64. **Germ cell tumor(s) of pediatric includes all except:** [PGI Nov. 09]
   a. Pure yolk sac tumor
   b. Leydig cell tumor
   c. Choriocarcinoma
   d. Embryonal cell carcinoma
   e. Endodermal sinus tumor

65. **Which statement(s) is/are true about neuroblastoma with respect to Wilms tumor?** [PGI Dec. 08]
   a. Neuroblastoma causes displacement of kidney inferolaterally without distortion of collecting system
   b. Stippled calcification is present in Wilms tumor
   c. Aortic and IVC invasion by neuroblastoma
   d. Neuroblastoma crossing midline
   e. Intraspinal extension by Wilms tumor

66. **True about childhood tumor are all except:** [PGI June 08]
   a. Wilm's tumor
   b. Neuroblastoma
   c. Retinoblastoma
   d. Embryonal rhabdomyoma
   e. Pleomorphic rhabdomyosarcoma

67. **Neuroblastoma originates from:** [PGI June 08]
   a. Adrenals
   b. Mediastinum
   c. Chest wall
   d. Peripheral nerves
   e. Neck

68. **Which of the following are associated with Wilms tumor?** [PGI 08]
   a. Aniridia
   b. Genitourinary abnormalities
   c. Cataract
   d. Hemihypertrophy
   e. Macroglossia

69. **Childhood malignancy producing proptosis is/are:** [PGI June 05]
   a. Neuroblastoma
   b. Hepatoma
   c. Retinoblastoma
   d. Germ cell tumor
   e. Nephroblastoma

70. **True about eosinophilic granuloma:** [PGI Dec. 04]
   a. M.C in 20-25 years of age
   b. More common in female
   c. Osteolytic lesion
   d. Skull is commonly affected
   e. Lung is commonly affected

71. **A 2-year-old boy suffering from leukemia, following are the x ray findings:** [PGI June 03]
   a. Osteolytic lesions in flat bones
   b. Metaphyseal osteoporosis
   c. Periosteal new bone formation
   d. Osteosclerosis of long bones
   e. Transverse line of dark band below the growth plate

72. **Treatment of ALL:** [PGI Dec. 02]
   a. Hydroxyurea
   b. All trans retinoic acid
   c. Prednisolone
   d. L-asparginase
   e. Vincristine

73. **True about Langerhans' histiocytosis 'X':** [PGI June 01]
   a. Can be associated with diabetes insipidus
   b. X-ray shows pathognomonic osteosclerotic lesions
   c. Birbeck's granules in Langerhans's cell
   d. Proliferation of antigen presenting cells
   e. Associated with specific HLA DR

74. **1-year-old child abdominal mass with calcification, possibilities are:** [PGI Dec. 2000)]
   a. Neuroblastoma
   b. Wilms tumor
   c. Nephronopthisis
   d. Pheochromocytoma

75. **X-ray features of leukemia in a 2 year old child is/are:** [PGI Dec. 00]
   a. Osteolytic lesions in flat bones
   b. Subperiosteal erosions
   c. Osteoporosis
   d. Thick line just below growth plate
   e. Metaphyseal infarcts

76. **Neuroblastoma-good prognostic factor is:** [PGI June 2000]
   a. N-myc amplification
   b. RAS oncogene
   c. Hyperdiploidy
   d. Translocation

77. **Commonest sarcoma in children is:** [PGI Dec. 99]
   a. Rhabdomyosarcoma
   b. Lipoma
   c. Angiosarcoma
   d. Fibrosarcoma

78. **Commonest tumor of face in children is:** [PGI Dec. 99]
   a. Rhabdomyosarcoma
   b. Sq. cell carcinoma
   c. Basal cell carcinoma
   d. Mixed parotid tumor

79. **Opsomyoclonus is encountered as C/F of:**
    [PGI Dec. 99]
    a. Meningioma
    b. Neuroblastoma
    c. Neurofibromatosis
    d. Excision

80. **Chloroma is due to:** [PGI 99]
    a. AML
    b. CLL
    c. ALL
    d. Non Hodgkin's lymphoma

81. **Treatment of choice of intracranial ALL is:** [PGI 99]
    a. Intrathecal methotrexate
    b. Vincristine and prednisolone
    c. Intrathecal vincristine
    d. Prednisolone

82. **Most of the ALLs have:** [PGI 98]
    a. B-cell origin
    b. T-cell origin
    c. NK cell origin
    d. None

83. **Histiocytosis X is seen in:** [PGI Dec. 97]
    a. Hand-Schuller-Christian disease
    b. Eosinophilic granuloma
    c. Letterer-Siwe disease
    d. Torres syndrome

84. **Non specific esterase is present in:** [PGI Dec. 97]
    a. Megakaryocytic leukaemia
    b. Lymphocytic leukaemia
    c. Erythroleukaemia
    d. AML

85. **Child coming with proptosis, multiple skeletal limb secondaries, sutural separation is having:**
    [PGI 95]
    a. Neuroblastoma   b. Medulloblastoma
    c. Retinoblastoma   d. None of the above

86. **Neuroblastoma is:** [PGI 87]
    a. Associated with mild hypertension
    b. Rare tumor to undergo regression
    c. Commonest tumor of adrenal cortex
    d. Treatment excision and postoperative radiotherapy

87. **A 1-year-old child presenting with abdominal mass and calcification on X-ray is suggestive of:**
    [PGI 86, 93]
    a. Teratoma   b. Neuroblastoma
    c. Wilm's tumor   d. Rhabdomyosarcoma

88. **In the case of CNS relapse in AML, chemotherapy would consist of intrathecal:** [UPSC 97]
    a. Methotrexate
    b. Methotrexate + cytosine arabinoside
    c. Prednisolone
    d. Adriamycin

QUESTIONS OF OTHER EXAMINATIONS

1. **Wilms tumor is associated with the following except:** [UPSC 10]
    a. Aniridia
    b. Horse-shoe kidney
    c. Hemihypertrophy
    d. Opsoclonus

2. **Deletion of chromosome 11 leads to:**
    a. Wilms tumor
    b. Neuroblastoma
    c. Retinoblastoma
    d. Osteosarcoma

3. **Which is not a tumor of the first decade of life?**
    [DPG 10, AIIMS 92]
    a. Rhabdomyosarcoma
    b. Neuroblastoma
    c. Ameloblastoma
    d. Retinoblastoma

4. **A family of child just diagnosed with acute lymphoblastic leukemia asks about the child's prognosis. Which of the following is a poor prognostic indicator?** [UPSC 09]
    a. Presence of mediastinal mass
    b. Age between 1 and 10 years

    c. Hyperploidy with more than 50 chromosomes
    d. WBC count less than 50,000/mm^3 at diagnosis

5. **Acute leukaemia in children is associated with all except:** [DPG 09]
    a. Down's syndrome
    b. Klinefelter's syndrome
    c. Marfan's syndrome
    d. Turner's syndrome

6. **Most common benign tumor during infancy is:**
    [UP 07]
    a. Lymphangioma   b. Hemangioma
    c. Cystic hygroma   d. Lipoma

7. **The most characteristic radiographic sign in a child with leukemia is:** [COMED 06]
    a. Osteosclerosis of metaphysis
    b. Metaphyseal translucencies
    c. Periosteal reaction
    d. Osteolytic lesions

8. **Genetic risk factors for leukaemia are all except:**
    [Kerala 04]
    a. Down syndrome   b. Bloom syndrome
    c. Ataxia telangiectasia d. Turner's syndrome

9. **Which of the following statements is true of brain tumors in children?** [SGPGI 04]
   a. Is rare form of malignancy
   b. Most tumors are below the tentorium
   c. Hemiparesis is frequent form of presentation
   d. Papilledema is infrequent

10. **All are associate with malignancy except:** [MP 2000]
    a. Down's syndrome   b. Fragile X syndrome
    c. Bloom syndrome   d. Fanconi's anemia

11. **Retinoblastoma gene is located on:** [TNPSC 2000]
    a. Chromosome 5   b. Chromosome 8
    c. Chromosome 13   d. Chromosome 16

12. **A 5-year-old child is admitted with headache and difficulty in walking. Physical findings include truncal ataxia, papilledema and left lateral rectus palsy. No finger to nose ataxia could be detected on the left side or right side. The most likely diagnosis:** [UPSC 99]

    a. Dandy-Walker syndrome
    b. Syringobulbia
    c. Arnold-Chiari malformation
    d. Medulloblastoma

13. **A 2-day-old newborn baby presented with microcephaly, macroglossia, visceromegaly and a blood glucose of 20mg/dl. What is the most likely diagnosis?** [Orissa 98]
    a. Prader-Willi syndrome
    b. Beckwith-Wiedeman syndrome
    c. Werner syndrome
    d. Cockayne syndrome

14. **The chemotherapeutic agent used in Wilms tumor is:** [DNB 90]
    a. Vincristine   b. Methotrexate
    c. Chlorambucil   d. Actinomycin D
    e. Busulfan

ANSWERS

1. **(b)** Medulloblastoma (Ref: Nelson 19th E/P1706)
   - **Chang staging** used for medulloblastoma is based on the foundation of **surgery.**

2. **(b)** Medulloblastoma (Ref: Rudolph 22nd E/P1659)
   Poor prognostic factors of medulloblastoma are:
   - Extracranial metastasis.
   - Location outside posterior fossa.
   - Age less than 3 years.

3. **(c)** Testicular involvement (Ref: Rudolph 22nd E/ P1621–22)
   - **CNS** and **testicular involvement** is associated with poor prognosis.

4. **(b)** Seen at eighty years of age (Ref: Nelson 19th E/ P1704)
   - Astrocytomas are primarily tumor of **posterior fossa** which can be classified as low grade astrocytomas and high grade astrocytomas.
   - Low grade astrocytomas are most common in **first two decades i.e. children and young adults.**
   - **Juvenile pilocytic astrocytoma** (grade I) is the most common type of astrocytoma, which is most commonly located in the **cerebellum.**
   - These are brain tumors with **best outcome** after resection followed by **radiotherapy** and **chemotherapy.**

5. **(c)** Cladribine (Ref: CPDT 19th E/P878)
   - Refractory histiocytosis can be treated with **cladribine,** interferon α and etarnecept.

6. **(d)** t(9:22), t(8:14), t(4:11) (Ref: Rudolph 22nd E/P 1621–22)
   - **Hypoploidy, t(1; 19), t(9; 22), t(4; 11)** are associated with poor prognosis in ALL.

7. **(a)** Bone (Ref: Nelson 19th E/P1729)
   - **Bone lesions** are the most common presentation of Langerhans cell histiocytosis seen in 80% of patients.

8. **(d)** Monosomy 7 (Ref: CPDT 19th E/P 858)
   - **Good prognostic factors** are **t (8; 21), inversion 16,** t (15; 17), CEBPα gene mutation, NPM mutations and association of Down syndrome.
   - **Bad prognostic factors** are **monosomy 7,** monosomy 5, deletion of 5q, FLT3 gene duplication and abnormalities of 11q chromosome.

9. **(a)** Acute promyelocytic leukaemia (Ref: CPDT 19th E/P857)
   - Arsenic trioxide can be used for treatment of resistant cases of promyelocytic leukaemia.

10. **(b)** An immature T cell phenotype (Tdt/CD34/CD37) (Ref: CPDT 19th E/P 854)
    - **Anterior mediastinal mass** can be seen due to thymic infiltration in case of **T cell ALL.**

11. **(c)** Promyelocytic leukaemia (Ref: CPDT 19th E/P857)
    - This patient has complaints of bleeding along with thrombocytopenia, decreased fibrinogen and an increased level of both PT and APTT. This is consistent with DIC.
    - **DIC** can be seen in M3, M4 and M5 subtypes of AML; however is more common in **AML M3 subtype.**

12. **(c)** CD 15/34 both seen in same cell (Ref: CPDT 19th E/P856–58)
    - AML M3 subtype is also called as Acute promyelocytic leukaemia which is caused by t (15; 17).
    - Retinoic acid is the drug of choice; however arsenic trioxide can be used for resistant cases.
    - Promyelocytic leukaemia is the most common type of AML associated with DIC.

13. **(a)** Retinoblastoma (Ref: Nelson 19th E/P1722)
    - 60% of neuroblastomaare acquired and the remaining **40% are hereditary.**

14. **(c)** Clear cell sarcoma (Ref: Nelson 19th E/P1711)
    - Clear cell sarcoma frequently metastasises to the bones.

15. **(a)** CD1a (Ref: Nelson 19th E/P1728)
    - The definitive diagnostic procedure for Langerhans cell histiocytosis is biopsy of the lesions and demonstrations of histiocytes which are **CD1a positive** and have **Bierbeck granules** of **tennis racket shape.**

16. **(c)** Langerhans cell histiocytosis (Ref: Nelson 19th E/P1729)
    - Osteolytic lesions of mastoid bone can lead to **chronic ear discharge.**
    - **Seborrheic dermatitis** of the scalp and diaper area **(diaper rash)** is seen.
    - Bone marrow dysfunction can cause pancytopenia and compensatory extramedullary hematopoesis can lead to **hepatomegaly** and **splenomegaly.**

17. **(b)** Craniopharyngioma (Ref: Nelson 19th E/P1707)
    - Craniopharyngiomas are solid tumor with **cysts** and **calcification** located in the suprasellar region.
    - It presents with symptoms of compression of hypothalamo-pituitary axis(short stature is common) and **optic tract (visual field defects);** and hydro-cephalus.

18. **(a)** Bierbeck granules in the cytoplasm (Ref: Nelson 19th E/P1728)
    - The definitive diagnostic procedure for Langerhans cell histiocytosis is biopsy of the lesions and demonstrations of histiocytes which are **CD1a positive** and have **Bierbeck granules** of **tennis racket shape.**

19. **(d)** Midline posterior fossa tumor (Ref: CPDT 19th E/P862)
    - This patient presents with symptoms of cerebellar involvement.
    - Out of the given options midline posterior fossa tumor i.e. medulloblastoma is the correct answer.

20. **(d)** Hypodiploidy (Ref: Rudolph 22nd E/P1621–22)
    - Hypoploidy is a poor risk factor of ALL
    - Female sex, WBC count <50,000 and age 1-10 years has a good prognosis.

21. **(c)** Same location (Ref: (Ref: Gupta Diagnostic radiology: Pediatric imaging P250–55)

22. **(d)** Medulloblastoma (Ref: CPDT 19th E/P862)
    - Medulloblastoma arises from **midline cerebellar vermis** and extends in to **4th** ventricle causing hydrocephalus.

23. **(b)** Rhabdomyosarcoma (Ref: Nelson 19th E/P1714)

24. **(a)** Juvenile CML (Ref: CPDT 19th E/P858)

25. **(c)** Neuroblastoma (Ref: Nelson 19th E/P1709)

26. **(a)** Craniopharyngioma (Ref: Nelson 19th E/P1707)

27. **(b)** Craniopharyngioma (Ref: Nelson 19th E/P1707)
    - Craniopharyngiomas are solid tumor with **cysts** and **calcification** located in the suprasellar region.

28. **(c)** Ameloblastoma (Ref: Ghai 7th E/P793)
    - Ameloblastoma is a bone tumor commonly seen in adults.

29. **(c)** t (9; 22), t (4;11), t (1;19) (Rudolph 22nd E/P1621–22)
    - **Hypoploidy**, **t(1; 19)**, **t(9; 22)**, **t(4; 11)** are associated with poor prognosis in ALL.

30. **(d)** Immediately start induction therapy (Ref: Ronald's paediatrics/P355)
    - Hyperleukocytosis i.e. WBC count >100,000/μl can cause hyperviscosity associated thrombosis and haemorrhage which can damage organs like CNS, kidney and lungs.
    - Treatment is started with **hydration (IV fluids without potassium)** and leukophoresis. After this induction chemotherapy should be started and rapid destruction of cells can cause tumor lysis syndrome.
    - Tumor lysis syndrome should be treated with **alkalinisation of urine** (IV sodium bicarbonate) and **allopurinol**.

31. **(c)** Lung metastasis are common (Ref: Nelson 19th E/1709)

- Neuroblastoma commonly metastasises to bones, lymphnodes and liver but lungs are seldom involved.

32. **(a)** i.e. International society of pediatric oncology (SIOP) (Ref: Rudolph 22nd E/P1645)
Staging of Wilms tumor are of two types based on the time of staging in relation to surgery and chemotherapy.
    - **NWTS (National Wilms Tumor Study)** staging is based on the principle that **first surgery and staging** is done followed by chemotherapy.
    - SIOP **(International Society of Pediatric Oncology)** staging is based on the principle that **first chemotherapy** is given followed by surgery and staging.

33. **(a)** Monosomy 7 (Ref: CPDT 19th E/P 858)
    - **Good prognostic factors** are **t (8; 21)**, **inversion 16**, **t (15; 17)**, CEBPα gene mutation, NPM mutations and association of Down syndrome.
    - **Bad prognostic factors** are **monosomy 7**, monosomy 5, deletion of 5q, FLT3 gene duplication and abnormalities of 11q chromosome.

34. **(d)** These tumors are common in females (Ref: Nelson 19th E/P1704)
    - Cerebellar a strocytomas most commonly seen in children are low grade astrocytomas.
    - These tumors have a very good prognosis.
    - Most commonly affected age group are first two decades i.e. in children and young adults.

35. **(d)** M6 (Ref: Daniel's Hematopathology P 1673–75)
    - Nonspecific esterase is positive in monoblasts **(AML M4 and M5)** and Promyelocytes **(AML M3)**.

36. **(a)** Leukemia (Ref: CPDT 19th E/P 853)
    - ALL is the most common malignancy of childhood overall and in age group of 1–15 years.
    - The 2nd most common are CNS tumors.
    - In infants, i.e. till 1 year of age neuroblastoma is the most common tumor.

37. **(c)** Precursor B cell ALL (Ref: Rudolph 22nd E/P1621–22)
    - **Precursor B cell ALL**, B cell ALL and T cell ALL has poor prognosis.

38. **(a)** Mature B cell (Ref: Nelson 19th E/P1694)

FAB classification of blast cells in ALL:

Blast type	Features
L1	<ul><li>Most common type</li><li>Good prognosis</li><li>Small cells with scant cytoplasm and small nucleoli</li></ul>
L2	<ul><li>2nd most common type</li><li>Poor prognosis</li><li>Large pleomorphic cells with abundant cytoplasm and prominent nucleoli</li></ul>
L3	<ul><li>Least common type</li><li>Poor prognosis</li><li>**Large cells derived from mature B cells**</li><li>ALL L3 is also called as Burkitt leukemia</li></ul>

39. (b) Within 10 days (Ref: Rath Radiation oncology 1st E/P 679)

40. (a) Stage of the disease (Ref: Rudolph 22nd E/P1647) There are various prognostic factors; however **tumor stage** at the time of diagnosis is the **best prognostic indicator.**
- Good prognostic factors are early stage disease i.e. stage I and II, favourable histology, age < 2 years and tumor <500 grams.
- Poor prognostic factors are anaplastic histology characterised by huge hyperchromatic nuclei and hyperdiploidy, age>2 years, tumor>500 grams, late stage disease (III and IV), loss of heterozygosity of 1p and 16q and; renal vessel and capsule invasion.

41. (b) Neuroblastoma (Ref: Nelson 19th E/P1709)
- Metastasis is commonly seen in **long bones** and **skull** which may present with **bone pain**, **sutural separation**, **orbital proptosis** and periorbital ecchymosis.

42. (b) Neuroblastoma (Ref: Nelson 19th E/P1709)
- Neuroblastoma is the **most common solid tumor of children** and **most common malignancy of infants.**

43. (a) As asymptomatic abdominal mass (Ref: Rudolph 22nd E/P1644)

" The classical presentation of a child with Wilms tumor is sudden discovery of a large abdominal mass by a parent while bathing or dressing the child."

44. (a) Diploidy (Ref: Rudolph 22nd E/P1650)
- Good prognostic factors for neuroblastoma are age <1year at the time of diagnosis, stage 1 and 2 of disease and **hyperdiploidy.**

45. (a) Acute leukemia (Ref: CPDT 19th E/P854)
- History fever on and off along with symptoms of thrombocytopenia (petechial spots), anemia (pallor) and extramedullary hematopoesis (splenomegaly) confirms the diagnosis of acute leukemia.
- In ITP and aplastic anemia splenomegaly is usually not seen.
- Hypersplenism may present with splenomegaly, anemia and thrombocytopenia but the history of fever on and off goes against it.

46. (d) Presence of t (8; 21) (Ref: CPDT 19th E/P858)
- Good prognostic factors of AML are **t(8; 21)**, inv 16, t (15; 17), CEBP β gene mutation, NPM mutations and association of Down syndrome.

47. (b) Down syndrome (Ref: Rudolph 22nd E/P1626) **Transient myeloproliferative disorder:**
- Transient myeloproliferative disorder is caused by mutation in GATA-1 gene. It is associated with **Down syndrome.**

- It presents with leucocytosis (>50,000/μl), hepatosplenomegaly and hydrops fetalis.
- There is increased risk of AML in these babies.
- It resolves spontaneously without treatment.

48. (c) Histiocytosis X (Ref: Nelson 19th E/P1729)
- Osteolytic lesions of mastoid bone can lead to **chronic ear discharge.**
- **Seborrheic dermatitis** of the scalp and diaper area (**diaper rash**) is seen.
- Bone marrow dysfunction can cause pancytopenia and compensatory extramedullary hematopoesis can lead to **hepatomegaly** and **splenomegaly**.

49. (a) Mostly infratentorial (Ref: Nelson 19th E/P1702)
- The most common location of CNS tumors is **infratentorial**; however it follows an unusual pattern according to age, i.e. infratentorial in age group of 1–10 years and supratentorial in <1 year and > 10 years
- ICT can be raised due to obstruction of CSF, which can cause hydrocephalus and papilledema; however papilledema is rare in infants due to open sutures that can absorb the pressure.
- Most common tumor in children are leukemias.

50. (b) Oligodendroglioma (Ref: Nelson 19th E/P1705)
- Oligodendroglioma is a tumor of cerebral cortex characterised by calcification.
- Medulloblastoma, Ependymoma and cystic astrocytoma are posterior fossa tumors.

51. (b) Lymphoma and leukemia (Ref: CPDT 19th E/P 853)
- **ALL** is the **most common malignancy of childhood overall** and in age group of 1–15 years.
- The 2nd most common are CNS tumors.
- **In infants** i.e. till 1 year of age **neuroblastoma is the most common tumor.**

52. (a) Lytic lesion in skull with suture diasthesis (Ref: Nelson 19th E/P1709)
- Neuroblastoma most commonly metastasises to long bones and skull which presents with lytic lesions and suture separation.

53. (b) Lymphoblastic leukemia (Ref: CPDT 19th E/P855)
- CNS relapse of lymphoblastic leukemia is characterised by headache, nausea, vomiting, photophobia and cranial nerve palsies.
- Since systemic therapy don't penetrate well to CNS, **intrathecal methotrexate** or a combination of methotrexate, cytarabine and hydrocortisone is given every 2–3 months.

54. (a) Craniopharyngioma (Ref: Nelson 19th E/P1707)

55. (c) Astrocytoma (Ref: Nelson 19th E/P1704)

56. (c) Cerebellar astrocytoma (Ref: Nelson 19th E/P1704)
- Cerebellar astrocytomas are grade I tumors with best prognosis.

- The other tumors are higher grade i.e. ependymoma is grade II and ; medulloblastoma and glioblastoma multiforme are grade IV tumors.

57. (a) Glioma (Ref: Nelson 19th E/P1704)

58. (c) ALL (Ref: CPDT 19th E/P 854)

- Chest X-ray in patients of ALL shows mediastinal widening or enlargement. It is more common in T cell ALL.

59. (a) ALL (Ref: CPDT 19th E/P855)

- **Intramuscular L-asparginase** is used for the induction phase of treatment in **ALL.**

60. (c) Philadelphia chromosome is positive (Ref: CPDT 19th E/P860)

- Philadelphia chromosome is positive in CML and not juvenile CML.

61. (c) Polycystic kidney (Ref: Nelson 19th E/P1711)

62. (a) Neuroblastoma (Ref: Nelson 19th E/P1709)

Clinical presentation of neuroblastoma:

- Paraneoplastic syndromes like **Vasoactive intestinal peptide (VIP) syndrome** is characterised by **secretory diarrhoea** and **increased catecholamine** secretions can cause hypertension, tachycardia, **sweating** and **flushing.**
- Metastasis is commonly seen in **long bones** and **skull** which may present with **bone pain, sutural separation, orbital proptosis** and periorbital ecchymosis.

63. (c) Neuroblastoma (Ref: Nelson 19th E/P1709)

64. (b) Leydig cell tumor (Ref: Nelson 19th E/P1724)

Germ cell tumors in children:

- Teratoma
- Germinoma
- Yolk sac tumor
- Embryonal carcinoma
- Choriocarcinoma

Nongerm cell gonodal tumors:

- Sertoli-Leydig cell tumor
- Epithelial carcinomas
- Granulosa cell tumor.

65. (a), and **(d)** Neuroblastoma causes displacement of kidney inferolaterally without distortion of collecting system and Neuroblastoma crossing midline (Ref: Gupta Diagnostic radiology: Pediatric imaging P250–55) (See Table 1)

66. (e) Pleomorphic rhabdomyosarcoma (Ref: Nelson 19th E/P1714)

There are 4 subtypes of rhabdomyosarcoma.

- Embryonal, botryoid and alveolar type is common in children.
- **Pleomorphic rhabdomyosarcoma** is an **adult form** which is rarely seen in children.

67. (a), (b) and **(e)** Adrenals, Mediastinum and Neck (Ref: Rudolph 22nd E/P1648–49)

- Most common site involved in neuroblastoma is **adrenal gland** followed by paravertebral ganglia of the abdomen, pelvis, **mediastinum** and **neck.**

68. (a), (b) and **(e)** Aniridia, Genitourinary abnormalities and Macroglossia (Ref: Nelson 19th E/P1711)

Increased incidence of Wilms tumor is seen with:

- WAGAR syndrome (Wilms tumor, Aniridia, **Genitourinary abnormalities** and mental retardation).
- Denys-Drash syndrome.
- Frasier syndrome.
- **Beckwith-Widemann syndrome** (large organs e.g. **macroglossia**).
- Simpson-Golabi-Behmel syndrome.
- Sotos syndrome.
- Perlman syndrome.
- **Hemihypertrophy.**
- Neurofibromatosis.
- Sporadic **aniridia.**
- von Wilebrand disease.

69. (a), (c) and **(e)** Neuroblastoma, Retinoblastoma and Nephroblastoma (Ref: Kalevar clinical ophthalmology/P416–17)

Causes of proptosis:

1. Tumors:
   - Primary Orbital tumors like **retinoblastoma.**
   - Extension of bone tumors from orbit like Paget's disease and fibrous dysplasia.
   - Metastasis from distant tumors like **neuroblastoma, Wilms tumor.**
2. Metabolic diseases like Hand-Schuller-Christian disease, xanthomatosis and amyloidosis.
3. Systemic diseases like leukaemia and thyrotoxicosis.
4. Miscellaneous causes like cysts, trauma, inflammation and vascular lesions of orbit like **orbital varix (it causes reducible proptosis).**

Table 1

Neuroblastoma	*Wilms Tumor*
• Arises from **adrenal gland** most commonly and **displaces kidney downwards without affecting the collecting system.**	• Arises in the **kidney** and **compresses the parenchyma and collecting system.**
• Ill-defined mass which **crosses the midline.**	• Well-defined mass that **does not cross the midline.**
• Midline mass can compress **trachea** and **esophagus** and **paraspinal mass can invade spinal cord.**	• Extends in to **IVC** → heart →lungs →aorta.
• **Lungs** are the **least common** site of **metastasis.**	• **Lungs** are the **most common** site of **metastasis.**
• CT scan shows **calcification.**	• CT scan shows **tumor necrosis** and **haemorrhage.**

Also know:

Bilateral proptosis	Intermittent proptosis	Pulsating proptosis
• Cavernous sinus thrombosis	• Orbital varix	• A-V fistula
• A-V fistula in cavernous sinus	• Hemangioma	• Aneurysm of ophthalmic artery
• Leukaemia	• Recurrent infection	• Hemangioma
• Thyrotoxicosis	• Recurrent emphysema	

70. **(c)** and **(d)** Osteolytic lesions and Skull is commonly affected (Ref: Robins 7th E/P701–2)
    - Eosinophilic granuloma is more common in age group of **5–15 years.**
    - **Osteolytic lesions** are commonly seen and the most common location is **skull.**

71. **(b), (c)** and **(e)** Metaphyseal osteoporosis, Periosteal new bone formation, Transverse line of dark band below the growth plate (Ref: CPDT 19th E/P854)
    - X-ray of chest shows mediastinal wideningand anterior mediastinal mass.
    - X-ray of long bone shows features of **osteoporosis, periosteal elevation, growth arrest lines** and compression of vertebral bodies.

72. **(c), (d)** and **(e)** Prednisolone, L-asparginase and Vincristine (Ref: CPDT 19th E/P855)
    - Anticancer therapy with **prednisolone, vincristine,** daunorubicin, **L-asparginase,** 6-mercaptopurine and methotrexate are used for induction and consolidation.

73. **(a), (c), (d)** and **(e) (Ref: Nelson 19th E/P1728)**
    - The definitive diagnostic procedure for Langerhans cell histiocytosis is biopsy of the lesions and demonstrations of **histiocytes (antigen presenting cells).**
    - These cells are **CD1a, s-100 positiveand MHC II (HLA-DR)** positive and have **Bierbeck granules** of **tennis racket shape.**
    - Pituitary involvement can lead to **diabetes insipidus** and growth hormone deficiency.

74. **(a), (b)** and **(d)** Neuroblastoma, Wilms tumor and Pheochromocytoma (Ref: Nelson 19th E/P1709)
    Causes of abdominal mass with calcification:
    - Neuroblastoma
    - Wilms tumor
    - Pheochromocytoma
    - Adrenal cysts
    - Adrenal cortical carcinoma

75. **(b), (c)** and **(d)** Subperiosteal erosions, Osteoporosis and Thick line just below growth plate (Ref: CPDT 19th E/P854)

X-ray findings of long bone in patients of ALL:
- **Osteoporosis.**
- **Periosteal elevation.**
- **Growth arrest lines.**
- Compression of vertebral bodies.

76. **(c)** Hyperdiploidy (Ref: Rudolph 22nd E/P1650)
    - Good prognostic factors of neuroblastoma are age<1year at the time of diagnosis, stage 1 and 2 of disease and **hyperdiploidy**.

77. **(a)** Rhabdomyosarcoma (Ref: Nelson 19th E/P1714)

78. **(a)** Rhabdomyosarcoma (Ref: Nelson 19th E/P1714)
    - Rhabdomyosarcoma is the most common soft tissue sarcoma in children.
    - Most common location of rhabdomyosarcoma is head and neck region.

79. **(c)** Neurofibromatosis (Ref: Nelson 19th E/P1709)
    - Paraneoplastic syndromes like **Opsomyoclonus-myoclonus-ataxia syndrome**, VIP syndrome and increased catecholamine secretion are commonly associated with neuroblastoma.

80. **(a)** AML (Ref: Rudolph 22nd E/P1627)
    - **Chloromas** (Myeloblastomas or granulocytic sarcomas) are solid tumors of myeloid cells seen in bones, CNS and soft tissue of head and neck. These are **more common with the M2 subtype**.

81. **(a)** Intrathecal methotrexate (Ref: CPDT 19th E/P855)
    - Intracranial ALL can be treated by **intrathecal methotrexate** or a combination of methotrexate, cytarabine and hydrocortisone.

82. **(a)** B-cell origin (Ref: Nelson 19th E/P1694)
    Origin of ALL:
    - **Progenitors of B cell – 85%**
    - T cells – 15%
    - B cells – 1%.

83. **(a), (b)** and **(c) Hand-Schuller-Christian disease, Eosinophilic granuloma, Letterer-Siwe disease (Ref: Nelson 19th E/P1728)**
    The different syndromes included in Langerhans cell histiocytosis are eosinophilic granuloma, Hand-Schuller-Christian disease and Letterer-Siwe disease.
    - **Eosinophilic granuloma** is a **localised disease** characterised by not only proliferation of histicytes but also other cells and predominantly eosinophils.
    - **Hand-Schuller-Christian disease** is characterised by triad of **Calvarine bone defects, diabetes insipidus** and **exophthalmos.**
    - **Letterer-Siwe disease** is characterised by involvement at **multiple foci and organs.**

84. **(d)** AML (Ref: Daniel's Hematopathology P 1673–75)
    - Nonspecific esterase is positive in monoblasts **(AML M4 and M5)** and Promyelocytes **(AML M3).**

85. **(a)** Neuroblastoma (Ref: Nelson 19th E/P1709)

86. **(a)** and **(b)** Associated with mild hypertension and Treatment excision and postoperative radiotherapy (Ref: Rudolph 22nd E/P1650)

87. **(b)** Neuroblastoma (Ref: Nelson 19th E/P1710)
   - **Computer tomography** is the imaging modality of choice for abdominal neuroblastoma which shows **calcification** and haemorrhage.

88. **(a)** and **(b)** Methotrexate and Methotrexate + cytosine arabinoside (Ref: Dutcher's Neoplastic diseases of the blood/ P362)
   - CNS relapse treatment by **intrathecal methotrexate or a combination of methotrexate and cytarabine** is advocated by some protocols; however the response is poor as compared to ALL CNS relapse.

QUESTIONS OF OTHER EXAMINATIONS

1. **(d)** Opsoclonus (Ref: Nelson 19th E/P1712)

2. **(a)** Wilms tumor (Ref: Nelson 19th E/P1712)

3. **(c)** Ameloblastoma (Ref: Ghai 7th E/P793)
   - Ameloblastoma is a bone tumor commonly seen in adults.

4. **(a)** Presence of mediastinal mass (Ref: Rudolph 22nd E/P1622)
   - Presence of mediastinal mass is associated with poor prognosis.

5. **(c)** Turner's syndrome (Ref: Ghai 7th E/P580)

6. **(b)** Hemangioma (Ref: Nelson 19th E/P2167)
   - Hemangioma is the most common benign tumor of infancy.

7. **(b)** Metaphyseal translucencies (Ref: CPDT 19th E/P854)

   X-ray of long bone in leukemia shows:
   - **Osteoporosis.**
   - **Periosteal elevation and new bone formation** caused by leukemic cells infiltration.
   - **Growth arrest lines (metaphyseal translucent lines) is characteristic for leukemia.**
   - Compression of vertebral bodies.

8. **(d)** Turner's syndrome (Ref: CPDT 19th E/P856)
   Increase incidence of AML is associated with:
   - **Down syndrome.**
   - Congenital bone marrow failure (Diamond-Blackfan anemia, Kostmann syndrome).
   - DNA repair defect (Fanconi anemia, **Bloom syndrome, ataxia telangiectasia**).
   - Neurofibromatosis 1.
   - Wiskott-Aldrich syndrome.
   - Li-Fraumeni syndrome.
   - Radiation.
   - Drugs (alkylating agents and topoisomerase II inhibitors).

9. **(b)** Most tumors are below the tentorium (Ref: Nelson 19th E/P1704)

10. **(b)** Fragile X syndrome (Ref: Ghai 7th E/P580)

11. **(c)** Chromosome 13 (Ref: Nelson 19th E/P1722)
   - Hereditary retinoblastoma is caused by inactivation of both alleles of **tumor suppressor gene (RB1)** located on **chromosome 13.**

12. **(d)** Medulloblastoma (Ref: Nelson 19th E/P1706)
   - Truncal ataxia is seen with cerebella tumor like medulloblastoma.

13. **(b)** Beckwith-Wiedeman syndrome (Ref: Nelson 19th E/P1712)
   - Beckwith-Wiedeman syndrome is characterised by **visceromegaly**, hemihypertrophy, omphalocele and **macroglossia.**
   - It is associated with an increased incidence of Wilms tumor, Portwine hemangioma, hepatoblastoma, rhabdomyosarcoma, neuroblastoma, medullary sponge kiney and adrenocortical cancer.
   - **Hypoglycemia** can be seen due to increased insulin secretion.

14. **(a)** and **(d)** Vincristine and Actinomycin D (Ref: Nelson 19th E/P1713)
   - Chemotherapy is given in all stages of Wilms tumor.
   - For stage I and II **vincristine** and **actinomycin D** is used whereas for stage III and IV doxorubicin is also added to the regimen.

16

Infectious Disease

BACTERIAL INFECTIONS

Sepsis

- A child with positive blood culture for pathogenic bacteria is said to have bacteraemia. The events following bacteraemia can be SIRS, Sepsis, severe sepsis and septic shock.
- **SIRS** — Systemic Inflammatory Response Syndrome.

Criteria for SIRS

a. Leukopenia or leucocytosis adjusted for age.
b. Hyperthermia (>38.5) or hypothermia (<36).
c. Tachypnea: 2SD> above normal.
d. Tachycardia: 2SD>above normal for age (or bradycardia if younger than 1 year).

Note: SIRS is defined as existence of two of the above criteria and one must be either a or b.

- Sepsis is defined as SIRS along with proven or probable infection.
- Septic shock is defined as sepsis along with cardiovascular dysfunction.
- According to the time of onset sepsis can be classified as early onset and late onset.

Early onset sepsis	*Late onset sepsis*
• Develop symptoms in **less than 72 hours**	• Develop symptoms **after 72 hours**
• **Most common** cause in India is **Klebsiella > *Staph aureus***	• **Most common** cause in India is **Klebsiella > *Staph aureus***
• **Most common** cause worldwide is *E.coli* > Group B Streptococcus	• **Most common** cause worldwide is **coagulase negative Staphylococcus** > Group B Streptococcus
• Most commonly manifests as **Pneumonia**	• Most commonly manifests as **sepsis, pneumonia or meningitis**
• Source of infection is the **maternal genital tract**	• Source of infection is the **external environment of the hospital or community**
• Mortality rate is higher	• Mortality rate is lower than early onset sepsis
• Predisposing factors are: 1. **Low birth weight** 2. **Premature or prolonged rupture of membranes** 3. Chorioamnionitis 4. Maternal UTI 5. Multiple per vaginal examinations 6. Prolonged labour 7. Meconium aspiration	• Predisposing conditions are: 1. Low birth weight 2. **Lack of breast feeding** 3. Poor cord care 4. Pyoderma and umbilical sepsis 5. Skin damage

- **Diagnostic markers of sepsis:**
  - ❖ Blood for culture should be taken before starting the antibiotic therapy.
  - ❖ Total leucocyte count — **Leukopenia** is seen.
  - ❖ Absolute neutrophil count below 1800/mm^3 i.e. **neutropenia** is the best predictor of sepsis.
  - ❖ **Immature/Total neutrophil ratio** of more than 0.2 is a sensitive marker.
  - ❖ **Increased CRP** of more than 1 mg/dl is found is neonatal sepsis.
  - ❖ **High microESR** is specific for neonatal sepsis but less sensitive.
- **Treatment:**
  - ❖ Supportive management aims at maintaining adequate tissue perfusion and oxygenation.
    1. **Adequate tissue perfusion** is maintained by administrating I/V fluids (ringer lactate or normal saline) in the dose of 10 mg/kg, dopamine and dobutamine.
    2. **Adequate oxygenation** is maintained by providing oxygen by mask or hood.
  - ❖ Antimicrobial therapy should be started immediately as delay is associated with increased mortality. Thus until culture is awaited empirical therapy should be started in the form of **ampicillin plus gentamicin or ampicillin plus cefotaxime**. If drug resistance is suspected then **vancomycin plus cefotaxime/ceftriaxone** should be given.

Pertussis (Whooping Cough)

- Pertussis is an acute respiratory disease transmitted via droplets and caused by aerobic gram negative coccobacilli Bordtella Pertussis.
- It is also called **'100 day cough'** which corresponds to the duration of illness.
- **Bacteriology:**
  - ❖ Bacterium attaches to the respiratory ciliated epithelial cells and produces various toxins and products that cause the disease i.e. it **does not cause invasive disease**.

Toxin	Effect
Pertussis toxin	Prevents migration of lymphocytes to the area of infection, inhibits the function of neutrophils, macrophages, monocytes and lymphocytes
Bacterial adenylate cyclase toxin	Downregulates immune cell function and cell surface proteins
Tracheal cytotoxin	Destroys ciliated epithelial cells
Filamentous hemagglutinin, Pertactin and fimbrial agglutinogens	Promote bacterial attachment to ciliated respiratory epithelium

- **Clinical features:**
  - ❖ Incubation period ranges from **7 to 14 days.**
  - ❖ Most commonly affects infants less than 6 months of age as passive immunity acquired by transplacental antibodies provide little protection.
  - ❖ The most common source of infection is adults with undiagnosed pertussis.
  - ❖ The disease progresses in 3 periods namely catarrhal, paroxysmal and convalescent stages:

Catarrhal stage	Paroxysmal stage	Convalescent stage

• **Most contagious phase**
 	
• Manifests as common cold with rhinorrhea, sneezing and mild cough
	• **Most complications occur in this phase**
	
	• Manifests as:
	  ▪ Forceful coughing followed by vomiting
	  ▪ Characteristic inspiratory whoop is seen at the end of paroxysm when air is sucked in through a partially closed glottis
		• Coughing may become louder but less distressing
		
		• Gradually paroxysms of cough and vomiting decrease in frequency

- **Complications associated with pertussis can be divided in to following subcategories:**
  - ❖ Immediate complications that can result from forceful coughing are **subconjunctival and scleral haemorrhages,** petechiae in upper part of body, umbilical and inguinal hernias, subcutaneous emphysemas, rib fractures and brain haemorrhages.

❖ Infectious complications can result from secondary infection. Otitis media and pneumonia are the most common secondary infections.

❖ Non-infectious complications are —
- ❑ Oesophageal tears, hematemesis and malena caused by posttussive emesis.
- ❑ Atelectasis, emphysema, pneumothorax and **bronchiectasis.**
- ❑ **Hypoxic encephalopathy** and seizures.
- ❑ Carotid artery aneurysms.
- ❑ Weight loss due to malnutrition.

- **Diagnosis:**
  - ❖ Gold standard for diagnosis is recovery of Bacillus Pertussis in culture.
  - ❖ The most appropriate way to collect the best desired specimen is **nasopharyngeal aspiration**. However if it is not available then the next best way is to collect by a **Dacron or calcium alginate pharyngeal swab.**
- **Treatment and prophylaxis:** Macrolides (**Erythromycin,** Clarithromycin and Azithromycin) are drug of choice for both treatment and prophylaxis. Prophylaxis is indicated for 14 days after the last contact and is indicated regardless of prior immunization.

Diphtheria

Diphtheria is an infection of nasopharynx and skin caused by an aerobic, nonencapsulated, nonmotile, nonsporulating bacillus Clostridium diphtheriae.The bacteria affects locally by producing a pseudomembrane and systematically by diphtheria toxin.

Clinical Features

Based on the site of location of infection it can have a wide range of presentation.
- Respiratory diphtheria.
- **Primary nasal diphtheria:** It is more common in young children and infants. It is the **mildest form** of diphtheria.
- **Tonsillopharyngeal diphtheria:** It is the **most common** type of diphtheria which appears as areas of yellow or dirty white exudate adjacent to tonsils which later join to form pseudomembrane on the mucous membranes of the pharynx, tonsils and uvula. After few days the pseudomembrane changes to **greyish colour** because of haemorrhage. Initially the patient presents with sore throat and fever but in later stages dysphagia, headache and voice change can be seen. The enlarged **lymph nodes** and soft tissue edema gives the appearance of **'bull neck'.**
- **Laryngotracheal diphtheria:** These patients have high chance to develop suffocation because of edema of soft tissue and dense cast of respiratory epithelium. Resection of pseudomembrane and establishment of artificial airway should be done.
- **Cutaneous diphtheria:** It is characterised by nonhealing, punched out ulcer with brown grey membrane. It is caused by nontoxigenic strains. Extremities are most commonly affected.
- Mucocutaneous sites like ear, eye and genital tract are rarely affected.

Complications of Diphtheria

- Airway obstruction by pseudomembrane is commonly seen.
- Isolated peripheral nerve palsies or a symptom complex mimicking Guillian-Bare syndrome and degenerative changes in the nervous system can be seen.
- Myocarditis, pneumonia, renal failure, encephalitis, cerebral infraction and pulmonary embolism also can be seen.

Treatment

- **Diphtheria antitoxin** is administered empirically based on the estimated amount of toxin present.
- **Penicillin G or Erythromycin** is generally given to render the patient noncontagious. Antibiotics do not affect the course of the disease.

Congenital Syphilis

Syphilis is a sexually transmitted disease caused by a motile spirochete **Treponema Pallidum.** Pregnant females can transmit this infection to developing fetus resulting in congenital morbidity and mortality like still birth, spontaneous abortion, nonimmune hydrops, **premature delivery**, perinatal death and early or late congenital syphilis.

- **Early congenital (prenatal) syphilis:** The signs appear generally **within 2 years** of birth.
  - ❖ Usually skin lesions are absent in live born syphilitic infants but if present they are **bullous lesions of the skin on palm and soles.**
  - ❖ **Snuffles** — It is a **rhinitis** producing a serous discharge. It is the **earliest manifestation** of congenital syphilis.
  - ❖ **Parrot paralysis** — Pain can cause pseudoparalysis of either an arm or leg.
  - ❖ **Bone inflammation** — It is the **most common presentation** of congenital syphilis. **Osteochondritis** at metaphyseal plate, periosteal elevation and symmetrical osteomyelitic leisons are seen. **Femur > Tibia** are most commonly affected bones and tibia has a characteristic **moth-eaten appearance**.
  - ❖ The other presentations can be hepatosplenomegaly, lymphadenopathy, Coombs negative haemolytic anemia, thrombocytopenia, leucocytosis and glomerulonephritis that presents as nephrotic syndrome.
- **Late congenital syphilis:** The signs are generally seen after 2 years of birth in the first 2 decades of life. It is usually due to the chronic inflammation of teeth, bone, cartilage and CNS.
  - ❖ **Rhagades** — It is postinflammatory scarring beneath the nose.
  - ❖ **Saddle nose deformity** — Involvement of nasal cartilage can result in depression in nose.
  - ❖ **Hutchinson triad** which was described in 19th century includes:
    1. **Hutchinson teeth** — Screwdriver or peg shaped deformity of the upper central incisors of the secondary dentition.
    2. Interstitial keratitis.
    3. 8th nerve deafness.
  - ❖ **Mulberry molars** – Molars with extra cusps.
  - ❖ Saber shins – Anterior bowing of midportion of tibia.
  - ❖ Olympian brow – Frontal bossing of forehead.
  - ❖ Juvenile paresis –A meningovascular infection presents in adolescence with focal seizures, behavioural changes and loss of intellectual function.
  - ❖ **Clutton joints** – Bilateral knee effusions.
- **Diagnosis:**
  - ❖ The best and most specific way of diagnosis is to isolate Treponema Pallidum from the lesions by dark ground microscopy.
  - ❖ If treponemas are not visible in the lesion then diagnosis is difficult in the early days. The status of maternal infection and her treatment, serologic tests and clinical findings in the infant and bone X-ray and CSF evaluation are evaluated to confirm the diagnosis.
  - ❖ **VDRL** or RPR should be done on infant blood for diagnosis; however these are not specific and reflect the activity of disease process.
  - ❖ Serological tests are more specific and aim at detecting the antitreponemal IgM antibodies in baby's serum. The various tests for IgM detection are **FTA-ABS 19S-IgM, IgM capture ELISA and western immunoblotting assay.**
- **Treatment:** Treatment of choice is **aqueous or procaine penicillin G** for 10 days.

Neonatal Tetanus

- Tetanus is an acute illness caused by a very potent neurotoxin produced by an **anaerobic**, spore forming, gram positive bacterium called as *Clostridium tetani*. *Clostridium tetani* is usually found in the intestines of horse, cattle and is also normal human faecal flora.
- **Neonatal (umbilical) tetanus** is still the **most common form** worldwide because of the practice of applying animal excreta to the umbilical stump for haemostasis. The bacterium in the umbilical stump produces tetanospasmin and tetanolysin. **Tetanospasmin** also called as tetanus toxin plays vital role in pathogenesis of disease. It is transmitted via **axonal transport** to the motor nuclei of cranial nerves and ventral horns of spinal cord and then it is transported to **GABAergic synapses** where it blocks the release of inhibitory neurotransmitter GABA. This induces susceptibility of the neurons to reflex spasms and convulsions.
- WHO defines neonatal tetanus as an illness occurring in a child who has the **normal ability to suck and cry in the first 2 days of life** but who loses this ability between **days 3 and 28** of life and becomes rigid with spasm.

Clinical Presentation

- The **incubation period is variable**; however the mean incubation period is 5–12 days. Usually short incubation periods are associated with higher mortality rates.

- Typical manifestation of neonatal tetanus is **progressive difficulty in feeding.**
- **Trismus (masseter muscle spasm or lock jaw) is the most common presentation.** The patient has difficulty in swallowing and sucking and body is in extreme hyperextension (opisthotonos).
- Risus sardonicus, i.e. sardonic smile of tetanus due to intractable spasm of facial and buccal muscles can be seen.
- Laryngeal and respiratory muscle spasm can also be seen and **respiratory failure is the most common cause of death.**

Diagnosis

It is usually diagnosed clinically.

Treatment

- Supportive care in a quiet and dark place is required.
- **Metronidazole** is the drug of choice for eradication of *Clostridium tetani.*

Rudolph 22nd E/P1104–05
Recent data indicate that treatment with metronidazole instead of penicillin G improves survival and decreases disease duration. Harrison 18th E/chapter 140 Metronidazole (400 mg rectally or 500 mg IV every 6 hours for 7 days) is the preferred drug.

- **Human tetanus immunoglobulin** in doses of 3000–6000 units is given I/M for neutralisation of tetanospasmin.
- Treatment of anxiety, seizure and spasms is done by diazepam.
- For autonomic instability alpha and beta blockers are used.

Tuberculosis in Children

- Tuberculosis is caused by an **acid fast**, rod shaped, **aerobic** bacterium called as *Mycobacterium tuberculosis.*
- Congenital tuberculosis is rarely seen as the most common manifestation of genital tuberculosis in females is infertility.
- **Infants and children under 5 years** of age are the **most common** victim of childhood tuberculosis, whereas children between 5–14 years of age are called favoured group as they have the lowest rate of tuberculosis disease.
- There is no gender predilection in childhood tuberculosis whereas in adults males are more commonly affected.

Clinical Presentation

Though pulmonary tuberculosis is the most common form of tuberculosis encountered, extrapulmonary tuberculosis cases have gone up with the spread of HIV infection.
- **Pulmonary tuberculosis:**
  ❖ **Primary pulmonary tuberculosis —**
    ❑ Initial infection with tubercular bacilli gives rise to **Ghon** focus which is generally located to the periphery.
    ❑ **Ghons complex** – The primary site of infection (Ghon focus) with or without paratracheal and mediastinal lymphadenopathy, overlying pleural reaction and thickening is called as Ghons complex.
    ❑ Non-productive cough and mild dyspnea are the most common symptoms in children.
    ❑ The severity of clinical presentation in children is less as compared to the radiological changes seen.
    ❑ **Pleural effusion** is commonly seen.
  ❖ **Secondary tuberculosis —**
    ❑ It is usually not seen in children.
    ❑ It is caused by endogenous reactivation of primary infection.
    ❑ Usually located in the **apical and posterior segments of upper lobe** because higher oxygen tension favours growth of tubercular bacilli.
    ❑ The disease can progress in various directions from **cavity formation** and caseating pneumonia to **fibrosis** and calcification.
- **Extrapulmonary tuberculosis:**
  ❖ **Tuberculous lymphadenitis —** Tuberculosis of the superficial lymphnodes (**scrofula**) is the **most common form** of extrapulmonary tuberculosis in children. Most commonly involved nodes are supra clavicular and posterior cervical.

❖ **CNS Tuberculosis** — It is the most serious complication of tuberculosis in children. Lymphohematogenous spread of tuberculosis leads to meningeal and cerebral metastatic caseous leisons which further pass the tubercular bacilli to subarachnoid space. **Gelatinous exudates** are produced that cause infarction of cerebral cortex by invading blood vessels and **communicating hydrocephalus** due to obstruction at basal cisterns

❖ Disseminated or military tuberculosis is most common in infants and malnourished or immunosuppressed patients.

❖ Other forms of extrapulmonary tuberculosis like genitourinary, skeletal and gastrointestinal are rarely seen in children.

- **Perinatal tuberculosis:** Perinatal tuberculosis can be prevented by early diagnosis and treatment of the mother and child. If the mother has evidence of active disease, ATT should be started for mother and neonate should be started on **isoniazid** until mother is sputum culture negative for at least 3 months. However, no separation of the neonate from mother is required and **breast feeding** can be continued.

Diagnosis

The diagnosis is made by assessing the tuberculin test, chest x-ray, physical examination, history of contact with patient of tuberculosis and various diagnostic methods like sputum smear examination, sputum culture, PCR and ELISA.

- **Mantoux tuberculin test:** It is done by injecting 0.1 ml containing 5 tubercular units (TU) of purified protein derivative (PPD). After 48–72 hours the diameter of the induration is measured in millimetres. The test is positive if specific conditions are associated with a particular size of induration.

Positive with induration > 5mm	*Positive with induration > 10 mm*	*Positive with induration > 15 mm*
• History of contact with known case of TB.	• **Infants and children ≤4 years of age.**	• Children > 4 years of age and older without any risk factors.
• Positive chest x-ray finding.	• Associated medical conditions like DM and renal disorders.	
• Associated immunosuppressive conditions.	• Frequent exposure to adults at high risk.	
• Patients on immunosuppressive therapy.	• Birth or recent immigration (<5 yr) from a high-prevalence country.	

Treatment

- The **first line antitubercular drugs** that are used in children are i**soniazid, rifampicin, pyrazinamide and ethambutol.**
- **Second line drugs** used in children are streptomycin, kanamycin, amikacin, capreomycin, ethionamide, cycloserine, linezolid, clarithromycin, ciprofloxacin, ofloxacin, PAS and thioacetazone.

VIRAL INFECTIONS

Measles

- Measles virus is a spherical, nonsegmented, single-stranded, **RNA virus** that belongs to the family of **Paramyxoviridae.**
- It is killed by UV light and heat and as measles vaccine retains these properties, it needs **cold chain** for transport and storage.
- **Secondary attack rate** is usually **90%.**

Clinical Features

Measles gradually progresses in 3 consecutive clinical phases.

- **Incubation phase:**
  ❖ This is the time from infection to clinical disease.
  ❖ It is approximately **10 days to the onset of rash and 14 days to the onset of fever.**
- **Prodromal phase:**
  ❖ It usually lasts 3–5days and is characterised by low grade fever, cough and coryza.
  ❖ **Steiner's line** — It is diagnostic of measles and is a **transverse line of conjunctival inflammation along the eyelid margin.**

❖ Children with vitamin A deficiency develop severe ocular disease with corneal ulcers, scarring and loss of vision. Hence WHO recommends **vitamin A** to all children suffering from measles in doses of
   ❑ **1 lakh IU** — Children less than 12 months
   ❑ **2 lakh IU** — Children more than 12 months
❖ **Koplik spots** — It is pathognomonic of measles and appears 24–48 hours before the onset of rash. It is a bluish white dot surrounded by a red rose areola located on the buccal mucosa opposite to lower molars.

- **Final stage :**
   ❖ It is characterised by fever, rash, lymphadenopathy and splenomegaly.
   ❖ **High grade fever of 40–41°C** associated with chills can be seen.
   ❖ **Rash** begins as discrete, irregular, erythematous macule **behind the ear, on the neck and along hairline**, which descends to other parts of body in next 24 hours.

Diagnosis

It is usually diagnosed on clinical basis. The CDC case definition for measles requires 3 criteria.
- A generalised maculopapular rash of atleast 3 days duration.
- Fever of atleast 38.3°C.
- Cough, Coryza or conjunctivitis.

Treatment

- There is no specific antiviral therapy.
- Supportive care and antipyretics should be given.
- Antibiotics should be administered in case of secondary bacterial infections.

Complication of Measles

- **Interstitial Pneumonia (Giant cell pneumonia)** and measles inclusion body encephalitis are usually seen in immunocompromised children.
- **Otitis media and pneumonia** are **most common secondary bacterial infections**.
- Acute myeloencephalitis is the most common neurological complication. It is rare in children younger than 2 years.
- **Subacute sclerosing panencephalitis (SSPE)** is a **very rare delayed complication** of measles. It is usually seen 6–8 years post measles infection in children. Children develop ataxia, progressive mental deterioration and extrapyramidal dyskinesia.
- Thrombocytopenic purpura and laryngotracheobronchiolitis (Croup) can also be seen.

Rubella

- Rubella virus is a single stranded, enveloped, RNA virus which belongs to the Togaviridae family.
- It is spread by oral droplets or transplacentally to the fetus, causing congenital infection.
- The incubation period is from **14 to 21** days.

Postnatal (Acquired) Rubella

- Most characteristic sign is **lymphadenopathy of postauricular, occipital and posterior cervical lymph nodes.**
- **Forchheimer spots** are rose-coloured spots on the soft palate that may coalesce in to a red blush.
- **Rash** starts as irregular **pink macules on the face** and then gradually descends to other parts of body. It is called as kaleidoscopic because of its changing pattern.
- Fever is low or usually absent in children.

Congenital Rubella

- This is the **most serious complication** of maternal rubella infection, which occurs when she gets infected during the first trimester. Most common complication is **IUGR.**

- As a result of virus induce vasculitis it can affect various organs and tissues.

Organ affected	Manifestation
Organ of corti	Sensorineural hearing loss
Heart	• **PDA**
	• **pulmonary artery stenosis**
	• **ASD**
	• **VSD**
Eye	• **Retinopathy** is most common ocular lesion
	• Pearly nuclear cataract is most characteristic ocular anomaly
	• Microopthalmia
Brain	• **Mental retardation**
	• spastic diplegia
	• Autism
	• Microcephaly
Pancreas	IDDM
Lung	Interstitial Pneumonitis

- Other clinical findings are thrombocytopenic purpura (characterised by lesions called as **"blueberry muffins"**), hepatosplenomegaly, haemolytic anaemia and bulging anterior fontanel.
- **Diagnosis:**
  - ❖ **Ig M antibodies in the serum** confirms diagnosis as it is not transferred from mother to baby.
  - ❖ **A four-fold rise in Ig G titre** is also confirmative of diagnosis.
  - ❖ The virus can be cultured from the infant's nasopharynx, urine or tissue.

Mumps

- It is an acute viral infection caused by a nonsegmented RNA virus, which belongs to the genus **Paramyxovirus.**
- The virus is usually spread by direct contact, airborne droplets, fomites contaminated by saliva, and urine.
- **Incubation period** ranges from **14–24 days.**
- Patients are most infectious **1–2 days before onset of clinical symptoms.**

Clinical Features

- The prodromal period is characterised by low-grade fever, malaise, myalgia, headache, and anorexia.
- **Parotitis** is the **most common** presentation of mumps. Usually both the parotid glands are involved. **Submaxillary and sublingual glands** are less commonly involved.
- **Epididymoorchitis** is the **second most common** manifestation of mumps. It usually occurs in postpubertal males but infertility is rarely seen.
- **Oophoritis** rarely associated with infertility or premature menopause. It may present with mastitis.
- **Meningoencephalomyelitis** can have variable presentation depending on the pathogenesis.
  - ❖ **Primary infection of neurons** — If this is the principal cause then **parotitis appears along with or after the onset of meningoencephalitis.**
  - ❖ **Post infectious encephalitis with demyelination** — In this case encephalitis follows parotitis by 10 days.
- Pancreatitis is usually difficult to diagnose as elevated serum amylase level is also associated with parotitis. Cranial nerve palsies may lead to various complications, e.g. deafness. Ocular complications like dacroadenitis and optic neuritis may be seen. Myocarditis, endocardial fibroelastosis, arthritis and thyroiditis are rarely seen.

Diagnosis

Demonstration of mumps Ig M antibodies or a fourfold rise in mumps Ig G titre is considered diagnostic.

Treatment

Usually supportive treatment is required in the form of antipyretics, bedrest, and local support for orchitis.

Chickenpox

- Chickenpox is a highly contagious disease caused by varicella zoster virus (VZV) which belongs to the family **Herpesviridae.**
- Secondary attack rate is nearly 70–90%.
- Children **5–9 years** are the most commonly affected age group.
- Incubation period is around **10–21 days**.
- Patients are infectious **48 hours before the onset of vesicular rash** till **the vesicles are crusted i.e. 2–7 days after onset of rash.**

Clinical Features

- Prodrome may be associated with fever, malaise, anorexia, headache and occasionally mild abdominal pain that may occur **24–48 hour before the rash appears.**
- Temperature is moderately elevated, usually from 100–102°F which persists during the first 2–4 days after the onset of the rash.
- **Rash:**
  - ❖ Rash is characterised by **maculopapules, vesicles and scabs** in various stages of evolution (**pleomorphic rash**). The rash is usually **centripetal** as compared to small pox where rash is distributed on face and extremities.
  - ❖ The lesions appear first on the scalp, face or trunk and then gradually involve other parts of body. The other common sites of involvement are the oropharynx, vagina, eye lids and conjunctiva, whereas cornea is rarely involved.

Diagnosis

- **VZV IgM antibodies** are not used for diagnosis as the currently available methods are not reliable.
- A fourfold increase in the titre of **VZV IgG** antibodies is diagnostic.
- **VZV DNA** can be detected by PCR.
- **Tzank smear** — Multinucleated giant cells can be seen in nonspecific stains but it has low sensitivity and specificity as it cannot differentiate between HSV and VZV infection.

Treatment

- Antiviral drug **Acyclovir** drastically changes the course of disease. It should be started within 24 hours of appearance of exanthem for better results. Generally it is given for 7 days or until no new lesions have appeared for 48 hours.
- VZ Ig postexposure prophylaxis is given to immunocompromised children, pregnant women, and newborns exposed to maternal varicella. The dosage is 1 vial (125 units) for each 10 kg increment (maximum: 625 units) given intramuscularly as soon as possible but within 96 hour after exposure.

Congenital and Neonatal Chickenpox

- **Neonatal chickenpox:**
  - ❖ It is associated with a high mortality rate when the mother is infected **within 5 days before delivery (as after 5 days sufficient maternal VZV antibodies will cross the placenta and protect the baby) or 2 days after the delivery.**
  - ❖ Newborns whose mothers develop varicella 5 days before to 2 days after delivery should receive one vial of VZ immunoglobulin.
  - ❖ As neonatal chickenpox is highly fatal acyclovir should be given.
- **Congenital varicella syndrome:**
  - ❖ The virus can cause a wide range of **congenital defects** depending on the time of infection.

Organ affected	Manifestation
Limb development is affected when mother is infected at 6–12 weeks of gestation.	**Limb hypoplasia.**
Skin	• **Cicatrix or zigzag scarring of skin in dermatomal distribution.** • Hypopigmentation.
Eye	• Microopthalmia • Cataracts • Chorioretinitis • Optic atrophy.
CNS	• Microcephaly • Hydrocephaly • Calcifications • Aplasia of brain.
Other	• Anisocoria • Horner syndrome • Anal/urinary sphincter dysfunction.

❖ **Acyclovir is not indicated** for treatment of congenital varicella syndrome because the damage caused by fetal VZV infection does not progress postpartum, i.e. there is no persistent viral replication.

Complications

- **Secondary bacterial infections** are the most common complication of chickenpox in children. **Pneumonia** is the **most severe complication.**
- **Neurological complications** like cerebellar ataxia, encephalitis and **Reye syndrome** can be seen. Other rare neurological complications are Guillian-Barre syndrome, transverse myelitis and **aseptic meningitis.**

Erythema Infectiosum or Fifth Disease

- **Erythema infectiosum** or **"fifth disease"** is the most common manifestation of **Parvo virus** B19 infection, which belongs to the genus erythrovirus and has tropism for the erythroid precursors.
- The most common age group affected are from **5 to 15 years**. Transmission is by respiratory route via droplets and seasonal peaks are seen in late winter and spring.
- The incubation period ranges from **4 to 28 days**. The prodromal phase starts with upper respiratory symptoms, headache and **low grade fever**. This is followed by a week-long asymptomatic phase before appearance of rash in 3 stages. Thus **rash appears after one week of defervescence** (disappearance of fever).
- The erythematous rash begins on the **face** as raised, red maculopapular lesions on the cheek that coalesce and is described as **"slapped cheek appearance"**. This is followed by spreading of diffuse macular erythema to **extremities**, primarily on the extensor surface with sparing of palms and soles. Further central clearing of macular lesions gives a **lacy, reticulated appearance**. The rash resolves spontaneously but **tends to persist for 1–3 weeks.**
- The most common complication Parvo virus B19 infection is **arthropathy** (follows rash and is more common in adult and adolescent females); however transient aplastic crisis, myocarditis, non-immune hydrops fetalis and PPGSS (popular-purpuric "gloves and socks" syndrome) can also be seen.
- **IVIG** has been of some value in treatment of immunocompromised patients.

Roseola Infantum or Sixth Disease

- **Roseola infantum** (exanthem subitum i.e. sudden onset of rash) or **sixth disease** is caused by **human herpesviruses (HHV 6 and 7)**, which are large double stranded DNA viruses.
- The source of infection is adult saliva; however transplacental transmission (HHV 6) and transmission via bone marrow and organ transplantation has been reported. Incubation period ranges from 5–15 days and the most common age group affected is 6–15 months, as maternal antibody prevents the disease for first 6 months.
- The prodromal period is usually asymptomatic or associated with **mild upper respiratory symptoms** and mild cervical > occipital lymphadenopathy. This is followed by high grade fever ranging up to 40°C, which lasts for 3–5 days and ceases suddenly.

- The **time of defervescence (disappearance of fever) or 12–24 hours after defervescence coincides with the onset of rash**. The **rash begins** as pink coloured, discrete, slightly raised and non-pruritic lesions **on the trunk**, which spreads to the neck, face and proximal extremities and spontaneously resolves within 1–3 days.
- The complications associated with Roseola infantum are febrile seizures, mononucleosis like illness, hepatomegaly, meningoencephalitis and ulcers at the uvulopalatal junction (**Nagayama spots**).
- Diagnosis can be established by Ig G seroconversion>Ig M determination. Viral culture is the most specific method; however determination of viral DNA by PCR can also be used.
- Ganciclovir, cidofovir and foscarnet can be used for HHV 6, whereas only the latter two can be used for HHV 7.

Human Immunodeficiency Type 1 Infection in Children

- HIV is a RNA virus that belongs to the family retroviridae.
- The paediatric population almost always acquires the infection from the mother during:
  - ❖ **Pregnancy and delivery** — Most common period of transmission from the mother to the foetus is **perinatal period.**
  - ❖ **Breast feeding** — The breast milk of infected mother contains both free and cell associated virus. Hence **ideally breast milk feeding should not be done in developed countries,** where other safer alternatives like infant formula feeds are available. However in **developing countries like India** where diarrhea, pneumonia, and malnutrition are responsible for greater infant mortality, **breast feeding should be done.**
- **Risk of mother-to-child transmissions are:**
  - ❖ **23–30% before birth.**
  - ❖ **50–65% during birth.**
  - ❖ 12–20% via breast-feeding.

Clinical Features

- The presentation varies widely among infants, adults and children.
- **Infants** usually present with lymphadenopathy **hepatosplenomegaly, failure to thrive, c**hronic or recurrent diarrhea, **interstitial pneumonia and o**ral thrush.
- **Children** present with symptoms that are more common than adults are mentioned below:
  - ❖ **Pneumocystis Jiroveci pneumonia** is the **most common AIDS defining disease in children** and adults.
  - ❖ **Recurrent bacterial infections** — *Streptococcus pneumonae* infection is most common in children with HIV.
  - ❖ **Lymphocytic interstitial pneumonitis (LIP),** chronic parotid swelling and early onset of progressive neurologic deterioration can also be seen.
  - ❖ Most common neoplasms among HIV-infected children are non-Hodgkin's lymphoma, primary central nervous system lymphoma, and leiomyosarcoma. **Kaposi sarcoma** is quite common in adults but **rare in children.**

Diagnosis

- A diagnosis of HIV infection can be made with two positive virological tests obtained from different blood samples.
- Viral diagnostic testing should be performed within the first 2 days of life, at 1–2 months of age, and at 4–6 months of age.
- **HIV infection can be reasonably excluded:**
  - ❖ If an infant has had at least two negative virological tests at age ≥1 month of age with at least one test performed at ≥4 month of age.
  - ❖ If in older children, two or more HIV antibody tests are negative with a time gape of at least 1 month apart past 6 months of age.
- **Young infants** — Viral diagnostic assays useful in young infants i.e. **1–6 months of age** are:
  - ❖ **HIV DNA PCR** — It is the most preferred method.
  - ❖ **HIV RNA PCR** — More sensitive than DNA PCR.
  - ❖ **HIV culture** — Equally sensitive as DNA PCR.
  - ❖ **HIV p24 antigen immune dissociated p24** — It is highly specific than all other tests but less sensitive.
- In infants older than **6 months** detection of **anti HIV Ig A antibodies by ELISA** is diagnostic of HIV.
- In infants older than 18 months demonstration of **anti HIV Ig G antibody by ELISA** establishes the diagnosis of HIV infection.

Treatment

- **Antiretroviral agents that are used can be divided in to six categories:**
  1. **Nucleoside/tide reverse transcriptase inhibitors — Zidovudine (AZT)**, Didaanosine, Zalcitabine, Stavudine, Lamivudine, Abacavir, Tenofovir.
  2. **Nonnucleoside reverse transcriptase inhibitor —** Efavirenz, **Nevirapine**, Delavirdine, Etravirine, Rilpivirine.
  3. **Protease inhibitors —** Saquinavir, Indinavir, Ritonavir, Nalfinavir, Amprenavir, Atazanavir, Darunavir.
  4. **Fusion inhibitors —** Enfuvirtide, Maraviroc.
  5. Cytokine receptor inhibitors.
  6. **Integrase inhibitors —** Raltregravir, Elvirtegravir.
- The most effective combinations are two NRTIs with a PI or NNRTI. These combinations are known as HAART.
- **Prevention of perinatal transmission of HIV from mother to child:**
  - ❖ **Nevirapine** is given once to women in labour and **once to the infant during the first 48-72 hour of life**. It reduces perinatal transmission of HIV by 50%.
  - ❖ **Zidovudine** is given to the pregnant woman starting at as early as 4 week of gestation and continued during delivery and in the newborn for the first 6 week of life. It decreases the rate of perinatal HIV-1 transmission to <8%.

Infectious Mononucleosis

- Infectious mononucleosis is caused by a double stranded DNA virus called as **Ebstein-Barr virus (EBV)**, which belongs to the family of Herpesviridae.
- The incubation period is 30–50 days in which the virus spreads to whole of the lymphoreticular system.
- EBV infects lymphocytes and transforms them in to continuously growing lymphoblastoid cell lines with EBV induced antigens on the cell surface that causes the cellular immune response to virus.

Clinical Features

- The characteristic triad of infectious mononucleosis is **fever, sore throat and posterior cervical lymphadenopathy.**
- Splenomegaly is seen in half of the cases whereas hepatomegaly is quite rare.
- Pharyngitis and petechiae at the junction of hard and soft palate are commonly seen.
- Maculopapularrash can be seen which is more common with the use of ampicillin or other beta-lactam antibiotics.

Diagnosis

- Leucocytosis of 10,000–20,000 cells/mm³ is seen. Atypical lymphocytes i.e. lymphoblastoid cells account for 20–40% of atypical lymphocytes.
- **Paul Bunnel test:** Transient heterophile antibodies seen in infectious mononucleosis, also known as Paul-Bunnel antibodies, are IgM antibodies detected by the Paul-Bunnel-Davidson test for sheep red cell agglutination.

Treatment

There is no specific therapy. Rest and symptomatic treatment is done.

PROTOZOAL INFECTIONS

Congenital Toxoplasmosis

Toxoplasma gondii is an obligate intracellular protozoan, which is usually acquired per orally by eating food contaminated with cysts.

Clinical Presentation

- The baby presents with a **characteristic triad of chorioretinitis, hydrocephalus and intracerebral calcification. Chorioretinitis is the most common presenting symptom in neonates.**

- The other important findings are CSF abnormalities, anemia, thrombocytopenia associated rash, petechiae and ecchymosis, convulsions, jaundice, lymphadenopathy, hepatosplenomegaly, nephrotic syndrome, microcephalus, microopthalmia, mental retardation, optic atrophy and pneumonitis.

Mnemonic: **TOKCOPLASMA**
T — Thrombocytopenia associated rashes
O — Optic atrophy
K — Kidney abnormalities like nephrotic syndrome
C — **Cerebral calcification, Chorioretinitis**
O — **Oedema of brain (Hydrocephalus)**
P — Pneumonitis
L — Lymphadenopathy
A — Anemia
S — Spleno-hepatomegaly
M — Microcephaly, Microopthalmia
A — Abnormal CSF

Diagnosis

The serological methods are the mainstay of diagnosis; however toxoplasma culture can also be done.
- The best tests for diagnosis of congenital toxoplasmosis are **Ig M ISAGA (immunosorbent agglutination assay), Ig A ISAGA and Ig A ELISA.**
- Ig G can be detected by Sabin-Feldman dye test, indirect fluorescent antibody test (IG-IFA) and ELISA; however **Sabin-Feldman dye test is gold standard for Ig G antibodies.**
- Ig M can be detected by Ig M IFA and ELISA; however the latter is more sensitive and specific.
- Ig A can be detected by ELISA in cases negative to Ig M ELISA and hence **Ig A ELISA is more sensitive than Ig M ELISA.**
- Avidity testing is done to establish the time of infection as antibody avidity increases with time. The **Ig M titre** should be compared with **Ig G titre** for avidity testing.
- The other tests that can be used are indirect hemagglutination test (IHA), enzyme linked immunofiltration assay (ELIFA), PCR and lymphocyte blastogenesis to toxoplasma.

Treatment

Spiramycin should be used to prevent the vertical transmission of toxoplasmosis and treatment of congenital toxoplasmosis.

MULTIPLE CHOICE QUESTIONS

1. **Congenital toxoplasmosis-False is:** [AIIMS May 10]
   a. Diagnosed by detection of IgM in cord blood
   b. IgA is more sensitive than Ig M for detection
   c. Dye is gold standard for IgG
   d. Avidity testing must be done to differentiate between IgA and IgM

2. **Most common cause of sepsis in India within 2 months:** [AIIMS Nov. 09]
   a. *H. influenzae*
   b. *E. coli*
   c. Coagulase positive *Staph. aureus*
   d. Group B streptococcus

3. **A child with complaints of cough. Characteristic inspiratory whoop. Sample for investigation is:** [AIIMS Nov. 09]

   a. Nasopharyngeal swab
   b. Tracheal aspiration
   c. Cough plate culture
   d. Sputum culture

4. **Most common cause of neonatal sepsis in hospitals in India is:** [AIIMS May 07]
   a. *Escherichia coli*   b. *Klebsiella*
   c. *Staph. aureus*   d. *Listeria monocytogens*

5. **Which drug is given to prevent HIV transmission from mother to child:** [AIIMS Nov. 06]
   a. Nevirapine   b. Lamivudnie
   c. Stavudine   d. Abacavir

6. **Which of the following does not establish a diagnosis of congenital CMV infection in a neonate?** [AIIMS May 06]

a. Urine culture of CMV

b. IgG CMV antibodies in blood

c. Intranuclear inclusion bodies in hepatocytes

d. CMV viral DNA in blood by polymerase chain reaction

7. **A 30 years old lady delivered a healthy baby at 37 weeks of gestation. She was a known case of chronic hepatitis B infection. She was positive for HBsAG but negative for HBeAG. Which of the following is the most appropriate treatment for the baby?** [AIIMS Nov. 05]

a. Both active and passive immunization soon after birth

b. Passive immunization soon after birth and active immunization at 1 year of age

c. Only passive immunization soon after birth

d. Only active immunization soon after birth

8. **Dengue shock syndrome is characterized by the following except:** [AIIMS May 05]

a. Hepatomegaly   b. Pleural effusion

c. Thrombocytopenia   d. Decreased hemoglobin

9. **Which of the following is true of mumps?** [AIIMS May 05]

a. Salivary gland involvement is limited to the parotids

b. The patient is not infectious prior to clinical parotid enlargement

c. Meningoencephalitis can precede parotitis

d. Mumps orchitis frequently leads to infertility

10. **All of the following strategies are effective in preventing mother to child transmission of HIV, except:** [AIIMS Nov. 03]

a. Zidovudine to mother and baby

b. Vaginal cleansing before delivery

c. Stopping breast feeding

d. Elective cesarean section

11. **All of the following methods are used for the diagnosis of HIV infection in a 2-months old child, except:** [AIIMS May 03]

a. DNA-PCR   b. Viral culture

c. HIV ELISA   d. p24 antigen assay

12. **An 8 years old female child following URTI developed maculopapular rash on the jaw spreading onto the trunk which cleared on the 3rd day without desquamation and tender post auricular and sub-occipital lymphadenopathy. The diagnosis is:** [AIIMS May 01]

a. Kawasaki disease   b. Erythema infectiosum

c. Rubella   d. Measles

13. **A child with fever and sore throat developed acute cervical lymphadenopathy, most likely investigation to be done is:** [AIIMS June 2000]

a. Open biopsy of node   b. Radical neck dissection

c. Neck x-ray   d. Complete hemogram

14. **A patient had fever and coryza for last 3 days developed maculopapular erythematous rash which lasted for 48 hours and disappeared without leaving behind pigmentation is most commonly due to:** [AIIMS June 00]

a. Measles   b. Typhoid

c. Roseola infantum   d. Fifth disease

15. **A child with fever and sore throat developed acute cervical lymphadenopathy most likely investigation to be done is :** [AIIMS June 00]

a. Open biopsy of node   b. Radical neck dissection

c. Neck X-ray   d. Complete hemogram

16. **In a 6 months old baby, floppy infant syndrome is seen commonly due to infection with:** [AIIMS June 00]

a. *Clostridium welchii*

b. *Clostridium tetani*

c. *Clostridium botulinum*

d. *Clostridium septicum*

17. **All are true about congenital rubella syndrome except:** [AIIMS 99]

a. Cardiac abnormality   b. Renal anomalies

c. Deafness   d. Cataract

18. **True about HIV in the neonate includes all the following except:** [AIIMS 99]

a. Cannot be diagnosed accurately by current methods

b. Failure to thrive may be presentation

c. Transmission rate during pregnancy exceeds 90%

d. Transmission vertically from mother

19. **HIV in children, characteristic finding is:** [AIIMS Dec. 98]

a. Kaposi sarcoma is common

b. Recurrent candidiasis

c. Recurrent chest infection

d. Cryptococcal diarrhea is common

20. **Regarding HIV transmission to fetus all are true except:** [AIIMS 98]

a. > 50% risk of transmission to fetus

b. Can present as failure to thrive

c. Greatest risk of transmission of in perinatal period

d. Cannot be diagnosed

21. **Erythema infectiosum is seen in:** [AIIMS Dec. 97]

a. Rubella   b. Fifth disease

c. Scarlet fever   d. Diphtheria

22. **Diarrhea syndrome in an AIDS patient can be d/t:** [AIIMS June 97]

a. Rota virus   b. Cryptospora

c. Adenovirus   d. E. coli

23. **Which of the following is not a feature of HIV infection in childhood?** [AIIMS Dec. 1994]

a. Failure to thrive

b. Hepatomegaly

c. Lymphoid interstitial pneumonitis

d. Kaposi sarcoma

24. **Which of the following is not a usual feature of Ascariasis?** [AIIMS 92]

   a. Abdominal pain   b. Urticaria

   c. Anemia   d. Loeffler syndrome

25. **The antibiotic of choice of pertussis is:**
   [AIIMS 79, AP 90]

   a. Ampicillin   b. Gentamicin

   c. Erythromycin   d. Penicillin

26. **Transplacental spread is least associated with:**
   [AI 11]

   a. HBV   b. Rubella

   c. HSV   d. HIV

27. **Vaccine with best efficacy:** [AI 09]

   a. TT   b. DPT

   c. Measles   d. Typhoid

28. **Which of the following intrauterine infections is associated with limb reduction defects and scarring of skin?** [AI 09]

   a. Varicella virus   b. Herpes virus

   c. Rubella   d. Parvo virus

29. **Resistant *Plasmodium falciparum* malaria in the pediatric age group should be treated by:** [AI 08]

   a. Chloroquine   b. Tetracycline

   c. Clindamycin   d. Doxycycline

30. **A premature baby of 34 weeks was delivered. The baby had a bullous lesion on the body and X-ray showed periostitis what will be the next diagnostic procedure :** [AI 07]

   a. VDRL of mother and baby

   b. ELISA for HIV

   c. PCR for Herpes

   d. HBsAg for mother

31. **All of the following statements are true about congenital rubella except:** [AI 05]

   a. It is diagnosed when the infant has IgM antibodies at birth

   b. It is diagnosed when IgG antibodies persist for more than 6 months

   c. Most common congenital defects are deafness, cardiac malformation and cataract

   d. Infection after 16 weeks of gestation results in major congenital defects

32. **A 10-month-old child presents with two weeks history of fever, vomiting and alteration of sensorium cranial CT scan reveals basal exudates and hydrocephalus, the most likely etiological agent is:** [AI 04]

   a. *Mycobacterium tuberculosis*

   b. *Cryptococcus neoformans*

   c. *Listeria monocytogens*

   d. *Streptococcus pneumoniae*

33. **Which one of the following hepatitis viruses have significant perinatal transmission?** [AI 03]

   a. Hepatitis E virus   b. Hepatitis C virus

   c. Hepatitis B virus   d. Hepatitis A virus

34. **A 45-day-old infant developed icterus and two days later symptoms and signs of acute liver failure appeared. Child was found to be positive for HBsAg. The mother was also HBsAg carrier. The mother's hepatitis B serological profile is likely to be:** [AI 03]

   a. HBsAg positive only

   b. HBsAg and HBeAg positivity

   c. HBsAg and anti-HBe antibody positivity

   d. Mother infected with mutant HBV

35. **A 5-year-old boy is detected to be HBs Ag positive on two separate occasions during a screening program for hepatitis B. He is otherwise asymptomatic. Child was given three doses of recombinant hepatitis B vaccine at the age of one year. His mother was treated for chronic hepatitis B infection around the same time. The next relevant step for further investigating the child would be to:** [AI 03]

   a. Obtain HBeAg and anti-HBe levels

   b. Obtain anti HBs levels

   c. Repeat HBsAg

   d. Repeat another course of Hepatitis B vaccine

36. **An 8-year-old boy presented with fever and bilateral cervical lymphadenopathy with prior history of sore throat. There was no hepatomegaly. The peripheral blood smear shows > 20% lymphoplasmacytoid cells. The most likely diagnosis is:**
   [AI 02]

   a. Influenza

   b. Tuberculosis

   c. Infectious mononucleosis

   d. Acute lymphoblastic leukemia

37. **Which of the following is not a common manifestation of congenital Rubella?** [AI 02]

   a. Deafness   b. PDA

   c. Aortic stenosis   d. Mental retardation

38. **Congenital syphilis can be best diagnosed by:**
   [AI 01]

   a. IgM FTA- ABS   b. IgG FTA-ABS

   c. VDRL   d. TPI

39. **Management of a newborn when mother has active tuberculosis and is taking ATT:** [AI 00]

   a. BCG + Rifampicin + INH + Breast feeding

   b. BCG +Isolation of baby

   c. BCG +INH for 6 week + Breast feeding

   d. BCG + INH + withhold Breast feeding

40. **Commonest complication of mumps is:** [AI 00]

   a. Orchitis and oophoritis

   b. Encephalitis

   c. Pneumonia

   d. Myocarditis

41. **A 7-day-old infant develops symptoms of neonatal septicemia. Most likely cause is:**   [AI 98]
    a. Local nursery environment
    b. Infection through umbilical cord
    c. Exclusively breast fed baby
    d. Infection by GIT bacteria

42. **Which of the following is the least common complication of measles?**   [AI 98]
    a. Diarrhoea   b. Pneumonia
    c. Otitis media   d. SSPE

43. **Least observed laboratory finding neonatal sepsis is:**   [AI 96]
    a. Increased C-reactive protein
    b. Neutrophilia
    c. Increased ESR
    d. Increased Immature Neutrophils

44. **All of the following are true about neonatal sepsis except:**   [AI 96]
    a. Preterm babies are predisposed to sepsis
    b. Late initiation of breast feeding is a predisposition
    c. Most common transmission of infection is through nursery personnel
    d. Premature rupture of membrane predisposes to sepsis

45. **Which heart diseases is most commonly associated with rubella infection?**   [AI 96]
    a. PDA   b. VSD
    c. ASD   d. Eisenmenger's syndrome

46. **Which of the following methods can be used to detect rubella infection in children?**   [AI 95]
    a. T$_4$ cell count
    b. Fetal haemoglobin
    c. IgM antibody in fetal serum
    d. IgA antibody in fetal blood

47. **Which of the following is true regarding typhoid in children?**   [AI 94]
    a. Leucocytosis is characteristic
    b. Encephalitis is common
    c. Mild splenomegaly is usual
    d. Urine culture is positive in 4 to 6 days

48. **Following are the complications of chickenpox except:**   [AI 93]
    a. Meningitis   b. Pneumonia
    c. Enteritis   d. Reyes syndrome

49. **Congenital Rubella syndrome in associated with anomalies?**   [PGI Nov. 09]
    a. VSD   b. ASD
    c. PDA   d. Coarctation of aorta
    e. Pulmonary stenosis

50. **True statement(s) regarding feeding of HIV infected child is/are:**   [PGI Dec. 08]
    a. Breast feeding for 4–6 months then start weaning
    b. Breast feeding for 1 year then start weaning

    c. Exclusive top feeding
    d. Breast feeding for 6 moths then rapid weaning

51. **Drugs used to prevent HIV from mother to child:**   [PGI Dec. 08]
    a. Zidovudine to mother
    b. Nevirapine to mother
    c. Nevirapine to baby up to 6 weeks
    d. Zidovudine to baby

52. **Perinatal prevention of HIV from mother to child, which of the following steps are useful:**   [PGI Dec. 08]
    a. Cleaning mothers vagina with antiseptic lotion
    b. Elective caesarean section
    c. Avoid breast feeding
    d. ART prophylaxis

53. **Vaccines contraindicated in HIV positive child:**   [PGI Dec. 08]
    a. OPV   b. MMR
    c. Rabies   d. Influenza
    e. Hepatitis

54. **A child presents with generalized petechiae. CSF shows gram negative diplococci. Treatment of choice:**   [PGI Nov. 07]
    a. IV ceftriaxone   b. IV cefotaxime
    c. IV penicillin G   d. IV ampicillin
    e. IV ofloxacin

55. **Child (girl) is suffering from varicella (fever, rash). And child's aunt is pregnant. When is it earliest that the child can meet her aunt:**   [PGI 2006]
    a. When the lesions have crusted
    b. Immediately
    c. Anytime as the child is aunt's favorite
    d. After the delivery of the baby

56. **Drugs included in ATT for children:**   [PGI June 06]
    a. Streptomycin   b. Ethionamide
    c. Ethambutol   d. Pyrazinamide
    e. Ofloxacin

57. **True about measles:**   [PGI Dec. 05]
    a. Rash appears first on leg
    b. Koplik spots are seen in retina
    c. Long-term complication follows in the form of SSPE
    d. Caused by RNA virus
    e. IP is 2–3 days

58. **First line ATT in children:**   [PGI June 05]
    a. Streptomycin   b. Pyrazinamide
    c. Ethionamide   d. Ethambutol
    e. Ofloxacin

59. **True about measles:**   [PGI June 04]
    a. Koplik spots appear in prodromal stage
    b. Fever stops after onset of rash
    c. Vaccine is given at 9 months
    d. It is not diagnosed when coryza and rhinitis is absent

60. **Which of the following is true about Roseola infantum?** [PGI Dec. 05]
    a. Defervescence follows the rash
    b. Caused by HHV 6 and 7
    c. Slapped cheek appearance is seen
    d. Otitis media is common complication
    e. Rash appears first on face and neck

61. **Which of the following is true about erythema infectiosum?** [PGI Dec. 05]
    a. Slapped cheek appearance seen
    b. Caused by parvovirus
    c. Defeverscence before rash
    d. Rash appears on head and neck

62. **True about neonatal sepsis:** [PGI June 03]
    a. Meningitis commonly occur lately
    b. Jaundice predisposes
    c. Fever
    d. Jaundice is a common feature

63. **SSPE (subacute sclerosing panencephalitis) is associated with:** [PGI June 01]
    a. Mumps
    b. Chickenpox
    c. Herpes
    d. Measles

64. **True about chickenpox:** [PGI June 01]
    a. I.P. 2–3 days
    b. Scabs are infective
    c. Centrifugal rash
    d. Rash appears on first day
    e. Rash can occur in axilla

65. **M/C complication of chickenpox in children:** [PGI June 00]
    a. Encephalitis
    b. Secondary bacterial infection
    c. Pneumonia
    d. Otitis media

66. **Cong. rubella manifestations are all except:** [PGI June 00]
    a. Rash appears first on trunk
    b. Pre-auricular lymph nodes
    c. Arthralgia
    d. Retinopathy

67. **Pertussis affects which age:** [PGI June 2000]
    a. 2–3
    b. <5
    c. 5–7
    d. > 10 years

68. **Measles is infectious during:** [PGI Dec. 98]
    a. After 4 days of rash
    b. 4 days before and 5 days after rash
    c. Throughout disease
    d. Only in incubation period

69. **Giant cell pneumonia is due to:** [PGI Dec. 98]
    a. CMV
    b. Measles
    c. Malaria
    d. P.Carinii

70. **Infant of HIV positive mother, which should be done:** [PGI June 98]
    a. BCG vaccine should not be given
    b. AZT therapy
    c. Separation from mother
    d. Other than BCG, all other vaccines are given

71. **Most common cause of HIV infection in infant is:** [PGI June 97]
    a. Perinatal transmission
    b. Breast milk
    c. Transplacental
    d. Umbilical cord sepsis

72. **Measles virus is:** [PGI 97]
    a. Paramyxovirus
    b. Orthomyxovirus
    c. Poxvirus
    d. Picorna virus

73. **Which of the following is the most common congenital viral infection?** [UPSC 10]
    a. Rubella
    b. Cytomegalovirus
    c. Herpes simplex
    d. HIV

74. **Incubation period of mumps is:** [MHCET 10]
    a. 5–7 days
    b. 8–15 days
    c. 14–24 days
    d. 24–30 days

75. **All of the following are features of mumps except:** [DPG 09]
    a. Caused by paramyxovirus
    b. Aseptic meningitis is a complication in children
    c. Orchitis is a complication in adults
    d. Incubation period is less than 2 weeks

76. **Which of the following is the common clinical manifestation of human parvovirus B 19 (HPV-B19) infection?** [UPSC 09]
    a. Aplastic crisis in hemolytic anemia patients
    b. Anemia in neonatal period
    c. Erythema infectiosum
    d. Hydrops fetalis

77. **Thrombocytopenia, macerated skin lesions, rash and periostitis in a newborn are seen in:** [COMED 09]
    a. Erythroblastosis fetalis
    b. Cytomegalovirus infection
    c. Syphilis
    d. HIV infection

78. **Which microorganism is responsible for classical presentation of hydrocephalus, chorioretinitis, intracerebral calcification?** [APPG 08]
    a. Toxoplasmosis
    b. Rubella
    c. Measles
    d. CMV

79. **Hutchison's triad is seen in:** [Manipal 06]
    a. Primary syphilis
    b. Congenital syphilis
    c. Secondary syphilis
    d. Tertiary syphilis

80. **The most common manifestation of congenital toxoplasmosis is:** [Manipal 06]
    a. Hydrocephalus
    b. Chorioretinitis

c. Hepatosplenomegaly

d. Thrombocytopenia

81. **Newborns have transplacentally acquired immunity against all of the following diseases except:**
[SGPGI 05]

a. Measles
b. Pertussis

c. Diphtheria
d. Poliomyelitis

82. **A 6-month-old baby was brought c/o difficulty in feeding. The child was found to be hypotonic with a weak gag. The chid is on breast milk and mother also gives honey to child during periods of excessive crying. The causative agent is:** [J and K 05]

a. Gram-positive aerobic coccus

b. Gram-positive anaerobic spre-suffering bacillus

c. Toxin produced by gram-positive anaerobic bacillus

d. Echovirus

83. **Which positive test does not necessarily indicate HIV infection in a newborn?** [KCET 04]

a. ELISA for HIV Ig G antibody

b. P24 antigen

c. Virus culture

d. ELISA for HIV Ig A antibody

84. **Roseola infantum is caused by:** [Kerala 04]

a. Herpes virus 6
b. Parvovirus B 19

c. Echovirus 19
d. All of the above

85. **In congenital infection with intracranial calcification most probable etiology is:** [JIPMER 03]

a. Toxoplasmosis

b. Cryptococcus meningitis

c. Cytomegalovirus infection

d. Cerebral abscess

86. **True about Roseola infantum:** [PGM June 03]

a. Also called 5th disease

b. Caused by HHV 6 and 7

c. Rash appear in trunk

d. During defervescence, rash appears

87. **10 years old child with 10 days continuous fever with soft, enlarged spleen, diagnosis is:**
[JIPMER 02]

a. Enteric fever
b. Malaria

c. Hodgkin's disease
d. Meningitis

88. **The etiological agent for roseola infantum is:**
[JIPMER 02]

a. Parvovirus
b. Human herpes virus 6

c. CMV
d. EBV

89. **The following age group is most severely affected by rubella infection:** [JIPMER 02]

a. Females aged 25–35 years

b. Young girls

c. Adolescent girls

d. Unborn child

90. **Which of the following is best used in the diagnosis of congenital syphilis?** [JIPMER 2000]

a. FTA-ABS
b. TPHA

c. IgM-FTA ABS
d. TPI

91. **The commonest route of transmission of HIV from mother to the baby is:** [UPSC 99]

a. Vertical transmission during pregnancy

b. During delivery through vagina

c. Breast milk

d. Constant touch and handling

92. **The risk of neonatal chickenpox is maximum if maternal infection occurs:** [UPSC 98]

a. During the first trimester

b. During the second trimester

c. Within five days of delivery

d. Within six weeks of delivery

93. **A 2-year-old child has a Mantoux test reading of 12 mm × 12 mm after 48 hours. In this case:**
[UPSC 98]

a. Anti TB drugs should be started even if x-ray chest and hemogram are normal

b. Treatment should be started only if x-ray cheat and hemogram are suggestive

c. One should wait till overt sign of TB appear

d. No treatment is required

94. **% of HIV infection in a child of HIV +ve mother is:**
[Kerala 97]

a. 20–30%
b. 10–20%

c. 70–80%
d. 100%

95. **The transmission of AIDS transplacentally is:**
[Kerala 97]

a. 10–20%
b. 20–30%

c. 30–40%
d. 40–50%

96. **Pleomorphic rash is a feature of:** [DPG 96]

a. Chickenpox

b. Smallpox

c. Erythema infectiosum

d. Erythema subitum

97. **In early congenital syphilis, which is not seen:**
[UP 96]

a. Keratitis
b. Vesicular rash

c. Chorioretinitis
d. Rhinitis

98. **Fever stops and rash begins is diagnostic of:**
[JIPMER 95]

a. Fifth disease
b. Roseola infantum

c. Measles
d. Toxic shock syndrome

99. **A line of conjunctival inflammation on the lower eyelid margin is diagnostic of:** [JIPMER 95]

a. Measles

b. Rubella

c. Kawasaki disease

d. Infectious mononucleosis

100. Complications of measles are all except:

[JIPMER 95]

a. Myocarditis   b. Appendicitis

c. SSPE   d. Pancreatitis

101. A poverty-stricken mother suffering from active tuberculosis delivers a baby. Which one of the following advises would be the most appropriate in her case?

a. Breast feeding and BCG immunization

b. Breast feeding and isoniazid administration

c. Expressed breast milk and BCG immunization

d. Stop feeds and isoniazid administration

102. Colour of diphtheric membrane is: [JIPMER 95]

a. Grey   b. White

c. Yellow   d. Cream

103. A child born with microcephaly, chorioretinitis and intracranial calcification. Most likely diagnosis is:

[JIPMER 90]

a. Congenital syphilis   b. Rubella

c. Toxoplasmosis   d. Trypanosomiasis

104. Which of the following is not transmitted transplacentally?   [TN 90]

a. Mumps   b. Syphilis

c. Rubella   d. Toxoplasma

105. Symptomatic neonatal CNS involvement is most commonly seen in which group of congenital intrauterine infection?

a. CMV and toxoplasmosis

b. Rubella and toxoplasmosis

c. Rubella and HSV

d. CMV and syphilis

ANSWERS

1. (d) Avidity testing must be done to differentiate between IgA and Ig M (Ref: Harrison 19th E/C214)

"Antibody avidity increases with time and can be useful in difficult cases during pregnancy for establishing when infection may have occurred. The serum IgM titre should be measured in concert with the IgG titre to better establish the time of infection."

- Sabin-Feldman dye test is gold standard for IgG antibodies.
- The IgA-ELISA is a more sensitive test than the IgM ELISA for detection of congenital infection in the fetus and newborn as well as for detection of acute infection in some pregnant women.
- Serologic diagnosis is based on the persistence of IgG antibody or a positive IgM titre after the first week of life (a time frame that excludes placental leak).

2. (c) Coagulase positive staph aureus (Ref: IJP vol 75, sepsis in the newborn, page 67)

Most common cause of sepsis:

- **India** — Most common cause of both early and late onset neonatal sepsis in India is *Klebsiella pneumoniae* followed by staphylococcus aureus.

IJP vol 75, sepsis in the newborn, page 67
"The database comprising 18 tertiary care neonatal units across India found sepsis to be one of the commonest causes of neonatal mortality contributing to 19% of all neonatal mortality. Among **intramural births Klebsiella pneumonae** was the most commonly isolated pathogen (32.5%) followed by *Staphylococcus aureus* (13.6%). Among **extramural (referred from community/other hospitals) neonates** *Klebsiella pneumoniae* (27%) was again the commonest organism followed by **staphylococcus aureus (15%)** and pseudomonas (13%)."

- **Worldwide** — Most common cause of early onset neonatal sepsis worldwide was Group B Streptococcus before introduction of antibiotics. But in today's era because of good antibiotic coverage *E.coli* has emerged as the **most common pathogen causing early onset neonatal sepsis worldwide**. Most common cause of **late onset neonatal sepsis worldwide** is **coagulase negative staphylococci.**

Neonatal sepsis: an international perspective S Vergnano, M Sharland, P Kazembe, C Mwansambo, P T Heath, page 220, 221
"Neonatal surveillance in developed countries generally identifies **GBS and** *E.coli* as the dominant EOS pathogens and **CONS the dominant LOS pathogen** followed by GBS and Staph aureus.↓" Faranoff and Martin's Neonatal perinatal medicine, 8th Edition"An increase in the incidence of *E.coli* and decrease in GBS has recently been found."

3. (a) Nasopharyngeal swab (Ref: Rudolph 22nd E/P1076, Ghai 7th E/P221)
"An alternative to aspirate is Dacron or Rayon nasopharyngeal swab."

Sample of choice in pertussis — Nasopharyngeal aspirate > Nasopharyngeal swab

4. (b) Klebsiella (Ref: IJP vol 75, sepsis in the newborn, page 67)

"The database comprising 18 tertiary care neonatal units across India found sepsis to be one of the commonest causes of neonatal mortality contributing to 19% of all neonatal mortality. Among **intramural births Klebsiella pneumonae** was the most commonly isolated pathogen (32.5%) followed by *Staphylococcus aureus* (13.6%). Among **extramural (referred from community/other hospitals) neonates** *Klebsiella pneumoniae* (27%) was again the commonest organism followed by staphylococcus aureus (15%) and pseudomonas (13%)."

5. (a) Nevirapine (Ref: Nelson 22nd E/P1120)
- **Nevirapine** given once to women in labour and once to the infant during the first 48–72 hour of life reduces perinatal transmission of HIV by 50%.
- Zidovudine given to the pregnant woman starting at as early as 4 week of gestation and continued during delivery and in the newborn for the first 6 week of life decreases the rate of perinatal HIV-1 transmission to <8%.

6. (b) Ig G CMV antibodies in blood (Ref: Nelson 29th E/P1068, Harrison 19th E/C182)

"**An Ig G antibody test** is of little diagnostic value because a positive result also reflects maternal antibodies, although a negative result excludes the diagnosis of congenital CMV infection."

Diagnosis of congenital CMVinfection:
- Virus isolation by culture from urine and saliva.
- Detection of viral DNA by PCR in amniotic fluid, blood and CSF (CMV encephalitis).
- Cytomegalic cells contain large intranuclear inclusions and smaller intracytoplasmic inclusions, and are pathognomonic for CMV infection.
- IgM antibodies are not used for diagnosis as they are neither specific nor sensitive for CMV.

7. (a) Both active and passive immunization after birth (Ref: Nelson 19th E/P1328)

"Infants born to HBsAg-positive women should receive **vaccine at birth, 1–2 mo, and 6 mo of age**. The first dose should be accompanied by administration of **0.5 mL of HBIG as soon after delivery** as possible, because the effectiveness decreases rapidly with increased time after birth."

8. (d) Decreased hemoglobin (Ref: Rudolph 22nd E/P1141, Nelson 19th E/P1093)
- Dengue virus can cause dengue fever, dengue hemorrhagic fever and dengue shock syndrome.
- There are 4 different antigenic types of dengue virus.
- **Pathology:**

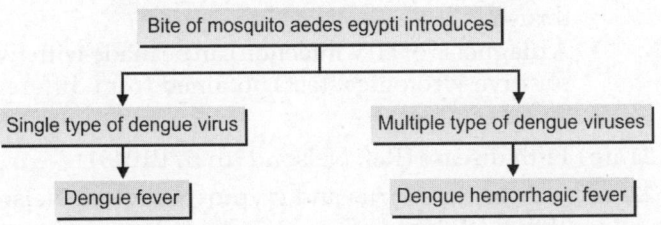

- **Dengue fever** is associated with fever, chills, retroorbital pain, myalgia, and arthralgia.
- **Dengue hemorrhagic fever** is characterized by **thrombocytopenia**, generalized bleeding and evidence of increased vascular permeability (hemoconcentration, pleural effusion, ascites and hypoalbuminemia).
- **Dengue shock syndrome** is advanced phase of dengue hemorrhagic fever, characterized by hypotension and a narrow pulse pressure.
- Pathological changes that can be seen are:
  - ❖ **Hepatomegaly** with fatty changes.
  - ❖ Focal hemorrhages in the lungs, liver, adrenals, and subarachnoid space.
  - ❖ Microscopically, there is perivascular edema in the soft tissues and widespread **diapedesis of red cells.**

9. (c) Meningoencephalitis can precede parotitis (Ref: Nelson 19th E/Chapter 227, Harrison 18th E/Chapter 194)

Meningoencephalomyelitis can have variable presentation depending on the pathogenesis:

- **Primary infection of neurons** — If this is the principal cause then **parotitis appears along with or after the onset of meningoencephalitis.**
- **Post infectious encephalitis with demyelination**— In this case encephalitis follows parotitis by 10 days.

10. (b) Vaginal cleansing before delivery (Ref: Nelson 19th E/P1111)

"A meta-analysis of more than 1,000 pregnancies demonstrated that **elective caesarean delivery** decreased transmission by 87% if used in conjunction **with zidovudine** therapy in the mother and infant."

- **Elective caesarean delivery** with **zidovudine** therapy decreases transmission by 87% if used in the mother and infant.
- Breast feeding is **contraindicated in developed countries** but not in developing countries as diarrhea, pneumonia and malnutrition substantially contribute to a high infant mortality.

11. (c) ELISA (Ref: Nelson 22nd E/P1116, Harrison 18th E/C189)
- **ELISA for anti HIV antibodies** cannot be used to establish a diagnosis of HIV in neonates till 6 months, because of passive transfer of maternal HIV antibody across the placenta during gestation.

Diagnosis of HIV:
- **Young infants** — Viral diagnostic assays useful in young infants i.e. 1–6 months of age are diagnosed by
  - ❖ **HIV DNA PCR** — It is the most preferred method.
  - ❖ **HIV RNA PCR** — More sensitive than DNA PCR.
  - ❖ **HIV culture** — Equally sensitive as DNA PCR.
  - ❖ **HIV p24** antigen immune dissociated p24 — It is highly specific than all other tests but less sensitive.
- In infants older than 6 months, detection of anti HIV Ig A antibodies by ELISA is diagnostic of HIV.
- In infants older than 18 months, demonstration of anti HIV Ig G antibody by ELISA establishes the diagnosis of HIV infection.

12. (c) Rubella (Ref: Nelson 19th E/P1032)

Postnatal (acquired) rubella:
- Most characteristic sign is **lymphadenopathy of postauricular, occipital and posterior cervical lymphnodes.**
- **Forchheimer spots** are rose-coloured spots on the soft palate that may coalesce into a red blush.
- **Rash** starts as irregular **pink macules on the face** and then gradually descends to other parts of body. It is called as kaleidoscopic because of its changing pattern.
- Fever is low or usually absent in children.

13. **(c)** Complete hemogram (Ref: Nelson 19th E/P1678)
   - The symptoms are consistent with infectious lymphadenopathy.
   - Hence complete hemogram should be done to differential between viral and bacterial causes.
   - Biopsy is done if there is persistent or unexplained fever, weight loss, night sweats, hard nodes, or fixation of the nodes to surrounding tissues.

14. **(c)** Roseola infantum (Ref: Nelson 19th E/P1070)
   - The prodromal period of roseola infantum is usually asymptomatic or associated **mild upper respiratory symptoms** and mild cervical>occipital lymphadenopathy. This is followed by high grade fever ranging up to 40°C, which lasts for 3–5 days and **ceases suddenly.**
   - The **time of defervescence (disappearance of fever) or 12–24 hours after defervescence coincides with the onset of rash**. The **rash begins** as pink coloured, discrete, slightly raised and non-pruritic lesions **on the trunk**, which spreads to the neck, face and proximal extremities and sponta-neously resolves within 1–3 days.

15. **(d)** Complete hemogram (Ref: Nelson 19th E/P1065)
   - The characteristic triad of **infectious mono-nucleosis** is:
     1. Fever
     2. Sore throat
     3. Posterior cervical lymphadenopathy
   - Hence this child is suffering from **infectious mononucleosis.**
   - Diagnosis of **infectious mononucleosis:**
     - ❖ **Leukocytosis** of 10,000–20,000 cells/mm³.
     - ❖ Atypical lymphocytes i.e. lymphoblastoid cells account for 20-40% of atypical lymphocytes.
     - ❖ **Paul Bunnel test** — Transient heterophile anti-bodies seen in infectious mononucleosis, also known as Paul-Bunnel antibodies are IgM antibodies detected by the Paul-Bunnel-Davidson test for sheep red cell agglutination.

16. **(c)** *Clostridium botulinum* (Ref: Harrison 19th E/C141)

17. **(b)** Renal anomalies (Ref: Rudolph 22nd E/P 1179, Nelson 19th E/chapter 226, Harrison 19th E/chapter 193) Kindly see text for details.

18. **(a)** and **(c)** Cannot be diagnosed accurately by current methods and Transmission rate during pregnancy exceeds 90% (Ref: Nelson 19th E/P1116, Harrison 18th E/C189)

"Viral diagnostic assays, such as **HIV DNA or RNA PCR, HIV culture, or HIV p24 antigen immune dissociated p24 (ICD-p24),** are considerably more useful in young infants, allowing a **definitive diagnosis in most infected infants by 1–6 month of age.**"

   - Maternal transmission to the fetus occurs most commonly in the perinatal period.

   - Risk of mother-to-child transmissions are:
     - ❖ 23–30% before birth
     - ❖ 50–65% during birth
     - ❖ 12–20% via breast-feeding.

19. **(c)** Recurrent chest infection (Nelson 19th E/1113, Rudolph 22nd E/P1165)

"**PCP** is the most common of the AIDS indicator diseases in children and adults and it previously affected one third of the affected children and adults."

   - **Kaposi sarcoma** is commonly seen in HIV-infected adults but is **uncommon in HIV-infected children.**
   - **Recurrent upper respiratory tract infections** such as otitis media and sinusitis are **very common.**

20. **(d)** Cannot be diagnosed (Ref: Nelson 19th E/P1116, Harrison 18th E/C189)
   - Maternal transmission to the fetus occurs most commonly in the perinatal period.
   - Risk of mother-to-child transmissions are:
     - ❖ 23–30% before birth
     - ❖ 50–65% during birth
     - ❖ 12–20% via breast-feeding.
   - Infant presents with lymphadenopathy, hepato-splenomegaly, **failure to thrive**, chronic or re-current diarrhoea, interstitial pneumonia or oral thrush.
   - A diagnosis of HIV infection can be made with two positive virological tests obtained from different blood samples.

21. **(b)** Fifth disease (Ref: Nelson 19th E/P1048)

22. **(a)** and **(b)** Rota virus and cryptospora (Ref: Nelson 19th E/P1115)

Causative agents of gastrointestinal disease in AIDS patients:

- *Salmonella*
- *Campylobacter*
- MAC
- *Giardia*
- ***Cryptosporidium***
- *Isospora*
- Microsporidia
- CMV
- HSV
- **Rotavirus**
- *Candida*

23. **(d)** Kaposi sarcoma (Ref: Nelson 19th E/P 1116)
   - Initial symptoms may be subtle, such as lympha-denopathy and **hepatosplenomegaly**, or nonspecific such as **failure to thrive**, chronic or recurrent diarrhea, interstitial **pneumonia** or oral thrush.
   - **Kaposi sarcoma** occurs frequently among HIV-infected adults but is exceedingly **uncommon among HIV-infected children.**

24. (c) Anemia (Ref: Nelson 19th E/P1156)

Clinical presentation of ascariasis:

- Most patients are asymptomatic due to moderate worm burden.
- Pulmonary involvement presents as **Loeffler syndrome**.
- Intestinal obstruction by worms can present as **abdominal distention and pain** and vomiting.
- Pancreatitis and cholecystitis can also be seen due to obstruction of ducts.
- Allergic symptoms, fever, rash and **urticaria** can be seen.

25. (c) Erythromycin (Ref: Rudolph 22nd E/P1077, Ghai 7th E/P 222)

26. (c) HSV (Ref: Field's Virology, Vol 1/P346)

- The order of transplacental spread of viral infections in the options, as per incidence can be graded as **HIV > Rubella > HBV > HSV.**

"Several human pathogens spread from the infected mother to the developing fetus via penetration of the placenta or during the birth process (21, 263, 405, 464, 510). These include HCMV (509, 510), **HIV (190, 665)**, **HBV (775)**, HCV (279), **Rubella virus (46, 464)**, **HSV (28)**, HPV (256, 263), VZV (464)."

27. (c) Measles (Ref: Parks 20th E/P 138)

Vaccine	Efficacy
Measles	95% after single dose
TT	80–90% after 2 doses
DPT	70–90 % after 3 doses
Typhoid	50–80%

28. (a) Varicella virus (Ref: Rudolph 22nd E/P1162, Nelson 19th E/P1059, Harrison 18th E/C180)

Organs affected in congenital varicella syndrome:

Organ affected	Manifestation
Limb development is affected when mother is infected at 6–12 weeks of gestation	Limb hypoplasia
Skin	• Cicatrix or zigzag scarring of skin in dermatomal distribution • Hypopigmentation
Eye	• Microopthalmia • Cataracts • Chorioretinitis • Optic atrophy
CNS	• Microcephaly • Hydrocephaly • Calcifications • Aplasia of brain
Other	• Anisocoria • Horner syndrome • Anal/urinary sphincter dysfunction

29. (c) Clindamycin (Ref: Nelson 19th E/P1141)

"The 3-day ACT regimens are all well tolerated, although mefloquine is associated with increased rates of vomiting and dizziness. As second-line treatments for recrudescence following first-line therapy, a different ACT regimen may be given; another alternative is a 7-day course of either artesunate or quinine plus tetracycline, doxycycline, or clindamycin. Tetracycline and doxycycline cannot be given to pregnant women or to children <8 years of age."

- *P. vivax*, *P. knowlesi*, *P. malariae*, and *P. ovale* should be treated with oral chloroquine but due to increasing drug-resistance to *P. falciparum*, Artemisinin combination treatment (ACT) regimens are now recommended as first-line treatment for falciparum malaria.
- In case of resistance to ACT regimen, artesunate or quinine plus tetracycline, doxycycline, or clindamycin should be given. However since only clindamycin is safe in children, it is preferred and is the answer of choice.

30. (a) VDRL for mother and baby (Ref: Rudolph 22nd E/P1102)

- The points in the question indicating towards congenital syphilis are:
  ❖ Premature delivery
  ❖ Bullous lesion
  ❖ Periostitis in X-ray
- Among the options provided only VDRL for mother and baby is the test for syphilis.

31. (d) Infection after 16 weeks of gestation results in major congenital defects (Ref: Rudolph 22nd E/P 1179, Nelson 19th E/P1033, Harrison 18th E/chapter 193)

- The most serious consequence of rubella virus infection can develop when a woman becomes infected during pregnancy, particularly during the first trimester.
- The resulting complications may include miscarriage, fetal death, premature delivery, or live birth with congenital defects.

32. (a) *Mycobacterium tuberculosis* (Ref: Rudolph 22nd E/P, Nelson 19th E/chapter 197)

CNS Tuberculosis:

It is the most serious complication of tuberculosis in children. Lymphohematogenous spread of tuberculosis leads to meningeal and cerebral metastatic caseous leisons which further pass the tubercular bacilli to subarachnoid space. Gelatinous exudates are produced that cause

1. Infarction of cerebral cortex by invading blood vessels.
2. Communicating hydrocephalus due to obstruction at basal cisterns.

33. (b) Hepatitis B virus (Ref: Rudolph 22nd E/P1144, Nelson 19th E/P1327)

Epidemiology of Hepatitis B infection:

> "Transmission occurs percutaneously, sexually, via mucous membranes, and **vertically from mother to infant**." "The most important risk factor for acquisition of **HBV in children is perinatal exposure to an HBsAg-positive mother**."

Transmission routes of other hepatitis viruses:

Hepatitis A virus	• **Fecal-oral route** — Most common route • Percutaneous • Transfusion of blood
Hepatitis B virus	• Percutaneous • Sexually • Via mucous membranes • **Vertically from mother to infant** — It is **most important** cause of hepatitis B in children
Hepatitis c virus	• **Blood transfusions or percutaneous** — Most common route • Sexual transmission – <5% cases • **Vertical transmission – 5% cases**
Hepatitis D virus	• Percutaneous • Sexually • **Vertical transmission** — Very rare
Hepatitis E virus	• Fecal-oral route

34. (b) HBs Ag and HBe Ag positivity (Ref: Nelson 19th E/P1327)

> "The most important risk factor for acquisition of HBV in children is perinatal exposure to an HBsAg-positive mother. The risk of transmission is greatest if the mother also is HBeAg positive; 70–90% of their infants become chronically infected if untreated."

35. (b) Obtain anti HBs levels (Ref: Nelson 19th E/P1328)

- HBs Ag is the first serological marker to appear after infection with Hepatitis B virus.
- The most important risk factor for acquisition of HBV in children is perinatal exposure to an HBs Ag-positive mother.
- Infants born to HBs Ag-positive mother should receive vaccine at birth, 1–2 months, and 6 months of age.
- Only anti-HBs Ag is present in persons immunized with hepatitis B vaccine, whereas anti-HBs Ag and anti-HBc Ag are detected in persons with resolved infection.
- Postvaccination testing for HBs Ag and anti-HBs should be at 9–15 months ideally:
  - ❖ If the result is positive for anti-HBs, the child is immune to HBV.
  - ❖ If the result is positive for HBs Ag only, the parent should be counselled and the child evaluated by a pediatric hepatologist.

- ❖ If the result is negative for both HBs Ag and anti-HBs, a second complete hepatitis B vaccine series should be administered, followed by testing for anti-HBs to determine if subsequent doses are needed.
- Hence the child should be tested for anti HBs levels and then managed accordingly as written above.

36. (c) Infectious mononucleosis (Ref: Rudolph 22nd E/P1155, Nelson 19th E/P1065)

The characteristic triad of infectious mononucleosis is:
1. Fever
2. Sore throat
3. Posterior cervical lymphadenopathy

37. (c) Aortic stenosis (Ref: Rudolph 22nd E/P 1179, Nelson 19th E/chapter 226, Harrison 19th E/chapter 193)

- **Pulmonary artery stenosis** is seen in CRS and not aortic stenosis.
- Kindly see text for details on manifestation of congenital rubella syndrome.

38. (a) IgM FTA-ABS (Reference: Rudolph 22nd E/P1102, Nelsons 19th E/P980)

> Nelson 19th E/P980
>
> Tests for IgM antibodies have been developed, including FTA-ABS 19S-IgM, IgM capture enzyme-linked immunosorbent assay, and Western immunoblotting assays, but these have been relatively insensitive and are not generally available.

39. (c) BCG +INH for 6 week + Breast feeding (Ref: Nelson 19th E/P971–72)

As per Nelson 19th edition this is the latest recommendation regarding drug therapy for infant of a mother born with active tuberculosis:

- If the mother's chest radiograph or acid-fast sputum smear shows evidence of current tuberculosis disease, INH treatment for the infant should be continued until the mother has been shown to be sputum culture negative for at least 3 months.
- INH therapy for newborns has been so effective that separation of the mother and infant is no longer considered mandatory. Hence breast feeding is not a problem.
- BCG is recommended for tuberculin skin test-negative infants and children who
  1. are at high risk of intimate and prolonged exposure to persistently untreated or ineffectively treated adults with infectious pulmonary tuberculosis and cannot be removed from the source of infection or placed on long-term preventive therapy or
  2. are continuously exposed to persons with tuberculosis who have bacilli that are resistant to INH and RIF.

- So the best answer in this question is **'c' i.e. BCG+INH for 6 weeks + Breast feeding**. It is not completely correct as INH is recommended for infant till mother has been shown to be sputum culture negative for at least 3 months.

40. (a) Orchitis and oophoritis (Ref: Rudolph 22nd E/P1175, Nelson 19th E/Chapter227, Harrison 18th E/Chapter 194)

41. (a) Local nursery environment (Ref: Rudolph 22nd E/P907, Ghai 7th E/P136)

"Late onset disease is variably defined as occurring after 72 hours in hospitalized infants to 6 days in neonates in the community. The bacteria causing late onset infection can be from the maternal genital tract, the hospital environment, or the community."

42. (d) SSPE (Ref: Rudolph 22nd E/P1172–73)
- The respiratory tract is involved most often, but severe gastroenteritis also occurs.
- Otitis media and Pneumonia are most common secondary bacterial infections.
- SSPE is a very rare complication seen in 1 in 10000 children.

43. (b) Neutrophilia (Ref: Ghai 7th E/P137)
Laboratory findings in sepsis:
- Neutropenia
- Increased immature neutrophils
- Raised CRP levels
- Raised Micro ESR.

44. (c) Most common transmission of infection is through nursery personnel (Ref: Rudolph 22nd E/P907, Ghai 7th E/P136)
Kindly see text for details.

45. (a) PDA (Ref: Rudolph 22nd E/P 1179, Nelson 19th E/chapter 226, Harrison 18th E/chapter 193)
Congenital rubella manifestations as per Harrison 19th E/Table193-1

Transient Manifestations	Permanent Manifestations
Hepatosplenomegaly Interstitial pneumonitis	Hearing impairment/deafness Congenital heart defects (**patent ductus arteriosus, pulmonary arterial stenosis**)
Thrombocytopenia with purpura/petechiae (e.g. dermal erythropoiesis, or "blueberry muffin syndrome") Hemolytic anemia Bony radiolucencies	Eye defects (cataracts, cloudy cornea, microphthalmos, pigmentary retinopathy, congenital glaucoma)
Intrauterine growth retardation Adenopathy	Microcephaly
Meningoencephalitis	Central nervous system sequelae (mental and motor delay, autism)

As per Nelson 19th E/Chapter226
"Other common findings include cataracts, bilateral or unilateral, which are frequently associated with microphthalmia; myocarditis and structural cardiac defects (e.g. **patent ductus arteriosus or pulmonary artery stenosis**)."
Only Rudolph mentions ASD and VSD as complications of rubella.
"**Patent ductus arteriosus and atrial and ventricular septal defects** are the most common cardiac lesions encountered."

46. (c) IgM antibody in fetal serum (Ref: Rudolph 22nd E/P 1179, Nelson 19th E/chapter 226, Harrison 19th E/chapter 193)

"The diagnosis is confirmed by finding **rubella-specific IgM antibody in the neonatal serum**, or by culturing rubella virus from the infant (nasopharynx, urine, or tissues)."

47. (c) Mild splenomegaly is usual (Ref: Nelson 19th E/P917)

48. (c) Enteritis (Ref: Rudolph 22nd E/P1163, Nelson 19th E/P1061, Harrison 18th E/C180)
Complications of chickenpox:

- **Secondary bacterial infections**
- **Pneumonia**
- Cerebellar ataxia
- Encephalitis
- Reye syndrome
- Guillian-Barre syndrome
- Transverse myelitis
- **Aseptic meningitis**

49. (a), (b), (c) and **(e)** (Ref: Rudolph 22nd E/P 1179, Nelson 19th E/chapter 226, Harrison 19th E/chapter 193)
- **Patent ductus arteriosus and atrial and ventricular septal defects** are the most common cardiac lesions encountered.
- Other common findings include cataracts, bilateral or unilateral, which are frequently associated with microopthalmia; myocarditis and structural cardiac defects (e.g. **patent ductus arteriosus or pulmonary artery stenosis**).

50. (c) and **(d)** (Ref: Rudolph 22nd E/P1170, Nelson 19th E/P1111)
- Breast feeding is associated with HIV 1 transmission.
- Hence in areas where safe alternatives to breast feeding are available (developed countries) substitution of **infant formula** for breast milk should be done.

- However in areas where safe alternative to breast feeding are not available (developing countries), **breast feeding should be done for six months and then discontinued as soon as possible** as the duration of breast feeding is positively related to the rate of HIV 1 transmission.
- It has been found that concurrent administration of breast milk and infant milk formula is associated with a higher rate of HIV infection. Hence in **developed countries baby should receive exclusively infant milk formula**, whereas **in developing countries exclusive breast feeding is preferred till 6 months.**

51. **(a), (b)** and **(d)** (Ref: Nelson 22nd E/P1120)
- **Nevirapine** given once to women in labour and **once to the infant** during the first 48–72 hour of life **reduces perinatal transmission of HIVby 50%.**
- **Zidovudine** given to the pregnant woman starting at as early as 4 week of gestation and continued during delivery and in the newborn for the **first 6 week of lifedecreases the rate of perinatal HIV-1 transmission to <8%.**

52. **(b)** and **(d)** (Ref: Nelson 19th E/P1111)

"A meta-analysis of more than 1,000 pregnancies demonstrated that **elective caesarean delivery** decreased transmission by 87% if used in conjunction **with zidovudine** therapy in the mother and infant."
"A meta-analysis of prospective studies found that the additional **risk of transmission** through **breast-feeding** in women with HIV infection before pregnancy was **14% compared with a 29% increase in breast-feeding women who acquired HIV postnatally**. However, the **WHO recommends that in developing countries** where other diseases (e.g. diarrhea, pneumonia, and malnutrition) substantially contribute to a high infant mortality rate, the benefit of breast-feeding outweighs the risk of HIV transmission, and **HIV-infected women should breast-feed their infants**."
Though breast feeding should be **avoided in developed countries** it is generally **indicated in developing countries like India.**

53. **(a)** OPV (Ref: Nelson 19th E/P1119)

"All HIV-exposed and infected children should receive standard pediatric immunizations. In general, live **oral polio vaccine** and live bacterial vaccines (e.g. **BCG**) should not be given."

54. **(c)** IV penicillin G (Ref: Harrison 18th E/C381)
- **Gram negative diplococci in CSF and generalized petechiae** confirm the diagnosis of meningococcal meningitis.

"Although ceftriaxone and cefotaxime provide adequate empirical coverage for *N. meningitidis*, penicillin G remains the antibiotic of choice for meningococcal meningitis caused by susceptible strains."

55. **(a)** When the lesions have crusted (Ref: Rudolph 22nd E/P1161, Nelson 19th E/P1057, Harrison 18th E/C180)
- Patients with varicella are contagious from 24–48 hr before the rash appears and until vesicles are crusted, usually 3–7 days after onset of rash.
- The child can meet when she is noncontagious i.e. when the vesicles are crusted.

56. **(a), (b), (c), (d)** and **(e)** (Ref: Nelson 19th E/P968–69)

"Ciprofloxacin and **ofloxacin** are quinolones with significant antituberculosis activity that are used commonly for drug-resistant tuberculosis in adults. These drugs are **generally contraindicated in children** because they cause destruction of growing cartilage in some animal models. However, they have been **used effectively in some cases** of multidrug-resistant tuberculosis in children when few other effective agents were available."

Kindly see text for other drugs.

57. **(c)** and **(d)** (Ref: Rudolph 22nd E/P1171–71)
Kindly See text for details.

58. **(b)** and **(d)** (Ref: Nelson 19th E/P968–69)
Kindly see text for details.

59. **(a)** and **(c)** (Ref: Rudolph 22nd E/P1171-72, Nelson 19th E/P1028)
- Koplik spots are seen in prodromal phase.
- Measles vaccine is given at 9 months of age.
- Nelson 19th E/Chapter 225

The **temperature rises abruptly as the rash appears** and often reaches 40°C or higher.

- The CDC case definition for measles requires:
  1. A generalised maculopapular rash of atleast 3 days duration
  2. Fever of atleast 38.3°C
  3. Cough, Coryza or conjunctivitis

60. **(b)** Caused by HHV 6 and 7 (Ref: Nelson 19th E/P1069)
- Roseola infantum (exanthem subitum i.e. sudden onset of rash) is caused by **human herpesviruses (HHV 6 and 7)**, which are large double stranded DNA viruses.
- The **time of defervescence (disappearance of fever) or 12–24 hours after defervescence coincides with the onset of rash**. The **rash begins** as pink coloured, discrete, slightly raised and non-

pruritic lesions **on the trunk**, which spreads to the neck, face and proximal extremities and spontaneously resolves within 1–3 days.

- The complications associated with Roseola infantum are febrile seizures, mononucleosis like illness, hepatomegaly, meningoencephalitis and ulcers at the uvulopalatal junction (**Nagayama spots**).
- **Slapped cheek appearance** is seen in **erythema infectiosum.**

61. **(a)**, **(b)** and **(c)** Slapped cheek appearance seen, Caused by parvovirus and Defeverscence before rash (Ref: Nelson 19th E/P1048–49)

Erythema infectiosum or Fifth disease:

- **Erythema infectiosum** or **"fifth disease"** is the most common manifestation of **Parvo virus** B19 infection, which belongs to the genus erythrovirus and has tropism for the erythroid precursors.
- The incubation period ranges from **4 to 28 days.** The prodromal phase starts with upper respiratory symptoms, headache and **low grade fever**. This is followed by a week-long asymptomatic phase before appearance of rash in 3 stages. Thus **rash appears after one week of defeverscence** (disappearance of fever).
- The erythematous rash begins on the **face** and is described as **"slapped cheek appearance"**. This is followed by spreading of diffuse macular erythema to **extremities**, primarily on the extensor surface with sparing of palms and soles. Further central clearing of macular lesions gives a **lacy, reticulated appearance.**

62. **(a) and (d)** Meningitis commonly occur lately and jaundice is a common feature (Ref: Rudolph 22nd E/P908, Ghai 7th E/P 136)

"Jaundice (direct hyperbilirubinemia) can indicate infection, especially when it occurs within the first 24 hours of life without Rh or ABO blood group incompatibility and when it is accompanied by an elevated bilirubin concentration."
"Late onset neonatal sepsis frequently is accompanied by meningitis, and usually is more insidious in clinical presentation than early onset disease."

63. **(d)** Measles (Ref: Rudolph 22nd E/P1173)

"A second form of measles encephalitis, subacute sclerosing panencephalitis, is a rare delayed complication of measles that occur in approximately 1 in 10000 cases."

64. **(e)** Rash can occur in axilla (Ref: Rudolph 22nd E/P1162, Nelson 19th E/P1057, Harrison 18th E/C180)

Rudolph 22nd E/P1162

The rash typically begins as "dew drops on rose petals", appearing on the face, trunk or scalp and eventually spreading to involve the entire body.

- The skin lesions of VZI include maculopapules, vesicles, and **scabs** in various stages of evolution
- **Scabs are crust** discharged from and covering a healing wound.
- Patients with varicella **are contagious from 24–48 hr before the rash appears and until vesicles are crusted**, usually 3–7 days after onset of rash.
- Incubation period is **10–21 days.**
- The distribution of the rash is predominantly central or **centripetal** in contrast to smallpox, where the rash is more prominent on the face and distal extremities.
- Fever, malaise, anorexia, headache, and occasionally mild abdominal pain may occur 24–48 hr before the rash appears.

65. **(b)** Secondary bacterial infection (Ref: Rudolph 22nd E/P1163, Nelson 19th E/P1061, Harrison 18th E/C180)

Rudolph 22nd E/P1163

"The most frequent complication in the young is the secondary bacterial infection of the skin."

- Most common clinical presentation is rash in the form of maculopapules, vesicles and scabs in various stages of evolution.
- Most common complication of VZI is secondary bacterial infection of skin caused by Streptococcus and Staphylococcus.
- Most common site of extracutaneous involvement in VZI is CNS, which is characterized by acute cerebellar ataxia and meningeal inflammation. Other less common CNS complications that can be seen are aseptic meningitis, encephalitis, transverse myelitis, and Guillain-Barre syndrome.
- Most serious complication of VZI is Varicella pneumonia which is more common in adults than children.

66. **(a)** and **(c)** (Ref: Rudolph 22nd E/P 1179, Nelson 19th E/P1032, Harrison 19th E/chapter 193)

- The rash first appears as irregular pink macules on face.
- Postauricular, occipital and posterior cervical lymph nodes are involved.
- Polyarthritis and polyarthralgia are common manifestations of rubella in women, less common in men and uncommon in children.
- Retinopathy is the most common ocular manifestation of rubella infection.

67. (b) <5 years (Ref: Nelson 18th E/P, Rudolph 22nd E/P1075)
- In the prevaccine era and countries with limited immunization the peak incidence of pertussis is in children 1–5 year of age.
- Now post vaccination and countries with good immunization coverage infants less than 6 month have the peak incidence of disease.
- Maximum mortality is seen in children less than 3 months.

68. (b) 4 days before and 5 days after rash (Ref: Harrison 19th E/chapter 192)

"Persons with measles are infectious for **several days before and after the onset of rash**, when levels of measles virus in blood and body fluids are highest and when cough, coryza, and sneezing, which facilitate virus spread, are most severe."

69. (b) Measles (Rudolph 22nd E/P1172, Nelson 19th E/P1027)
- Interstitial Pneumonia (Giant cell pneumonia) — It is a fatal complication of measles usually seen in immunocompromised children.

70. (a) and **(b)** BCG vaccine should not be given and AZT therapy (Ref: Nelson 19th E/P1118)

"All HIV-exposed and infected children should receive standard pediatric immunizations. In general, live oral polio vaccine and live bacterial vaccines (e.g. BCG) should not be given."

- Live oral polio vaccine and other live bacterial vaccination like **BCG should not be given**.
- All other **standard childhood vaccination** should be given.
- **Zidovudine (AZT)** is given to the newborn for the first 6 wk of life.
- Breast feeding is contraindicated in developed countries but child is not separated from mother.

71. (a) Perinatal transmission (Ref: Nelson 19th E/P1111, Harrison 18th E/C180)
- Maternal transmission to the fetus occurs **most commonly in the perinatal period**.
- **Breast milk is the least common route** of vertical transmission in developed countries.

72. (a) Paramyxo virus (Ref: Rudolph 22nd E/P1171) Kindly see text for details.

73. (b) Cytomegalovirus (Ref: Field's Virology, Vol. 1/P346)

"Several human pathogens spread from the infected mother to the developing fetus via penetration of the placenta or during the birth process (21, 263, 405, 464, 510). These include **HCMV (509, 510)**, HIV (190, 665), HBV (775), HCV (279), Rubella virus (46, 464), HSV (28), HPV (256, 263), VZV (464)."

74. (c) 14–24 days (Ref: Nelson 19th E/P1035)

75. (d) Incubation period is less than 2 weeks (Ref: Nelson 19th E/P1035)

76. (c) Erythema infectiosum (Ref: Nelson 19th E/P1049)

"The **most common manifestation of parvovirus B19 is erythema infectiosum**, also known as fifth disease, which is a benign, self-limited exanthematous illness of childhood."

77. (c) Syphilis (Ref: Nelson 19th E/P979)

78. (a) Toxoplasmosis (Ref: Nelson 19th E/P1148)

79. (b) Congenital syphilis (Ref: Rudolph 22nd E/P1102)
- **Hutchinson triad** which was described in 19th century as a presentation of **late congenital syphilis includes:**
  1. **Hutchinson teeth** — Screwdriver or peg shaped deformity of the upper central incisors of the secondary dentition.
  2. Interstitial keratitis.
  3. 8th nerve deafness.

80. (b) Chorioretinitis (Ref: Nelson 19th E/P1148)

81. (b) Pertussis (Ref: Ghai 7th E/P221)

82. (c) Toxin produced by gram positive anaerobic bacillus (Nelson 19th E/P947)
- This is a case of botulism caused by consumption of honey.
- Botulism is caused by C. botulinum, a gram positive, spore forming obligate anaerobe.

83. (d) ELISA for HIV Ig G antibody (Ref: Ghai 7th E/P203)

84. (a) Herpes virus 6 (Ref: Nelson 19th E/P1069)

85. (a) Toxoplasmosis (Ref: Nelson 19th E/P1148)
Manifestations of congenital toxoplasmosis:
- **Intracranial calcifications**
- **Hydrocephalus**
- **Chorioretinitis** — Most common manifestation
- Cataract
- **Microcephaly**
- Mental retardation
- Convulsions
- Rash
- Hepatosplenomegaly
- Lymphadenopathy.

86. (b), (c) and **(d)** Caused by HHV 6 and 7, Rash appear in trunk, During defervescence, rash appears (Ref: Nelson 19th E/P1069–72)
- **Roseola infantum** (exanthem subitum i.e. sudden onset of rash) or **sixth disease** is caused by **human herpesviruses (HHV 6 and 7)**, which are large double stranded DNA viruses.

- The **time of defervescence (disappearance of fever) or 12–24 hours after defervescence coincides with the onset of rash**. The **rash begins** as pink coloured, discrete, slightly raised and non-pruritic lesions **on the trunk**, which spreads to the neck, face and proximal extremities and spontaneously resolves within 1–3 days.

87. (a) Enteric fever (Ref: Ghai 7th E/P222)

88. (b) Human herpes virus 6 (Nelson 19th E/P1069)

89. (d) Unborn child (Ref: Nelson 19th E/P1032)

90. (c) IgM-FTA ABS (Ref: Nelson 19th E/P980)

91. (a) Vertical transmission during pregnancy (Ref: Ghai 7th E/P203)

   Risk of mother-to-child transmission of HIV is:
   - 23–30% before birth
   - **50–65% during birth**
   - 12–20% via breast-feeding

92. (c) Within five days of delivery (Ref: Nelson 19th E/P1058)

93. (a) Anti TB drugs should be started even if x-ray chest and hemogram are normal (Ref: Nelson 19th E/P962)
   - This induration is of 12 mm i.e. >10 mm in a child of 2 years i.e. <4 years. Thus this is a positive tuberculin test and hence treatment should be started even if other investigations are normal. Have a look at the table given below for assessment of tuberculin test (See Table 1).

94. (a) 20–30 % (Ref: Ghai 7th E/P203, Park 20th E/P302)

95. (b) 20–30 % (Ref: Ghai 7th E/P203, Park 20th E/P302)

96. (a) Chickenpox (Ref: Ghai 7th E/P186)

97. (a) Keratitis (Ref: Nelson 19th E/P979)

98. (b) Roseola infantum (Ref: Nelson 19th E/P1070)

99. (a) Measles (Ref: Nelson 19th E/P1028)

100. (d) Pancreatitis (Ref: Nelson 19th E/P1029)

101. (b) Breast feeding and isoniazid administration (Ref: Nelson 19th E/P972)

102. (a) Grey (Ref: Ghai 7th E/P227)

103. (c) Toxoplasmosis (Ref: Nelson 19th E/P1147)

104. (a) Mumps (Ref: Field's Virology, Vol 1/P346)

105. (c) Rubella and HSV (Ref: Rudolph 22nd E/P902-07, Nelson 19th E/P1146)

Congenital intrauterine infection:

- Almost one-third of all neonates with **HSV infection** are categorized as having **CNS infection**. Clinical manifestations of CNS disease includes seizures, lethargy, irritability, tremors, poor feeding, temperature instability and bulging anterior fontanel.

- **Meningoencephalitis** is a **common finding in congenital rubella** infection.

- Almost all congenitally infected individuals manifest signs or symptoms of toxoplasmosis, such as chorioretinitis by **adolescence** if they are not treated in the newborn period. Predilection to predominant involvement of the **CNS** and eye **in congenital infection has not been fully explained.**

- Babies born with **congenital CMV infection** may have neurologic sequalae and psychomotor retardation. However **majority of infants remain asymptomatic.**

- Kindly see text for symptoms of congenital syphilis.

Table 1

Positive with induration>5mm	Positive with induration>10 mm	Positive with induration>15 mm
• History of contact with known case of TB	• Infants and children ≤4 years of age	• Children >4 years of age and older without any risk factors
• Positive chest x-ray finding	• Associated medical conditions like DM and renal disorders	
• Associated immunosuppressive conditions	• Frequent exposure to adults at high risk	
• Patients on immunosuppressive therapy	• Birth or recent immigration (<5 yr) from a high-prevalence country	

1. **Which of the following will make you suspect developmental delay:**
   a. Cannot sit at 9 months
   b. Cannot walk up and down stairs at 30 months
   c. No pincer grasp at 9 months
   d. Cannot talk 2 words phrases at 18 month

2. **Among the following, the least common cause of neonatal sepsis in India is:**
   a. *Staphylococcus aureus*
   b. *E.coli*
   c. Klebsiella
   d. Group B Streptococcus

3. **Premature baby weight 1000 grams are less likely to suffer from:**
   a. Cataract   b. Glaucoma
   c. ROP   d. Retinal detachment

4. **An 18-year-old primigravida complained of decreased fetal movements. She delivered a baby weighing 2000 grams at 30 weeks of gestation. The APGAR scores of the baby were 4 and 5 at 1 and 5 minutes respectively. The baby died in an hour. Post-mortem examination revealed multiple, peripheral, radially arranged cysts in the kidney. Most common associated finding in the baby would be:**
   a. Holoprosencephaly
   b. Hepatic cysts and hepatic fibrosis
   c. Ureteral agenesis
   d. Medullary sponge kidney

5. **A newborn female child weight 3.5 kg, delivered by uncomplicated delivery, developed respiratory distress immediately after birth. On chest X-ray ground glass appearance was seen. Baby put on mechanical ventilation and was given surfactant but condition of the baby deteriorates and increasing hypoxemia was present. History of 1 week old female sibling died before present. ECHO is normal. Usual cultures are negative. Your diagnosis is:**
   a. Total anomalous pulmonary vein connection
   b. Meconium aspiration syndrome
   c. Neonatal pulmonary alveolar proteinosis
   d. Dissemination HSV infection

6. **Newborn babies are able to breathe and suck at the same time due to:**
   a. Wide short tongue
   b. Short soft palate
   c. High position of larynx
   d. Short pharynx

7. **Preterm baby with PDA which is least likely finding:**
   a. CO_2 washout
   b. Pulmonary hemorrhage
   c. Necrotizing Enterocolitis
   d. Bounding pulses

8. **Child with croup, well hydrated, feeding well, consolable. T/t is:**
   a. Racemic epinephrine
   b. Dexamethasone
   c. Nasal washing for influenza and RSV
   d. Antibiotics

9. **A child with abdominal mass and elongated right upper and lower limb is suffering from:**
   a. Wilm's tumor
   b. Neuroblastoma
   c. Nephroblastoma
   d. Angiosarcoma

10. **An 8-year-old child presents with muscle tightness, creatinine kinase level has been falling as the age is increasing. Which is the most likely abnormality:**
    a. Dystrophin absent
    b. Myelin deficiency
    c. Hereditary myopathy
    d. Congenital myopathy

11. **Rett's syndrome, not seen is:**
    a. Macrocephaly   b. Mental retardation
    c. Gait disorder   d. Seizure

AIIMS NOVEMBER — 2012

1. A neurosurgeon dropped his kid to the school, then there he saw a child with uncontrollable laughing and precocious puberty. When he again went to the school in capital parent teacher meeting, he talked to the father of that boy and advised him to get an MRI done and the diagnosis was confirmed. What is the most probable diagnosis:
   a. Hypothalamic hamartoma
   b. Pineal germinoma
   c. Pituitary adenoma
   d. Craniopharyngioma

2. A child presented to the casualty with seizures. On examination an oval hypopigmented macules were noted on the trunk, along with subnormal IQ. Probable diagnosis of the child is:
   a. Neurofibromatosis   b. Sturge Weber
   c. Tuberous sclerosis   d. Incontinentia pigmenti

3. A child is able to dress herself, knows her gender, feeds without spilling. What is her age?
   a. 2 years   b. 3 years
   c. 4 years   d. 5 years

4. A preterm 32 week newborn baby with respiratory rate 86/min with presence of grunting. On examination there was no nasal flaring, abdomen behind in movement than chest, minimal intercostal retraction and no xiphisternal retraction. The silverman scoring for the neonate shall be:
   a. 3   b. 4
   c. 5   d. 6

5. Which of the following in the natural course of disease has no reversal of the shunt?
   a. ASD   b. VSD
   c. TOF   d. PDA

6. A peterm infant with poor respiration at birth starts throwing seizures at 10 hours after birth. Anti-epileptic of choice shall be:
   a. Leveteracetam   b. Phenytoin
   c. Phenobarbitone   d. Lorazepam

7. Which of the following finding in newborn suggests RDS?
   a. Develop 6 hours after birth
   b. Air bronchogram seen
   c. Receipt of antenatal steroids
   d. Term gestation

8. A 7-year-old girl with falling grades and complaints by the teacher that she is inattentive in class to her parents and has bad school performance. On hyperventilation her symptoms increased and showed the following EEG findings. Diagnosis is (graph is given):
   a. Myoclonic epilepsy   b. Myoclonus
   c. Absence seizure   d. Juvenile myoclonic epileps

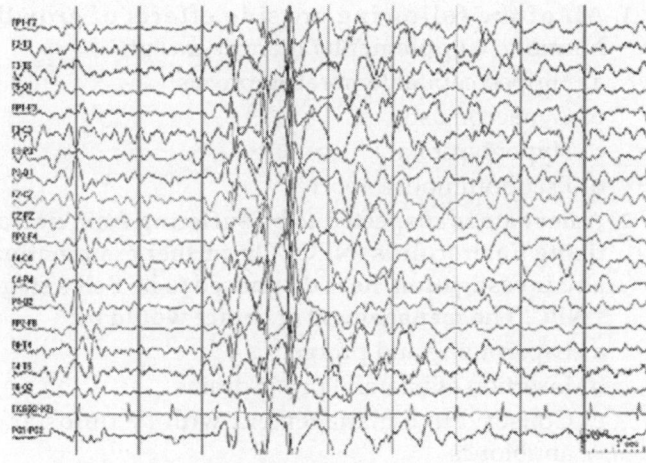

Fig. 1

9. One of the parents has a balanced translocation between chromosome 15 and 21. What advice will you provide to the couple to prevent a child being born with Down's syndrome:
   a. Prenatal diagnosis and advice abortion
   b. Artificial insemination with donor's semen
   c. Adoption
   d. No need to worry as there is no increased risk

10. About trisomy 13 which of the following is true statement?
    a. Bilateral microopthalmia
    b. Neurofibroma
    c. Rocker bottom feet
    d. Dermoid cyst

11. A child with hypoglycemia is not able to utilize glucose from glycogenolysis or gluconeogenesis. Which of the following enzyme is deficient in the child?
    a. Fructokinase   b. Glucokinase
    c. Glucose-6-phosphatase d. Transketolase

12. A child presents with Seborrheic dermatitis, sinusitis and chronically draining ears. On examination child has failure to thrive with hepatosplenomegaly and exophthalmos. Probable diagnosis is:
    a. Histiocytosis X
    b. Wegener's granulomatosis
    c. Chronic granulomatous disease
    d. Chediak-Higashi syndrome

13. Most common organism causing neonatal sepsis:
    a. Staphylococcus   b. *E.coli*
    c. *Hemophilus influenzae* d. Klebsiella

14. Which of the following is not a sign of PDA in preterm baby?
    a. Apnea
    b. Tachycardia
    c. Necrotising enterocolitis
    d. Narrow pulse pressure

AIIMS MAY — 2012

1. **All of the following are side effects of growth hormone (supplements) therapy except:**
   a. Slipped capital femoral epiphysis
   b. Gynaecomastia
   c. Hypoglycemia
   d. Pseudotumourcerebri

2. **A neonate is suspected to be suffering from necrotizing Enterocolitis (NEC). On further examination and investigation, he is diagnosed to be Bell's stage I NEC. The management of choice would be:**
   a. Laparotomy and proceed
   b. Insertion of bilateral pelvic drains
   c. Conservative management with IV fluids and antibiotics
   d. Initial conservative management and laparotomy after 24 hours

3. **Cancer management in which of the following malignancies has dramatically increased the survival?**
   a. Esophagus carcinoma
   b. Glioblastoma multiforme
   c. ALL in children
   d. Cholangiocarcinoma

4. **A 10-year-old male child was presented to the paediatrician for evaluation of a seizure disorder. On examination a vascular plaque was found along the ophthalmic and maxillary divisions of the trigeminal nerve. The mother informed the paediatrician that the lesion was present since birth and there was no change in morphology. The most likely possibility is:**
   a. Sturge Weber syndrome
   b. Infantile hemangioma
   c. Congenital hemangioma
   d. Proteus syndrome

5. **Which of the following finding in newborn suggests RDS?**
   a. Develop 6 hours after birth
   b. Air bronchogram seen
   c. Receipt of antenatal steroids
   d. Term gestation

6. **Most common clinical presentation in juvenile myoclonic epilepsy:**
   a. Generalised tonic clonic seizures in sleep
   b. Generalised tonic clonic seizures in awake state
   c. Myoclonus
   d. Absence seizures

7. **Which of the following statements is true?**
   a. Chronic myeloid leukemia occurs beyond 50 years of age
   b. Hairy cell leukemia in less than 50 years of age has a good prognosis
   c. Acute lymphoid leukemia in less than 1 year has a poor prognosis
   d. Chronic lymphocytic leukemia occurs in less than 50 years of age

8. **A newborn baby presented with profuse bleeding from the umbilical stump after birth. Rest of the examination and PT, APTT are within normal limits. Most probable diagnosis is:**
   a. Factor X deficiency
   b. Glanzmann thrombasthenia
   c. von Willebrand disease
   d. Bernard soulier disease

9. **Which of the following is associated with an intrinsic defect in the RBC membrane?**
   a. Autoimmune hemolytic anemia
   b. Hereditary spherocytosis
   c. Microangiopathic hemolytic anemia
   d. Thermal injury anemia

10. **A boy is suffering from acute pyelonephritis. Most specific urinary finding will be:**
    a. W.B.C casts
    b. Leucocyte esterase test
    c. Nitrite test
    d. Bacteria in Gram stain

AIIMS NOVEMBER — 2011

1. Which of the following is the most appropriate investigation for a leaking meningomyocele?
   a. Blood culture
   b. Wound culture
   c. Urine culture
   d. Rectal Swab

2. The important fatty acid present in breast milk which is important for growth?
   a. Docosahexaenoic acid
   b. Palmitic acid
   c. Linoleic acid
   d. Linolenic acid

3. NESTROFT test is used in screening of:
   a. Thalassemia
   b. Autoimmune hemolytic anemia
   c. Spherocytosis
   d. G6PD deficiency

4. A newborn presents with congestive heart failure, on examination has bulging anterior fontanel with a bruit on auscultation. Transfontanellar USG shows a hypoechoic midline mass with dilated lateral ventricles. Most likely diagnosis is:
   [AIIMS Nov. 06, AI 07]
   a. Medulloblastoma
   b. Encephalocele
   c. Vein of Galen malformation
   d. Arachnoid cyst

5. PGE causes worsening in infant with?
   a. PS without VSD
   b. Hypoplastic left heart syndrome
   c. Obstructive TAPVC
   d. Obstruction in aorta

6. Premature baby of 34 weeks was delivered. Baby had bullous lesions on the body. X-ray shows periostitis. What is the next investigation?
   a. VDRL for mother and baby
   b. ELISA for HIV
   c. PCR for TB
   d. Hepatitis surface antigen for mother

7. A downs child mentally retarded, a/e:
   a. Deleted 21
   b. Trisomy 21
   c. Robertsonian translocation
   d. Mosaic

8. Episodic anemia + jaundice since birth except:
   a. G6PD
   b. Sickle cell anemia
   c. Paroxysmal nocturnal Hemoglobinuria
   d. Hereditary spherocytosis

9. All the following can occur in a neonate for heat production except: [AIIMS Nov. 06]
   a. Shivering
   b. Breakdown of brown fat with adrenaline secretion
   c. Universal flexion like a fetus
   d. Cutaneous vasoconstriction

10. What is the diagnosis in a patient who has situs inversus and sinusitis?
    a. Kartagener's syndrome
    b. Goodpasture syndrome
    c. Cystic fibrosis
    d. William Campbell syndrome

11. Short child with low T4 and raised TSH and swelling of pituitary, what is the diagnosis?
    a. Pituitary tumor
    b. Primary hypothyroidism
    c. TSH secreting pituitary adenoma
    d. TSH resistance

12. Karyotyping of fetus can be done in all except:
    a. Chorionic villus sampling
    b. Cordocentesis
    c. Amniocentesis
    d. Fetal skin biopsy

13. The most common gene defect in idiopathic steroid resistant nephrotic syndrome (SRNS):
    a. ACE
    b. NPHS 2
    c. HOX 1
    d. PAX

14. Which of the following is not true?
    a. William syndrome consists of precocious puberty, mental retardation and obesity
    b. In absence of sunlight daily requirement of vitamin D is 400–600 IU
    c. 1 alpha hydroxylation occurs in kidney
    d. 25 alpha hydroxylation occurs in liver

15. Which of the following is not a limb girdle dystrophy?
    a. Sarcoglycan dystrophy
    b. Dystrophin dystrophy
    c. Dysferlin dystrophy
    d. Calpain dystrophy

16. The first centres of ossification appear during which month of pregnancy?
    a. At the end of 2nd month of pregnancy
    b. At the beginning of 3rd month of pregnancy
    c. At the end of 3rd month of pregnancy
    d. At the end of 4th month of pregnancy

AIPGE — 2012

1. All of the following statements regarding jaundice in a newborn are true except:
   a. Physiological jaundice usually peaks after 48 hours
   b. Breast milk jaundice usually peaks after day 7
   c. High levels of conjugated bilirubin may cause kernicterus
   d. All of the above are true

2. A child has vocabulary of 4–6 words however the mode of communication and social interaction continues to be non-verbal. What is the most likely developmental age of child:
   a. 12 months   b. 15 months
   c. 18 months   d. 24 months

3. The most common bacterial cause for diarrhoea in children in India is:
   a. Enterotoxigenic *E.coli* (ETEC)
   b. Enteropathogenic *E.coli* (EPEC)
   c. Enterohemmorhagic *E.coli*
   d. *Vibrio cholerae*

4. A child is brought to the pediatric OPD with fever of 24 hours duration. History reveals 3 episodes of chest infection and passage of foul smelling bulky stools. The most probable diagnosis is:
   a. Cystic fibrosis
   b. Maple syrup disease
   c. Bilirubin conjugation defect
   d. Criggler Najjar syndrome

5. A child with an obvious rash presents with recurrent infections. Investigations revealed decreased platelet count and reduced Ig M. Which of the following is most likely diagnosis?
   a. Idiopathic thrombocytopenic purpura
   b. Thrombotic thrombocytopenic purpura
   c. Wiskott-Aldrich syndrome
   d. Di-George anomaly

6. A 7-year-old child presents to the pediatric clinic with ambiguous genitalia increasing with age. On examination her height, weight and blood pressure were recorded within normal limits. Labia appeared bifid with two separate perineal openings, phallic length was 2.5 cm and no palpable gonads were noted in inguinal region. USG shows presence of mullerian structures. The most probable diagnosis is:
   a. Classic salt-wasting 21 hydroxylase deficiency
   b. Simple virilising congenital adrenal hyperplasia
   c. Complete androgen insensitivity syndrome
   d. 5-alpha reductase deficiency

7. A child with decreased levels of LH, FSH and testosterone presents with delayed puberty. Which of the following is the most likely diagnosis?
   a. Klinefelter's syndrome
   b. Kallman's syndrome
   c. Androgen insensitivity syndrome
   d. Testicular infection

8. Which of the following is the most common tumor of the fetus and the newborn?
   a. Neuroblastoma
   b. Wilm's tumor
   c. Leukemia
   d. Sacrococcygeal teratoma

9. Which of the following hormones are raised in Prader-Willi syndrome:
   a. Growth hormone (GH)
   b. Leutinizing hormone (LH)
   c. Follicle stimulating hormone (FSH)
   d. Ghrelin

10. Which of the following is treatment of choice for stage I Wilm's tumor?
    a. Laparoscopic nephrectomy
    b. Open nephroureterectomy
    c. Chemotherapy
    d. Observation

11. A large for gestational age baby delivered at 40 weeks was observed to be lethargic. The blood sugar was measured to be 35 mg/dl. The management is:
    a. Fortified breast milk   b. 10% IV dextrose
    c. Oral glucose solution   d. Normal saline

12. Parenteral nutrition to supply fatty acids is being considered for a neonate. When comparing a 10% intralipid solution to a 20% solution, the 10% solution has all of the following except:
    a. High phospholipid/triglyceride ratio
    b. Less energy/caloric content
    c. Low serum triglyceride concentrations
    d. High serum phospholipid concentrations

ANSWERS

AIIMS MAY — 2013

1. (a) Cannot sit at 9 months (Ref: Nelson 19th E/P36)
- The mentioned milestones in the options can be developed at the following age:
  - ❖ Sits without support — 8 months.
  - ❖ Walk upstairs — 30 months.
  - ❖ Walk downstairs — 4 years.
  - ❖ Pincer grasp — Starts developing at 9 months and matures at 12 months.
  - ❖ Talk 2 word phrases — 24 months.
  - ❖ Hence developmental delay should be suspected if the child cannot sit at 9 months.

2. (d) Group B Streptococcus (Ref: IJP vol 75, sepsis in the newborn, page 67)
  Most common cause of sepsis:
- **India** — Most common cause of both early and late onset neonatal sepsis in India is *Klebsiella pneumoniae* followed by *Staphylococcus aureus.*

> **IJP vol 75, sepsis in the newborn, page 67**
> "The database comprising 18 tertiary care neonatal units across India found sepsis to be one of the commonest causes of neonatal mortality contributing to 19% of all neonatal mortality. Among **intramural births** *Klebsiella pneumonae* was the most commonly isolated pathogen (32.5%) followed by staphylococcus aureus (13.6%). Among **extramural (referred from community/other hospitals) neonates** *Klebsiella pneumoniae* (27%) was again the commonest organism followed by *Staphylococcus aureus* **(15%)** and Pseudomonas (13%)."

- **Worldwide** — Most common cause of early onset neonatal sepsis worldwide was Group B Streptococcus before introduction of antibiotics. But in today's era because of good antibiotic coverage *E.coli* has emerged as the **most common pathogen causing early onset neonatal sepsis worldwide**. Most common cause of **late onset neonatal sepsis worldwide** is **coagulase negative staphylococci.**

> Neonatal sepsis: an international perspective S Vergnano, M Sharland, P Kazembe, C Mwansambo, P T Heath, page 220, 221
> "Neonatal surveillance in developed countries generally identifies **GBS and E coli** as the dominant EOS pathogens and **CONS the dominant LOS pathogen** followed by GBS and Staph aureus."
> Faranoff and Martin's Neonatal perinatal medicine, 8th Edition.
> "An increase in the incidence of *E.coli* and decrease in GBS has recently been found."

3. (c) ROP (Ref: Nelson 19th E/P553)
  Complications associated with prematurity: Low birth weight and premature infants lack maturity and coordination of certain body systems that manifest as various derangements.
- Metabolic derangements like hypoglycemia, hyperglycemia and hypocalcemia can be seen:
  - ❖ **Hypoglycemia** is seen due to low hepatic glycogen stores.
  - ❖ **Hyperglycemia** is seen due to immature glucose utilising mechanisms.
  - ❖ **Hypocalcemia** — Early onset is usually asymptomatic but late onset hypocalcemia presents as neonatal tetany and seizures.
- **Jaundice** can be seen as the preterm has larger RBC volume for body weight and immature hepatic enzymes and hepatic excretory capacity.
- Hematological abnormalities like **polycythemia** and **anemia** (Due to rapid destruction of fetal RBCs) can be seen.
- Immature organ systems can lead to various disorders:
  - ❖ **Intraventricular haemorrhage** can be seen due to fragile blood vessels.
  - ❖ **Retinopathy of prematurity** develops because of high oxygen saturation used during resuscitation.
  - ❖ **Osteopenia of prematurity** is caused by low levels of calcium, vitamin D and phosphorous.
  - ❖ **Respiratory distress syndrome** can be associated due to lack of surfactant.
- **Hypothermia** is seen due to **higher surface area to body weight ratio**, **low subcutaneous fat** and low glycogen store.

4. (b) Hepatic cysts and hepatic fibrosis (Ref: Nelson 19th E/P1749–50)
  Autosomal recessive polycystic kidney disease: Autosomal recessive polycystic kidney disease (ARPKD) is caused by mutation of **PKHD1 gene** which results in transformation of collecting ducts in to **fusiform cysts**.
  Clinical presentation:
- The patient has **bilaterally enlarged kidneys** and associated extrarenal involvement.
- **Liver** is the most common extrarenal site of involvement characterised by **fibrosis and cysts**; however cysts of **pancreas**, **spleen** and biliary tree (Caroli disease) can also be seen.

- Lung underdevelopment leads to oligohydramnios and potter facies.
- Complications like portal hypertension, urinary tract infection, hypertension, growth retardation and ascending cholangitis can be seen.

Diagnosis:

- Prenatal USG shows a **salt and pepper appearance** of the kidney.
- MRI of kidney shows **radially arranged fusiform dilated collecting ducts**.

Treatment:

- The treatment of complications, dialysis and transplantation of cystic organs (liver and kidney) is the most that can be done.

5. **(c)** Neonatal pulmonary alveolar proteinosis (Ref: Nelson 19th E/P1453–54)

Pulmonary alveolar proteinosis (PAP):

- PAP is characterised by accumulation of surfactant in the alveoli because of increased production or decreased clearance.
- Congenital PAP is characterised by early onset, grave prognosis and **positive family history**. The baby presents with **severe respiratory distress after birth**. It can be caused by inherited deficiency of surfactant protein B. Other factors that may play a role are abnormalities in production of GM-CSF, IL 4 and surfactant protein D.
- In older children the symptoms of respiratory distress develop gradually. Males are more commonly affected than female.
- Gold standard for diagnosis is histopathological examination of lung biopsy. BAL fluid can be examined for surfactant in adults.
- Recurrent BAL is done to remove the accumulated surfactant.

6. **(c)** High position of larynx (Ref: Rudolph 22nd E/P1329)

- In infants the superior border of larynx is located at the level of first cervical vertebrae. This **high location of larynx** elevates epiglottis to the level of palate and facilitates nasal breathing.
- Further during breast feeding the forward thrust of tongue further elevates larynx and facilitates baby's nasal breathing while feeding.

7. **(a)** CO_2 washout (Ref: Nelson 19th E/P1510–12)

Clinical presentation of PDA:

- A small PDA is usually asymptomatic, but large PDA may result in **CHF** due to volume overload of right and left ventricle and left atrium. **CHF** is the **most common cause of death in adolescents**, however they may present with other frequent complications like **infective endocarditis**, pulmonary or systemic embolism and **pulmonary hemorrhage**. Infective endocarditis is more common with **smaller lesions** and hence requires early closure.

- **Bounding peripheral arterial pulses** can be seen because of increased stroke volume (increased systolic B.P). **Wide pulse pressure (Pulse pressure = systolic B.P – Diastolic B.P)** is seen due to passage of blood into the pulmonary artery during diastole and reflex peripheral vasodilation (decreased diastolic BP).
- A prominent apical pulse and systolic thrill is maximally seen in the 2nd left interspace.
- **Machinery like or thunder rolling murmur** because of continuous passage of blood from aorta to pulmonary artery. The patient has other features like resting **tachycardia, CO_2 retention, frequent apnoea** and a hyperactive precordium.
- **Differential cyanosis** can be seen when PDA is associated with severe pulmonary hypertension or reversal of shunt.
- **Prematurity** is an important cause of necrotizing Enterocolitis.

8. **(b)** Dexamethasone (Ref: Nelson 19th E/P1405–06)

Laryngotracheobronchiolitis (Croup):

- This is the most common infectious cause of stridor in children. The most common cause is **parainfluenza type I virus**; however RSV, adenovirus, influenza virus, rubeola virus and mycoplasma pneumonae can also cause croup.
- The characteristic presentation is a harsh cough called as "**barking seal or dog**". X ray of neck shows **steeple sign** caused by tapering of subglottic airway.
- **Mild cases i.e. no stridor at rest** and seen on **crying**, no agitation and activity can be treated with **hydration** and **corticosteroids (I/M dexamethasone or inhaled budesonide)**.
- Treatment of moderate and severe cases i.e. stridor at rest consists of **oxygenation, nebulization with epinephrine** and **corticosteroids (I/M dexamethasone or inhaled budesonide)**. Nebulization with epinephrine is used to relieve the acute symptoms of upper airway obstruction.
- The **mainstay of treatment is corticosteroids** which not only decrease the symptoms but also improve the outcome.

9. **(a) and (c)** Wilm's tumor and Nephroblastoma (Ref: Nelson 19th E/P1712)

- **Wilms tumor or nephroblastoma** is the second most common abdominal tumor. The three classical component of Wilms tumor are epithelium, blastema and stroma. It is associated with **deletion of 11p chromosome** containing WT1 gene, imprinting loss of IGF2, mutation of β catenin gene and loss of heterozygosity of 1p and 16q.
- Increased incidence of Wilms tumor is seen with WAGAR syndrome (Wilms tumor, Aniridia, **Genitourinary abnormalities** and mental

retardation), Denys-Drash syndrome, Frasier syndrome, **Beckwith-Widemann syndrome** (large organs e.g. **macroglossia, hypoglycemia**), Simpson-Golabi-Behmel syndrome, Sotos syndrome, Perlman syndrome, **hemihypertrophy**, genitourinary anomalies (**horse-shoe kidney**, duplication of collecting system, cryptorchidism, hypospadias) neurofibromatosis, sporadic **aniridia** and von Wilebrand disease.

- This is a case of Wilms's tumor with hemihypertrophy.

10. **(a)** Dystrophin absent (Ref: Nelson 19th E/P2061)

Duchenne muscular dystrophy:

DMD is an X linked recessive disorder characterised by mutation of the dystrophin gene responsible for production of a **sarcolemmal protein dystrophin**. It is **most common** inherited neuromuscular disease.

- **Clinical presentation:**
  - ❖ **Muscle weakness** — The **proximal muscles** of limbs are more affected, which gives a characteristic **Trendelenburg** or **waddling gait**. Because of proximal muscle weakness of leg (thigh muscles), the compensatory overuse of **calf muscle** leads to **hypertrophy**. Weakness of the respiratory (pulmonary infections, decreased respiratory reserve) and pharyngeal muscles (aspiration) can also be seen. Extraocular muscles are spared.
  - ❖ **Cardiomyopathy** is seen in majority of patients and is an important cause of mortality after respiratory failure.

- ❖ Other features that can be seen are skeletal abnormalities (scoliosis), epilepsy and mild mental retardation (almost in all patients).
- **Clinical signs:**
  - ❖ **Gower sign** — The child uses hand support to push themselves in to upright position from sitting because of proximal muscle weakness of legs.
- **Diagnosis:**
  - ❖ **CPK levels are elevated many fold** than the normal level (<160 IU/L) but **gradually decreases as the age progresses** due to decrease in muscle mass.
  - ❖ Blood PCR for the dystrophin gene mutation is the definite diagnosis.
  - ❖ Muscle biopsy show characteristic changes of myopathy; however it is less preferred as it is an invasive method.
- **Treatment:** Apart from supportive treatment, prednisolone has been seen to improve the muscular strength.

11. **(a)** Macrocephaly (Ref: Nelson 19th E/P94)

Rett syndrome:

- Rett syndrome is usually seen in **females**.
- These children develop normally till 6–18 months of age followed by rapid regression in language and hand skills, repetitive hand movements, decreased rate of head growth (**microcephaly), ataxia**, breathing dysfunction, bruxism, scoliosis, and profound **mental retardation.**
- Diagnosis is confirmed by DNA analysis for methyl CpG-binding protein 2 (MECP2).

AIIMS NOVEMBER — 2012

1. (a) Hypothalamic hamartoma (Ref: Nelson 19th E/ P1865–66)

   Hypothalamic hamartoma:
   - Hypothalamic hamartoma is congenital presence of ectopic neural tissue releasing gonadotropin releasing hormone.
   - It is characterised by rapidly progressive sexual precocity associated with unnatural crying or laughing (gelastic seizures).
   - MRI is the diagnostic method of choice, which shows a small pedunculated mass or a sessile mass, which remains static in size over years.
   - Treatment is usually done with GnRh agonists. Surgical management is not preferred, except in case of refractory seizures.

2. (c) Tuberous sclerosis (Ref: Nelson 19th E/P2017)

   Tuberous sclerosis:
   Tuberous sclerosis (Bourneville's disease) is caused by mutation of TSC genes. TSC1 gene is located in **9th** chromosome and TSC2 gene in **16th** chromosome. The clinical findings in tuberous sclerosis can be classified as major and minor findings.
   - **Major clinical findings:**
     - ❖ **Skin lesions** — The different skin lesions that can be seen are **hypopigmented macules (ashleaf macules), sebaceous adenomas**, shagreen patches and subungual or periungual fibromas.
     - ❖ Retinal lesions like mulberry tumors and hamartomas can be seen.
     - ❖ **CNS manifestations — Seizures** (infantile spasms, myoclonic epilepsies), **cognitive and behavioural impairment** can be seen (autism).
     - ❖ **Tumors — Malignant astrocytoma**, rhabdomyosarcoma of heart, renal angiomyolipoma and pulmonary lymphangiomyomatosis can be seen.
   - Minor clinical findings like bone and renal cysts, rectal polyps, confetti skin lesions and neuronal migrational defects can be seen.
   - **Diagnosis** —For diagnosis either 2 major findings or 1 major plus 1 minor is required.

3. 3 years (Ref: Nelson 19th E/P39, CPDT 19th E/P73)
   - Baby can **feed with spoon without spilling** at 2 years of age.
   - Baby helps in **dressing (unbuttoning clothes, puts on shoes)** and **Knows full name and gender** by 3 years of age.
   - Hence the best answer is 3 years.

4. (Ref: Kulkarni Manual of neonatology/P267)

Silverman's score:

Signs	0	1	2
Thoraco abdominal movement in respiration	Significant	Thoracic lag	See-Saw
Nasal flaring	Nil	Mild	Severe
Lower intercostal retraction	Nil	Mild	Severe
Xiphoid retraction	Nil	Mild	Severe
Grunting	Nil	Audible with stethoscope	Audible without stethoscope

Inference of scores:
- 1–3 — Mild RDS
- 4–7 — Moderate RDS
- 7–10 — Severe RDS

- Putting the values for the signs in the question:
  - ❖ Absent Nasal flaring – 0.
  - ❖ Audible grunting – 2.
  - ❖ Abdomen lagging – 1.
  - ❖ Intercostal retraction– 1.
  - ❖ Xiphoid retraction absent – 0.
- Hence the Silverman's score is 4 and the child is having moderate RDS.

5. (c) TOF (Nelson 19th E/P1549–51)

   Pathophysiology of acyanotic heart diseases:
   (See Flowchart 1)

   Eisenmenger syndrome:
   It is defined as an increase in the pulmonary vascular resistance by a ratio of pulmonary to systemic ratio of **more than 1**. It is **usually seen in patients with VSD** but can be associated with **ASD, PDA** or any aorto-pulmonary connection.
   - **Clinical presentation:** Patients become symptomatic usually after 3rd decade of life with initial mild presentations like cyanosis, fatigue and dyspnea which can progress to heart failure. The clinical findings can be a right ventricular heave, **loud single or narrow split S₂, loud P₂** and murmurs of tricuspid regurgitation and pulmonary insufficiency (early decrescendo diastolic murmur or **Ghram steel murmur**).
   - **Diagnosis:**
     - ❖ X-ray shows a prominent pulmonary artery, **enlarged pulmonary vessels in the hilar areas which taper down at the periphery.**
     - ❖ Echocardiographical **"W" sign** is the characteristic sign of early midsystolic closure of the pulmonary valve.

Flowchart 1

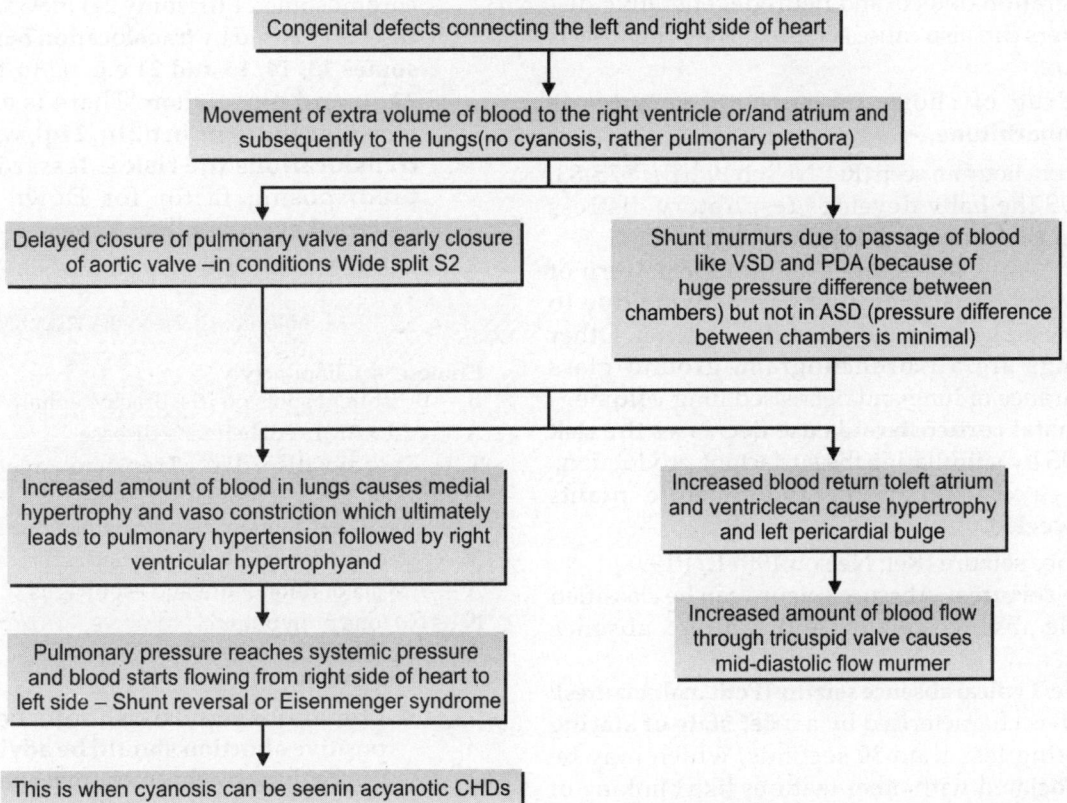

Congenital defects connecting the left and right side of heart

Movement of extra volume of blood to the right ventricle or/and atrium and subsequently to the lungs(no cyanosis, rather pulmonary plethora)

Delayed closure of pulmonary valve and early closure of aortic valve –in conditions Wide split S2

Shunt murmurs due to passage of blood like VSD and PDA (because of huge pressure difference between chambers) but not in ASD (pressure difference between chambers is minimal)

Increased amount of blood in lungs causes medial hypertrophy and vaso constriction which ultimately leads to pulmonary hypertension followed by right ventricular hypertrophyand

Increased blood return toleft atrium and ventriclecan cause hypertrophy and left pericardial bulge

Pulmonary pressure reaches systemic pressure and blood starts flowing from right side of heart to left side – Shunt reversal or Eisenmenger syndrome

Increased amount of blood flow through tricuspid valve causes mid-diastolic flow murmer

This is when cyanosis can be seenin acyanotic CHDs

❖ **Pulmonary capillary wedge pressure is usually normal.**

- **Treatment:** The best way of treatment is to prevent it in infancy by surgical approach. However once it has developed the patient is given symptomatic (phlebotomy with volume replacement for polycythemia), medical (calcium channel blocker and prostacyclin analogue i.e. epoprosterenol) and/or surgical (combined heart-lung or bilateral lung transplantation) treatment.

6. **(c)** Phenobarbitone (Ref: Nelson 19th E/P2037)
Neonatal Seizures:

Neonatal seizures can be classified based on their presentation as focal, multifocal, myoclonic, tonic and **subtle seizures (most common type). Subtle seizures** are characterised by movements of upper limb ("swimming", "boxing" or "hooking") and lower limb ("bicycling"); sucking, lip smacking and apnoea. These are caused by a wide range of pathological abnormalities and hence require a multidimensional approach for management.

- **Causes of neonatal seizures:**
  ❖ **Hypoxic ischemic encephalopathy** is the **most common cause of neonatal seizures** and is associated with **worst prognosis**. Seizures develop within first 24 hours because of cerebral edema.

❖ In neonatal period various metabolic abnormalities can cause seizure:
  ❑ **Hypoglycemia** — It develops within 24 hours after birth and **Seizure with mental retardation** can be seen.
  ❑ **Hypocalcemia** — It can be early onset hypocalcemia (within 72 hours) and late onset hypocalcemia. Seizures are usually caused by early onset hypocalcemia and are associated with a **better neurological outcome**.
  ❑ Hypo and hypernatremia.

❖ Metabolic diseases like galactosemia, hyperglycinemia and urea cycle disorders can cause seizures.

❖ Benign familial neonatal seizures start at 2nd-3rd day of life, but most commonly present on 5th day (**Fifth day fits**). It is associated with a favourable outcome.

❖ **Pyridoxine** dependent seizures are seen shortly after birth, which are resistant to anticonvulsants. Pyridoxine deficiency leads to depletion of inhibitory neurotransmitter GABA, which is the primary cause for seizure. The best treatment is pyridoxine replacement.

❖ Withdrawal of certain drugs like barbiturates, benzodiazepines and opioids can cause seizure.

- ❖ Congenital brain abnormalities like neuronal migration defects and neurodegenerative disorders can also cause seizures. The prognosis is poor.
- The drug of choice for neonatal seizures is **phenobarbitone**.

7. (b) Air bronchogram seen (Ref: Nelson 19th E/P575–83)

- In RDS the baby develops respiratory distress **within first 6 hours of birth.**
- Chest X-ray shows reticulogranular pattern of increased density of lung parenchyma due to miliary atelectasis and interstitial edema. Other findings are **air bronchogram**, ground glass appearance of lung and decreased lung volume.
- **Antenatal corticosteroids use decreases the risk of RDS** by stimulating the surfactant production.
- RDS is a common disorder of **premature infants (<34 weeks).**

8. (c) Absence seizure (Ref: Nelson 19th E/P1997)

Absence seizures: Absence seizure can be classified as simple absence seizure and complex absence seizure.

- **Simple/Typical absence seizure (Petit mal seizures):**
  - ❖ SAS is characterised by a **brief state of staring** lasting less than 30 seconds, which may be associated with other features like blinking of eyes, upward deviation of eyes and slackening of facial muscles. Most of the times it can be **precipitated by hyperventilation.**
  - ❖ It is seen in **children after 5 years of age** and is more common in female child. Most of the times these children have **poor school performance** due to intermittent episodes during classes.
  - ❖ It is not associated with falls, aura or **postictal confusion.**
  - ❖ EEG shows a characteristic **3 Hz spike wave discharge.**
- **Complex/Atypical absence seizure:**
  - ❖ Apart from the general features of SAS, CAS also has myoclonic movements of face, fingers or extremities and loss of body tone.
  - ❖ **Rolandic spikes** (centrotemporal spikes) are characteristic.
- **Treatment** — The most preferred drug for treatment of absence seizures is **sodium valproate**. However because of its increased risk of hepatotoxicity in **children less than 2 year, ethosuximide** is more preferred in this age group.

9. (a) Prenatal diagnosis and advice abortion (Ref: Nelson 19th E/P386)

The chances of Down syndrome in t(15, 21) is 1 in 8 and hence prenatal diagnosis should be done and if positive abortion should be advised.

Down syndrome:

- Down syndrome is the **most common form of trisomy as well as chromosomal disorder** which is caused by **maternal meiotic nondisjunction** of chromosome 21 **(trisomy 21)** in 95% cases. Rest 5% cases are caused by **translocation between chromosomes 13, 14, 15 and 21 e.g. t(13q,15q) and t(21q, 21q); and mosaicism.** There is a **100% risk of Down's syndrome** in t(21q, 21q), whereas in **other translocations the risk is lesser i.e. 1 in 8.** The predisposing factor for Down syndrome is **maternal age more than 35 years.**
- **Clinical findings:**

Mnemonic: Chinese **BATSMAN**

Chinese — Clinodactyly
B — Brushfield spots on iris, Brachycephaly
A — ALL>AML, Alzheimer's disease
T — Thyroid disorders, Transient myeloproliferative syndrome
S — Sandal gap, Simian crease, Septal defects (ASD, VSD)
M — Mental retardation, Mongolian slant
A — Atresia of duodenum and esophagus
N — No tone or hypotonia

- **Diagnosis:**
  - ❖ Prenatal diagnosis should be done and if positive **abortion should be advised**. Diagnosis can be done by chromosomal analysis of amniocentesis or chorionic villous sample and USG, which shows **nuchal fold thickening, absent nasal bone**, short femur and other systemic congenital anomalies.
  - ❖ **Triple screening test** can also be done for diagnosis, which involves a **low maternal serum α fetoprotein** and **unconjugated estriol;** and **high HCG.** The other maternal markers for diagnosis of Down syndrome are an increased serum inhibin A and **decreased serum PAPPA** (pregnancy associated plasma proteins).

10. (a) Bilateral micropthalmos (Ref: Nelson 19th E/P404)

Patau syndrome:

- Patau syndrome or **trisomy 13** is more common in females.
- The babies present with failure to thrive, growth retardation, apnoeic spells, seizures, deafness and a characteristic facies with bulbous nose and low set malformed ears. Other abnormalities associated are midline cleft lip, cleft palate, scalp defects, microcephaly, polydactyly or syndactyly and hypoplastic or absent ribs.
- Disorders of CNS (holoprosencephaly and arrhinencephaly), CVS (VSD) and eye (**micropthalmia**, colobomas and hypertelorism) can be seen.

11. (a) Glucose-6-phosphatase (Ref: Nelson 19th E/P469-70)

- **Type Ia GSD or Von Gierke's disease** is caused by deficiency of **glucose-6-phosphatase.**

- The specific findings are hyperuricemia, hyperlipidemia, lactic acidosis, platelet adhesion and aggregation defect, PCOD, growth retardation, hepatic adenomas, renal disorders with an enlarged kidney and pulmonary hypertension.
- **Type Ib GSD** is caused by defective glucose-6-phosphate transporter. Apart from the features of type Ia, **neutropenia** is also seen in type Ib.
- Diagnosis is based on the laboratory findings as well as test that demonstrate **no rise in glucose level after administration of glucagon or epinephrine** because of **defective glycogenolysis and gluconeogenesis**.

12. **(a)** Histiocytosis X (Ref: Nelson 19th E/P1727–30)

Langerhans cell histiocytosis:

Langerhans cell histiocytosis or histiocytosis X is a reactive proliferation of the dendritic cells. The different syndromes included are eosinophilic granuloma, Hand-Schüller-Christian disease and Letterer-Siwe disease. **Eosinophilic granuloma** is a **localised disease** characterised by not only proliferation of histiocytes but also other cells and predominantly eosinophils. **Hand-Schüller-Christian disease** is characterised by triad of **calvarine bone defects, diabetes insipidus** and **exophthalmos. Letterer-Siwe disease** is characterised by involvement at **multiple foci and organs**.

- **Clinical presentation:**
  ❖ Incidence of LCH is evenly distributed among adults and children, i.e. 50% in both. It is commonly seen in children of 1–2 year age group.
  ❖ Localised disease is characterised by **osteolytic bony lesions** which is **most common presentation**. Most common bone involved is **skull** and mastoid involvement can lead to **chronic ear discharge.**
  ❖ **Seborrheic dermatitis** of the scalp and diaper area (**diaper rash**) is seen.
  ❖ Bone marrow dysfunction can cause **pancytopenia** and compensatory extramedullary hematopoesis can lead to **hepatomegaly** and **splenomegaly.**
  ❖ Cystic lesions in the lung (**honeycomb lung**) can be seen and these lesions if rupture can cause pneumothorax.
  ❖ Pituitary involvement can lead to hormonal disorders like **diabetes insipidus** and **growth hormone deficiency.**
- **Diagnosis:** The definitive diagnostic procedure is biopsy of the lesions and demonstrations of **histiocytes (antigen presenting cells)**. These cells are **CD1a, s-100 positive**and **MHC II (HLA-DR)** positive and have **bierbeck granules** of **tennis racket shape.**

- **Treatment:**
  ❖ Localised lesions are treated with intralesional corticosteroids, radiation and curettage.
  ❖ Multifocal diseases are treated with agents like vinblastine or etoposide with prednisolone.
  ❖ Refractory cases can be treated with stem cell transplantation and drugs like **cladribine**, interferon α and etarncept.

13. **(d)** Klebsiella (Ref: IJP vol 75, sepsis in the newborn, page 67)

Most common cause of sepsis:

- **India** — Most common cause of both early and late onset neonatal sepsis in India is *Klebsiella pneumoniae* followed by *Staphylococcus aureus*.

IJP vol 75, sepsis in the newborn, page 67

"The database comprising 18 tertiary care neonatal units across India found sepsis to be one of the commonest causes of neonatal mortality contributing to 19% of all neonatal mortality. Among **intramural births** *Klebsiella pneumonae* was the most commonly isolated pathogen (32.5%) followed by *Staphylococcus aureus* (13.6%). Among **extramural (referred from community/other hospitals)** neonates *Klebsiella pneumoniae* (27%) was again the commonest organism followed by *Staphylococcus aureus* **(15%)** and Pseudomonas (13%)."

14. **(d)** Narrow pulse pressure (Ref: Nelson 19th E/P1510–12)

Clinical presentation of PDA:

- A small PDA is usually asymptomatic, but large PDA may result in **CHF** due to volume overload of right and left ventricle and left atrium.**CHF** is the **most common cause of death in adolescents**, however they may present with other frequent complications like **infective endocarditis**, pulmonary or systemic embolism and **pulmonary hemorrhage**. Infective endocarditis is more common with **smaller lesions** and hence requires early closure.
- **Bounding peripheral arterial pulses**can be seen because of increased stroke volume (increased systolic B.P). **Wide pulse pressure (Pulse pressure = systolic B.P – Diastolic B.P)** is seen due to passage of blood into the pulmonary artery during diastole and reflex peripheral vasodilation (decreased diastolic BP).
- A prominent apical pulse and systolic thrill is maximally seen in the 2nd left interspace.
- **Machinery like or thunder rolling murmur** is heard because of continuous passage of blood from aorta to pulmonary artery. The patient has other features like resting **tachycardia, CO_2 retention, frequent apnoea** and a hyperactive precordium.
- **Differential cyanosis** can be seen when PDA is associated with severe pulmonary hypertension or reversal of shunt.
- **Prematurity** is an important risk factor for necrotizing Enterocolitis.

AIIMS MAY — 2012

1. (c) Hypoglycemia (Ref: Nelson 19th E/P1852) (See Table 1)

2. (c) Conservative management with IV fluids and antibiotics (Nelson 19th E/P591)

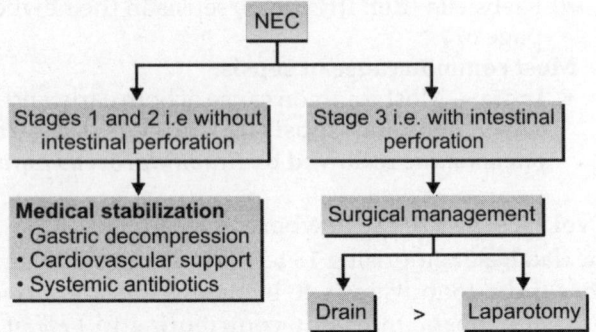

3. (c) ALL in children (Ref: Nelson 19th E/P1695–96)
Treatment of ALL in children:
- Medical management is the mainstay of treatment which is divided in to three phases i.e. induction, consolidation and maintenance. Anticancer therapy with **prednisolone**, **vincristine**, dauno-rubicin, **L-asparginase**, 6-mercaptopurine and **methotrexate** are used for induction and consolidation. Mainte-nance phase is administration of these drugs at regular intervals. Maintenance therapy for **prophylaxis of CNS complications** consists of **intrathecal methotrexate or a combination of methotrexate, cytarabine and dexamethasone**.
- Bone marrow transplantation can be done but is less preferred than medical management.
- **Intensive chemotherapy** along with **bone marrow transplantation** has significantly **increased the survival and decreased the relapse rate** in patients of ALL in recent years.

4. (a) Sturge Weber syndrome (Ref: Nelson 19th E/P2018)

Sturge Weber syndrome:
- **Port-wine stain (facial nevus)** — This is a capillary malformation characterised by unilateral pink-purple macular lesion seen on the **ophthalmic and maxillary distribution of trigeminal nerve** in the head and neck region (**upper face and eyelid is always involved**) and at times in mucous membranes. This is a **permanent lesion**, which in adulthood can give cobblestone appearance. These lesions should be distinguished from salmon patch which is a **transient vascular lesion**. The best treatment is **flashlamp-pumped-pulse dye laser**.
- **Seizures** — Focal tonic-clonic seizures are seen opposite to the side of nevus. If seizures are refractory to medication, hemispherectomy is done.
- Transient stroke like episodes can be seen due to cortical vein thrombosis.

5. (b) Air bronchogram seen (Ref: Nelson 19th E/P575–83)
- In RDS the baby develops respiratory distress **within first 6 hours of birth.**
- Chest X-ray shows reticulogranular pattern of increased density of lung parenchyma due to miliary atelectasis and interstitial edema. Other findings are **air bronchogram**, ground glass appearance of lung and decreased lung volume.
- **Antenatal corticosteroids use decreases the risk of RDS** by stimulating the surfactant production.
- RDS is a common disorder of **premature infants (<34 weeks).**

6. (c) Myoclonus (Ref: Nelson 19th E/P1998)
Juvenile myoclonic epilepsy (Janz syndrome):
- JME begins in the age group of 12–16 years with bilateral **myoclonic jerks (myoclonus)** in **early morning period** which later progress to **GTCS and absence seizures in only 25% of patients**. It can be precipitated by sleep deprivation.

Table 1

Uses of growth hormone	Side effects and contraindications of growth hormone
S — Small for gestational age babies	C — CTS
M — Malabsorption associated with short bowel syndrome	H — **Hyperglycemia**
A — AIDS related wasting syndrome	I — ICP is raised } Side effects
L ⎤	L — Leukemia
L ⎦ — Length decreased in various syndromes	D — Dislodgement of femoral epiphysis
(Prader-Willi, Turner, Noonan)	R ⎤ — Retinopathy
	E ⎦ } Contraindications
	N — Neoplasia

- Family history of epilepsy is common and the gene locus for JME is chromosome 6p21.
- EEG shows a **4–6 Hz irregular spike and wave discharges (fast spikes)** enhanced by photo stimulation. **Neurological examination is normal**.
- Out of all drugs that block the thalamic calcium channels JME responds best to **valproate** but recurrence rate is very high on discontinuation. This makes the therapy mandatory for **lifelong**. Other drugs which are effective in treating JME are **topiramate, zonisamide and lamotrigine.**

7. **(c)** Acute lymphoid leukemia in less than 1 year has a poor prognosis (Nelson 19th E/P1696)

Good prognostic factors of ALL:

Mnemonic: **Good Females Tried Less Hyper-man AT 1221**
Good — Good prognosis **Females** — Females **Tried** — Trisomy 4, 17, 10 **Less** — Less than 50,000 leucocytes, 5% blasts and 0.1% MRD **Hyper-man** — Hyperploidy **AT** — After 1 year till 10 year **1221** — Translocation (12; 21)

8. **(b)** Glanzmann thrombasthenia (Ref: Pedro Neonatal Hematology/P95, Nelson 19th E/P1673–74)
   - Since PT and APTT are normal coagulation disorder like factor X deficiency and von Willebrand disease can be easily ruled out. Out of the bleeding disorders Glanzmann thrombasthenia is associated with bleeding in the newborn period.

Bernard soulier syndrome
"Inspite of its severity, newborns with this disorder do not bleed."

Glanzmann thrombasthenia
"In the neonate, generalised purpura or petechiae and bleeding from the circumcision are the most common manifestations." (See Table 1)

9. **(b)** Hereditary spherocytosis (Ref: Nelson 19th E/P1620)

Hereditary spherocytosis:
Hereditary spherocytosis is an AD condition caused by frame shift mutation of various RBC proteins like ankyrin, spectrin, band 3 and band 4.2. This leads to **loss of some part of the RBC membrane with same cytoplasm** and it assumes a shape to accommodate maximum volume i.e. sphere. This spheroid RBC which is inflexible undergoes sequestration in the spleen.
- **Clinical presentation:** The patient presents with anemia, pallor, jaundice and splenomegaly. Gallstones are frequently seen in case of spherocytosis. Patients are at high risk of **parvovirus infection and resultant aplastic crisis.**

Table 2

Bernard soulier syndrome	*Glanzmann thrombasthenia*
• It is an AR disorder	• It is an AR disorder
• Cause by defect of VWF or GP Ib receptor	• Caused by defect of GP IIb-IIIa receptors
• **Thrombocytopenia** is seen and **bleeding time is prolonged. PT** and **aPTT** are normal	• **Thrombocytopenia** is seen and **bleeding time is prolonged. PT** and **aPTT** are normal
• Despite of severe thrombocytopenia, **bleeding is not seen in newborns**	• **Newborns** present with generalised purpura and **bleeding from the umbilical stump**. Older children present with nose bleeds, easy bruising and menorrhagia
• **Platelet aggregation in response to ristocetin is absent;** however is **present with other agonists like ADP,** epinephrine, **collagen**, and thrombin	• Platelet aggregation is seen only in response to ristocetin
• **Platelets are of large size**	• Platelets are of normal size
• **Desmopressin** is used to treat acute bleeding episode **Platelet transfusion** is done to maintain homeostasis. In case of resistance due to antiplatelet antibody production, **recombinant factor VIIa** is given	• **Desmopressin** is used to treat acute bleeding episode. **Platelet transfusion** is done to maintain homeostasis. In case of resistance due to antiplatelet antibody production, **recombinant factor VIIa** is given

- **Diagnosis:**
  - ❖ **MCV is normal** and **MCHC is increased.**
  - ❖ Peripheral smear shows spherocytes and reticulocytes.
  - ❖ **Osmotic fragility test (pink test)** — Osmotic fragility is increased if there is a relative decrease in the RBC membrane circumference as compared to the RBC volume. It is **increased** in hereditary spherocytosis but is not specific as it can be positive in other conditions with spherocytes like haemolytic anemia. Osmotic fragility is decreased in thalassemia, iron deficiency anemia and splenomegaly.
- **Treatment:** Splenectomy is the mainstay of treatment. Folic acid is advised prophylactically to maintain an effective erythropoiesis.

10. **(a)** WBC cast (Ref: Nelson 19th E/P1785)

Diagnosis of UTI:
- Urine sample is collected for both microscopic analysis and culture. In older children midstream clean catch is sufficient but in **infants suprapubic aspiration should be done** as it is the most uncontaminated urine specimen.

- Microscopic analysis showing pyuria i.e. **>5 W.B.Cs/hpf** is suggestive of infection; however it is **not confirmatory** as **pyuria can be seen without infection** and **infection can be present without pyuria**.
- **Deep stick test for nitrite** and **leucocyte esterase** can add to diagnosis but are **not specific** for UTI. **WBC casts are specific for pyelonephritis,** as casts are seen only if renal parenchyma is involved.
- Microscopic examination of urine showing **1 bacterium per oil-immersion field on gram stain** is also a **specific test** as it equals to 100,000 bacteria/ml of urine.
- Urine culture is the mainstay of diagnosis. For diagnosis **>100,000 colonies** or >10,000 colonies with symptomatic child is required.
- **VCUG** should be done to rule out the obstructive lesions. It is indicate in a **male child with more than one UTI** and a **female child with more than two UTIs within 6 months.**
- **DMSA** scan can be done to confirm the diagnosis of pyelonephritis.

AIIMS NOVEMBER — 2011

1. **(b)** Wound culture (Ref: David Pediatric neurosurgery/ P371)

   Myelomeningocele:
   - This is the **most severe form of NTD** characterised by herniation of the meninges along with the spinal cord. The most common site of location is **lumbosacral region**. The clinical presentation depends on the site of location.
   - Lower sacral lesions cause **bladder** and **bowel incontinence** with perineal anaesthesia.
   - Midlumbar lesions cause **flaccid paralysis of lower limbs**, constant urinary dribbling, **laxed anal sphincter** and a higher incidence of lower limb deformities like club feet and subluxation of hip joint.
   - **Hydrocephalus** can be seen in 80% cases and is commonly associated with **type II Chiari defect**.
   - Treatment comprises of early surgical repair (within 3 days) of the defect to prevent infection. This is followed by shunt placement for hydrocephalus. Broad spectrum antibiotic from birth till closure is indicated.
   - The most common postoperative complication is **wound dehiscence** which can be followed by CSF leak if a shunt is not placed. The baby is at a high risk of fecal contamination of the wound and in case of CSF leak, meningitis is unavoidable. In this case a **CSF study should be done with biochemical parameters and culture**.
   - Since CSF culture is not in options wound culture is the best answer.

2. **(a)** Docosahexaenoic acid (Ref: Rudolph 22nd E/P100)

   "Some studies demonstrated **improved neurodevelopmental in infant fed human milk, which contains higher concentrations of DHA than cow milk formulas,** leading many formula companies to add arachidonic acid and DHA directly to formulas."

3. **(a)** Thalassemia (Ref: IAP textbook of pediatrics 4th E/P799)

   NESTROFT (Naked eye single tube red cell osmotic fragility test):
   - In one tube 2ml of 0.36% buffered saline solution is taken and in another 2ml of distilled water is taken. A drop of blood is added to both tubes and left undisturbed for 20 minutes. Both the tubes are shaken and then held against a white paper on which black line is drawn. Normally the line is clearly visible through the second tube containing distil water. If the line is clearly visible through the first tube, the test is negative. If line is not clearly visible then test is positive.
   - The principle is that normocytic normochromic cells undergo lysis when put in hypotonic solution. In thalassemia trait the cells are hypochromic and microcytic which are resistant to hemolysis due to decreased osmotic fragility.
   - A **negative test negates the possibility of beta thalassemia trait**, however it is not specific as it can also be seen in alpha thalassemia trait, iron deficiency anemia, Hb E, Hb S and in hereditary persistence of fetal hemoglobin.
   - This test has a high sensitivity of 95% and negative predictive value of 98%. However due to poor precision, intertechnician variability and low specificity, it is not done routinely.

4. **(c)** Vein of Galen malformation (Ref: Ronald Clinical Paediatric Neurology/P375)

   Vein of Galen malformation (VGAM):
   - VGAM is a misnomer as it is malformation of the precursor of vein of Galen i.e. median prosencephalic vein of Markowsky. So the vein of Galen never forms in a VGAM.
   - This is a large midline arterio-venous malformation that shunts a significant amount of blood in to the venous circulation. It is more common in **males.**
   - **Clinical presentation:**
     - ❖ **CHF** — It is the most common presentation in neonates because of increased venous return to the right side of heart. It begins as right sided heart failure but later biventricular failure develops.
     - ❖ **Hydrocephalus** — It develops because of the venous hypertension which decreases the CSF absorption (non-communicating hydrocephalus). In neonates it presents with fullness of fontanels. Communicating hydrocephalus can be rarely seen because of aqueductal stenosis.
     - ❖ **Cerebral calcification and haemorrhage** can be seen in some cases.
   - **Diagnosis:**
     - ❖ CECT or MRI shows **enlargement of lateral and 3rd ventricles** if there is aqueductal stenosis.
     - ❖ X-ray chest shows an enlarged heart with a normal shape.
     - ❖ A **cranial bruit** can be heard on auscultation.
   - **Treatment: Embolization of VGAM** is the current treatment of choice.

5. **(c)** Obstructive TAPVC (Ref: ???)
   - Patients condition may worsen if Pg E1 is given in TAPVC, as pooling of blood is seen in the right

side of heart and subsequently to lungs with compromised left side and systemic circulation. In this case if DA is patent then it will shunt blood from left to right side and further compromise the systemic circulation.

Ductus dependent cardiac leisons:

Ductus dependent pulmonary blood flow	Ductus dependent systemic blood flow
• Pulmonary atresia with intact. ventricular septum. • Tricuspid atresia. • Critical pulmonary stenosis. • TOF.	• Coarctation of aorta. • Aortic arch interruption. • Hypoplastic left heart syndrome.

Pg E1 analogues (misoprostol and alprostadil) are used to maintain patency of ductus arteriosus in some CHDs. (Remember: **P**rostaglandin maintains **P**atency)

6. **(a)** VDRL for mother and baby (Ref: Nelson 19th E/P978–82)
   - Bullous lesions on X-ray and periostitis on X-ray are sufficient for diagnosis of congenital syphilis.
   - **Diagnosis of congenital syphilis:**
     ❖ The best and most specific way of diagnosis is to isolate Treponema Pallidum from the lesions by dark ground microscopy.
     ❖ If treponemas are not visible in the lesion then diagnosis is difficult in the early days. The status of maternal infection and her treatment, serologic tests and clinical findings in the infant and bone X-ray and CSF evaluation are evaluated to confirm the diagnosis.
     ❖ **VDRL** or RPR should be done on mother and infant blood for diagnosis; however it is not specific and reflects the activity of disease process.
     ❖ Serological tests are more specific and aim at detecting the antitreponemal Ig M antibodies in baby's serum. The various tests for Ig M detection are **FTA-ABS 19S-IgM, IgM capture ELISA and western immunoblotting assay.**

7. **(a)** Deleted 21 (Ref: Nelson 19th E/P386)
   - Down syndrome is the **most common form of trisomy as well as chromosomal disorder** which is caused by **maternal meiotic nondisjunction** of chromosome 21 **(trisomy 21)** in 95% cases.
   - Rest 5% cases are caused by **translocation e.g. t(13q,15q) and t(21q, 21q); and mosaicism.**

8. **(b)** Sickle cell anemia (Ref: Nelson 19th E/P1624–28)
   Sickling of RBCs depend on multiple factors like:
   - **Hb S concentration** — Increased Hb S concentration of >50% precipitates sickling.

- **Hb F and Hb A concentration** — Increased Hb F and Hb A (Hb F > Hb A) concentration prevents polymerisation of Hb S. Since Hb F concentration is high **till 6 months of life, babies are asymptomatic till this period.**
- **Intracellular pH** — Decreased pH decreases tendency of binding of Hb to oxygen. Deoxygenation precipitates sickling.
- **RBC passing time through microvasculature** — Increase time of presence in microvascular can cause deoxygenation and sickling.

9. **(c)** Universal flexion like a fetus (Ref: Rudolph 22nd E/P171)

> Rudolph 22nd E/P171
> "Heat production postnatally is the result of **shivering and nonshivering** thermogenesis. In general nonshivering thermogenesis is thought to be more important than shivering thermogenesis in newborn. Although under usual circumstances nonshivering thermogenesis may be the primary means by which heat is generated in the newborn, at least some capacity for **shivering** may exist."

As per text the other mechanisms of heat production are:
- Vasoconstrition.
- Nor epinephrine induced beta oxidation of brown fats.

10. **(a)** Kartagener's syndrome (Ref: Nelson 19th E/P1451)
    Primary ciliary dyskinesia:
    - Cilia motility is required for clearance of secretions and foreign body from the upper and lower respiratory tract.
    - Most common ciliary disorder associated with immotility is absence of one or both dynein arms. Dyenin gene DNAH5 is located in chromosome 5 and this disorder is AR in inheritance. This is the defect found in most patients of Kartagener's syndrome.
    - **Kartagener's syndrome** is characterised by:
      1. Situs inversus
      2. **Chronic sinusitis** and otitis
      3. Bronchiectasis
      4. Male infertility
    - Other less common ciliary disorder associated with immotility are defects in radial spoke linkages, with disorientation of the central microtubular doublets and absence of the central microtubular doublet and replacement by a doublet from the outer ring.
    - Primary ciliary dyskinesia is associated with recurrent or chronic otitis media, sinusitis, rhinitis, nasal polyposis and bronchiectasis. Male patients may have immotile spermatozoa.

- In 50% of patients, embryonic ciliary immotility is associated with situs inversus.
- The diagnosis is made by electron microscopy of cilia obtained by nasal scrapings or mucosal biopsy. In older patients diagnosis can be made by measuring the clearance rate of technetium labelled albumin microspheres.
- Treatment is same like bronchiectasis.

Ciliary structure

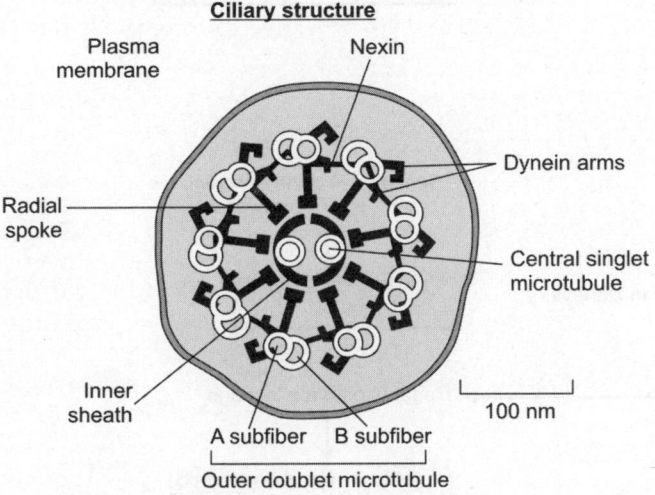

11. **(b)** Primary hypothyroidism (Ref: Rudolph 20th E/P2064)
- Raised TSH, low T4 and pituitary swelling are sufficient to make a diagnosis of primary hypo-thyroidism.
- In primary hypothyroidism the defect in thyroid hormone production lies in the thyroid gland itself. Hence there is compensatory increased production of thyrotropin releasing hormone (TRH). TRH stimulates the thyrotrophs in the pituitary and leads to increased production of TSH.
- Continuous stimulation of the thyrotrophs can lead to hyperplasia and pituitary enlargement.

12. **(d)** Fetal skin biopsy (Sinuhe Fetal cells and fetal DNA in maternal blood/P22)

"A variety of different ultrasound guided sampling techniques to obtain cells for fetal karyotyping are available. They include conventional **amniocentesis, chorionic villus sampling (CVS)**, placental biopsy (late CVS) and **fetal blood sampling.**"

13. **(b)** NPHS 2 (Ref: Nelson 19th E/P1755-57, Robin's 8th E/P927)

Primary nephrotic syndrome:
- Primary nephrotic syndrome consists of 3 clinical entities named **minimal change disease (MCD) or lipoid nephrosis**, mesangial proliferation and **focal segmental glomerulosclerosis (FSGS).**

- It is more common in males.
- **Minimal change disease** is the **most common cause of nephrotic syndrome in children** and is the **most responsive of all to steroids**. It is characterised by **fusion of foot processes or podocytes** in electron microscopy.
- **Mesangial proliferation** is associated with Ig A and Ig M deposition and effacement of podocytes.
- **Focal segmental glomerulosclerosis** is the **most common cause of steroid resistant NS**. It is an AR disorder characterised by mutation of **NPHS2 gene** which codes for slit diaphragm protein podocin. It shows Ig M and C3 deposition and scarring of the glomerular tuft.

14. **(a)** William syndrome consists of precocious puberty, mental retardation and obesity (Ref: Nelson 19th E/P216)
- **William's syndrome:**
  - ❖ William's syndrome is caused by microdeletion in chromosome 7 and since these are new deletions, parents are unaffected.
  - ❖ The younger children usually have **mental retardation** and older children have an **outgoing "cocktail party" personality.**
  - ❖ In infants a typical facies with periorbital fullness, broad nasal bridge, anteverted nares, long philtrum, open mouth, and full cheeks can be seen. Older children have an elongated face and thicker lips.
  - ❖ The most common CVS defect seen is **supra-valvular aortic stenosis.**
  - ❖ Hypercalcemia is seen in most cases due to abnormal metabolism of vitamin D; however resolves spontaneously.
- **Metabolism of vitamin D:** (See Flowchart 1)

15. **(b)** Dystrophin dystrophy (Ref: Nelson 19th E/P2066–67)

Limb-Girdle Muscular dystrophy:
- This is a group of muscular dystrophies which have predominantly AR inheritance and are caused by mutation of several sarcolemmal protein that decreases production of several proteins like adhalen, **dysferlin, caveolin-3 or calpain-3, sarco-glycans (α, β, γ, σ),** fukutin, titin **and** telethronin.
- It usually presents in the late childhood i.e. towards the end of first decade.
- **Clinical presentation:**
  - ❖ **Muscle weakness** — Apart from hip and shoulder girdle muscles, the neck muscles are also universally involved.
  - ❖ Other features like **cardiac involvement** and **MR are usually not seen.**

Flowchart 1

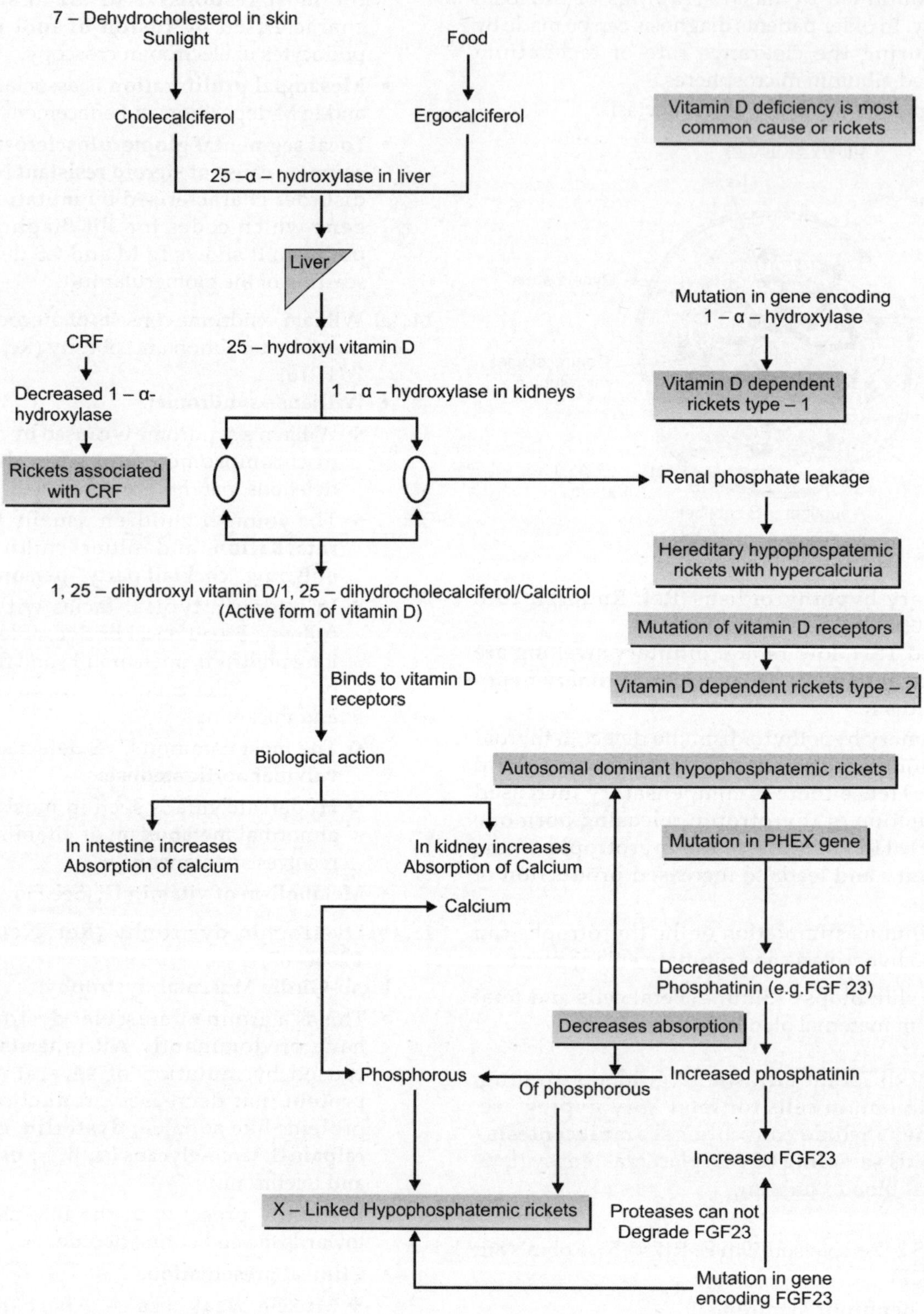

7 – Dehydrocholesterol in skin
Sunlight

Food

↓

↓

Cholecalciferol

Ergocalciferol

| Vitamin D deficiency is most common cause or rickets |

25 –α – hydroxylase in liver

↓

Liver

Mutation in gene encoding
1 – α – hydroxylase

↓

CRF

25 – hydroxyl vitamin D

| Vitamin D dependent rickets type – 1 |

Decreased 1 – α-hydroxylase

1 – α – hydroxylase in kidneys

↓

| Rickets associated with CRF |

→ Renal phosphate leakage

↓

| Hereditary hypophospatemic rickets with hypercalciuria |

1, 25 – dihydroxyl vitamin D/1, 25 – dihydrocholecalciferol/Calcitriol
(Active form of vitamin D)

| Mutation of vitamin D receptors |

↓

| Vitamin D dependent rickets type – 2 |

Binds to vitamin D receptors

↓

| Autosomal dominant hypophosphatemic rickets |

Biological action

| Mutation in PHEX gene |

In intestine increases
Absorption of calcium

In kidney increases
Absorption of Calcium

Decreased degradation of
Phosphatinin (e.g.FGF 23)

→ Calcium

| Decreases absorption |

Phosphorous ← Of phosphorous ← Increased phosphatinin

↓

Increased FGF23

| X – Linked Hypophosphatemic rickets |

Proteases can not
Degrade FGF23

Mutation in gene
encoding FGF23

16. (a) At the end of 2nd month of pregnancy (Ref: Reddy's Forensic 29th E/P65)

Developmental events during fetal life:

Events	Age in weeks
Taste bud appears	7
First centres of ossification appear	8
Muscle contraction first appear	8
Breathing and swallowing	13-14
Grasp reflex appears	17
Grasp reflex is well developed	27
Suckling movements	24

Eye opening	26
Appearance of lanugo hair	20
Testes descend in to internal inguinal ring	28
One testicle descends to scrotum	36
Disappearance of lanugo hair	36
Both testicles descend in to scrotum	40
Posterior fontanel is closed	40
Fetal movement felt	20
Primary ossification centres are present	12
*Gender of external genitals are clearly distinguishable	12

*Nelson 19th E/P27

AIPGE — 2012

1. **(c)** High levels of conjugated bilirubin may case kernicterus (Ref: Ghai 7th E/P147)
   - **Unconjugated bilirubin is toxic to nervous system** and its toxic symptom in newborn period due to accumulation in basal ganglia and brain stem nuclei is called as acute bilirubin encephalopathy.
   - Kernicterus is the term used for severe form of bilirubin toxicity caused by **unconjugated bilirubin**, which leads to permanent neurologic damage. The infant may develop delayed motor skills, movement disorder (**cheroathetosis**, ballismus and tremor), **upward gaze,** paralytic palsies, intellectual deficits and **sensorineural hearing loss.**

   Causes of jaundice: (See Flowchart 1)

2. **(b)** 15 months (Ref: Nelson 19th E/P38)

Milestones at 15 months
- **Walks alone**
- Creeps upstairs
- Imitates scribbling
- Tower of 2 blocks
- Hugs parents
- Indicates some desires or needs by pointing
- **Jargon (non-verbal communication)**
- **4–6 words vocabulary**

3. **(a)** Enterotoxigenic *E.coli* (ETEC) (Ref: Ghai 7th E/P261)
   - Most common cause of bacterial diarrhoea in India is ETEC.
   - Most common cause of diarrhoea in India is rota virus.

4. **(a)** Cystic fibrosis (Ref: Nelson 19th E/P1437–50)
   Cystic fibrosis:
   Cystic fibrosis is an **autosomal recessive** disorder caused by mutations of the **cystic fibrosis transmembrane regulator (CFTR) gene** located in chromosome 7. CFTR is a pump which controls movement of salt and water through the epithelial cells of various systems.

   Clinical presentation:
   - **Meconium ileus** is a characteristic finding seen in newborns with cystic fibrosis.
   - **Pulmonary involvement** is characterised by occlusion of the airway and an increased predisposition to infection with pseudomonas, staphylococcus and H.influenzae. The patient presents with productive cough, wheeze, hemoptysis and dyspnea.
   - **Pancreatic insufficiency** can be seen which presents with **steatorrhea with bulky, foul smelling stools**, deficiency of fat soluble vitamins and hyperglycemia.
   - Delay in sexual development and azoospermia can be seen in males.
   - Loss of chloride ion in sweat can present as hypochloremic alkalosis.

   Diagnosis:
   - **Sweat chloride testing** — Pilocarpine induced sweating and measurement of chloride ion in the sweat is the initial diagnosis of choice. **More than 60 mEq/L** of chloride in the sweat along pulmonary or pancreatic findings or positive family history is diagnostic.
   - **Nasal epithelial potential difference test** — Loss of the nasal epithelial potential difference on application of amiloride is used for diagnosis **in case sweat chloride test is normal**.
   - DNA mutation for **CFTR genes(F-508)** can be done for diagnosis.

   Treatment:
   - Bronchodilators, corticosteroids and mucolytics (human recombinant DNase and N-acetyl cysteine) are given by inhalational route for symptomatic relief.

Flowchart 1

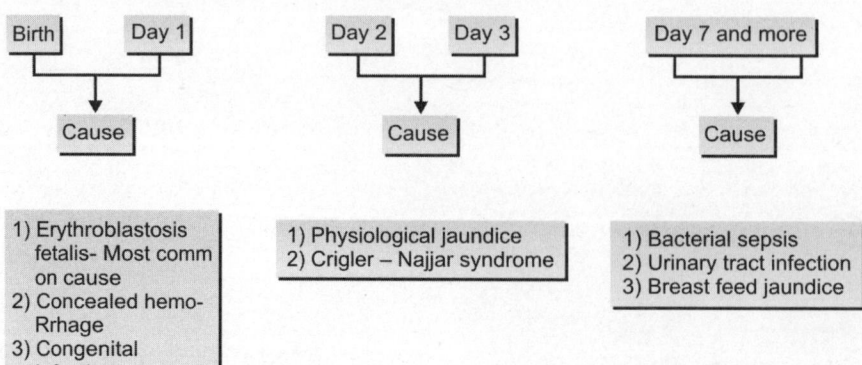

- Antibiotic therapy is indicated for the pulmonary infections associated with cystic fibrosis.

5. **(c)** Wiskott-Aldrich syndrome (Robins Pathology 8th E/P235)

Wiskott-Aldrich syndrome:

- Wiskott-Aldrich syndrome is an X-linked recessive disorder characterised caused by mutation in the Wiskott-Aldrich syndrome protein (WASP) gene in chromosome 11.
- The WASP is required for anchoring the membrane receptors to the cytoskeletal elements and plays an integral role in regulating the cytoskeletal architecture of both platelets and T lymphocytes in response to receptor-mediated cell signalling.
- The presenting symptoms are:
  ❖ **Thrombocytopenia.**
  ❖ **Eczema.**
  ❖ **Recurrent infections due to immunodeficiency characterised by T lymphocyte depletion and decreased Ig M.**
- There is progressive depletion of lymphocytes in the blood and lymphnodes, however thymus is usually normal.
- Antibody production in response to antigens is blunted. There is decreased Ig M production; however Ig G production is normal. The levels of Ig A and E is increased.
- Bone marrow transplantation is the treatment of choice.

6. **(b)** Simple virilising congenital adrenal hyperplasia (Ref: Nelson 19th E/P1911)

21β hydroxylase deficiency:

Deficiency of 21β hydroxylase leads to partial abolition of the mineralocorticoid and glucocorticoid pathways but the sex steroid pathway is completely potentiated. This can present clinically in two forms i.e. classical and non-classical.

- **Classical form:** Classical form or salt wasting form is associated with decrease in glucocorticoids and mineralocorticoids, whereas sex steroids are increased.
  ❖ Decreased aldosterone leads to **hyponatremia, hypotension** and **hyperkalemia.** Decreased cortisol can cause **hypoglycemia.**
  ❖ DHES, androstenadione and testosterone is increased.
    ❑ **Males** — Increased sex hormones cause **precocious puberty,** virilisation and rapid growth.
    ❑ **Females** — Increased sex hormones cause **ambiguous genitalia (pseudohermaphroditism), virilisation** and rapid growth.
  ❖ If there is history of 21 hydroxylase deficiency, prenatal diagnosis can be done by DNA analysis of **chorionic villous sample** obtained in late 1st or 2nd trimester. Once diagnosis is confirmed **dexamethasone** should be started **at 6 weeks of gestation,** which would normalise the sex hormone pathway.

- ❖ Since 21 hydroxylase deficiency accounts for 90% of cases of CAH, newborn screening can be done for increased level of **17-hydroxyprogesterone** in blood obtained by heel-stick.

- **Non-classical form:**
  ❖ **Non-classical form or simple virilising form of CAH** is associated with normal levels of glucocorticoids and mineralocorticoids with selective increase in sex steroids.
  ❖ Hence these patients present only with symptoms of increased DHES, androstena-dione and testosterone.
  ❖ **Males** — Increased sex hormones cause **precocious puberty,** virilisation and rapid growth.
  ❖ **Females** — Increased sex hormones cause **ambiguous genitalia (pseudohermaphroditism), virilisation** and rapid growth.

7. **(b)** Kallman's syndrome (Ref: Nelson 19th E/P1928) This is a case of **hypogonadotrophic hypogonadism** as there is decrease in both LH and FSH, which is secondarily causing testosterone deficiency.

Delayed puberty in males:

- In males delayed puberty is characterised by absence of secondary sexual characteristics by 14 years of age. The **most common cause of delayed puberty is constitutional growth delay;** however other causes of growth delay like **hypothyroidism** and growth hormone deficiency can also delay puberty.
- Testicular failure (Hypergonadotrophic hypogonadism) due to **infection (mumps orchitis), Klinefelter syndrome, radiation,** trauma and tumor can delay puberty in males.
- Decreased GnRH secretion (Hypogonadotrophic hypogonadism) due to **Kallman syndrome,** CNS disorders like infection, trauma, tumours; Prader-Willi syndrome and **Laurence-Moon syndrome** may also delay puberty.

8. **(d)** Sacrococcygeal teratoma (Ref: Narain Textbook of Neurosurgery 3rd E/P1220)

"**Sacrococcygeal teratoma,** the **most common congenital tumor,** is a very rare tumor occurring congenitally, with an incidence of approximately one in 40,000 births."

9. **(d)** Ghrelin (Ref: Nelson 19th E/P1845, CPDT 19th E/P995)

Prader-Willi syndrome:
- Prader willi syndrome is caused most commonly by **genomic imprinting** i.e. inactivation of **paternal gene of 15q11** chromosome. The least common cause is **maternal disomy** i.e. if both the genes of 15q11 chromosome are derived from the mother.
- The baby is born with hypotonia and a characteristic facies i.e. almond-shaped eyes and strabismus. **Growth hormone deficiency** can lead to short stature, obesity, hypogenitalism, small hands and feet.
- There is compensatory **increase in Ghrelin levels** due to decrease in GH. Ghrelin is secreted by the stomach> arcuate nucleus of hypothalamus, which stimulates growth hormone releasing hormone (GHRH) receptor in the somatotroph cells of pituitary and increases GH release.
- Hypogonadotrophic hypogonadism, due to impaired GnRH secretion can be seen which is associated with a **decreased LH and FSH release**.
- Obsessive hyperphagia and DM can be commonly seen.

10. (b) Open nephroureterectomy (Ref: Nelson 19th E/P1713)

Treatment of Wilm's tumor:
- **Surgical removal** of the tumor is the mainstay of treatment. An **open anterior surgical approach** is used to explore the abdomen for spread of disease to other organs and both the kidneys. This is followed by **nephrectomy** i.e. an en-block resection of the tumor.

- Chemotherapy is given in all stages. For stage I and II **vincristine** and **actinomycin D** is used whereas for stage III and IV **doxorubicin** is also added to the regimen.
- **Radiation therapy** is reserved for the advanced stages i.e. stage III and IV, which should be started **within 10 daysof surgery.**

11. (b) 10% IV dextrose (Ref: Nelson 19th E/P518)
Management of hypoglycemia: (See Flowchart 2)

12. (b) Less energy/caloric content (Ref: Neonatal Formulary: Drugs used in pregnancy and first year of life/P134)

Intralipid:
- Intralipid is an emulsion of soyabean oil, which is stabilized with egg phospholipid.
- The different components of intralipid are:
  - ❖ Linoleic acid — 52%
  - ❖ Oleic acid — 22%
  - ❖ Palmitic acid — 13%
  - ❖ Linolenic acid — 8%
- It is approximately isotonic and available in 10% and 20% solution with same energy/caloric content i.e. 4.18 KJ/Kcal. However the Kcal/ml content is lesser in 10% solution due to lesser triglycerides. (10% solution provides 1.1 Kcal/ml and 20% solution provides 2 Kcal/ml).
- The 20% intralipid has less phospholipid content and hence is better tolerated than 10% intralipid.
- It is the most caloric rich intravenous fluid.
- Use of intralipid is associated with infections like Malassezia and coagulase negative Staphylococcus.

Flowchart 2

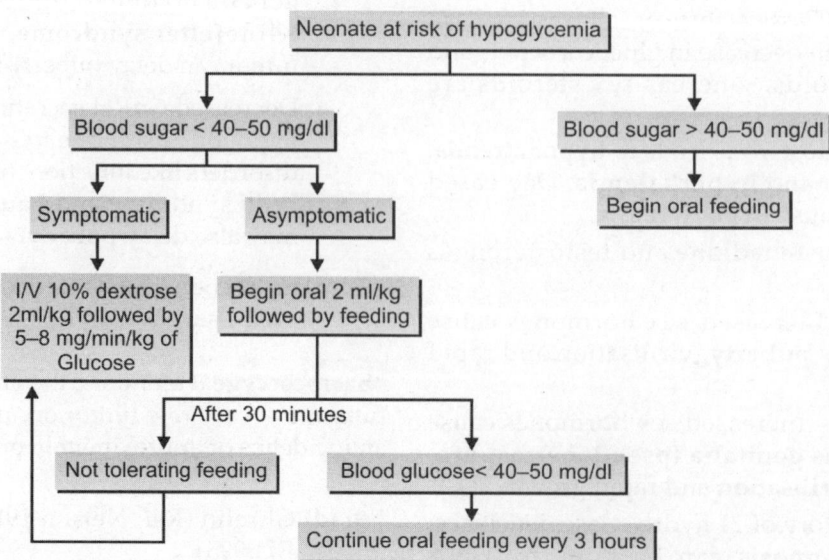